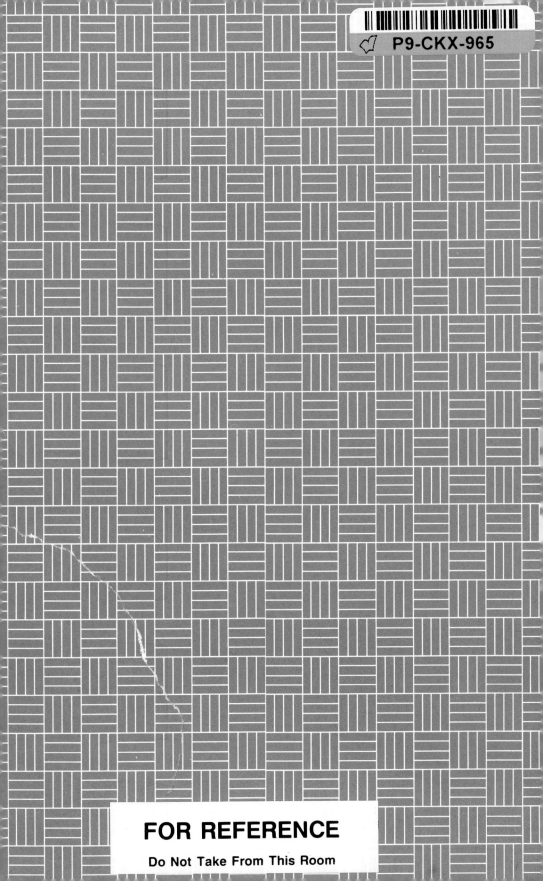

COMPANION ENCYCLOPEDIA
OF THE
HISTORY OF MEDICINE

COMPANION ENCYCLOPEDIA
OF THE
HISTORY OF MEDICINE

Volume 1

Edited by

W. F. BYNUM AND ROY PORTER

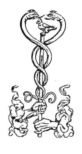

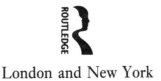

London and New York

First published in 1993
by Routledge
11 New Fetter Lane, London EC4P 4EE

Simultaneously published in the USA and Canada
by Routledge
a division of Routledge, Chapman and Hall, Inc.
29 West 35th Street, New York, NY 10001

Selection and editorial matter © 1993 W. F. Bynum and R. Porter
The chapters © 1993 Routledge

Phototypeset in 10/12½ Ehrhardt Linotronic 300 by Intype, London
Printed in England by Clays Ltd, St Ives plc
Paper manufactured in accordance with the proposed ANSI/NISO Z 39.48–199X
and ANSI Z 39.48–1984

British Library Cataloguing in Publication Data

A catalogue record for this book is available from the British Library

Library of Congress Cataloging-in-Publication Data

A catalog record for this book is available on request.

ISBN 0–415–04771–4 (set)
ISBN 0–415–09242–6 (Volume 1)
ISBN 0–415–09243–4 (Volume 2)

CONTENTS

NOTES ON CONTRIBUTORS

THE EDITORS

W. F. Bynum is head of the Academic Unit at the Wellcome Institute for the History of Medicine and Professor of the History of Medicine at University College London. He has published widely on many aspects of the biomedical and life sciences from the seventeenth century to the present and, with Roy Porter, is General Editor of the Wellcome Institute for the History of Medicine Series.

Roy Porter is Reader in the Social History of Medicine at the Wellcome Institute for the History of Medicine. He is currently working on the history of hysteria. Recent books include *Mind Forg'd Manacles. Madness in England from the Restoration to the Regency* (Athlone, 1987); *A Social History of Madness* (Weidenfeld & Nicolson, 1987); and *Health for Sale. Quackery in England 1660–1850* (Manchester University Press, 1989). Also, he co-authored with Dorothy Porter: *In Sickness and in Health. The British Experience, 1650–1850* (Fourth Estate, 1988); and *Patient's Progress* (Polity Press, 1989).

CONTRIBUTORS

William Randall Albury completed his Ph.D. degree in the history of science and a post-doctoral fellowship in the history of medicine at the Johns Hopkins University. He is currently Professor of History and Philosophy of Science in the School of Science and Technology Studies at the University of New South Wales, Sydney, Australia.

David Armstrong is Reader in Sociology as applied to Medicine at the

United Medical and Dental Schools, London University, and is an Honorary Consultant in Public Health Medicine at Guy's Hospital. He is the author of a standard textbook in medical sociology, *An Outline of Sociology as Applied to Medicine* (Bristol, John Wright, 1989, 3rd edn), as well as co-author of a text on research methods in primary health care. His monograph, *Political Anatomy of the Body* (Cambridge University Press), published in 1983, was one of the first books to elucidate the sociology of the body; it also served to introduce the work of Michel Foucault to a wider medical sociology audience.

David Arnold has been Professor of South Asian History at the School of Oriental and African Studies, London, since 1988. He formerly taught at the University of Dar es Salaam, Tanzania, and the University of Lancaster in England, and has worked on various aspects of the political and social history of modern India. His latest book, *Colonizing the Body: State Medicine and Epidemic Disease in Nineteenth-Century India*, is to be published by University of California Press in 1993. Previous publications include *Police Power and Colonial Rule: Madras, 1859–1947* (Delhi, Oxford University Press, 1986); *Famine: Social Crisis and Historical Change* (Oxford, 1988); and (ed.) *Imperial Medicine and Indigenous Societies* (Manchester, Manchester University Press, 1988).

Robert Baker is Professor and Chair at the Department of Philosophy, Union College, Schenectady, New York. He graduated from City College of New York, earned a Ph.D. from the University of Minnesota, and did a one-year post-doctoral fellowship at the Albany Medical College. He has taught at the University of Iowa, Wayne State University, and the New York University Medical School. His most recent books are (with M. Stosberg and J. Weiner) *Rationing America's Health Care* (The Brookings Institution, 1992) and (with D. and R. Porter) *The Codification of Medical Morality* (Vol. I, 1993).

Christopher Booth graduated in medicine at St Andrews University in 1951. He was Professor of Medicine at the Royal Postgraduate Medical School, London, from 1966 to 1977, subsequently becoming Director of the Clinical Research Centre at Northwick Park Hospital. Since 1989, he has been Harveian Librarian at the Royal College of Physicians of London.

Nick Bosanquet is currently Professor of Health Policy at Imperial College/ St. Mary's Hospital Medical School. He was formerly a special adviser to the House of Commons Select Committee on Social Services. His publications include *Family Doctors and Economic Incentives* (Dartmouth Publishing,

1989, and *A Smoke-Free Europe in the Year 2000: Wishful Thinking or Realistic Strategy?*

Brian Bracegirdle worked in industry before heading the science department in a college of education for many years, during which time he published a dozen books on industrial archaeology, photography, and microscopy. Following a doctorate in the history of medicine, he wrote the standard text on the development of microscopical preparation methods, *A History of Microtechnique* (London, Heinemann, 1978), and set up the Wellcome Museum of the History of Medicine at the Science Museum, London. He took early retirement from his administrative duties, and is working on a catalogue of the Science Museum's extensive microscopical collections, while continuing to publish other books and papers on the history of microscopy.

Allan M. Brandt is Amalie Moses Kass Professor of the History of Medicine at Harvard Medical School. He is the author of *No Magic Bullet: a Social History of Venereal Disease in the United States since 1880* (rev. edn, Oxford, 1987). In recent years, he has written about the history of public health as it relates to AIDS policy, and is currently writing a social history of cigarette smoking in the United States.

Francesca Bray read Chinese Studies at Cambridge, then worked with Joseph Needham for several years, contributing Vol. VI, Part 2: *Agriculture*, to his series *Science and Civilisation in China*. She now teaches anthropology at the University of California at Los Angeles. Her current research interests include the history of technology and the history and anthropology of medicine in China.

Gert H. Brieger is William H. Welch Professor and chair of the Department of the History of Science, Medicine and Technology at the Johns Hopkins University. He has worked mainly on American medicine, public health, and surgery of the nineteenth and twentieth centuries. He is presently completing a book on the history of pre-medical education in America.

William H. Brock is Reader in the History of Science at the University of Leicester. He has written extensively on the history of chemistry, the development of scientific education, and the history of scientific periodicals.

Theodore M. Brown teaches in the Division of Medical Humanities and in the Departments of History and Community and Preventive Medicine at the University of Rochester, New York. He is interested in the intellectual history of medicine, psychiatry, and psychosomatic medicine; in European and American health policy and politics; and in twentieth-century American efforts to reform medical education. He is currently co-editing a book of essays on the life and work of Henry E. Sigerist.

David Cantor is a Research Associate at the Institute of the History of Medicine, Johns Hopkins University. His Ph.D. thesis was on the history of radiobiology in Britain in the 1920s and 1930s. Subsequently, he worked on the history of rheumatology and rheumatism charities. His current project is a study of the representations of rheumatoid arthritis and its associated disablements.

Arthur Caplan, formerly Associate Director of the Hastings Center, is currently Director of the Center for Biomedical Ethics at the University of Minnesota. He is also a professor of philosophy and a professor of surgery. He is the author or editor of fifteen books, including *If I were a Rich Man Could I Buy a Pancreas?* (Indiana University Press, 1992), *Which Babies Shall Live?* (Humana, 1985), *The Sociobiology Debate, Concepts of Health and Disease,* and *In Search of Equity.*

Kenneth J. Carpenter has been a professor in the Department of Nutritional Sciences at the University of California at Berkeley, since 1977. Previously, he was Reader in Nutrition at the University of Cambridge. His research has been on the effect of processing (including traditional cooking practices) on nutrient availability in foods. He is the author of *The History of Scurvy and Vitamin C* (Cambridge, 1986), and other historical studies.

Lawrence I. Conrad is Historian of Arab-Islamic Medicine at the Wellcome Institute for the History of Medicine. His particular research interests are the history of medicine in the early medieval Near East, and problems of historiography and source criticism. He is currently working on the history of epidemic disease.

Harold J. Cook, an associate professor of the history of medicine and history of science at the University of Wisconsin-Madison, has published many articles and a book (*The Decline of the Old Medical Regime in Stuart London,* 1986) on seventeenth-century English medicine. He is currently embarked on studies regarding medicine and natural history in the seventeenth century, with special reference to the Netherlands.

Roger Cooter is a senior research officer at the Wellcome Unit for the History of Medicine, University of Manchester. He has published articles on various aspects of the social history of science and medicine, and is the author of *The Cultural Meaning of Popular Science* (1984), *Phrenology in the British Isles* (1989), and *Surgery and Society in Peace and War* (1993). He has also edited *Studies in the History of Alternative Medicine* (Macmillan, 1988) and *In the Name of the Child: Health and Welfare, 1880–1940* (1991). Until recently, he was one of the editors of *Social History of Medicine*.

Catherine Crawford studied history at the universities of British Columbia, Sussex, and Oxford, taking her D.Phil. in 1987. She taught history of science at the University of Leeds, and was a research fellow at the Wellcome Institute for the History of Medicine before joining the history department at the University of Essex in 1990. She is the co-editor of *Legal Medicine in History* (Cambridge University Press, 1993), and is writing a book on the history of medical testimony.

Debórah Dwork is a historian of children and childhood and an associate professor at the Child Study Center, Yale University. Her publications include: *War is Good for Babies and Other Young Children: a History of the Infant and Child Welfare Movement in England, 1898–1918* (Tainstock, 1987) and *Children with a Star: Jewish Youth in Nazi Europe* (Yale University Press, 1991). She is currently working on a historical study of the plight of refugee children, entitled *Flight from the Reich: Jewish Refugee Youth*.

Daniel M. Fox became President of the Milbank Memorial Fund in 1990. Prior to that, he was Professor of Social Sciences and Humanities in Medicine and Director of the Center for Assessing Health Services at the State University of New York at Stony Brook, having previously taught at Harvard University. He has also served in state government in Massachusetts and on the staff of several federal agencies. He has written numerous articles on public policy, the history of medicine, health affairs, and photography; and several books, which include the prize-winning *The Discovery of Abundance* (1967), *Economists and Health Care* (1979), *Health Politics, Health Policies: the Experience of Britain and America 1911–65* (1986), and (with C. Lawrence) *Photographing Medicine: Images and Power in Britain and America since 1840* (London, Greenwood Press, 1988), and *Power and Illness: The Failure and Future of American Health Policy*.

Roger French completed his D.Phil. at Oxford, and then taught history and philosophy of science in the universities of Leicester and Aberdeen. He is now Director of the Wellcome Unit for the History of Medicine in the University of Cambridge, and his special interests are natural philosophy and medicine in the Middle Ages and Renaissance.

Toby Gelfand is Hannah Professor of History of Medicine at the University of Ottawa, where he holds a joint appointment in the Medical Faculty and the Department of History. His current research deals with Charcot's Salpêtrière school. He is collaborating on a new biography of Charcot, and is co-editor of, *Freud and the History of Psychoanalysis* (Analytic Press, 1992). He has taught at the universities of Minnesota and Princeton. His publications focusing on the history of French medicine include *Professionalizing Modern Medicine: Paris Surgeons and Medical Science and Institutions in the Eighteenth Century* (Greenwood Press, 1980).

Norman Gevitz is Associate Professor of the History of Medicine, University of Illinois College of Medicine, Chicago. He is the author of *The D.O.'s: Osteopathic Medicine in America* (Johns Hopkins University Press, 1983), and editor of *Other Healers: Unorthodox Medicine in America* (Johns Hopkins University Press, 1988). He has written widely in the areas of education for the health professions, health-care licensure, and early American medicine. He recently received a Fellowship from the National Endowment for the Humanities supporting a long-term project on the history of domestic medicine in the United States.

Johanna Geyer-Kordesch is Director of the Wellcome Unit for the History of Medicine at Glasgow University. She has published on eighteenth-century German medicine, medical education, medicine and Pietism; and is currently working on the history of case histories. She has also published a number of articles on the entry of women into professional medicine in the nineteenth century. She is currently working on the entrance of women into medicine and its impact on higher education in Scotland, 1860–1920.

Sander L. Gilman is the Goldwin Smith Professor of Humane Studies at Cornell University and Professor of the History of Psychiatry at the Cornell Medical College. During 1990–1, he was Visiting Historical Scholar at the National Library of Medicine, Bethesda, Maryland. A member of the Cornell faculty since 1969, he is an intellectual and literary historian and the author or editor of over twenty-seven books, among the most recent are *Sexuality: an Illustrated History* (John Wiley & Sons, 1989) and *The Jew's Body* (Routledge, 1992). He is the author of the basic study of the visual stereotyping of the mentally ill, *Seeing the Insane* (John Wiley & Sons, 1982).

Jan Goldstein is Professor of History at the University of Chicago, where she specializes in modern European intellectual history. Her book *Console and Classify: the French Psychiatric Profession in the Nineteenth Century* (Cambridge University Press, 1987) received the Herbert Baxter Adams Prize of the

American Historical Association. She had edited and contributed to a forth-coming volume, *Foucault and the Writing of History*, and is working on a book about competing psychological theories and the politics of selfhood in nineteenth-century France.

Lindsay Granshaw was, until recently, Historian of Modern Medicine at the Wellcome Institute for the History of Medicine. She is the author of *St Mark's Hospital London: a Social History of a Specialist Hospital* (London, King's Fund, 1985), and co-editor (with Roy Porter) of *The Hospital in History* (Routledge, 1989). She has written various articles on hospitals, surgery, nursing, and the National Health Service.

Caroline Hannaway is currently Historical Consultant to the National Institute of Health Historical Office, Bethesda, Maryland. She is editing books on the Paris Clinical School of the nineteenth century and on the history of tropical and colonial medicine.

Colin Jones is Professor of History at Exeter University. He is the author of *Charity and 'Bienfaisance': The Treatment of the Poor in the Montpellier Region 1740–1815* (1983); *The Longman Companion to the French Revolution* (1989) and *The Charitable Imperative: Hospitals and Nursing in Ancien Régime and Revolutionary France* (Routledge, 1989). He edited (with M. Newitt and S. K. Roberts) *Politics and People in Revolutionary England* (Blackwell, 1986); and (with Jonathan Barry) *Medicine and Charity Before the Welfare State* (Routledge, 1991).

K. F. Kiple took a Ph.D. in history and Ph.D. certificate in Latin American Studies at the University of Florida. He is currently Professor of History at Bowling Green State University, Ohio. He is the author of numerous articles and four books, among them *The Caribbean Slave: a Biological History* (Cambridge University Press, 1984); and the editor of *The Cambridge World History of Human Disease* (Cambridge, 1993).

Arthur Kleinman is Professor of Psychiatry and Chair of the Department of Social Medicine at Harvard Medical School, and Professor of Anthro-pology in the Faculty of Arts and Sciences at Harvard University. His research and teaching involve studies of the effect of the social context on the course of chronic illness (that is, medical and psychiatric disorders) in China, Taiwan, and the United States. His books include *Patients and Healers in the Context of Culture* (University of California Press, 1980), *Social Origins of Distress and Disease: Neurasthenia, Depression and Pain in Modern China* (Yale University Press, 1986), *The Illness Narratives: Suffering, Healing and the*

Human Condition (Basic Books, 1988), and *Rethinking Psychiatry: From Cultural Context to Personal Experience* (Free Press, 1988).

Stephen Kunitz is a physician and sociologist, with an MA in the history of medicine. His interests are in the historical and cross-cultural study of morbidity and mortality. He is currently a professor in the Department of Community and Preventive Medicine at the University of Rochester, New York.

Gerald V. Larkin is Professor of Sociology and Head of Applied Social Sciences in the School of Health and Community Studies at Sheffield Hallam University. He has also held lectureships at Kingston University and the University of Leeds. He is the author of a wide range of publications on both historical and contemporary issues related to a number of health professions, and his research interests include the history and sociology of the professions, particularly as exemplified in the evolution of the medical division of labour.

Murray Last is Reader in Social Anthropology at University College London, where he started research in medical anthropology in 1968 after completing a Ph.D. in history. He has carried out a long-term study of the non-Muslim Maguzawa and their medicine in northern Nigeria, and has continued writing on Nigeria's pre-colonial history. Currently, he is directing a five-year collaborative project on youth and health in Kano, and organizing a volume of essays on 'healing the wounds of war'. In 1986, he edited (with G. L. Chavunduka), *The Professionalisation of African Medicine* (Manchester University Press for IAI). Since 1987, he has been the editor of *Africa*, the journal of the International African Institute.

Ghislaine Lawrence qualified in medicine from St Mary's Hospital, London, in 1975, working in hospital and general practice before joining the Science Museum in 1979. There, she became involved in the creation of the Wellcome Galleries of the History of Medicine, and is now Senior Curator of Clinical Medicine. Her research interests lie in the technologically oriented medical specialities of the nineteenth and twentieth centuries, and in cognitive issues involved in scientific and medical exhibitions generally.

Susan C. Lawrence is Assistant Professor in the Department of History and Medical Historian in the College of Medicine at the University of Iowa. Among her publications are 'Private enterprise and public interests: medical education and the Apothecaries' Act, 1780–1825', in *British Medicine in the Age of Reform* (Routledge, 1991); and 'Educating the senses: students, teachers and medical rhetoric in eighteenth-century London', in *Medicine and the Five*

Senses (Cambridge, 1993). She is currently working on *Charitable Knowledge: Hospital Practitioners and Pupils in Eighteenth-Century London.*

Irvine S. L. Loudon qualified in medicine in 1951. From 1952 to 1981 he worked as a general practitioner in Wantage, Oxfordshire, including obstetrics in the local maternity unit. He became interested in historical research in 1970, and resigned from general practice in 1981 to take up a second career as a medical historian. He was Research Associate and Wellcome Research Associate at the Wellcome Unit for the History of Medicine 1979–81 and 1986–9, and Wellcome Research Fellow from 1981 to 1985. His interests include the history of medical practice, historical epidemiology, and the history of childbirth. His publications include papers on these subjects, *Medical Care and the General Practitioner, 1750–1850* (Oxford University Press, 1986 and, he is currently completing a book entitled *Death in Childbirth. An International Study of Maternal Care and Maternal Mortality, 1800–1950* (1992).

Françoise Loux is Director of Research at the Centre National de la Recherche Scientifique, and works at the Centre d'Ethnologie Française situated at the Musée des Arts et Traditions Populaires in Paris. She conducts research into the anthropology of the body in complementary directions: images and representations of the body in traditional French society, infancy and knowledge about the body, popular medicine, the transfer of knowledge about the body and identity, and anthropology and nursing care. She has written ten books in this field.

Carol MacCormack is Katharine McBride Professor in Anthropology at Bryn Mawr College, having previously taught at Cambridge University and the London School of Hygiene and Tropical Medicine. Since the 1960s, she has done research primarily in West Africa, and also in East Africa, Asia, and the Caribbean. Her publications are on anthropology and tropical public health.

Christopher Maggs, a state registered nurse, registered mental nurse and registered clinical nurse teacher, earned a Ph.D. in economic and social history and now has his own consultancy. He is Professor of Nursing Research at the University of Wales College of Medicine, and has taught history, supervised postgraduate students, and advised radio and television companies on the history of health care and nursing. He has written extensively on nursing history, social policy, and continuing education, and his current work includes a history of the Royal College of Midwives and a biography of Sir Henry Burdett.

Harry M. Marks graduated from Hofstra University, the University of Wisconsin, and the Massachusetts Institute of Technology. He taught history and health policy for several years at the schools of Medicine and of Public Health at Harvard University. He is presently an assistant professor at the Department of the History of Science, Medicine and Technology, Johns Hopkins University, where he is working on a book on the history of therapeutic drug experimentation and regulation.

Russell C. Maulitz is a physician and medical historian in Philadelphia, Pennsylvania. His monograph on the pathological tradition, *Morbid Appearances* (Cambridge University Press, 1987), explores at greater length some of the questions addressed in his chapter in this encyclopedia. More recently, he has edited two books: *Grand Rounds* (1988), on the history of internal medicine; and *Unnatural Causes* (Rutgers, 1989), on the three leading causes of mortality in the United States. He has translated (with Jacalyn Duffin) Mirko Grmek's landmark *History of AIDS* (1990). His current research concerns the history of medical workers.

Michael Neve is a lecturer in the history of medicine at the Wellcome Institute for the History of Medicine. He teaches the history of the life sciences, the history of psychiatry, and degeneration in nineteenth-century European writing.

Malcolm Nicolson is Research Fellow at the Wellcome Unit for the History of Medicine, University of Glasgow. He works on a number of topics in the history and sociology of eighteenth- and twentieth-century medicine and science, and is currently engaged, with David Smith, in a study of the 'Glasgow School' of chemical physiology. His recent publications include: 'Henry Allan Gleason and the individualistic hypothesis: the structure of a botanist's career', *Botanical Review* 1990, 56: 91–161; and 'The social and the cognitive: resources for the sociology of scientific knowledge', *Studies in the History and Philosophy of Science*, 1991, 22: 1–23.

Vivian Nutton, formerly a Fellow of Selwyn College, Cambridge, has been a senior lecturer at the Wellcome Institute for the History of Medicine since 1977. He specializes in the history of the Graeco-Roman medical tradition, and his books include *From Democedes to Harvey* (1988) and *Galen: On Prognosis* (1979). He has been joint editor, with W. F. Bynum, of *Medical History* since 1980.

Robert C. Olby was formerly Reader in the History of Science in the Division of the History and Philosophy of Science at the University of Leeds.

He is currently Mellon Research Fellow at the Rockefeller University. His research interests lie in the interface between neurobiology, AI, and molecular biology. He is completing a study of the establishment of Mendelian genetics in Britain, and is preparing a text on the history of biology for the general reader.

Margaret Pelling is Deputy Director of the Wellcome Unit for the History of Medicine, University of Oxford. Her book, *Cholera, Fever and English Medicine 1825–1865* (1978), is concerned with theories of disease and sanitary reform. Latterly, her main research interest has been medical practice and social conditions in early modern England. Her recent publications include (ed., with R. M. Smith) *Life, Death and the Elderly: Historical Perspectives* (Routledge, 1991).

Dorothy Porter is Wellcome Research Lecturer at Birkbeck College. She has written (with Roy Porter) *In Sickness and in Health: the British Experience 1650–1850* (Fourth Estate, 1988, Basil Blackwell, 1989), and *Patient's Progress* (1989). She is currently writing *A Political History of Public Health* Routledge, forthcoming; editing an essay collection on *The History of Health and the Modern State: National Contexts Compared* (University of Pennsylvania Press, forthcoming); and researching a study of *The Pursuit of Social Pathology: Medicine, Social Science and the Visible College in Britain in the Twentieth Century.*

Stanley Joel Reiser is the Griff T. Ross Professor of Humanities and Technology in Health Care at the University of Texas Health Science Center at Houston. His recent publications include *The Machine at the Bedside: Strategies for Using Technology in Patient Care* (Cambridge University Press, 1984), and *Divided Staffs, Divided Selves: a Case Approach to Mental Health Ethics* (Cambridge University Press, 1987).

Guenter B. Risse is Professor and Chair, Department of the History of Health Sciences, University of California, San Francisco. A physician-historian, he is the author and editor of several books and numerous articles. His work *Hospital Life in Enlightenment Scotland, Care and Teaching at the Royal Infirmary in Edinburgh* (Cambridge, 1986) won the 1988 Welch Medal of the American Association for the History of Medicine. He is presently completing a historical synthesis dealing with the evolution of the hospital, and preparing a book on bubonic plague in San Francisco during 1900–10.

Milton I. Roemer has been a professor in the School of Public Health at the University of California, Los Angeles, since 1962. He taught previously at Cornell and Yale universities. He earned the MD degree in 1940, and also holds master's degrees in sociology and in public health. He has served at all levels of health administration – county, state, national, and international (with the World Health Organization). He has published thirty-two books and 400 articles on the social aspects of health care. As an international consultant, Dr Roemer has studied health-care organization in sixty-one countries, and in 1977 received from the American Public Health Association (APHA) the International Award for Excellence in Promoting and Protecting the Health of People. In 1983, the APHA awarded him its highest honour, the Sedgwick Memorial Medal for Distinguished Service in Public Health.

Edward Shorter, currently Hannah Professor in the History of Medicine at the University of Toronto, took his Ph.D. at Harvard University in 1968, and has worked at the University of Toronto ever since. He has written eight books, the latest being *From Paralysis to Fatigue: a History of Psychosomatic Illness in the Modern Era* (Free Press, 1992).

Richard Smith is Director of the Wellcome Unit for the History of Medicine and Reader in the History of Medicine at the University of Oxford, and a Fellow of All Souls College. He has published extensively on the demographic history of Britain and Europe from the Middle Ages to the twentieth century. He is currently working on the medical provisions of the English Poor Law, and directs a collaborative project on the epidemiological history of the southern North Sea basin.

Christine Stevenson studied the history of art and architecture in Victoria (British Columbia), Helsinki, Copenhagen, and London. Formerly Deputy Editor of the journal *Medical History*, and now Honorary Editor of *Architectural History*, she lectures at Reading University on seventeenth- and eighteenth-century architecture. She has published articles about the history of industrial design, painting, and architecture (including lunatic asylums), and is writing a book about the history of hospital building.

Tilli Tansey studied neurotransmitters in *Octopus* brain for her Ph.D., after which her research ranged from invertebrate neuropharmacology to the physiology and biochemistry of demyelination. In 1986, she became a Research Fellow at the Wellcome Institute for the History of Medicine, working on the history of neurotransmission; and in 1990, she completed a Ph.D. thesis on the early scientific career of Sir Henry Dale FRS. She is currently Historian of Modern Medical Science at the Wellcome Institute for the History of Medicine, and is Honorary Archivist of the Physiological Society.

Pat Thane is Reader in Social History, University of London, and teaches in the Department of Social Policy and Politics, Goldsmith's College, University of London. She has written numerous books and articles on the history of ageing, of social welfare, of women, and of the labour movement, mainly in nineteenth- and twentieth-century Britain. She is currently writing a book on the History of old age in Britain.

Ulrich Tröhler, formerly a physician, is currently Professor and Chairman of the Institute for the History of Medicine at the University of Göttingen. Among his works on the history of surgery is a biography of the Nobel Prizewinner, T. Kocher (1841–1917). Other major contributions and research interests concern the history of obstetrics, clinical statistics, human and animal experimentation, as well as antivivisection and medical education (including social and ethical aspects).

Andrew Wear lectures in the history of medicine at University College London and the Wellcome Institute for the History of Medicine. He has research interests in Renaissance medicine and in the social history of medicine in early modern England.

Miles Weatherall has been Professor of Pharmacology at the London Hospital Medical College and a director at the Wellcome Research Laboratories at Beckenham, near London. He has served as a Privy Council nominated member of the Council of the Pharmaceutical Society, and as a Medicines Commissioner. After retiring, he wrote a widely acclaimed account of the history of the discovery of drugs, *In Search of a Cure* (Oxford University Press, 1990), and has been engaged in other studies of pharmacological history.

Paul Weindling is Senior Research Officer at the Wellcome Unit for the History of Medicine, University of Oxford. He is the author of *Health, Race and German Politics between National Unification and Nazism, 1870–1945* (Cambridge University Press, 1989), and *Darwinism and Social Darwinism in Imperial Germany: the Contribution of the Cell Biologist Oscar Hertwig (1849–1922)* (Stuttgart, 1991); and has co-edited *Information Sources for the History of Science and Medicine* (London, 1983).

Richard Burkewood Welbourn was educated at Cambridge and Liverpool universities and the Mayo Foundation. Now retired, he has been Professor of Surgical Science at Queen's University of Belfast, and Professor of Surgery and Surgical Endocrinology at the Royal Postgraduate Medical School, London. He is the author of *Clinical Endocrinology for Surgeons* (1963) and

Medical and Surgical Endocrinology (1975) (both with D. A. D. Montgomery), and *The History of Endocrine Surgery* (Praeger, 1990).

Lise Wilkinson graduated in pharmacy, then did postgraduate work in plant physiology at Copenhagen and Berkeley, California. Her thesis and papers were on the path of carbon (the role of glycolic acid) in photosynthesis, and the fate of pre-formed chlorophyll in germinating seeds. She has written many papers and, with A. P. Waterson, wrote a history of the study of viruses and of the later development of the scientific discipline of virology. She is based at the Department of Virology at the Royal Postgraduate Medical School, and the Wellcome Institute for the History of Medicine. Her current interests include the development of scientific veterinary and comparative medicine, and the history of the London School of Hygiene and Tropical Medicine.

Leonard G. Wilson was educated in biology at the University of Toronto and pursued postgraduate study at University College London and the University of Wisconsin. He has taught at Mount Allison University in Sackville, New Brunswick, the University of California at Berkeley, Cornell University, and Yale University. He has been Professor of the History of Medicine at the University of Minnesota since 1967. He is the author or editor of several books and numerous articles on the history of medicine and the biological sciences, and from 1973 to 1982 served as Editor of the *Journal of the History of Medicine and Allied Sciences*.

Michael Worboys is Wellcome Reader in the History of Medicine at Sheffield Hallam University, and Associate Fellow at the Wellcome Unit for the History of Medicine at the University of Manchester. He has worked on the history of science and British colonial imperialism, and the history of tropical medicine, and is currently working on germ theories and bacteriology in the period 1870–1940. He has recently published on sanatoriums, vaccine therapy, and veterinary responses to germ theories and practices.

Dominik Wujastyk has been on the staff of the Wellcome Institute for the History of Medicine since 1982 and is responsible for cataloguing the Institute's large Sanskrit manuscript collection. He has published the first volume of a *Handlist* of this collection, as well as books, articles and reviews on Sanskrit linguistics, the history of Indian science and medicine, codicology, and computing.

NOTE TO THE READER

Cross-references between chapters in this work are indicated in parentheses, for example: (➤Ch. 19 Fevers; Ch. 11 Clinical research). Cross-references are given only when referral will provide further information concerning the subject under discussion: they are not included automatically merely to indicate that a separate entry exists.

Dates of birth and death have been included at the first mention of individuals in the text of each chapter. Despite careful research, it has not been possible to discover these dates in all cases: occasionally, only the birth or death date or a time-span of known activity (for example, *fl.* 1780–1810) can be provided.

ACKNOWLEDGEMENTS

The idea and inspiration for this volume came from Jonathan Price of Routledge. We are grateful to him for having given us the opportunity to undertake the venture and for having provided us with his full encouragement. At every stage, Routledge have been supportive and efficient in providing the facilities vital for a huge collaborative volume such as this. In addition, we would like to thank Shan Millie and her colleagues at Routledge. Both copyeditor and indexer, Jean Runciman has, as ever, exercised her exemplary care on the finished product. And, throughout the planning, commissioning, and revision of the chapters, the services of Sally Bragg have been both indispensable and immaculate. Without her unflagging administrative and secretarial skills, without her boundless energy and tireless commitment, it is no exaggeration to say that this volume would never have been completed. Caroline Prentice has coped admirably with the checking of dates and references, and has been of invaluable assistance in the preparation of the final manuscript. Our thanks to all these special helpers.

Our thanks, too, to many other people at the Wellcome Institute, especially Andy Foley, for a variety of back-up services, efficiently and cheerfully provided. No finer academic environment could be imagined than the Wellcome Institute. Our thanks, as always, to Sir Henry Wellcome and his Trustees, whose forethought and generosity have provided over the years a workplace so congenial to scholarship.

INTRODUCTION

1

THE ART AND SCIENCE OF MEDICINE

Roy Porter and W. F. Bynum

The seventy-two essays that follow speak for themselves. Beyond argument, they comprise the best and biggest body of expert research and interpretation in the history of medicine currently available, the fruits of the learning of scholars from many nations and a host of specialities, co-operating to provide numerous rich perspectives upon medicine in its widest connotations.

The discipline of the history of medicine has been growing with extraordinary rapidity over the last generation. It has not merely increased in size but has changed its scope and nature. Alongside traditional approaches – the history of epidemics, of medical theory and practice, surgery and therapeutics, and of medical science, all of which are themselves studied in greater depth than ever – the history of medicine now draws increasingly upon the techniques and findings of often-new sister-disciplines (demography is one instance) and is more broadly integrated within the wider histories of science and society.

There is greater attention to the whole range of medical personnel and healers than in the days when the medical historian's attention focused principally on 'great doctors'. There is a new sensitivity to the profound moral and philosophical questions that medicine has raised and continues to raise; for example, the recent emergence of medical ethics as a field of medicine testifies to the ways in which current concerns illuminate once-neglected historical dimensions, the past and the present fruitfully interacting. The once-common assumption of the essential benignity and triumphal progress of medicine has found its critics, resulting in a greater concern to dispassionately scrutinize the social and cultural roles that the medical profession has played in the past, in respect, for instance, to the law or to minority groups (infants, the insane, and so forth). Not least, and thanks in part to the emergence of a new social history, the dynamic personal and professional relations of patients and practitioners, and of the various inter-locking ranks within the medical profession itself, are now receiving the historical attention they long lacked but richly deserve.

With growing interest in the history of medicine, both within and beyond the academy, it is high time for the appearance of works synthesizing these deep and diverse researches. We do not pretend that the present work is the last word: it is an overview, a stock-taking which we hope will serve as a springboard for future investigations. But we do feel confident that it com-prises by far the best broad survey of the development of medicine and the healing arts as understood by medical historians today, and also the finest instance of the intellectual commitments and working practice of medical historians of many hues and schools and types of technical expertise.

Hence, as editors, our advice to the reader is: read on. To a large degree, the chapter headings will make it perfectly evident where discussion relevant to the reader's interests may be found, be it 'Chinese medicine' (Ch. 32), 'Tropical diseases' (Ch. 24), 'Drug therapies' (Ch. 39), or 'Nursing' (Ch. 54). Cross-referencing within each chapter, and the copious index, provide further internal maps and signposts.

It might, however, be useful to make a few preliminary points about the aims, scope, and organization of this work, emphasizing what has been included and what, principally for reasons of space, has had to be left out. We have decided upon an encyclopedia rather than a dictionary or a com-panion. In this work there are to be found no brief accounts of individual diseases, no potted biographies of great individuals or histories of famous institutions, no quick guides to breakthroughs. To some extent, reference works already exist which adequately fulfil such functions. For instance, Roderick E. McGrew's *Encyclopedia of Medical History* (New York, McGraw-Hill, 1985) is a useful compendium of historical information, principally arranged by an alphabetical sequence of entries on individual diseases and medical specialities; and the more recent volume edited by Kenneth Kiple, *The Cambridge World History of Human Disease* (New York and Cambridge, Cambridge University Press, 1993), provides a new synthesis of current understanding of diseases. *The Oxford Companion to Medicine*, edited by John Walton, Paul Beeson, and Ronald Bodley Scott (2 vols, Oxford and New York, Oxford University Press, 1986) is more contemporary in its focus but also contains much historical material. At the close of this introductory essay will be found a list of helpful reference works in the history of medicine.

The history-of-medicine cake may be cut in various ways. We have chosen to carve it into large slices – essays ranging from around 6,000 to some 12,000 words – so as to give plentiful scope for detailed and wide-ranging analysis and the opportunity to authors to offer the larger perspective and a view of interconnections. And we have tried to divide the whole into portions that reflect real historical problems, fields, and disciplinary specialities. We have elected not to provide entries upon individual diseases as presently labelled (tuberculosis, smallpox, malaria, and so forth), because delving into the strata of history by this means will inevitably obscure as much as it illuminates: as the essay on 'Nosology' (Ch. 19) underscores, medical theory and practice in the past frequently did not recognize diseases or divide the disease terrain as we do today. Other ways of categorizing diseases ('holism', fevers, etc.) have tended to apply in earlier centuries and previous intellectual traditions; and, in our conceptual divisions of the material, we have sought to avoid, whenever feasible, grossly Whiggish or anachronistic categorizations.

Yet avoidance of hindsight naturally has its limits in practice, above all in a practical handbook such as this. We have a chapter titled 'The physiological tradition' (Ch. 7). Strictly speaking, it is anachronistic to speak of physiology or biology before the nineteenth century; earlier investigations carried such names as *anatomia animata*, but it would be merely finicky in this kind of work to put 'animal economy' and 'physiology' in separate chapters. Doubtless a heading such as 'Nutritional diseases' (Ch. 22) also smacks somewhat of hindsight, being primarily a twentieth-century category: in the eighteenth century, after all, a complaint like scurvy was viewed as a disease of putrescence rather than a consequence of dietary deficiency. On the other hand, it is the historian's task not merely to recover the intellectual universes of the past, but also to trace long-term chains of connection and the transformations of scientific paradigms; and so longitudinal studies, taking broad themes over many centuries, are also rewarding, even at the risk of a certain degree of organizational artificiality and anachronism.

Dividing the history of medicine into some seventy segments thus poses conceptual and practical problems. It is possible to go back to Hippocrates (*c*.460–370 BC) for guidance and inspiration. *'Ars longa'*, begins the most famous of his aphorisms: the art is long; life is short; the occasion fleeting; experience fallacious, and judgement difficult. It is remarkable how much that is pregnant of the whole of later medicine is contained in this and other prescient maxims of the father of Western medicine. The art has indeed proved long. By that, Hippocrates meant that the individual practitioner could acquire medical skills only by patient observation and by training. But it has proved long in another sense. For perhaps two thousand years after Hippocrates, ebbing and flowing within the broad channels carved out by the Hippocratics and the later Galenists, medicine developed its well-established structures, cognitive, therapeutic, professional. Numerous chapters in this volume focus, at least in their initial pages, upon the traditions of medical thought and practice thereby entrenched: see the contributions on 'The anatomical tradition' (Ch. 5), 'Humoralism' (Ch. 14), 'The art of diagnosis' (Ch. 35),

'Medical care' (Ch. 4), 'Physical methods' (Ch. 40), Traditional surgery' (Ch. 47), and so forth.

Yet, although medicine became organized and established as a healing art, it remained equivocal as an enterprise. Other chapters – 'Medicine and demography' (Ch. 71), 'Ecology of disease' (Ch. 18), 'Medicine, mortality, and morbidity' (Ch. 72) – demonstrate at length that for all the efforts of practitioners in the two thousand years after Hippocrates, disease and death still hold centre stage. Indeed, it is for this reason that it has seemed to us that the history of medicine, at least before the last few hundred years, must primarily be contextualized in terms of far wider themes: the histories of the vulnerable human body, its elementary conceptualization and experiences ('Pain' (Ch. 67), 'Medicine and religion' (Ch. 61), and, beyond Europe, in 'Non-Western concepts of disease' (Ch. 29)), and the life cycle ('Childbirth' (Ch. 44), 'Geriatrics' (Ch. 46)); basic disease experiences ('Nutritional diseases' (Ch. 22), 'Tropical diseases' (Ch. 24), 'Diseases of civilization' (Ch. 27)), and non- and pre-professional medicine ('Folk medicine' (Ch. 30), 'Unorthodox medical theories' (Ch. 28), 'Medicine and women' (Ch. 38), 'Personal hygiene' (Ch. 53)). For most of the history of civilization, any primary concentration upon the history of professional medicine, to the exclusion of a far wider range of belief systems and healing practices, would be deeply distorting.

Furthermore, medicine itself, throughout most of its recorded history, must be seen more as an art than a science. 'Medicine is an art', insisted Plato, (c.427-c.347 BC), 'and attends to the nature and constitution of the patient, and has principles of action and reason, in each case.' The two terms, art and science, are not, of course, mutually exclusive; and, as we shall emphasize below, even today one of the distinctive, complicating but fascinating features of medicine remains its special union of basic scientific knowledge with craft skill and individual experience, its integration of theory and practice, its dedication to understanding ('Clinical research' (Ch. 11), 'Pathology' (Ch. 9), etc.) and application (the broad realm of 'Medical care' (Ch. 4)). But it is important to emphasize that pre-modern medicine was personal and traditional in its modes of education, training, and organization, with emphasis upon received wisdom, book-learning, and apprenticeship (Ch. 48). It set great store by highly personal clinical relationships between the doctor and the patient (Ch. 34), and emphasized personal experience in diagnosing and treating the individual case as the royal road to successful healing ('The art of diagnosis' (Ch. 35); 'Humoralism' (Ch. 14); 'Medical care' (Ch. 4)). A similar emphasis upon medicine as an art may be found in traditional Islamic, Chinese and Indian medicine, and, arguably, in the discussion of non-Western theories of disease (Chs 29, 31, 32, 33).

That preoccupation has never waned. A line of notable physicians right down to the present day has continued to insist that medicine, because its basic rationale is the healing of the individual sick person, must ever remain an art. But an increasingly defensive tone in some of these pronouncements signals an important shift. For the distinctive feature of European and Euro-American medicine over the last few hundred years (as is pointed out in 'What is specific to Western medicine?' (Ch. 2)) is its ever-increasing aspirations to be a science as well as an art, or a science-based art.

This is not to say that Galen (AD 129-*c*.200/210) or Rhazes (AD *c*.854–925) did not think of medicine as a science. But it is to stress that medicine was not traditionally pigeon-holed primarily as a science, or that the business of the good physician was seen as essentially a scientific skill. 'Medicine is not only a science,' Paracelsus (1493–1541) insisted in the Renaissance, 'it is also an art.' The great clinician Thomas Sydenham (1624–89) thought much the same in the next century: 'the art of medicine was to be properly learned only from its practice and its exercise.' And it is to draw attention to change. Since the broad Scientific Revolution of the sixteenth and seventeenth centuries, which introduced a New Philosophy of matter in motion and privileged mechanism and mathematics, medicine has always pursued, and sometimes realized, a new dream of making its intellectual foundation more secure, and its practices better grounded, by enlarging basic scientific understanding in such fields as physiology, pathology, nosology, biochemistry, and so forth. By the nineteenth century, the ideological vindication of the newly reformed medical profession was increasingly judged to be its scientific grounding (or 'pretensions', as critics pointed out, leading to hostility to orthodox medicine amongst religious sectaries, literary critics, naturopaths, and others for whom the vain claims of scientificity were anathema).

A radical transformation of medicine rapidly occurred from the latter part of the eighteenth century. Medical education came increasingly to depend upon a groundwork in basic science. As the essay on 'The hospital' (Ch. 49) demonstrates, that institution was transformed from a place of charity and care into a *machine à guérir*, a site of pathological anatomy where patients were observed in sufficient numbers to permit eventual reclassifications of disease in terms of the normal and the pathological (see 'The concepts of health, illness and disease' (Ch. 12), and 'Ideas of life and death' (Ch. 13)). In turn, the laboratory joined the hospital as the place of medical investigation, and Clinical research (Ch. 11) gathered momentum. 'Medicine is a science in the making', suggested François Magendie (1783–1855) early in the nineteenth century. By the late twentieth century, many would consider that infant science to be fully grown.

Alongside certain basic and applied sciences, medicine generated its own technologies, often deployed in a new science of diagnosis (Ch. 36). The 'Microscopical tradition' (Ch. 6) came early; in the twentieth century, it has been supplemented with the massive diagnostic and intensive-care equipment discussed in 'Medical technologies' (Ch. 68), and echoed in 'Medicine and architecture' (Ch. 64). And one major consequence of all such thrusts has been the vast increase in the division of medical labour and, above all, the emergence of new medical specialities. Chapters such as 'Constitutional disorders' (Ch. 20), 'Mental diseases' (Ch. 21), 'Endocrine diseases' (Ch. 23), 'Cancer' (Ch. 25) and 'Sexually transmitted diseases' (Ch. 26) and, above all, 'Clinical research' (Ch. 11), trace the intimate interplay between new specialized forms of understanding (highly dependent upon basic science and technological breakthroughs) and the swiftly growing range of clinical interventions. Modern surgery (Ch. 42) is barely recognizable as the offspring of the primitive and modest practices of a century and a half ago (Ch. 41); the same is equally true of 'Drug therapies' (Ch. 39), with their intense research orientation and sophisticated clinical trials. New realms of medicine flourish today (such as 'Geriatrics' (Ch. 46)), that were virtually unheard of in former centuries. Whereas two hundred years ago there were few intraprofessional divisions within medicine – indeed, the very term 'general practitioner' had just come into vogue – today (as the chapters on 'Paramedical professions (Ch. 55) and 'Psychiatry' (Ch. 56) clearly demonstrate) the medical profession possesses an infinitely intricate structuring.

The inevitable consequence of this development of specialized, high-science and high-tech medicine over the last century or so is that it has become institutionally extraordinarily complex, requiring massive funding, and interlocking at innumerable points with society at large. The chapters on 'Health economics' (Ch. 57) and 'Medical philanthropy' (Ch. 63) trace the staggering increase in costs that have accompanied the advances in modern medicine, and explore the diverse ways in which different political systems have chosen to underwrite those charges. More broadly, the growing presence and power, but also potential dangers, of modern interventionist medicine have to the maturation of 'Public Health' (Ch. 51), the revolutionizing of 'Epidemiology' (Ch. 52), the invention of new areas of activity ('Medicine and colonialism' (Ch. 58), and the notable new problems of jurisprudence explored in 'Medical ethics' (Ch. 37) and 'Medicine and the law' (Ch. 69). The chapter on 'Medical institutions and the state' (Ch. 50) explores the inexorable extension of the claims of the modern polity upon medicine and of medicine upon the state. If, in some sense, traditional medicine as an art focused upon the clinical encounter between patient and practitioner, medicine as a science embraces the whole of society.

Powerful yet problematic, medicine has come under intense academic scrutiny during the last century, the interest in medical history itself being one manifestation of this. As the relationships between 'Medicine and literature' (Ch. 65) demonstrate, writers have used the mirror of medicine to throw light on their own worlds, while also exploring the doctor's dilemma. Above all, such disciplines as 'Medical sociology' (Ch. 70), and 'Medical anthropology' (Ch. 60) have partaken of the scientific drive that has informed medicine itself, while seeking to analyse its theory and practice. They have helped fuel a continued nagging critique. 'Harvey's discovery of the circulation of the blood', Thomas Jefferson (1743–1826) remarked to Edward Jenner (1749–1823), 'was a beautiful addition to our knowledge of the animal economy, but on a review of the practice of medicine before and since that epoch, I do not see any great amelioration which has been derived from that discovery.' The ambiguities of medicine as art and science, measured against the discrepancies of aspiration and achievement, have ever been present. Medicine is only as scientific as the most recent patient cured, but doctors have always pronounced cures, even while invoking the healing power of nature.

If medicine forms the core of this volume, it is medicine in the broadest sense, encompassing understanding of the body in sickness and in health, the parts played by morbidity and mortality in shaping human destinies, the multiform interactions between patients, doctors, medical institutions, and the wider world. 'The art has three factors:' judged Hippocrates in the *Epidemics*, 'the disease, the patient, the physician. The physician is the servant of the art. The patient must co-operate with the physician in combating the disease.' Hippocrates identified the elements; he postulated a solution; the consequences of this view of the healing process form the subject of this volume.

FURTHER READING

Each contribution to this volume contains notes and 'Further Reading' suggestions, and important trends in history of medicine scholarship are reviewed in the essay on 'Medical historiography' (Ch. 3). Here, we merely give the briefest list of major surveys of the history of medicine and some other classic works in the field, an indication of other bibliographical guides to the history of medicine, and some relevant works of reference.

Ackerknecht, Erwin H., *A Short History of Medicine*, Baltimore, MD, Johns Hopkins University Press, 1968.

——, *Therapeutics from the Primitives to the Twentieth Century*, New York, Hafner, 1973.

Brieger, Gert H., 'History of medicine', in Paul T. Durbin (ed.), *A Guide to the Culture of Science, Technology and Medicine*, New York, Free Press, 1980, pp. 121–94.

Bynum, W. F., 'Health, disease and medical care', in G. S. Rousseau and R. Porter (eds), *The Ferment of Knowledge*, Cambridge, Cambridge University Press, 1980, pp. 211–54.

Castiglioni, Arturo, *A History of Medicine*, trans. and ed. by E. B. Krumbhaar, New York, Alfred A. Knopf, 1941.

Clarke, Edwin, (ed.), *Modern Methods in the History of Medicine*, London, Athlone Press, 1971.

Garrison, Fielding H., *An Introduction to the History of Medicine*, 4th edn., Philadelphia, PA, and London, W. B. Saunders, 1929, 1960.

Howells, John G. and Osborn, M. Livia, *A Reference Companion to the History of Abnormal Psychology*, 2 vols, Westport, CT, and London, Greenwood Press, 1984.

Jordanova, L. J., 'The social sciences and history of science and medicine', in P. Corsi and P. Weindling (eds), *Information Sources in the History of Science and Medicine*, London, Butterworth Scientific, 1983, pp. 81–98.

McGrew, Roderick E., *Encyclopedia of Medical History*, New York, McGraw-Hill, 1985.

Morton, L. T., *A Medical Bibliography (Garrison and Morton): an Annotated Checklist of Texts Illustrating the History of Medicine*, 4th edn., Aldershot, Hants, Gower, 1983.

Neuburger, Max, *History of Medicine*, trans. by Ernest Playfair, 2 vols, London, H. Frowde, 1910–25.

Olby, R. C., Cantor, G. N., Christie, J. R. R. and Hodge, M. J. S. (eds), *Companion to the History of Modern Science*, London, Routledge, 1989.

Pelling, Margaret, 'Medicine since 1500', in P. Corsi and Paul Weindling (eds), *Information Sources in the History of Science and Medicine*, London, Butterworth Scientific, 1983, pp. 379–407.

Shryock, Richard H., *The Development of Modern Medicine: an Interpretation of the Social and Scientific Factors*, 2nd edn., New York, Alfred A. Knopf, 1947; reprinted Madison, WI, University of Wisconsin Press, 1980.

Sigerist, Henry E., *Civilization and Disease*, Ithaca, NY, Cornell University Press, 1943; reprinted Chicago, University of Chicago Press, 1962.

——, *A History of Medicine*, Vol. I, *Primitive and Archaic Medicine*, New York, Oxford University Press, 1951.

——, *A History of Medicine*, Vol. II, *Early Greek, Hindu and Persian Medicine*, New York, Oxford University Press, 1961.

Singer, Charles and Underwood, E. Ashworth, *A Short History of Medicine*, Oxford, Clarendon Press, 1928; 2nd edn., New York, Oxford University Press, 1962.

Stevenson, Lloyd G. and Multhauf, Robert P. (eds), *Medicine, Science and Culture, Historical Essays in Honor of Owsei Temkin*, Baltimore, MD, Johns Hopkins University Press, 1968.

Temkin, O., *The Double Face of Janus and Other Essays in the History of Medicine*, Baltimore, MD, and London, Johns Hopkins University Press, 1977.

Walton, John, Beeson, Paul B. and Scott, Ronald Bodley (eds), *The Oxford Companion to Medicine*, 2 vols, Oxford and New York, Oxford University Press, 1986.

Webster, Charles, 'The historiography of medicine', in P. Corsi and P. Weindling (eds), *Information Sources in the History of Science and Medicine*, London, Butterworth Scientific, 1983, pp. 29–43.

Contemporary research in the history of medicine is comprehensively listed in two ongoing publications:

Bibliography of the History of Medicine, Bethesda, MD, National Library of Medicine, 1965-. Annual with quinquennial cumulations.

Current Work in the History of Medicine. An International Bibliography, London, Well-come Institute for the History of Medicine, 1954. Quarterly.

A cumulation of *Current Work*, plus most secondary literature of the twentieth century until 1977, is listed in Wellcome Institute for the History of Medicine, *Subject Catalogue of the History of Medicine*, 18 vols (subject section, 9 vols; biographical section, 5 vols; topographical section, 4 vols), Munich, Krays International, 1980. Material since 1977 is held in card files in the Wellcome Library, 183 Euston Road, London NW1 2BE.

PART I

THE PLACE OF MEDICINE

2

WHAT IS SPECIFIC TO WESTERN MEDICINE?

Arthur Kleinman

THE FORMS OF MEDICINE

A coherent structure of health beliefs and the institutionalization of decisive therapeutic practices are so widespread around the globe, that *medicine*, so defined, is surely a universal in human organizations. If suffering can be said to be a defining quality of the experience of being human, so too is medicine, as organized therapeutic practice (the process of care), fundamental to the lived flow of human experience within cultural worlds. At this high level of abstraction, it is even possible, by drawing on a large array of cross-cultural sources, to distinguish several characteristics which would appear to be shared by nearly all social systems of healing, be they forms of small-scale, pre-literate societies or of peasant or even industrialized states. These shared characteristics include, among other things: categories by which illness is diagnosed; narrative structures that synthesize complaints into culturally meaningful syndromes; master metaphors, idioms, and other core symbolic forms that conduce to the construction of aetiological interpretations of pathology so as to legitimate practical therapeutic actions; healing roles and careers; rhetorical strategies that healers deploy to move patients and families to engage in therapeutic activities; and an immense variety and number of therapies, combining, almost seamlessly, symbolic and practical operations, whose intention is to control symptoms or their putative sources.[1]

Of course, even more impressive differences distinguish the healing traditions of different societies from each other. So much variety, indeed, is usually apparent even within the same society that to talk of 'Western medicine' or 'traditional healing' as if these terms denominate homogeneous social realities would be a serious misapprehension of ethnographic descriptions. The same therapeutic technologies – say, for example, particular pharmaceuticals or surgical equipment – are also perceived and employed in different ways in local worlds. Thus, in cross-cultural perspective it is as valid to talk about the cultural processes of *indigenization* of biomedicine, as to implicate the Westernization of local therapeutic traditions. (➤ Ch. 60 Medicine and anthropology; Ch. 30 Folk medicine)

Nonetheless, there is something special about biomedicine and its Western roots, something fundamentally distinctive from most other healing systems cross-culturally – for example, the great literate systems of traditional Chinese, Hindu, or Islamic medicine and, of course, the vast array of local healing activities described by ethnographers (➤ Ch. 32 Chinese medicine; Ch. 33 Indian medicine; Ch. 31 Arab-Islamic medicine; Ch. 29 Non-Western concepts of disease) – so that it is appropriate to essay an answer to the question put to me by the editors of the *Encyclopedia*: namely, what is specific to Western medicine?

I shall employ the term *biomedicine* in place of Western medicine, however, because it emphasizes the established institutional structure of the dominant profession of medicine in the West, and today worldwide, while also conjuring the primacy of its epistemological and ontological commitments, which are what is most radically different about this form of medicine.[2] Thus, I will not concern myself with Western religious healing; nor will I deal with other local folk and popular therapeutic practices that are indigenous to the West. The focus on biomedicine will also exclude alternative Western therapeutic professions or heterodox movements among professionals, such as osteopathy, homoeopathy, chiropractic, naturopathy, or, most recently, 'holistic medicine'. (➤ Ch. 28 Unorthodox medical theories)

Furthermore, I will primarily deal with the biomedicine of knowledge-creators (researchers, textbook authors, teachers) and of the high-technology tertiary care institutions that dominate medical training and which represent high status in the profession. While recognizing that the working knowledge of the ordinary practitioner in the community is more complex and open to a wider array of influences, I wish to emphasize the scientific paradigm that is at the core of the profession's knowledge-generating and training system.

MONOTHEISM AND MEDICINE

The historian of Chinese medicine, Paul Unschuld,[3] claims that the monotheism of the Western tradition has had a deterministic effect on biomedicine, even as it is practised in non-Western societies, that distinguishes it in a fundamental way from Asian medical systems. The idea of a single god legitimates the idea of a single, underlying, universalizable truth, a unitary paradigm. Tolerance for alternative paradigms is weak or absent. The development of concepts is toward proof of the validity of a single version of the body, of disease, and of treatment. Alternatives may persist in the popular culture or at the professional fringe, but they are anathematized as false beliefs by the profession as a whole, not unlike the accusation of heresy in the Western religious traditions. (➤ Ch. 61 Religion and medicine) At least, this is the way biomedicine looks from the non-Western world, inasmuch as Chinese and Ayurvedic medical traditions tolerate alternative competing paradigms, and are more pluralistic in their theoretical orientations and therapeutic practices.[4] Thus, *yin yang* theory, the macrocosmic–microcosmic correspondence theory of the Five Elemental Phases (*wu xing*), and specific views of the body in acupuncture and practical herbology exist simultaneously, and are made compatible in the practitioner's practice. Even biomedical concepts and practices are accorded a legitimate place in traditional Asian medical systems. Indeed, in India and Sri Lanka, traditional practitioners of Ayurveda often integrate biomedicine into their practice. No viewpoint ever dies out completely; alternatives are never totally discredited.[5]

The entailments of monotheism foster a single-minded approach to illness and care within biomedicine that has the decided advantages of pushing medical ideas to their logical conclusion, uncovering layers of reality to establish with precision what is certain and fundamental, and establishing criteria against which orthodoxy and orthopraxy can be certified. Indeed, from the point of view of Asian medical systems, the uniqueness of biomedicine lies in its method (of controlling existing data within its theory, and the resultant predictions and determinations based on past facts).[6] While the more fluid complementary paradigms of Asian medical systems appear weak in methodological rigour and not conducive to empirical testing, their categories do represent active categories of relationships and have produced many positive practical results. The Chinese approach, for example, is grounded within the phenomenological constraints of time, place, and phase. Though excessive flexibility limits its function as a science, it presents a serious attempt to codify complex, subtle, and interactive views of experience into therapeutic formulations that claim contextual rather than categorical application. Chinese medicine attempts to account for psychological and moral and even ecological as well as corporeal phenomena through the use of dynamic, dialectical, process-oriented methods of clinical appraisal.[7]

Biomedicine differs from these and most other forms of medicine by its extreme insistence on materialism as the grounds of knowledge, and by its discomfort with dialectical modes of thought. Biomedicine also is unique because of its corresponding requirement that single causal chains must be used to specify pathogenesis in a language of hard structural flaws and mechanical mechanisms as the rationale for therapeutic efficacy. And particularly because of its peculiarly powerful commitment to an idea of *nature* that excludes the teleological, biomedicine stands alone. This medical value orientation is, ironically, not nearly as open to competing paradigms or intellectual play of ideas as is 'hard' natural science, whose ways of approaching problems in cosmology and theoretical physics seem more flexible and tolerant than the anxious strictness of the 'youngest science', though ultimately natural science, too, discloses certain of the same consequences of monotheism.

In the biomedical definition, nature is physical. It is knowable independent of perspective or representation as an 'entity' that can be 'seen', a structure that can be laid bare in morbid pathology as a pathognomonic 'thing'. Thus, special place is given to the role of seeing in biomedicine, which continues a powerful influence of ancient Greek culture. Biology is made visible as the ultimate basis of reality which can be viewed, under the microscope if need be, as a more basic substance than complaints or narratives of sickness with their psychological and social entailments. The psychological, social and moral are only so many superficial layers of epiphenomenal cover that disguise the bedrock of truth, the ultimately natural substance in pathology and therapy: biology as an architectural structure and its chemical associates. The other orders of reality are by definition questionable.

This radically reductionistic and positivistic value orientation is ultimately dehumanizing. That which has been such a successful blueprint for a biochemically oriented technology in the treatment of acute pathology places biomedical practitioners into a number of extremely difficult situations when it comes to the care of patients with chronic illness; situations which, as I review below, offer obdurate resistance to affirmation of the patient's experience of the illness; to understanding of social, psychological and moral aspects of physiology; and ultimately to the humane practice of medicine. These extreme situations are not created, at least with the same regularity and intensity, by other healing traditions described in the cross-cultural record.

DISEASE WITHOUT SUFFERING/TREATMENT WITHOUT HEALING

Through its insistence on the primacy of definitive materialistic dichotomies (for example, between body/mind (or spirit), functional/real diseases, and highly valued specific therapeutic effects/discredited non-specific placebo effects) biomedicine presses the practitioner to construct disease, disordered biological processes) as its object of study and treatment. There is hardly any place in this narrowly focused therapeutic vision for the patient's experience of suffering. The patient's and family's complaints are regarded as subjective self-reports. The physician's task, wherever possible, is to replace these biased observations with objective data: the only valid sign of pathological processes because they are based on verified or verifiable measurements. Thus, doctors are expected to decode the untrustworthy story of illness as experience for the evidence of that which is considered authentic, disease as biological pathology. In the process, they are taught to regard experience, at least the experience of the sick person, as fugitive, fungible and therefore discreditable and invalid. Yet by denying the patient's and family's experience, the practitioner is also led to discount the moral reality of suffering – the experience of bearing or enduring pain and distress as a coming to terms with that which is most at stake, that which is of ultimate meaning, in living – while affirming objective bodily indices of morbidity. The result is a huge split between the constructed object of biomedical cure – the dehumanized disease process – and the constructed object of most other healing systems – the all-too-humanly narrated pathos and pain and perplexity of the experience of suffering. (➤ Ch. 12 Concepts of health, illness, and disease; Ch. 67 Pain and suffering)

Thus, biomedicine constructs the objects of therapeutic work without legitimating suffering. Physicians are correspondingly hedged in by their role as healers. Providing a meaningful explanation for the illness experience is something physicians (and especially those in marginal sub-disciplines such as psychiatry and family medicine) undertake, so to speak, with both hands tied behind the back. They may succeed in using their personality and communicative skills to assist patients; yet they do so, as it were, against the consequences of biomedical orientations for their training and the care they give. Meaning itself is not configured as a central focus or task of medicine. Because it eschews teleology, the very idea of a moral purpose to the illness experience is a biomedical impossibility. That illness involves a quest for ultimate meaning is disavowed. Because of its distrust of qualitative interpretations and concomitant emphasis on quantitative data, biomedicine accords no legitimacy to values. Hence, the practitioner of biomedicine must struggle to practise competent biomedicine, while at the same time searching for some extra-biomedical means to authorize an empathic response to the patient's and family's moral needs to have a witness to the story of suffering, to find support for the experience of illness, and to receive a meaningful interpretation of what is at stake for them in their local world. It should not be at all surprising then that hospitals and clinics are frequently criticized in the current period of consumer interest in patient-centred care for their dehumanizing ethos. Indeed, it is a tribute to the stubborn humanity of practitioners and to the recalcitrant influence of extra-professional cultural traditions that these institutional settings are not routinely experienced as suCh. (➤ Ch. 34 The history of the doctor–patient relationship)

That practitioners of Western medicine are trained in a radically sceptical method that ought to diminish the placebo response in their care is another curious corollary of this peculiar healing tradition, whose many positive aspects also must not go underemphasized. Although there is no other healing tradition that possesses a significant fraction of the specific therapeutic interventions for serious disorders that biomedicine includes, there is also no other tradition that so distrusts and chooses not to elaborate non-specific therapeutic sources of efficacy that are associated with the rhetorical mobilization of the charismatic powers of the healer–patient relationship that persuade patients and families to believe in successful outcomes and thereby create such scenarios of efficacy.

And yet, the anti-placebo scepticism of the current phase of biomedicine must also be balanced by its associated anti-authoritarianism, which contrasts strikingly with the paternalism of most traditional forms of healing. Egalitarianism, demystification of medical terminology and concern for patient rights, in cross-cultural perspective, are also rather peculiar to the contemporary Western tradition of biomedicine. The virtues, such as they are, which Max Weber (1864–1920) attributed to bureaucratic rationality – namely, generalizability, quantification, prediction, efficiency, quality control – are now ingrained in the professional structure of biomedicine. Their absence in folk healing systems makes those practices problematic. The rub, of course, is the iron cage of technical rationality which, as Weber also saw, would come to replace sensibility and sensitivity. Sadly, though tellingly, the professionalization of Asian medical systems has not infrequently led in the same direction.[8]

THE PROGRESSIVE SEARCH FOR POWERFUL OPERATIONS

Biomedicine instantiates the Western tradition's idea of progress. The profession's self-portrait is of a scientific, technological programme that is continuously progressing in acquisition of knowledge and especially in deployment of powerful therapeutic operations. Even in spite of limited progress over the past decade in the treatment of the chronic diseases that contribute most significantly to morbidity and mortality indices, biomedicine's self-image emphasizes awesome technological capacity to operate on the patient's organ systems. There is only a poorly articulated notion of an absolute limit to that progress. Organs can be transplanted; limbs can be reimplanted; life-support systems even 'prevent' death. It is not surprising, then, that therapeutic hubris is commonplace. Physicians are not educated to feel humble in the face of sources of suffering that cannot be reversed or to place limits on the utilization of powerful technologies. (➤ Ch. 68 Medical technologies: social contexts and consequences)

Whereas in traditional Chinese medicine, as in many other indigenous non-Western healing systems, and even earlier within healing professions in the West, the idea of progress is balanced by the idea of regress, and suffering and death are viewed as expectable and necessary, biomedicine again represents a radical therapeutic departure. Powerful actions – from purging and bleeding to stopping and starting the heart, delivering a short sharp shock to brain matter, or changing the genes of cells to enhance anti-cancer drugs – not restraint or negative capability, iconically represent biomedicine's imagery of efficacy. Where Asian medical systems invoke weak treatments as virtuous because they are held to be 'natural' and non-iatrogenic, biomedi-cine's therapeutic mandate, for which all pathology is natural, emphasizes decidedly 'unnatural' interventions. The sub-specialities, like family medicine or psychiatry, that employ weaker therapeutic operations are near the bottom of the intraprofessional hierarchy of status and financial reward. The historic Western interest in nature's healing powers has passed out of the mainstream of the profession and into the New Age fringe. (➤ Ch. 56 Psychiatry)

The burden on the practitioner of the idea of progress and the expectation of powerful opertions is considerable, not least through the astonishing claim that ultimately death itself can be 'treated', or at least 'medically managed'. Another aspect of this ideological influence is the euphemization of suffering, which becomes medicalized as a psychiatric condition, thereby transforming a moral category into a technical one. The consequence is a further transvalu-ation of therapeutic values.[9] As a result, practitioners of biomedicine are in a situation unlike that of most other healers: they experience a therapeutic environment in which the traditional moral goals of healing have been replaced by narrow technical objectives.

One other curious particularity to biomedicine, at least in its present-day form, is its anti-vitalism.[10] Traditional Chinese medicine, like many traditional systems of healing, centres on the idea of a vital power – in this instance, *qi* (energy that is associated with movement) – at the centre of health and disease. The source of disease is not traced to a particular organ, but to the disharmony of *qi* circulating in the body. Nor is the pulse and circulation of the blood understood only in the physical anatomical sense of the beating heart, but in terms of inspiration and expiration – and the techniques of breath control, *qigong*, 'the work of breath *qi*'. Ayurvedic medicine and ancient Greek medicine shared a somewhat similar conception. Vitality, efficacy, power – all capture the idea of a force of life that animates bodies/selves. Biomedical materialism decries a vital essentialism. Things are simply things: mechanisms that can be taken apart and put back together. It is a thoroughly disenchanted world-view. There is no mystery, no quiddity. Therapy does not, cannot, work by revitalizing devitalized networks – neuronal or social. There is no magic at the core; no living principle that can be energized or creatively balanced. Thus, though depression feels like soul-loss to many persons around the globe, there is no possibility for a lost soul in psychiatry. Psychotherapy, in like fashion, whatever else it is, cannot be construed as a quest for the spirit, though that is what its felt experience is for many.[11] (➤ Ch. 43 Psychotheraphy)

The attention of biomedicine is also focused on the body of the individual sick person because of Western society's powerful orientation to individual experience. That illness infiltrates and deeply affects social relations is a difficult understanding to advance in biomedicine. Population- and community-based public health orientations run counter to the dominant biomedical orientation, which takes for its subject the isolated and isolatable organism. In contrast, African healing systems see illness as part of kinship networks and healing as a kinship or community effort.[12] The foundation of biomedical psychiatry is also a single self in a single body. The presence of alternative selves or dissociated mental states, measured against this norm, is interpreted as pathology. Trance and possession, which are ubiquitous cross-cultural processes that serve social purposes and can be adaptive, are invariably cast by biomedical nosologies as pathology. In contrast, the sociocentric orientation of non-biomedical forms of healing will strike many as a more adequate appreciation of the experiential phenomenology of suffering cross-culturally.

To be sure, much that we have associated with biomedicine at present can also be discussed in other institutions in technologically advanced societies. To that extent, the sources of these qualities may be societal rather than strictly medical. Yet, these attributes are not only absent in many non-Western healing traditions, but also are far less significant in most other healing traditions in the West. In this sense, at least, biomedicine is, like all forms of medicine, both the social historical child of a particular world with its particular pattern of time and an institution that over time develops its own unique form and trajectory.

NOTES

1   A. Kleinman, *Patients and Healers in the Context of Culture*, Berkeley, University of California Press, 1978, pp. 207–8; Kleinman, *Rethinking Psychiatry*, New York, Free Press, 1988, pp. 114–16.

2   M. Lock and D. Gordon (eds), *Biomedicine Re-examined*, Hingham, MA, Kluwer, 1988.

3   P. U. Unschuld, seminar presentation given to the Medical Anthropology Program, Harvard University, 1988.

4   F. Zimmermann, *Le Discours des remèdes au Pays des Épices. Enquête sur la médecine Hindone*, Paris, Payot, 1989.

5   P. U. Unschuld, *Medicine in China: a History of Ideas*, Berkeley, University of California Press, 1985.

6   S. Nakayama, *Academic and Scientific Traditions in China, Japan, and the West* trans. by J. Dusenberg, Tokyo, Tokyo University Press, 1984.

7   Ibid.
8   C. Leslie (ed.), *Asian Medical Systems*, Berkeley, University of California Press, 1976.
9   J. Bottéro, 'La magie et la médecine règnent à Babylone', *L'Histoire*, [n. d.], 74: 12–23.
10 G. Canguilhem, *The Normal and the Pathological*, New York, Zone Press, 1989; orig. pub. 1966.
11 R. A. Schweder, 'Menstrual pollution, soul loss and the comparative study of emotions', in A. Kleinman and B. Good (eds), *Culture and Depression*, Berkeley, University of California Press, 1985, pp. 182–215.
12 J. Janzen, *The Quest for Therapy in Lower Zaire*, Berkeley, University of California Press, 1978.

FURTHER READING

Canguilhem, G., *The Normal and the Pathological*, New York, Zone Press, 1989; orig. pub. 1966.

Janzen, J., *The Quest for Therapy in Lower Zaire*, Berkeley, University of California Press, 1978.

Kleinman, A., *Patients and Healers in the Context of Culture*, Berkeley, University of California Press, 1980.

——, *Rethinking Psychiatry*, New York, Free Press, 1988.

—— and Good, B. (eds), *Culture and Depression*, Berkeley, University of California Press, 1985.

Leslie, C. (ed.), *Asian Medical Systems*, Berkeley, University of California Press, 1976.

Lock, M. and Gordon, D. (eds), *Biomedicine Re-examined*, Hingham, MA, Kluwer, 1988.

Nakayama, S., *Academic and Scientific Traditions in China, Japan, and the West*, trans. by J. Dusenberg, Tokyo, Tokyo University Press, 1984.

Unschuld, P. U., *Medicine in China: a History of Ideas*, Berkeley, University of California Press, 1985.

——, seminar presentation given to the Medical Anthropology Program, Harvard University, 1988.

Zimmermann, F., *Le Discours des remèdes au Pays des Épices. Enquête sur la médecine Hindone*, Paris, Payot, 1989.

3

THE HISTORIOGRAPHY OF MEDICINE

Gert Brieger

The historiography of medicine has greatly expanded in scope in the last twenty-five years. New directions in the field will be the main focus of this section, and some of these developments will be discussed below. What follows, however, is in no sense a review of all the pertinent literature in the history of medicine. Not even all pertinent literature in the history of medicine. Not even all pertinent categories of historiographic changes can be included here.[1]

Similar changes may be seen in other fields of history as well.[2] Like the history of science, the history of medicine was long dominated by a simple, positivist point of view. The great doctors and the great ideas were often portrayed as a march of the intellect, devising new explanations of disease and techniques for curing the ills of humankind. By the middle of this century, scientific medicine had also become increasingly effective; thus it should not be surprising that its history was so often being written in triumphalist terms. Progress and triumph over disease were the implicit messages, and as was also often true for the history of science, the history of medicine was frequently written by doctors for the service of the profession. While this is now justly considered an old-fashioned way to write any kind of history, the older works should not simply be ignored or dismissed. Earlier historians of medicine, such as Karl Sudhoff (1853–1938), Julius Pagel (1851–1912), Charles Daremberg (1817–72), Charles Singer (1876–1960), Max Neuburger (1868–1955), and Fielding Garrison (1870–1935) accomplished much, began to build a discipline, and often provided a basis for the work of the next generation of medical historians.

A word of explanation about the basis for much of this earlier work may be helpful. From antiquity to the early twentieth century, medical history was dominated by a doxographic approach. Physicians have always been eager to learn about the opinions of their predecessors. This was a hallmark of history in the service of medicine. The obvious questions are: why did so many medical writers refer to the work and opinions of their predecessors? And, as a corollary, why is doxography no longer a prominent part of medical historiography? Were earlier generations of physicians less confident of their own opinions? Possible explanations for this waning of interest include the increasing certainty and confidence afforded by the advances in science that have helped to explain basic mechanisms of disease and therapy, the causal precision afforded by new methods used by historians, and the fact that much more history of medicine is now being written by historians who are not themselves physicians.

It is a mistake, however, to dismiss the earlier history of medicine as mere hagiography. In the training of physicians, from the time of Hippocrates (c.460–370 BC) to our own day, much of medical knowledge is transmitted through the opinions, experiences, and ways of the elders. It should not be surprising that the value of such opinions and experiences was reflected in the history that these physicians wrote.

In contrast to the historiography of science, the historiography of medicine lacks such striking landmarks as Boris Hessen's famous 1931 paper on the social and economic roots of *Newton's Principia* or Thomas Kuhn's *Structure of Scientific Revolutions*.[3] Instead, our field has been marked by a number of programmatic statements made by an earlier generation that included Henry Sigerist, Richard Shryock, and George Rosen, who articulated the problems and prospects of the history of medicine that today we have come to take almost for granted. While a previous generation may have voiced some of the concerns and proposed some of the new methods, it is only in the last two to three decades that they have become so widely accepted.

The credo for the change and expansion of the historiography of medicine was clearly set forth twenty-five years ago by George Rosen, who urged his colleagues to a more extensive study of people, disease, and emotion. Since the work of his own mentor, Henry Sigerist, led to the recognition for the need to interpret the medical past from a broader point of view, Rosen wrote in 1967: 'A shift in the angle of vision not infrequently reveals new facets of a subject, and this has happened to the history of medicine. By taking the social character of medicine as a point of departure, the history of medicine becomes the history of human societies and their efforts to deal with problems of health and disease.'[4] New questions result, and new emphases appear.

That more of our work in the history of medicine should take into consideration the experiences of patients has by now assumed the status of a cliché. Yet it is only quite recently that the idea has achieved that status. Nearly fifty years ago, Sigerist emphasized the importance of the patient, but few followed his lead. Witness, for instance, what Sigerist wrote in the preface to his last book, *Landmarks in the History of Hygiene*:

> A review of my first volume [published in 1951], alleged that I was devoting too much space to the description of man's environment, yet we know well enough that next to heredity a man's physical and social environment is primarily responsible for his illnesses, and our efforts as physicians tend to readjust him to this very environment from which he has dropped out as a result of illness. Another reviewer stated that I was looking at the history of medicine from the angle of the patient rather from that of the physician, and this I consider a great compliment, as the patient, or rather man in health and illness, is the object of all the physician's actions.[5]

In recent years, Roy Porter has been especially articulate in calling for a history of medicine from the patient's perspective.[6] What is different in the present generation is that many of Porter's colleagues have heard and heeded the call.

This new, more mature social history of medicine of recent decades has better managed to keep both the individual doctor and the patient as well as their society in proper view, as Andrew Wear and others have pointed out.[7] Like social history in general, the newer history of medicine has been more problem-oriented as well as more interdisciplinary than the earlier work in the field. Medical historians are now also more concerned with aggregates of people, more with private matters rather than merely with public figures and public affairs. In this newer history of medicine it is not the play that is the thing, but rather the playgoer.

The greater maturity of this new social history of medicine also stems from its increasingly empirical or at least experiential researCh. Thus it is less based upon dogma, assertion, or mere impression, as was formerly so often the case.

If anything may be said with certainty about recent trends in scholarship in the humanities and social sciences generally, and medical history more specifically, it is that we are witnessing an increasing amount of interdisciplinary work. The crossing of traditional boundaries that once separated history, literature, sociology, and anthropology is now commonplace in those fields, as it is in ours. While in a previous generation the fields ancillary to the history of medicine were philology, palaeography, and epigraphy, now linguistics, anthropology, sociology, and demography have taken their place. The studies that have resulted from such interdisciplinary work have been formulated with broader questions of economic development, modernization, industrialization, food supplies and their consumption, and their broad relationships to the health of the people.

Why, we must ask, did medical historians not heed the call to a social history voiced so eloquently by Sigerist and Rosen, and practised so successfully by Richard Shryock? For the answer to why it took still another generation for us to embark on the new social history of medicine we might look to the field of history in general. As John Higham has written, 'Social history had accumulated over the decades, but it had been contained. It had never seemed powerful. Now an earthquake split the dam and released a flood of waters across the entire terrain of scholarship.'[8] Thus in the wake of the many social issues such as the unpopular war in Vietnam, the rights of blacks and of women, and a renewed concern for the environment, historians turned from the lives of the 'great men' who waged wars to the story of the common people – men, women, children, and the minorities who too often in the past histories had remained invisible. So too in medical history we turned from those who waged war on disease – the 'great doctors' – to those who suffered, and to the legion of workers, men and women, who for so long had waged the daily battle against the ravages of ill health, but who, in the histories of medicine, were as anonymous as their counterparts in society had been in the general histories.

It is not surprising, then, that in the last twenty-five years, as societies in the so-called First World began to spend increasing amounts of their gross national products on matters of health, the public was increasingly interested in seeing just what all this money was really buying for them. As increasing sums were expended on prevention and treatment of sickness, there was some question about increasing benefits to be derived. This questioning, even mistrust, of those responsible for such huge expenditure has been fairly widespread in the last few decades. So it should not surprise us that it is also reflected in the current, much more probing, histories of medicine. (➤ Ch. 57 Health economics)

In addition to these forms of the social history of medicine, a new cultural history of medicine has also evolved. Turning to language, symbols, and discourse of the art and the science of medicine, this new historical approach has brought linguists and literary scholars to join anthropologists. The French historians of the *Annales* School have been especially prominent, as can be readily seen in the volumes of essays translated by Orest Ranum and Robert Forster.[9]

In the 1960s and 1970s, the French philosopher Michel Foucault's influence on historians of medicine was notable. His *Histoire de la Folie* (1961) became available in a shorter, English translation as *Madness and Civilization* in 1965. This extended discussion of the mad and the sane was widely read and cited, but had somewhat less influence on the history of psychiatry than did *Naissance de la clinique* on the history of modern medicine more generally. Published in 1963, it became available a decade later in English as *The Birth of the Clinic*. Its subtitle, *An Archaeology of Medical Perception*, was the important thread that ran through all of Foucault's work. If, for some, seeing is believing, for Foucault seeing or perceiving is also knowing. Probably his most lasting influence has been his stress on language and its uses in medicine to constitute the text as well as the context of medical events. While most historians of medicine have continued to focus their attention on the genesis and meaning of those events, since the work of Foucault we can no longer ignore the discourse surrounding them.

Like the emphasis on social and cultural aspects, explicit concern for questions of historiography is a fairly recent phenomenon in the history of medicine. For several centuries, medical historians have been interested in the history of the history of medicine, and periodically we have reviewed our own historical literature. While one definition of historiography is bound to the history of writing history, in this section the main emphasis will be on the recent development of historical styles and the scope of the history of medicine rather than upon either its history or its development as a discipline. Each historian of medicine might answer the question 'What is this field called medical history?' differently, but a historiographical essay can at least begin to formulate a generally acceptable view of the field.

There are many windows through which we may glance at the current state of medical history. Some are decades old, and others are more recent, but only some will be discussed below. Perspectives include new ways of studying the history of diseases and the private and public responses they have evoked; the history of the care of the mentally ill; the history of the roles of women in the health professions and the changing nature of women's health care; the role of science in the professionalization of medicine, the general scientific enterprise, and the role of the laboratory sciences of medicine; the role of medicine and public health in the history of the Third World; the varieties of local history, including institutions such as medical schools and hospitals; and the relationship of the history of medicine to anthropology and biohistory.

Historians have recently come to consider the Enlightenment as the period from about 1650 to 1820, referring to it as 'the long eighteenth century', and to consider the five centuries from the twelfth through the sixteenth as the 'long Renaissance'. Along with the expanded time-frame has come a far broader view of the medicine of those periods. Just as the study of classical medicine has become more than merely the study of the theory of medicine set forth in the ancient writings, medievalists and Renaissance scholars (often one and the same when it comes to the history of medicine) have increasingly turned their attention to health and disease, medical beliefs of patients and the attitudes of their physicians, and public health. Thus the social history of medicine, now so securely established for recent studies of the eighteenth and nineteenth centuries, has played a much more prominent part in the history of earlier medicine as well.

The recently expanded scope of the history of medicine is especially apparent in the medieval and Renaissance periods. A generation ago, a series of essays on medical learning during these periods would have been far more narrowly conceived than is true today. Witness, for instance, the issue of *Osiris*, which features articles on topics ranging from the intellectual to the social. The assessments of Avicenna (by Nancy Siraisi) and Fracastoro (by Vivian Nutton) are but two examples of the new attention to social context.[10] Moreover, although the writings of Avicenna (980–1037) and Fracastoro (1478–1553) were known and discussed by earlier historians, ideas about their subsequent influence were far more speculative than they are today. What distinguishes the work of recent scholars on medieval and Renaissance medicine from that of earlier generations is the far greater reliance by the former on rich archival sources. Thus the work of Katharine Park on doctors and the medical market-place in Florence, or of Ann Carmichael on plague in that city, and several studies by Carlo Cipolla on public health and responses to disease, to cite but a few examples, all show clearly the possibilities of such imaginative use of legal and administrative as well as medical records.[11]

THE HISTORY OF DISEASE

The history of disease has been discussed from many perspectives. The broad approach of earlier scholars such as August Hirsch (1817–94) and Charles Creighton (1847–1927) resulted in what was conveniently called the history and geography of disease. Part clinical, part epidemiological, and part social historical, the writings of these pre-germ-theory historians struggled to account for causes as well as effects, but the social and biological impact of disease was described in less specific detail than today. A major collaborative effort is *The Cambridge World History of Human Disease* (1993), under the editorship of Kenneth Kiple. This multi-volume work serves, at the end of the twentieth century, as a comprehensive summary of current understanding of the historical, geographical, and social dimensions of the diseases of the world, much as did the three-volume work of Hirsch over a century ago. It surely is a comment on the burgeoning of knowledge, and on the specialization of our time, that what Hirsch accomplished alone now requires well over a hundred scholars in history, geography, and anthropology to produce. (➤ Ch. 18 The ecology of disease)

Illnesses, and people's responses to them, have shaped human history in biological as well as cultural ways. We are what we eat as well as what our genetic endowments have programmed for us. Thus the Hippocratic dictum that the broad basis of medicine includes the patient, the physician, and the disease has endured. In the historiography of medicine emphases have changed as new sources became available, as more imaginative techniques of analysis were applied, and as new questions were posed. But the link between disease, medicine, and human culture, as David Landy has stressed, has been both intimate and inexorable.[12]

Many of the recent histories of disease have moved the narrative as well as the analysis beyond biological events and their physical or emotional effects to the broader social construction of disease. This is merely to say that our entire culture is the construct we have erected to explain and to understand our world. To view illness as a part of that cultural construct is to broaden the basis of analysis of its causes, progress, and effects.[13]

The richness of more recent work is illustrated by books such as Paul Slack's *The Impact of Plague in Tudor and Stuart England* or Richard Evans's *Death in Hamburg*.[14] Here, one realizes immediately the enlarged scope and the more minute descriptions of the reactions of the various segments of the population to the onslaught of such serious epidemic diseases as plague and cholera. Slack is quite correct in concluding that 'What plague did do was exaggerate features of the demographic scene which would not without it have been so obvious. It emphasized distinctions in health and morality between different sources of settlement and different social groups.' (➤ Ch. 52 Epidemiology)

From the social, cultural, and economic perspectives of disease have come a series of studies by historians who have generally been able to paint an even broader picture of the responses to disease by the populations afflicted by them. Besides the books of Slack and Evans, others are *The Cholera Years* of Charles Rosenberg, followed by a series of other books about the cholera epidemics of the nineteenth century:[15] Allan Brandt on syphilis in *No Magic Bullet*;[16] Elizabeth Etheridge on pellagra in *The Butterfly Caste*;[17] and John Ettling on hookworm in *The Germ of Laziness*.[18]

On the other hand, to deny the biological basis of disease seems to me, as a medically trained historian, to lead us astray. We can readily agree that by viewing disease and medicine as a whole, as socially constructed, we are widening our gaze upon the development of medical knowledge and medical practices, but to claim, as François Delaporte does, that disease does not exist, and that what does exist is only practices, is to deny too muCh.[19] With a somewhat different emphasis, a number of valuable histories of single diseases have appeared in the last two decades. Examples of this genre – besides the earlier, well-known *Rats, Lice and History* (typhus) of Hans Zinsser,[20] and *The White Plague* (tuberculosis) of Jean and René Dubos,[21] both of which are of broad cultural scope – are J. F. D. Shrewsbury's *A History of Bubonic Plague in the British Isles*,[22] John R. Paul's *A History of Poliomyelitis*,[23] Daphne Roe's *A Plague of Corn* (pellagra),[24] Donald R. Hopkins's *Princes and Peasants* (smallpox),[25] and Kenneth Carpenter's *The History of Scurvy and Vitamin C*.[26] All these authors generally pay more attention to the biological bases of these diseases, despite what they may have said in prefaces or subtitles. This emphasis does not necessarily diminish their value as contributions to our understanding of the history of these diseases.

A model study in the history of disease since its publication in 1945, Owsei Temkin's *The Falling Sickness* is not an epidemiological or clinical history of a disease, but a history of the evolution of ideas about epilepsy: its cause, its implications for the lives of sufferers, and ideas about its treatment.[27] Temkin thus used epilepsy to say much about ancient, medieval, and Renaissance concepts of health and disease and the role of medicine during those eras, much as Rosenberg used cholera to describe nineteenth-century urban America's response to epidemics, and Ettling and Etheridge used hookworm and pellagra to describe the social and health conditions of the American South in the early twentieth century. Thus, again and again, disease has served the historians of medical ideas or the social historians of medicine as a useful sampling device.

The synergistic relationship of illnesses has been extensively probed by the Indiana University demographic historian, James Riley. Using records of occupational groups such as the employees of an Antwerp printing-house from 1654 to the 1780s and of members of nineteenth-century British Friendly Societies, Riley has been able to focus on the historical problems of sickness in large groups.[28] Sickness, as he points out, is a slippery phenomenon. Roy and Dorothy Porter and others have begun to describe individual reactions to illness, but the problem of morbidity in populations is far more difficult for the historian and for the epidemiologist than is the study of mortality. (➤ Ch. 67 Pain and suffering; Ch. 72 Medicine, mortality, and morbidity)

Riley has postulated a concept of synergy that he calls insult accumulation. Most episodes of illness are not now, and probably were not in the past, resolved by death. But each episode of illness, followed by recovery, will leave a certain residue of damage or weakening of the organism. Future episodes of sickness will then, in a cumulative manner, lead to death. Thus he postulates that each insult leaves the individual more susceptible to disease in the future. He further postulates that cohorts of the population who enjoy better health early in their lives will have longer life-spans and greater vigour at subsequent ages. These are intriguing hypotheses that have stimulated Riley and others to further work in determining the causes of the shift in the patterns of disease. (➤ Ch. 70 Medical sociology; Ch. 71 Demography and medicine)

In bringing together the recent work in population history, in biohistory, in the history of public health, and in the study of diseases in past times, it is important to invoke the name of Thomas McKeown. Beginning in the 1950s with articles, and from his first book on the rise of human population to his last on the origins of human diseases, McKeown brought the biological events of history to the foreground of his analysis of the roles that medicine and public health have played in the changes of the world's demographic patterns.[29] While he has been criticized by historians for using their craft merely to make his points while ignoring contrary or expanded data, he did play an important role in the changing historiography of medicine during the last quarter of a century. His focus upon fertility and mortality patterns, on the illnesses of populations as different as the nomadic hunter-gatherers to the sedentary, highly industrialized, and his attempt to relate changes to nutrition, sanitation, and the general standard of living, has stimulated much important work in the history of medicine. (➤ Ch. 51 Public health)

MEDICAL RECORDS

Medical records, now an important aspect of our medical and legal world, were much sparser in earlier centuries. Increasingly, historians of medicine have used a variety of records to probe the evolutuion of medical practices, aetiologic and therapeutic theories, and the changing nature of the relationships between doctors and their patients. (➤ Ch. 34 History of the doctor–patient relationship) Guenter Risse's imaginative use of the records of the Royal Infirmary of Edinburgh enabled him to describe medical practices and medical education in eighteenth-century Scotland.[30] Martin Pernick and John Warner have used nineteenth-century American hospital records to describe in much richer detail than their predecessors the use of anaesthesia and a wide variety of therapeutic practices.[31] Similarly, Joel Howell has focused attention on the use of hospital records to ascertain the uses made of diagnostic techniques based upon the technological developments of the early decades of this century. The electrocardiograph, for instance, became a diagnostic instrument while also serving a broader role in the increasing specialization of medicine.[32] Thus it is important to note that the books by Pernick and Warner and the paper by Howell all contribute to our understanding of the process of professionalization of medicine in America and Britain in the nineteenth century.[33] (➤ Ch. 47 History of the medical profession; Ch. 36 The science of diagnosis: diagnostic technology)

While quantitative methods of the new social history have been used increasingly by historians of diseases and of demography, as well as by those who focus upon aggregates of clinical records in hospitals or dispensaries, individual practitioners have also, on occasion, left a rich store of their clinical cases. In earlier centuries, extensive case-notes were not routine, so that Saul Jarcho's use of the clinical records of Giovanni Battista Morgagni (1682–1771), Ippolito Francesco Albertini (1662–1738), and Francesco Torti (1658–1741) make the volumes that resulted all the more useful for other scholars.[34]

Three other books that were derived from an extensive use of a physician's case-notes are those by Michael MacDonald, Nancy Tomes, and Barbara

Duden. MacDonald, in *Mystical Bedlam*, used the extensive collection of case-books from the practice of Richard Napier (1559–1634), an astrological physician.[35] Napier's records of over two thousand cases of mental disorders allowed MacDonald to explore the rich social history of the world of Napier's patients between 1597 and 1634. The resulting picture of the contemporary beliefs about illness, attitudes toward the sick, and practices of their physicians provides a far more richly textured portrait of early seventeenth-century medicine than previously. (➤ Ch. 21 Mental diseases)

In using the notes, records, and journals of Thomas Kirkbride (1809–93), a nineteenth-century American leader in the care of the mentally ill, Tomes has been able to portray the social context of asylum treatment.[36] Barbara Duden's book concerns a German physician of 1730 and his women patients.[37] Duden describes not only the medical theories and practices of Dr Johannes Storch (1681–1751), but is able also to trace in rich detail the emerging views of the human body.

EPIDEMIOLOGY

Recent historical work to unravel the enigma of yellow fever – its origins, disappearance, and absence in Asia and Australia – is a good example of the new history of disease. (➤ Ch. 24 Tropical diseases) American historians such as Martin Pernick and Margaret Humphreys have clearly related the responses to this disease to political and economic conditions, and John Duffy has drawn a careful social profile of one outbreak in 1853 in New Orleans.[38] James Goodyear has connected ten outbreaks in American and French cities, but especially in nineteenth-century Caribbean island communities, to the presence of sugar-cane cultivation, refining, or shipping. This 'sugar connection' seems very plausible since the small containers used to process sugar in the nineteenth century offered favourable breeding conditions for mosquitoes.[39] (➤ Ch. 58 Medicine and colonialism; Ch. 19 Fevers)

For the history of epidemiology, William Coleman's *Yellow Fever in the North* was a landmark.[40] It is of particular importance because he traced the history of epidemiology, in this case in the era prior to the germ theory, by studying the theories of disease that were applied in three epidemics of yellow fever: in Gibraltar in 1828, Saint-Nazaire in 1861, and Swansea in 1865. Coleman's contribution does not merely further the discussion of contagion versus non-contagion, but focuses our attention on the dimensions of epidemiology, and on the evolution of epidemiologic thinking and how it was evoked to explain disease. Except for John Eyler's fine book about William Farr (1807–83) and his methods, and a slim symposium volume edited by Abraham Lilienfeld, very little has been published about the development of epidemiology as a discipline.[41] (➤ Ch. 16 Contagion/germ theory/specificity)

This lack of understanding of epidemiology by both historians and physicians has, until recent decades, left a telling gap. Epidemiology is the basis for the study of population medicine. It has been necessary to shift our gaze from the individual cases of illness to the broader issues of the health of the public. John Graunt (1620–74), Sir William Petty (1623–87), William Farr, and Major Greenwood (1880–1949) notwithstanding, it is only quite recently, as the work of social historians and demographers such as Arthur Imhof have clearly shown, that historians have fully appreciated the rich variety of things that fall upon the people, the true meaning of *epi demos*.

BIOLOGICAL FACTORS IN HISTORY (BIOHISTORY)

The importance of the biological element in history has long been acknowledged, but only recently has a real biohistory begun to emerge. The task of the historian, George Rosen noted in 1957, is to analyse where, how, and when human culture and biology have interacted, and to assess the effects. Stephen Boyden has called attention to the importance of this interplay, and he referred to this broadening of the conventional historical approach as biohistory.[42]

In this biological variety of social history, or 'anthropomedical historiography', as it has also been called, the focus is upon ecology in its broadest sense. Alfred Crosby, one of the most prominent of this group of biohistorians, has used such an approach in his books *The Columbian Exchange*,[43] and *Ecological Imperialism*.[44] Crosby explored the relationship of migration, foods, flora, and fauna to diseases. Migration, he claimed, brought diseases to new populations. Those who were isolated the longest suffered the most in the so-called virgin-soil epidemics that were the consequence of diseases introduced to highly susceptible populations.

William McNeill's *Plagues and Peoples* was devoted to micro- and macro-parasitism and their effects upon empires.[45] The microscopic disease agents and the aggression of human beings against their fellows have each had profound consequences for the course of history. McNeill's book was a call to his fellow historians to pay more attention to the biological factors in history, especially the role of disease. His was, by necessity, still a fairly speculative book. It will be up to his successors to confirm or to disprove such generalizations as the importance of the lopsided impact of disease upon the indigenous population in the Spanish conquest of America.

An important work that defies easy classification is Mirko Grmek's *Diseases in the Ancient Greek World*.[46] In a vast compilation of literary and archaeological sources, Grmek has stressed the environmental approach to explaining disease spread. Admittedly, Grmek notes, diseases generally occur at the intersection of two causal chains, one genetic, the other external. Thus most diseases, he concludes, result from a conjunction of an innate weakness and a wide array of environmental factors. In a long chapter on findings from the fields of palaeopathology and palaeodemography, he clearly utilizes the biohistorical approach. He discusses population density, nutrition, height and stature, and life-spans of ancient populations. Although disease is featured in the title, this book is not merely a history of disease, but a rich view of the complex ecology of disease in ancient Greece. (➤ Ch. 15 Environment and miasmata)

NUTRITION AND HEALTH

The role of diet has always been a part of the concern of the historian of medicine. A more direct exploration of the role of nutrition may be found in *Height, Health and History*.[47] The authors, Roderick Floud, Kenneth Wachter, and Annabel Gregory, assess the nutritional status of the British people in the period 1750 to 1980 by using data from military recruits. They are able thereby to throw light upon the health and nutritional status of the people, but in addition they can also draw some conclusions about the British economy. There was a time when the upper classes could literally look down upon those less fortunate. Recent data show that the social-class disparities in height have disappeared as general nutritional status has improved. The historical approach, and the sources used by Floud *et al.*, demonstrate the potential for this newer form of biological history. Their data are confined to one country and mostly to the records of young men, but their results show clearly that the historiography of medicine can no longer be narrowly defined.

French historians were among the earliest to probe the complex relationships of nutrition and health. Demographers and economic historians have more recently joined the list. While famine and pestilence have long been associated, it still is not entirely clear how and at what stage malnutrition compromises the immunological response. Histories of diet in various national contexts have also long been available. In fact, it is well to recall that according to the author of the Hippocratic text *Ancient Medicine*, one of the earliest histories of medicine known, medicine as an organized activity had its beginning when it was noted that those who were sick required a different diet from those who were well.

In relating disease, diet, and history, as Andrew Appleby and others have now amply demonstrated, the interdisciplinary character of the newer work in the history of medicine is very clearly evident.[48] This newer work is also related to demographic studies, and to the newer forms of biohistory. The concern about nutritional factors as explanation for major disease outbreaks, or, on the other hand, for improvements in health, has for over a quarter of

35

a century been the focus of the studies of Thomas McKeown. John Post is another historian who has long been at work to assess the relative influence of climatic changes and nutritional status, and their effects upon morbidity and mortality. In his 1985 book, *Food Shortage, Climatic Variability, and Epidemic Disease in Pre-industrial Europe,* he discusses the marked demographic and epidemiological changes around 1740.[49] An important and related question that has concerned numerous historians is to find an explanation for the disappearance of bubonic plague from Europe in the late seventeenth century. Post concludes that the nutritional status of western Europeans around 1740 cannot be invoked to explain the various epidemics of that time. The synergy between under-nutrition and infection is a still-unresolved problem. Ann Carmichael has pointed out that poverty and hunger are added environmental strains, but that the synergy between multiple infections may be of greater importance than the synergy between hunger and disease.[50] Perhaps the most useful review of all these developments is in the long introductory essay by John Walter and Roger Schofield in their edited volume, *Famine, Disease, and the Social Order in Early Modern Society.*[51] (➤ Ch. 22 Nutritional diseases)

PUBLIC HEALTH – INTERNATIONAL HISTORIOGRAPHY

One of the roots of the newer history of public health is the revival in the 1950s of interest in the problems of international health. With economic recovery of the Western nations after the Second World War, they began to turn once again to the concerns of the Third World. In today's scholarly world, the role of medicine in the building of colonial empires, the extension of medicine's authority through the medicalization of many aspects of life and death, as well as the use of medicine and its related sciences to combat the world's diseases, have all led to an expansion of historical work. As the world of medicine has slowly and somewhat grudgingly accepted the even broader universe of public health, so have historians turned increasing attention to the study of populations and societies rather than continuing to focus on doctors and their individual patients. Neither in medicine nor in its history has the population approach entirely won the day, yet in the history of public health it is more broadly conceived than mere sanitary legislation and clean-ups, and it is in the rich new studies of tropical medicine that exciting new historiography is appearing.

The newly developing field of medical anthropology had part of its roots in the international health movement of the time. And it was the medical anthropologists who most clearly and forcefully showed once again what medical writers from Hippocrates to Rudolph Virchow (1821–1902) had also stressed: health and disease are as much social and cultural phenomena as biological.[52]

Historians working on colonialism and imperialism quickly realized that disease was an important element in their story. Medical geography has been subsumed by tropical medicine in the last hundred years, but tropical medicine, as Ackerknecht has shown, really meant colonial medicine.[53] And it is in this venerable field that much work is now progressing. Its recency is underscored by the comment of two Africanists, Hartwig and Patterson, who could say in 1978 that their colleagues 'have generally neglected the study of past health conditions – as well as the role of disease, health care, and medicine in history – despite the obvious importance of the disease burden on the African continent.'[54] Even though hardly more than a decade has elapsed, much exciting new work on the socio-political and cultural impacts of disease in the history of the Third World has appeared.

LaVerne Kuhnke uses the clash between the ontologic and the physiologic conceptions of disease and its aetiology to elucidate the battle over quarantine practices in nineteenth-century Egypt as a means of more widely assessing health developments in that country.[55] The argument, of course, goes well beyond the familiar disputes over contagionism versus non-contagionism, because it also takes into account the tensions between Western and indigenous medicine, and between urban and rural needs.

Regional studies such as Kuhnke's, or Nancy Gallagher's work on Tunisia in the nineteenth century and Egypt in the twentieth,[56] or the award-winning study of cholera in Hamburg by Richard Evans (see note 14), all describe a socio-political process in which disease or the threat of its coming played a role in the governmental responses to a range of civic issues beyond just those of health. Evans provides an important glimpse into the changing structure of the city's government and its responses to civic problems. Thus medical theory and the threat of disease or its actual occurrence serve in Hamburg, as they do in other parts of the world, as convenient probes for a wider understanding of society, its institutions and its culture. As Gallagher has shown, the three major analytic approaches to the history of epidemics all lead to wider understanding of the historical forces at work. Epidemics may be viewed as causative agents in history, as in the work of Michael Dols or William McNeill,[57] or epidemics may serve as mirrors reflecting social processes, as in Rosenberg's *The Cholera Years*, and epidemics may help us to understand changing medical theories, as in Margaret Pelling's work on cholera in the early nineteenth century (see note 15).

As I have already indicated, the definitions of tropical medicine have not been precise. For many years the standard work on its history was a two-volume work by H. H. Scott, a teacher of tropical medicine in London.[58] Scott, whose *A History of Tropical Medicine* appeared in 1939, admitted to difficulty with defining his field. Was it concerned with those diseases restricted to the tropics themselves – that is, to just a few degrees either side of the equator? He did realize that the impetus for early improvements in the treatment of such diseases was spurred by the wish to keep European settlers and military forces as healthy as possible. Interestingly, Scott said that he deliberately left the subject of tropical sanitation 'severely alone'.

The subjects covered in recent collected works such as *Disease, Medicine and Empire*, edited by Roy Macleod and Milton Lewis, and *Imperial Medicine and Indigenous Societies*, edited by David Arnold, range along several themes.[59] These include the introduction of European medicine to tropical countries, especially public-health practices, the role of disease and their effects on colonial populations as compared to the indigenous peoples, and the role of disease in the colonial process itself. In African studies, as Gwyn Prins has pointed out, the importance of reviewing the consequences of illness and therapy in the colonial context, the history of the interaction of pathogens and politics, and the necessity of moving from a Western, doctor-centred account to a patient-centred one have all been well recognized by recent scholars.[60] Philip Curtin has made good use of military statistics in his book *Death by Migration*.[61]

Thus for historians in Africa, Asia, and Latin America, the study of the history of diseases, their treatment and prevention, and their broad cultural effects on the politics and economy of those regions will help to integrate the regional histories into a broader world history. (➤ Ch. 59 Internationalism in medicine and public health)

CONCLUSION

Henry Sigerist pointed out that there is no such thing as a definitive history, because interpretation and evaluation change over time.[62] At the close of the twentieth century, new topics and new approaches beckon. Important current and future topics in the history of medicine include, in addition to those already discussed, the science of medicine and the investigative enterprise; the history of medical institutions, particularly hospitals; a new view of the care of the mentally ill; and, perhaps most important, a growing body of literature about women's health and women's roles in the health professions. The subject of women's history is among the broadest in scope, as it overlaps with the history of psychiatry, with literature on professionalization, and with the history of therapeutics. (➤ Ch. 38 Women and medicine)

The two most important tasks for medical historians are now to concentrate on comparative and on synthetic studies. We need comparisons across cultural, national, and social lines. In this type of endeavour, medical anthropologists have thus far been ahead of medical historians. But if it is to continue to expand its approaches to the medical past, the field of medical history must also pause significantly to begin to synthesize. Despite the changing emphases in interpretation and evaluation, the time has come for more attempts to sum up what historians of medicine now believe they do know about medicine's past. Much of that knowledge has been gained in quite recent decades, and more is surely to come. Taking stock is nevertheless helpful in setting priorities for future research. This encyclopedia is one such effort to take stock of what we know, what we think we know, and what we ought to know about the history of medicine.

NOTES

1 Three very useful review articles are William F. Bynum, 'Health disease and medical care', in G. S. Rousseau and Roy Porter (eds), *The Ferment of Knowledge. Studies of the Historiography of Eighteenth-Century Science*, Cambridge, Cambridge University Press, 1980, pp. 211–53; Margaret Pelling, 'Medicine since 1500', in P. Corsi and P. Weindling (eds), *Information Sources in the History of Science and Medicine*, London, Butterworth Scientific, 1983, pp. 379–407; and Gert H. Brieger, 'History of medicine', in Paul Durbin (ed.), *A Guide to the Culture of Science, Technology and Medicine*, New York, Free Press, 1984, pp. 121–94.

2 Lynn Hunt (ed.), *The New Cultural History*, Berkeley, University of California Press, 1989; Oliver Zunz (ed.), *Reliving the Past. The Worlds of Social History*, Chapel Hill, University of North Carolina Press, 1985.

3 Roy MacLeod, 'Changing perspectives in the social history of science', in Ina Spiegel-Rösing and Derek de Solla Price (eds), *Science, Technology and Society*, Beverley Hills, CA, Sage Publications, 1977, pp. 149–95.

4 George Rosen, 'People, disease and emotion. Some newer problems for research in medical history', *Bulletin of the History of Medicine*, 1967, 4: 5–23.

5 Henry E. Sigerist, *Landmarks in the History of Hygiene*, Oxford, Oxford University Press, 1956, p. vii.

6 Roy Porter, 'The patient's view. Doing medical history from below', *Theory and Society*, 1985, 14: 167–74; Roy Porter and Dorothy Porter, *In Sickness and in Health. The British Experience 1650–1850*, London, Fourth Estate, 1988; Dorothy Porter and Roy Porter, *Patient's Progress. Doctors and Doctoring in Eighteenth-Century England*, Cambridge, Polity Press, 1989.

7 Andrew Wear, 'Interfaces: perceptions of health and illness in early modern England' in Roy Porter and Andrew Wear (eds), *Problems and Methods in the History of Medicine*, London, Croom Helm, 1987, pp. 230–55.

8 John Higham, 'Introduction', in John Higham and Paul Conkin (eds), *New Directions in American Intellectual History*, Baltimore, MD, Johns Hopkins University Press, 1979, p. xiii.

9 Alain Corbin, *The Foul and the Fragrant. Odor and the French Social Imagination*, trans. by Miriam Kochan, Cambridge, MA, Harvard University Press, 1986; Toby Gelfand, 'The *Annales* and medical historiography. *Bilan et perspectives*', in Porter and Wear, op. cit. (n. 7), pp. 15–39; Robert Forster and Orest Ranum (eds), *Biology of Man in History*, Baltimore, MD, Johns Hopkins University Press,

1975; Forster and Ranum, *Medicine and Society in France*, Baltimore, MD, Johns Hopkins University Press, 1980. See also Jean Pierre Goubert, *The Conquest of Water. The Advent of Health in the Industrial Age*, trans. by A. Wilson, Princeton, NJ, Princeton University Press, 1989.

10   Nancy Siraisi, *Medieval and Early Renaissance Medicine. An Introduction to Knowledge and Practice*, Chicago, IL, University of Chicago Press, 1990. This book is one of the very few examples of the kinds of syntheses so much needed. See also Michael McVaugh and Nancy Siraisi (eds), *Renaissance Medical Learning. Evolution of a Tradition* (*Osiris*, 1990, vol. 6), especially the introduction by McVaugh and Siraisi. See also two review articles and an editorial by Siraisi: 'Some recent work on western European medical learning, *ca.*1200–*ca.*1500', *History of Universities*, 1982, 2: 225–38; 'Some current trends in the study of renaissance medicine', *Renaissance Quarterly*, 1984, 37: 585–600; [editorial], 'Medieval and Renaissance medicine. Continuity and diversity', *Journal of the History of Medicine*, 1986, 41: 391–4. For a convenient summary of the state of ancient medicine see Wesley D. Smith, 'Notes on ancient medical historiography', *Bulletin of the History of Medicine*, 1989, 63: 73–109. For an extensive review that ties together medieval medicine and women's studies, see Monica Green, 'Women's medical practice and health care in medieval Europe', *Signs: Journal of Women in Culture and Society*, 1989, 14: 434–73.

11   Katharine Park, *Doctors and Medicine in Early Renaissance Florence*, Princeton, NJ, Princeton University Press, 1985; Ann G. Carmichael, *Plague and the Poor in Renaissance Florence*, Cambridge, Cambridge University Press, 1986; Carlo M. Cipolla, *Cristofano and the Plague. A Study in the History of Public Health in the Age of Galileo*, Berkeley, University of California Press, 1973; Cipolla, *Public Health and the Medical Profession in the Renaissance*, Cambridge, Cambridge University Press, 1976.

12   David Landy (ed.), *Culture, Disease and Healing. Studies in Medical Anthropology*, New York, Macmillan, 1977; see also Charles Leslie (ed.), *Asian Medical Systems. A Comparative Study*, Berkeley, University of California Press, 1976.

13   See especially the introductory essay by Charles Rosenberg in Charles Rosenberg and Janet L. Golden (eds), *Framing Disease: Studies in Cultural History*, New Brunswick, NJ, Rutgers University Press, 1992.

14   Richard J. Evans, *Death in Hamburg. Society and Politics in the Cholera Years 1830–1910*, Oxford, Oxford University Press, 1987; Paul Slack, *The Impact of Plague in Tudor and Stuart England*, Oxford, Oxford University Press, 1985.

15   Charles Rosenberg, *The Cholera Years*, Chicago, IL, University of Chicago Press, 1962; Roderick E. McGrew, *Russia and the Cholera, 1823–1832*, Madison, University of Wisconsin Press, 1965; R. J. Morris, *Cholera 1832. The Social Response to an Epidemic*, New York, Holmes & Meier, 1976; Margaret Pelling, *Cholera, Fever and English Medicine, 1825–1865*, Oxford, Oxford University Press, 1978.

16   Allan M. Brandt, *No Magic Bullet. A Social History of Venereal Disease in the United States since 1880*, New York, Oxford University Press, 1985.

17   Elizabeth W. Etheridge, *The Butterfly Caste. A Social History of Pellagra in the South*, Westport, CT, Greenwood Press, 1972.

18   John Ettling, *The Germ of Laziness. Rockefeller Philanthropy and Public Health in the New South*, Cambridge, MA, Harvard University Press, 1981; for a discussion

of health and disease in early nineteenth-century France see William Coleman, *Death is a Social Disease. Public Health and Political Economy in Early Industrial France*, Madison, University of Wisconsin Press, 1982.

19 François Delaporte, *Disease and Civilization. The Cholera in Paris, 1832*, Cambridge, MA, MIT Press, 1986.

20 Hans Zinsser, *Rats, Lice and History*, Boston, MA, Atlantic Monthly Press, 1934.

21 René and Jean Dobos, *The White Plague. Tuberculosis, Man and Society*, Boston, MA, Little Brown, 1952; reprinted with new introductions, New Brunswick, NJ, Rutgers University Press, 1987.

22 J. F. D. Shrewsbury, *A History of Bubonic Plague in the British Isles*, Cambridge, Cambridge University Press, 1970.

23 John R. Paul, *A History of Poliomyelitis*, New Haven, CT, Yale University Press, 1971.

24 Daphne A. Roe, *A Plague of Corn. A Social History of Pellagra*, Ithaca, NY, Cornell University Press, 1973.

25 Donald R. Hopkins, *Princes and Peasants. Smallpox in History*, Chicago, IL, University of Chicago Press, 1983.

26 Kenneth J. Carpenter, *The History of Scurvy and Vitamin C*, Cambridge, Cambridge University Press, 1986.

27 Owsei Temkin, *The Falling Sickness. A History of Epilepsy from the Greeks to the Beginnings of Modern Neurology*, 2nd edn, Baltimore, MD, Johns Hopkins University Press, 1971.

28 See especially two articles and a book by James Riley: 'Disease without death. New sources for a history of sickness', *Journal of Interdisciplinary History*, 1987, 18: 537–63; Riley and George Alter, 'Frailty, sickness and death. Models of morbidity in historical populations', *Population Studies*, 1989, 43: 25–45; Riley, *Sickness, Recovery and Death. A History and Forecast of Ill Health*, Iowa City, University of Iowa Press, 1989.

29 Thomas McKeown, *The Modern Rise of Population*, New York, Academic Press, 1976; McKeown, *The Role of Medicine. Dream, Mirage or Nemesis?*, Princeton, NJ, Princeton University Press, 1979; McKeown, *The Origins of Human Disease*, Oxford, Basil Blackwell, 1988.

30 Guenter B. Risse, *Hospital Life in Enlightenment Scotland. Care and Teaching at the Royal Infirmary of Edinburgh*, Cambridge, Cambridge University Press, 1986.

31 Martin S. Pernick, *A Calculus of Suffering. Pain, Professionalism and Anesthesia in Nineteenth-Century America*, New York, Columbia University Press, 1985; John Harley Warner, *The Therapeutic Perspective. Medical Practice, Knowledge and Identity in America 1820–85*, Cambridge, MA, Harvard University Press, 1986.

32 Joel D. Howell, ' "Soldier's heart": the redefinition of heart disease and speciality formation in early twentieth-century Great Britain', in W. F. Bynum, C. Lawrence and V. Nutton (eds), *The Emergence of Modern Cardiology, Medical History*, suppl. 5, 1985, pp. 34–52; see also Christopher Lawrence, 'Moderns and ancients. The new cardiology in Britain 1880–1930', ibid., pp. 1–33.

33 Besides Risse's work on Scotland, for England see especially M. Jeanne Peterson, *The Medical Profession in Mid-Victorian London*, Berkeley, University of California Press, 1978; and Irvine Loudon, *Medical Care and the General Practitioner, 1750–1850*, Oxford, Clarendon Press, 1986.

34 Saul Jarcho (trans.), *The Clinical Consultations of Giambattista Morgagni*, Boston, MA, Francis A. Countway Library of Medicine, 1984; Jarcho, *Clinical Consultations and Letters by Ippolito Francesco Albertini, Francesco Torti and Other Physicians*, Boston, MA, Francis A. Countway Library of Medicine, 1989.

35 Michael MacDonald, *Mystical Bedlam. Madness, Anxiety and Healing in Seventeenth-Century England*, Cambridge, Cambridge University Press, 1981.

36 Nancy Tomes, *A Generous Confidence. Thomas Story Kirkbride and the Art of Asylum-Keeping, 1840–1883*, Cambridge, Cambridge University Press, 1984.

37 Barbara Duden, *The Woman Beneath the Skin. A Doctor's Patients in Eighteenth-Century Germany*, trans. by Thomas Dunlap, Cambridge, MA, Harvard University Press, 1991.

38 Martin S. Pernick, 'Politics, parties and pestilence. Epidemic yellow fever in Philadelphia and the rise of the first party system', *William and Mary Quarterly*, 1972, 29: 559–86; Margaret Humphreys, *Yellow Fever and the South*, New Brunswick, NJ, Rutgers University Press, 1992; John Duffy, *Sword of Pestilence. The New Orleans Yellow Fever Epidemic of 1853*, Baton Rouge, LA, LSU Press, 1966.

39 James D. Goodyear, 'The sugar connection', *Bulletin of the History of Medicine*, 1978, 52: 5–21.

40 William Coleman, *Yellow Fever in the North. The Methods of Early Epidemiology*, Madison, University of Wisconsin Press, 1987.

41 John M. Eyler, *Victorian Social Medicine. The Ideas and Methods of William Farr*, Baltimore, MD, Johns Hopkins University Press, 1979; Abraham M. Lilienfeld (ed.), *Times, Places and Persons. Aspects of the History of Epidemiology*, Baltimore, MD, Johns Hopkins University Press, 1980.

42 Stephen Boyden, *Western Civilization in Biological Perspective. Patterns in Biohistory*, Oxford, Clarendon Press, 1987.

43 Alfred W. Crosby, *The Columbian Exchange. The Biological and Cultural Consequences of 1492*, Westport, CT, Greenwood Press, 1972.

44 Crosby, *Ecological Imperialism. The Biological Expansion of Europe, 900–1900*, Cambridge, Cambridge University Press, 1986.

45 William H. McNeill, *Plagues and Peoples*, New York, Anchor, 1977.

46 Mirko D. Grmek, *Diseases in the Ancient Greek World*, trans. by M. Muellner and L. Muellner, Baltimore, MD, Johns Hopkins University Press, 1989; see also Mark Nathan Cohen, *Health and the Rise of Civilization*, New Haven, CT, Yale University Press, 1989, in which the author used prehistoric evidence to assess the influence of civilization on health.

47 Roderick Floud, Kenneth Wachter and Annabel Gregory, *Height, Health and History. Nutritional Status in the United Kingdom, 1750–1980*, Cambridge, Cambridge University Press, 1990.

48 Andrew Appleby, *Famine in Tudor and Stuart England*, Stanford, CA, Stanford University Press, 1978; Appleby, 'Epidemics and famine in the little ice age', *Journal of Interdisciplinary History*, 1980, 10: 643–63; Massimo Livi-Bacci, *Population and Nutrition. An Essay on European Demographic History*, trans. by Tania Croft-Murray, Cambridge, Cambridge University Press, 1991; Robert I. Rotberg and Theodore K. Rabb (eds), *Hunger and History. The Impact of Changing Food Production and Consumption Patterns on Society*, Cambridge, Cambridge University Press, 1983; John Komlos, *Nutrition and Economic Development in the Eighteenth-*

Century Hapsburg Monarchy. An Anthropometric History, Princeton, NJ, Princeton University Press, 1989.

49 John D. Post, *Food Shortage, Climatic Variability and Epidemic Disease in Pre-industrial Europe. The Mortality Peak in the Early 1740s*, Ithaca, NY, Cornell University Press, 1985.

50 Ann G. Carmichael, 'Infection, hidden hunger and history', *Journal of Interdisciplinary History*, 1983, 14: 249–64.

51 John Walter and Roger Schofield (eds), *Famine, Disease and the Social Order in Early Modern Society*, Cambridge, Cambridge University Press, 1989.

52 George M. Foster and Barbara G. Anderson, *Medical Anthropology*, New York, John Wiley, 1978.

53 Erwin H. Ackerknecht, *History and Geography of the Most Important Diseases*, New York, Hafner, 1972.

54 Gerald W. Hartwig and K. David Patterson (eds), *Disease in African History. An Introductory Survey and Case Studies*, Durham, NC, Duke University Press, 1978, p. 3.

55 LaVerne Kuhnke, *Lives at Risk. Public Health in Nineteenth-Century Egypt*, Berkeley, University of California Press, 1990.

56 Nancy Gallagher, *Medicine and Power in Tunisia, 1780–1900*, Cambridge, Cambridge University Press, 1983; Gallagher, *Egypt's Other Wars. Epidemics and the Politics of Public Health*, Syracuse, NY, Syracuse University Press, 1990.

57 Michael W. Dols, *The Black Death in the Middle East*, Princeton, NJ, Princeton University Press, 1977.

58 H. Harold Scott, *A History of Tropical Medicine*, 2 vols, Baltimore, MD, Williams & Wilkins, 1939.

59 Roy Macleod and Milton Lewis (eds), *Disease, Medicine and Empire. Perspectives on Western Medicine and the Experience of European Expansion*, London, Routledge, 1988; David Arnold (ed.), *Imperial Medicine and Indigenous Societies*, Manchester, Manchester University Press, 1988; see also Norman G. Owen (ed.), *Death and Disease in Southeast Asia. Explorations in Social, Medical and Demographic History*, Oxford, Oxford University Press, 1987.

60 Gwyn Prins, 'But what was the disease? The present state of health and healing in African studies', *Past and Present*, 1989, no. 124, pp. 159–79.

61 Philip D. Curtin, *Death by Migration. Europe's Encounter with the Tropical World in the Nineteenth Century*, Cambridge, Cambridge University Press, 1989; see also Curtin's important earlier articles: 'Epidemiology and the slave trade', *Political Science Quarterly*, 1968, 83: 190–216; and 'The white man's grave. Image and reality, 1780–1850', *Journal of British Studies*, 1961, 1: 94–110.

62 Henry E. Sigerist, *A History of Medicine*, Vol. I: *Primitive and Archaic Medicine*, New York, Oxford University Press, 1951, p. 12.

FURTHER READING

Evans, Richard J., *Death in Hamburg. Society and Politics in the Cholera Years 1830–1910*, Oxford, Oxford University Press, 1987.

Granshaw, Lindsay and Porter, Roy (eds), *The Hospital in History*, London and New York, Routledge, 1989.

Lawrence, Christopher (ed.), *Medical Theory, Surgical Practice. Studies in the History of Surgery*, London, Routledge, 1992.

Leslie, Charles (ed.), *Asian Medical Systems. A Comparative Study*, Berkeley, University of California Press, 1976.

Ranger, Terence and Slack, Paul (eds), *Epidemics and Ideas. Essays on the Historical Perception of Pestilence*, Cambridge, Cambridge University Press, 1992.

Rosenberg, Charles, *The Care of Strangers. The Rise of America's Hospital System*, New York, Basic Books, 1987.

Siraisi, Nancy, *Medieval and Early Renaissance Medicine. An Introduction to Knowledge and Practice*, Chicago, IL, University of Chicago Press, 1990.

Slack, Paul, *The Impact of Plague in Tudor and Stuart England*, Oxford, Oxford University Press, 1985.

Walter, John and Schofield, Roger (eds), *Famine, Disease and the Social Order in Early Modern Society*, Cambridge, Cambridge University Press, 1989.

Wear, Andrew, 'Interfaces: perceptions of health and illness in early modern England', in Roy Porter and Andrew Wear (eds), *Problems and Methods in the History of Medicine*, London, Croom Helm, 1987, pp. 230–55.

—— (ed.), *Medicine in Society. Historical Essays*, Cambridge, Cambridge University Press, 1992.

4

MEDICAL CARE

Guenter B. Risse

THE HEALING FRAMEWORK

History reveals that, in every society, people have suffered physical and emotional distress for which they promptly sought assistance from specific categories of individuals devoted to healing. Traditionally, the care of the sick has been an important societal arena, with knowledge, skills, institutions, and remedies perennially provided by and contested by several groups, from families and folk practitioners to professional physicians. Past healing schemes not only provided explanations and human resources for caring efforts, they also regularly furnished particular remedies and techniques designed to achieve recovery, thus helping the sick re-integrate into their communities.

For historians interested in the phenomenon of healing, the fact of illness raises a number of important questions about the manner in which the sick have coped with pain and disability. Perhaps the first issue to be addressed is that of *definition*. What, for example, was meant by a fever? Why and by whom was this suffering categorized as sickness? Once a problem had been identified, what options were available to ameliorate it? Often, those who felt sick relied on themselves for help. A cold cloth on the forehead could perhaps stanch a fever. If that was not enough, the sick sought social organizations and resources that routinely handled their complaints. The final choice of healer and the negotiating process involved in this selection are equally important components of the therapeutic dynamic.

Because of social, political, and economic determinants, healing is and has been a local expression of culture and society. Care continues to be a complex transaction involving a variety of individuals in distinctive sick and caring roles. One speaks about an 'ecology' of medical care that focuses on the factors and circumstances influencing those who feel ill enough to adopt sick roles, as well as the actions of their selected healers.[1]

To assist people who feel or are said to be sick, all healing frameworks provide a number of distinct functions, all of them intended to contribute to the relief of suffering and perhaps the restoration of health. Foremost, answers may be provided to questions about the nature of the presenting dysfunction, perhaps even furnishing a definition of the problem. Is sickness trivial or life threatening, brief or long lasting, routine or unusual? Such distinctions have been based on contemporary health-related knowledge embedded in cultural beliefs and social values, historically creating patterns of meaning that could be labelled and classified. The naming or diagnosis of a given sickness such as 'a fever' is still an important step in the healing process. Both for the sick and for those living close to them, it reduces some of the psychological uncertainty caused by manifestations of the presenting disorder. (➤ Ch. 67 Pain and suffering)

All definitions of sickness are based on principles and theories derived from the observation of many sufferers, theories which are interpreted within culturally accepted frameworks of analysis. Through inference, comparison, and speculation, both the sick and their healers perennially seek an *explanation*, hoping to unravel the reasons and causes of specific dysfunctions. As an example, it was conjectured that fever was caused by excessive combustion within the body. (➤ Ch. 19 Fevers)

Historically, all explanatory models were periodically constructed and reconstructed as societies and their healers made new linkages between phenomena. As with definitions, the ability to explain events surrounding sickness, and perhaps even arrive at causal explanations, has therapeutic value. Such explanations, organized into increasingly more complex medical theories, have traditionally provided guidelines and rationales for therapeutic action.[2] (➤ Ch. 12 Concepts of health, illness, and disease.)

Culturally acceptable definitions and causal explanations of disability allow healers to name and sanction the health problem. This certification places sufferers into acceptable sick roles with particular privileges, obligations, and stigmas. *Validation* remains critical for the identification and possible separation of sick individuals from their immediate surroundings, and makes them eligible for further care efforts. Similarly, the official determination diminishes confusion and fear, reducing potential social tensions caused by the occurrence of illness in a given family or community.

Finally, before or after being defined, explained, and validated, sickness is routinely subjected to *therapy*. Deliberate measures and techniques aimed at coping with the key manifestations of ailments are provided by members of various healing groups. In the past, their actions have ranged widely from dietary adjustments to the administration of specific drugs, and from psychological reassurance to physical procedures such as massage and surgery. These activities, whether initiated by the sick themselves, their immediate families, or members of specific healing organizations, are likewise set in prevailing cultural values and norms and depend on particular community relationships and institutional settings for their execution. All therapeutic outcomes, in turn, are similarly evaluated in terms of culturally determined beliefs, expectations, and behaviour.[3]

Congruent with assumptions governing various healing systems, the therapeutic process underlying care has traditionally consisted of a series of interactions occurring within specific contexts. One cannot overemphasize the dynamic nature of these transactions, which involve choices and decisions carefully negotiated between those who represent the sick and their selected healers. The perception of events surrounding sickness, as well as actual diagnosis and prognosis of a disease, plays a decisive role in shaping the therapeutic response. Verbal and non-verbal communication between healers and the ill is a critical vehicle for establishing a relationship. (➤ Ch. 34 The history of the doctor–patient relationship)

Each diagnostic and therapeutic determination triggers and shapes successive stages of the healing process, modifying the range of treatment options, and ultimately affecting the final outcome. Cognitive and behavioural components often influence that result. One is the so-called placebo effect, originally meant to represent a pleasing or soothing healing measure employed when no cures could be expected. Although later condemned as fraudulent, the placebo is still used for its beneficial psychological effect or to eliminate observer bias in experimental conditions.[4]

Most societies have historically managed sickness through a set of different but coexisting and interconnected levels of care. Many conditions were handled by the sick persons themselves, with the aid of families, folk healers, or organizations offering more specialized aid. With the advent of complex civilizations, another level of care appeared, offering greater diagnostic and prognostic skills while promising more effective therapies. At any given moment, the sick selected a particular category of care because of its promise to provide an acceptable meaning as well as treatment for the illness in question. Proximity, personal preference, knowledge, cost, type of illness, and speciality of the healer played major roles in such choices. In times of illness, however, all healing groups in their own way functioned as valuable therapeutic resources and networks. While overlapping significantly, each system has had its own set of definitions, explanations, validations, and treatments for illness. In practice, the sick usually resorted to one or all sectors at once, indiscriminately alternating between them until a final resolution or cure was perceived.[5]

EARLY HEALTH CARE

In pre-literate societies before 4000 BC, self-help and folk healing prevailed. To this day, domestic healing is still the level at which ill health is first recognized, defined, and treated. Self-diagnosis and treatment, often in consultation with immediate family members, other relatives, close friends, neighbours, and workmates, remains the basis of medical care. If the sickness is deemed more complex, care activities shift to other identifiable persons believed to possess special expertise.

In the past, both the sick and those involved in domestic healing shared similar assumptions and beliefs about bodily structure and function in health and sickness. Indeed, they mutually attempted to validate their problems, frequently entering into informal and often-reciprocal healing relationships. Since care took place among people already linked by ties of kinship, friendship, or membership in religious organizations, the therapeutic actions failed to follow fixed rules of behaviour, nor did they require formal settings. Many such transactions occurred in a family setting. The main providers were usually women: wives, mothers, grandmothers, and friends. These persons all shared in basic knowledge concerning common ailments and popular remedies.

The habitual 'kitchen' medicine prominently featured a jumble of magical and empirical measures such as the use of charms and amulets, dietary changes, or the use of specially prepared botanicals that were not always harmless. Behavioural changes such as seclusion, rest, and fasting were supplemented with special rituals, prayers, and confession. Midwifery was also practised in the popular sector of health care, where birth attendants were experienced mothers of the community helping their friends and neighbours.

An examination of contemporary societies of hunter-gatherers and early agriculturalists provides tantalizing hints about the health-related activities of our distant ancestors, allowing tentative reconstructions of such events. In their efforts to survive in a potentially hostile environment, such groups constructed a world divided into spiritual and physical realms and adopted a number of techniques to cope with the problems of human suffering. Common illness was viewed in purely naturalistic ways, its effects treated in practical terms by drawing on the shared problem-solving experiences of families and groups. Knowledge of available dietary measures and simple drug therapy was empirical, communal, and orally transmitted.

Because of their perceived threat to social cohesion, dramatic and severe episodes of sickness required greater and more spectacular efforts involving the manipulation of a perceived supernatural realm. To this day, specialized individuals are consulted who are believed to be endowed with effective methods for battling invisible forces with the use of magic and religious measures. Although quite a heterogeneous group, all folk healers, from diviners to herbalists, share the basic world-views of the cultures they serve. Moreover, they work in close contact with the sick, their families, and surrounding community members, thus helping to articulate and reinforce societal values. This folk-healing approach is always sacred and holistic, bringing together treatments that address the physical, psychological, and social dimensions of sickness involving the affected individuals and the entire social group. (➤ Ch. 30 Folk medicine)

Historically, folk healers have addressed health concerns that were ascribed to either a divine or natural agency, often operating in both supernatural and natural realms. In the former setting, they acted as clairvoyants, shamans, diviners, charmers, or priests, capable of dealing with transcendental forces presumed to be responsible for illness. Other secular healers were generally identified and consulted for their empirical expertise in particular therapeutic roles, from herbalists to midwives, and from bone-setters to tooth-extractors. Even today, folk healers usually operate as individuals or members of informal caring networks. Traditionally, their healing powers are said to be acquired through inheritance, especially in cases involving the supernatural, or by apprenticeship, and personal experience.[6]

The worldwide phenomenon of shamanism can be seen as a particular and early historical model of folk healing. While past pre-literate groups probably differed greatly in their particular beliefs and social organizations, they all adhered to a supernatural view of illness. An often invisible realm of powers and forces was constructed to understand the effects of a potentially hostile natural environment. Shamanism, therefore, remains a form of religious belief and activity aimed at protecting a society from the destructive actions of divine entities. Its roots can be traced back at least to the palaeolithic age. Through a continuing relationship with the spiritual world, its practitioners attempted to avoid conflict and sickness as well as ensure fertility, thereby bolstering the confidence and harmony of the community they served. (➤ Ch. 60 Medicine and anthropology)

When sickness was blamed on supernatural agents, shamans played important roles in the diagnosis, validation, and therapy of the person found to be ill. Identification of the responsible agent was usually made through divination procedures such as dreams, the scattering of bones and pebbles, or impressions gathered in a trance, often induced by hallucinogenic drugs. Among the major causes observed in contemporary societies are the ingestion or penetration of harmful objects into the body, soul loss, spirit intrusion, and breach of taboo. Once such a causal determination has been made, removal of the illness becomes the shaman's fundamental task.

Shamanistic curing is a social and cultural phenomenon. Healing occurs along a symbolic pathway of words and songs, feelings and expectations. The art of interpreting and controlling the supernatural world depends on the shaman's status, image, costume, and the use of objects and procedures, including masks, rattles, drums, incantations, and prayers. Issues of social control and cultural identity are paramount in such ceremonies. Shamans are frequently selected because of their special qualities and undergo years of rigorous apprenticeship. Widely scattered on all continents, shamanistic care continues to be a very significant form of folk healing that demonstrates the tremendous power of faith and suggestion.

In neolithic times, social transition to more agrarian societies not only expanded the realm of domestic healing, but stimulated the creation of new levels of specialized care and the establishment of additional folk-healing functions and techniques. As hunters, warriors, and farmers learned more about trauma caused by accidents and warfare, they developed specific wound-healing and bone-setting skills. Certain gatherers became more knowledgeable about particular healing plants as well as the dietary and medicinal effects of domesticated animal products. Experienced women continued to assist with childbirth. Magicians and wise men interpreted omens and offered charms as magical protection.[7]

Since their inception around 4000 BC, civilizations of greater complexity and division of labour in the Near and Far East expanded their own care frameworks. In addition to the usual local self-help schemes, folk healing changed dramatically as organized religions with their pantheons of gods and goddesses provided sufferers with a coherent, mythical system of explanations to account for all natural phenomena, including the appearance of illness. In some countries, specific individuals of the official priesthood were even identified with shamanistic healing skills, such as ancient Mesopotamia's magical expert, the *ashipu*, Egypt's *wab* or priest healer, India's exorcist, the *blisaj*, and China's *wu*, diviner and wizard. In addition, both ancient Mesopotamia and Egypt also created special and communal rituals which took place in temples dedicated to gods of healing such as the Babylonian goddess Gula and, later, the Egyptian architect-scribe Imhotep.

Early empires in Mesopotamia and Egypt also organized care systems headed by lay healers. These individuals elaborated comprehensive explanations of illness, and took advantage of their ability to preserve and disseminate medical knowledge through the use of writing. Anatomical understanding and clinical skills were acquired through cumulative individual experiences and written down on clay tablets and papyrus leaves. By naming body parts, illnesses, and remedies, a technical medical language emerged.

Professionally, the new healers were usually trained by apprenticeship and formed part of a literate élite that began to occupy positions of privilege and status equivalent to those held by the established priesthood and bureaucracy. Expected to combine magical and naturalistic problem-solving, practitioners such as ancient Mesopotamia's *asu* (he who has healing skills) and ancient Egypt's *swnw* (the knife and mortar expert) also apropriated valuable healing knowledge from the domestic sector.

Faced with intensified military operations and monumental construction projects, these healers improved the management of trauma through better wound drainage, sutures, and cauterization. New extraction and preparation techniques yielded an expanded materia medica of compounded drugs containing plant, animal, and mineral ingredients. Together, these measures offered further opportunities for successful treatment. The same can be said of roles played by the Ayurvedic practitioner in ancient India and China's Confucian *i*. In the latter two cultures, minerals and particularly metals assumed greater importance in therapeutics, especially from the eleventh century onward, as alchemical yogis began to experiment with such drugs in their search for immortality.[8] (➤ Ch. 32 Chinese medicine; Ch. 33 Indian medicine)

CLASSICAL GREECE AND ROME

Well before 400 BC, ancient Greece possessed extensive networks of domestic medicine and folk healing. One was the Greek *iatromantis* who combined sacred and secular functions, employing magical procedures such as divination together with drug treatments. As a logical consequence of sustained warfare with its battlefield trauma, essential wound healing techniques were known to the combatants themselves, spawning a new generation of technical experts and leading to the gradual establishment of a surgical craft. At the same time, the demands of athletic competition created specialists in the art of dietetics and physical fitness, who eventually focused on broader life-style issues such as exercise, bathing, and massage in addition to the regulation of food and drink.

These domestic and folk-healing traditions in ancient Greece ostensibly contributed to the creation of a healing craft or *techne iatriche* around 500 BC. This system consciously sought to define its own intellectual approach to sickness while formulating a new methodology and rationale for medical care. The foremost representative of classical Greek medicine was Hippocrates (*c*.450–370 BC), a prominent practitioner and teacher. Followers and rivals of this physician focused exclusively on physical factors related to health and disease, paying special attention to the ill person's immediate environment and life-style as important factors in causing and shaping sickness. For some, health was viewed as a state of balance of bodily humours, including blood, phlegm, and yellow and black bile. Each humour had a specific bodily source and possessed a pair of fundamental qualities. Sickness occurred when the humoral balance was upset through lack of proper nourishment, or imperfect production, circulation, and elimination of the humours. (➤ Ch. 14 Humoralism)

Within a century of Hippocrates's death, unknown disciples and competing groups composed nearly sixty treatises on medical subjects, creating a body of knowledge usually known as Hippocratic.

The modest goal of a Greek healing practitioner was the restoration of a healthy balance through attention to natural or internal bodily factors together with the so-called non-naturals or external, environmental influences such as food and drink, sleep and exercise. A specific regimen was prescribed which included diet and exercise, together with a limited number of drugs capable of aiding the natural healing powers of the human organism. Indeed, classical Greek medical art was conservative and expectant, modelled on the concept that nature possessed health-giving and healing powers. The healer's identification as merely a 'follower of nature' reflected the tenuous social position of the often itinerant Hippocratic practitioner, who was entirely dependent on his personal reputation to earn a living. To this end, he tried above all else to avoid iatrogenic harm. As stated in the Oath, 'I will use my power to help the sick to the best of my ability and judgement; I will abstain from harming or wronging any man by it.'[9]

In direct imitation of the natural bodily discharges, such as bleeding, defecating, vomiting, and sweating, that frequently occurred during acute illnesses, the ancient Greek healer employed a number of remedies and physical methods to accomplish similar depletions. This approach was congruent with the tenets of humoralism, which viewed the eliminations as nature's way of removing harmful fluids believed to be responsible for the imbalance. In their competition for patients, Greek healers hoped to discover a universal remedy or panacea, capable of curing a wide range of ailments. Favourable therapeutic results helped to legitimate theoretical frameworks, build credibility, and persuade those who recovered to furnish career-building testimonials about the physicians who had cured them. (➤ Ch. 40 Physical methods)

With no obligations to society at large, the personalized nature of Hippocratic medical care was quite compatible with Sophist philosophy. While lacking a formal process of education and training, the ancient Greek physician formulated an occupational ethos often taken as an oath that placed prudent limits on medical intervention and created rules to regulate contact with patients. Unfettered by religious and legal barriers, the *techne iatriche* prospered in the ensuing centuries within the flexible framework of the humoral doctrine, a cultural system articulated by philosophers and widely shared by the sick and their healers.[10]

Similar linkages were established with a Greek religious healing scheme that began in the third century BC: the cult of Aesculapius, the Greek god of healing. In this scheme, the sick travelled to shrines consecrated to the god and participated in a number of rituals and ceremonies. Central among them was incubation, the act of going to sleep in the sacred temple precincts and being visited in person by the god who, often in a dream, provided reassurance and advice. As in other Near Eastern cultures, Greek temple medicine appealed to the mystical and emotional aspects of healing, and was a refuge for the disabled who, placed in an optimistic atmosphere of the divine, sought succour in mass worship. The gradual spread of this cult throughout Greece, and its eventual importation into Rome after 293 BC, converted the earlier shrines into recreational spas with hostels, baths, theatres, and gymnasia with large staffs of priests and attendants. In time, Aesculapius was increasingly depicted as a physician, recommending enemas and bloodletting, preparing useful drugs, even displaying surgical instruments. The popularity of Greek temple medicine came to reside in its ability to provide a synthesis of sacred and secular care that continued to have broad cultural appeal among the masses.[11]

In subsequent centuries, however, the provision of Hippocratic medical care remained mostly an individually negotiated arrangement between practitioners and their patients. In their struggle to acquire greater authority, two early weaknesses were progressively overcome by the Greek *techne iatriche*: meagre theoretical and clinical knowledge about the phenomena of health and disease, and limited transmission of that knowledge to new apprentices. Gradually, a substantial corpus of writings and commentaries, emanating from small networks of practitioners in Cos, Cnidus, Rhodes, and Sicily, diffused through the Mediterranean world and was subsequently collected in several urban centres, including libraries at Alexandria, Pergamon, Smyrna, and finally Rome. Paradoxically, the often contradictory content of that knowledge and the increasingly greater competition among Hippocratic practitioners for upper-class patronage and compensation generated serious debates about the value of medical theory and bedside expertise. The ensuing epistemologic fragmentation of classical Greek healing in the Hellenistic period and formation of opposing sects such as the dogmatists and empiricists decisively conspired against further efforts to establish a truly independent medical profession.[12]

With the emergence of the Roman Empire, both domestic and folk healing flourished. Indeed, the Romans traditionally stressed the role of the *pater familias* in the provision of medical advice. Healing was viewed as a popular skill practised by slaves and foreigners. In Imperial Rome, the cult of Aesculapius reached its highest level of diffusion and popularity. Greek healing practitioners were often mistrusted and provided care only to a narrow tier of aristocratic households.[13] In this regard, the efforts of Galen (AD 129-c.200/210) to create a cadre of learned and experienced physician-philosophers were meant to remedy the perceived epistemological and practical deficiencies. In his words, Galenic practitioners needed to employ 'the science of reasoning to the way of choosing foods, general treatments and drugs.'[14]

Yet Rome also provided the first clear example of state-sponsored medical care for a privileged sector of the population: its soldiers. Away from make-shift tent facilities near the battlefield, the Romans established so-called *valetudinaria* or regional military hospitals for the care of wounded and sick legionnaires.[15]

THE MIDDLE AGES

The advent of Christianity dramatically altered previous patterns of care. Physical welfare became secondary to spiritual salvation. Although sickness could be viewed alternately as an expression of punishment for sins or an expression of divine grace, the body as a repository of the immortal soul remained a legitimate object for caring efforts. According to St Matthew's gospel, 'Jesus went about all Galilee teaching in their synagogues, and preach-ing the gospel of the kingdom, and healing all manner of sickness and all manner of disease among the people.' Healing the sick, therefore, was viewed as a divine gift not solely restricted to trained practitioners, but shared by people with strong Christian faith. Indeed, caring and curing became a popular religious vocation, an act of conscious humility and thus a vital component of Christian *caritas* or good works. Within this ideology, Christ became the ultimate god of healing, replacing the hitherto popular but pagan Aesculapius, whose temples were systematically destroyed and replaced during the fourth century by Christian churches and shrines.[16] (➤ Ch. 61 Religion and medicine)

In the midst of the ensuing social and political turmoil following the disintegration of the Roman Empire, most health-related knowledge remained in the possession of families, folk healers, and religious orders. While dom-estic healing retained its basic practical and familiar orientation, a new level of magical and empirical Christian folk medicine developed in the early centuries of our era, featuring a number of saints whose relics and shrines became the focus of mass worship. At several monasteries in the Latin West, the followers of Benedict of Nursia (AD *c*.480–547) created working communities that cared for their own sick brethren as well as visitors and transients. As St Benedict declared, 'Before all things and above all things care is to be had of the sick. Let it be therefore the abbot's greatest care that they suffer no neglect.'[17] Other groups established so-called hospitals or small inns, located near cathedrals or on roads leading to places of pilgrimage. Their purpose was to admit tired and ill Christian travellers converging from all over Europe.[18]

In Byzantium, the provision of shelter and food extended to physical care in hostels called *xenones* and *nosokomeia*, or places for the sick, which were created after AD 400. Clerical medicine provided free assistance in monastic infirmaries, hospices, and shelters, combining religious procedures such as prayers, exorcisms, laying-on of hands, and miracles with certain herbal and physical treatments. Instead of medical care, hospitality and spiritual revival were emphasized.[19] This contrasted with conditions in contemporary Islamic hospitals, where by the seventh century early Byzantine models had already led to the foundation of secular *bimaristans* in the major urban centres of the Islamic empire. Endowed with a clear medical focus, these institutions were staffed by physicians, surgeons, and apothecaries and equipped with well-stocked pharmacies and medicinal herbal gardens.[20]

In spite of frequent tensions with Christian healing schemes, remnants of the Hippocratic craft tradition also flourished in Byzantium and Islam. This sector worked hard at standardizing its body of knowledge, with practitioners such as Oribasius (AD 325–400), Alexander of Tralles (AD 525–605), and Paul of Aegina (AD 925–90) compiling and preserving classical medical knowledge. With the help of Christian scholars, the Abbasid rulers in Baghdad sponsored translations of medical texts into Arabic around AD 800, setting the stage for the systematic arrangement of Graeco-Roman humoralism, the *Canon* by Ibn Sina's (Avicenna, AD 980–1037). Provided at the cost of high honoraria, Hippocratic care was mostly restricted to selected upper-class individuals. Following the classical model, it advocated both a preventive regimen based on a prudent management of the so-called 'six things non-natural', and a curative strategy based on the restoration of basic humoral balances.

After the twelfth century, Europe's burgeoning population witnessed an expansion of its different care systems. As before, domestic networks continued to prosper, their knowledge base now enriched by widespread cultural and commercial exchanges with other parts of the globe. New drugs from the Mediterranean trade prompted creation of *apothecas* or import/export depots for the blending and sale of these products. Its owners, the pharmacists or apothecaries, began supplying these drugs to practitioners and the public, often in mixtures of increasing complexity and price. In addition, a phalanx of mostly itinerant folk healers roamed the fledgling urban centres as well as the countryside, peddling amulets, charms, and cure-alls. On the basis of an increasing fragmentation and specialization of healing skills, intense competition ensued between folk 'empirics', including herbalists, bone-setters, barbers, diviners, bladder-stone removers, those responsible for the reduction and management of hernias, tooth-extractors, and those couching cataracts. For a fee, midwives continued to preside over the birthing event. All popular healers stressed practical problem-solving and many of their techniques remained secret, communicated only to other family members.[21]

As part of the church-sponsored healing activities, particular groups cared for the sick as the principal focus of their charitable work. In this respect the Knights of St John, the Teutonic Knights, and the Augustinian brother-hoods all played important roles, especially during the Crusades.[22] Local rulers, bishops, and even kings sponsored the founding of numerous hospitals staffed by monastic orders. Their expanded services included physical care for the indigent, ageing, infirm and sick. An extensive network of leprosaria was created in western Europe to isolate and house lepers away from population centres.[23] (➤ Ch. 62 Charity before c.1850)

At the same time, medieval society signalled a willingness to bestow on specific groups of individuals the exclusive right to practise medicine and surgery. In order to practise medicine locally, a small number of physicians for the first time acquired academic degrees in medicine and thus were able to claim greater learning and competence. Because of the vast collection and translation efforts of the Islamic Empire, an essential body of medical literature was reintroduced into the Western university curriculum for commentary and memorization. (➤ Ch. 31 Arab-Islamic medicine) The addition of medicine to European university studies, together with the widespread establishment of local licensing regulations in southern Europe, dramatically solidified the professional character of the classical Graeco-Roman *techne iatriche*. The mechanism used for such licensing was the guilds, which were thus effectively awarded a monopoly on professional healing.[24] (➤ Ch. 48 Medical education)

To this day, professional healers are offered higher status and prestige because they are believed to possess greater theoretical knowledge, better diagnostic and prognostic skills, and can provide seemingly more effective therapies. Often, individual sick persons consult with them after experiencing therapeutic failures at both the domestic and folk-healing levels. Like the Hippocratic practitioners, their emphasis is generally on physical disease, with reference to social and behavioural contexts. Both the definitions and explanations of sickness are said to be 'rational', logical inferences from principles and theories constructed on the basis of pre-existing philosophical and scientific knowledge as well as on information derived from the systematic observation of the sick.

Professional systems place great value on status, autonomy, credentials, and specialized skills. For protection and self-policing, their members come together in collegial types of organizations with hierarchically arranged healing roles, each with its own rights and obligations. Professional knowledge is preserved, transmitted, and updated in numerous texts provided to new members who must rely on memory and practical experience to be successful. For this purpose, healing professionals undergo a rigorous process of education and training within institutional settings that are controlled by the profession itself.[25] (➤ Ch. 47 History of the medical profession)

Since medical education in medieval universities emphasized theory and rhetoric while encouraging philosophical speculation, some practical aspects of healing were initially excluded, especially surgery. Clinical evidence was often disregarded if prevailing theories could not justify it. Medieval medical-care schemes remained firmly wedded to humoralism, with the physician continuing to rely on regimen and the healing power of nature to re-establish healthy balances. Patients were usually members of the upper class, a very small sector of the population. Obedience to prevailing social relations and cultural taboos ensured the use of traditional therapeutic measures. Yet, within the Christian framework, university-trained physicians found themselves characterized as agents of divine will with God-given skills and powers to heal. They made sure that patients' souls received the critical cleansing that promised life after death, and they were seen merely as the purveyors of divine remedies.[26]

THE RENAISSANCE

During the Renaissance, the sick continued to rely for care on domestic networks and a variety of folk healers, both magical healers and 'empirics', with their special powers and practical skills. This group included astrologers and exorcists, bone-setters and tooth-extractors, as well as the usual assortment of herbalists, barbers, and birth-attendants. Given the limited capacity of learned institutions and the high cost of education, university-trained physicians remained scarce. Apprenticed surgeons gradually improved their knowledge and skills by attending university courses and by performing anatomical dissections. (➤ Ch. 5 The anatomical tradition) While the church continued its own healing schemes, local and national authorities sponsored a number of care plans involving these physicians and surgeons. In larger cities, religious hospitals increasingly shifted to secular jurisdiction. Because of the prevalence of plague, local authorities in Italy and elsewhere set up numerous lazarettos or pest-houses aimed at isolating and caring for those infected with the disease.[27]

In all urban areas of Europe, a small cadre of university-trained physicians and surgeons soon positioned themselves at the top of what was fast becoming a hierarchy of professional healers. In such places, a separate, organized, autonomous occupation began to thrive, with its own particular world-view, value system, and rules of behaviour. Among credentials which lent legitimacy and status were lineage, diploma, citizenship, and often a local licence, awarded by bishops or secular authorities. Colleges or corporations, in turn, received authority to control and regulate the profession, formulating codes of occupational ethics.

Continued use of Latin and a growing number of specialized, technical terms put distance between such professionals and other healers. Some became salaried, employed by municipal governments to function on public health boards or to care for the poor in secular and religious hospitals, prisons, and pest-houses. Others cared for personnel on naval and commercial vessels. Most were in private practice on fixed retainers, providing personal services to secular and religious dignitaries. Therapy, however, retained its classical *modus operandi*: strategies were designed to remove corrupt and excessive humours through the employment of traditional drugs and physical methods.[28]

By the sixteenth century, growing disagreements about the theoretical underpinnings of professional healing ensued, prompting changes in the provision of medical care. The widespread acceptance of Vesalian anatomy not only popularized dissections, but also weakened the classical medical models of disease. New explanations incorporated the recent findings of pathological anatomy uncovered during autopsies.[29] The emergence of a chemical theory of human physiology and pathology articulated by Paracelsus (1493–1541) led to a revolutionary shift from an almost exclusively plant-based materia medica to the extensive administration of chemical remedies. In Paracelsian terms, God was the premier apothecary, his universe an immense pharmacy. Through careful observations, practitioners could discover and alchemically manipulate such natural chemical treasures for the benefit of the sick. 'The man who desires to teach men must derive his learning from God and from nature', he wrote.[30] For many, however, Paracelsian therapeutics were deemed aggressive and even dangerous, fraught with potential iatrogenic effects that violated the traditional Hippocratic precept of avoiding harm. Yet, in the case of the dreaded syphilis, large doses of mercury quickly became the treatment of choice.[31] (➤ Ch. 7 The physiological tradition; Ch. 9 The pathological tradition)

Especially important at this time were the innovations in surgery, including new techniques to treat gunshot wounds that were pioneered by Ambroise Paré (1510–90). His methods and instruments profoundly influenced contemporary surgical craft, replacing ancient authority with new procedures and tools to deal with a variety of novel lesions caused by modern warfare. (➤ Ch. 41 Surgery (traditional)) While still lacking effective anaesthetic agents and antisepsis, many surgeons nevertheless gradually improved their lower status, distancing themselves professionally from barbers and bleeders. A new level of powerful patrons, upper-class warriors suffering life-threatening bullet wounds, eagerly sought their services.[32]

THE SEVENTEENTH CENTURY

By the seventeenth century, Europe had not only retained but had expanded its domestic, folk, and professional healing schemes. Such pluralism in care was certainly not novel, and the diverse treatment options were not easily categorized according to vocational or educational criteria. The overlap between the three care sectors persisted, with the public continuing to be governed in its selection of practitioners by each group's distinct ability to define, explain, validate, and treat illness. In England, the domestic arena at this time featured unpaid gentlewomen healers, scattered through the country-side, who were essential components of the Jacobean care system. Some possessed far-ranging reputations that rivalled those of folk healers and even of licensed physicians. Not surprisingly, their numerous remedies were often identical to those prescribed by representatives of learned medicine.

Midwifery in Jacobean England remained the exclusive domain of women, who continued to orchestrate birth as a ritualized social event. Their expanded knowledge and skills came to include related instances of female sexual pathology. Other healers operating at that folk level were local specialists who dispensed drugs, let blood, or set bones. 'Cunning' men and women, also known as strokers, performed magical rituals including exorcisms and the prescription of amulets. In flamboyant advertisements linked with public entertainment, itinerants offered universal panaceas. From a respectable social position, clergymen-healers effected treatment through the use of domestic and professional measures while claiming access to special curative powers.[33]

Among the most popular contemporary folk-healing schemes in all of Europe was astrological medicine, a theory and practice based on the assumption that sickness was caused by influences emanating from the stars and planets. Although its origins were in early Near Eastern cultures, a more systematized astrology in the service of health-related problems now promised greater certainty in the diagnosis and treatment of diseases.[34]

In European medical circles, the seventeenth century became a turning-point as the classical assumptions of humoralism were openly challenged. In close association with a changing world-view, a functional view of the human body emerged, with claims made that it operated as a machine governed by physical principles. The dual nature of the Cartesian human, a physical body ruled by universal laws of matter and motion, linked to an immaterial soul, spawned new theories of physiology and pathology. The discovery by William Harvey (1578–1657) of blood circulation dramatically demonstrated, to phys-icians at least, the usefulness of a scientific approach to problems of human physiology. If the body could be interpreted as a machine, physicians reasoned that they should be able to control its mechanisms through internal adjust-ments. Novel sets of physical and chemical explanations of bodily function confronted the sick, replacing the traditional humours and their qualities. Some practitioners explained and justified their interventions on such engin-eering principles. However, they remained at a loss when challenged to apply the new knowledge in therapy. Physicians, with support from their patients, continued to employ traditional depleting measures based on humoral corruption and displacement, but recast them as logical and rational procedures to be used within the new theoretical scaffolding.[35]

These fissures in professional medicine's theoretical underpinnings had an impact on care. Top establishment physicians practising in Europe's cities continued to benefit from royal and aristocratic patronage, devoting most of their conservative healing efforts to individuals of the upper classes. Alongside traditional botanical agents, chemical remedies had been used with more frequency since Paracelsian times. Prominent practitioners were members of exclusive colleges or academies, and protected their absolute control over a small but very lucrative medical market. Yet, even those physicians with licences failed to achieve sufficient power to dictate or even control their patients' therapeutic preferences. Many eagerly followed the call by Thomas Sydenham (1624–89) to bring order to the available clinical information, distinguishing particular ailments and classifying them accordingly. Such knowledge was seen as critically important for diagnosis, leading perhaps to the future prescription of specific remedies to cure distinct diseases. Wrote Sydenham: 'I conceive that the advancement of medicine lies in . . . a history of the disease [and] a *praxis* or *methodus* respecting the same, and this must be regular and exact.'[36]

While many surgeons remained at the lower level of barbers and phlebotomists, others continued their gradual professional ascent, receiving a university education as well as special postgraduate hospital training, especially in France. Some specialized in certain operations such as amputation, trephining, the removal of bladder-stones and the care of hernias, ulcers, and fistulas with the help of new instruments and techniques. With the popularization of chemical remedies, apothecaries and their suppliers, the druggists and chemists, also came into greater demand and thus attained a higher status. As before, many of the drugs were imported from afar, requiring vast mercantile supply networks. Apothecaries displayed a keen knowledge of the composition and action of these compounds. In the transition from servants to prescribing physicians, apothecaries were valuable partners in the exchange of therapeutic information, and fierce competitors in the provision of medical care to the lower and middle classes.[37] (➤ Ch. 39 Drug therapies)

THE EIGHTEENTH CENTURY

Enlightenment ideology set the stage for a more optimistic outlook concerning the role and benefits of medicine. Among the newly perceived requirements of national power was a healthy and expanding population. Thus, European governments increasingly sought to develop social policies that included the promotion of physical well-being for all citizens. Greater emphasis was placed on environmental health, infant and maternal welfare, military and naval hygiene, and the mass treatment of the poor in newly erected hospitals. Society could be medicalized with the help of physicians who considered themselves experts in health-related matters. A comprehensive system of health preservation sought to portray sickness as an avoidable evil that endangered both individuals and the community. While most domestic-care networks could easily be compelled to serve the new professional programme, folk healing declined in the face of a dramatic expansion of the professional sphere of medical care.[38]

Yet, for many, sickness remained a mysterious and unavoidable event resulting from fate or divine retribution. The goal of Enlightenment medical practitioners, however, was to displace such pessimism in favour of more optimistic models. Happiness could be promoted if physical health was protected and restored. 'The appropriate means of conserving life consists in the apt usage of the things necessary to the body such as hygiene and diet which must be observed for their best possible effect when carried out in the prescribed manner', wrote one author in the French *Encyclopédie*.[39] (➤ Ch. 53 History of personal hygiene)

Indeed, for the first time in history, physicians began to play more prominent medical roles in European society. By assuming a range of responsibilities under the auspices of local and national governments, practitioners now broadened their mission and achieved a near-monopoly on care. Gone were the days when their services were restricted to a small élite on top of the social pyramid. A growing bourgeoisie eagerly joined the upper classes in demanding medical services. Physicians became steadily involved in private and public health for all levels of society. They attended the sick poor in hospitals, dispensaries, and polyclinics. Moreover, they took care of mothers and children, soldiers and sailors, all within officially sanctioned arrangements.[40]

Although frequently Utopian in outlook, a popular bureaucratic scheme was the 'medical police', a plan that in various European countries instituted inclusive, cradle-to-grave programmes of health education and medical assistance. Such programmes were most clearly articulated within the framework of German mercantilism, assuming a comprehensive albeit paternalistic character consonant with political systems of enlightened despotism. The goal was to persuade the lower classes that health could be attained if they submitted to governmental advice and control in matters ranging from personal hygiene to public water supplies, education, job training, marriage, child-rearing, and even burial.[41] (➤ Ch. 51 Public health; Ch. 50 The medical institutions and the state)

In Britain, by contrast, voluntary and private medical schemes predominated, leading to the establishment of educational and institutional facilities partially supported by private philanthropy. Indeed, British *laissez-faire* created a bustling medical market-place where among other domestic and folk advice, professional services could be easily obtained according to the laws of supply and demand. Lacking state and professional protection, physicians, surgeons, apothecaries, and chemists openly competed with each other in the healing business. Individual reputation and patronage often determined advancement; entrepreneurial skills and social manners sometimes mattered more than medical knowledge. In the end, paying patients retained their power to choose their healers, purchasing cures as they did other commodities.[42]

Such conditions favoured the fusion of two professional groups of lesser status, the surgeons and apothecaries, who gradually became Britain's general practitioners, blurring the traditional tripartite division that had separated them from physicians and each other. Another development in the professional sector was the emergence of the man-midwife, who displaced the female birth attendant of the folk sector. More thoroughly trained in anatomy and instructed in the use of a new technology – the forceps – male midwives first appealed to the wealthy with claims of greater competence and safety, proposing to lower the perils of assisted births. (➤ Ch. 44 Childbirth) By the end of the eighteenth century, the sick in Europe drew more heavily on professional healing services than at any previous time in history. Other remaining traditional folk healers such as itinerant cure-all peddlers, magicians, hernia-operators, and cataract-couchers were repeatedly discredited and branded as quacks by the regular medical profession.[43]

Within the new medical-care programme, hospitals occupied an important place. Their transformation from undifferentiated welfare establishments into strictly medical institutions started in Britain and gradually spread through Europe. British infirmaries as well as French and German general hospitals became facilities exclusively devoted to care of the sick poor. For the medical profession, the rise of such hospitals had truly momentous consequences. (➤ Ch. 49 The hospital) Opportunities for observing large numbers of patients and systematically performing post-mortem dissections allowed for a dramatic improvement in the understanding of disease. Physicians constructed patterns of sickness and established correlations between symptom sequences and diseased bodily organs. For the first time, trials with traditional treatments also planted the seeds for future therapeutic scepticism. The new hospital medicine, as epitomized in France, established a clinically oriented medical science that became pre-eminent throughout Europe in the early 1800s.[44]

Clearly in ascendance, medical healing sought to influence the basic health beliefs of the laity. Physicians endeavoured to share and popularize their knowledge and practices, forcing self-help to conform with the basic tenets of the Enlightenment. In retrospect, this was to be the final wholesale demystification of medicine designed by experts to bring medical information to educated Europeans. Practitioners depended on the ability and willingness of their patients to provide the necessary information for making a diagnosis. At this point, patient and physician power had reached a balance. Subsequent developments in medical knowledge placed professionals in charge of the healing relationship. (➤ Ch. 35 The art of diagnosis: medicine and the five senses)

A plethora of health manuals and pamphlets, many written by prominent physicians, became widely available. This literature was targeted at city and country laity, many of them engaged in dangerous self-dosing from a variety of patented medicines. Composed in the vernacular, such publications embodied the contemporary ideals of human progress and popular education. Medical practitioners believed that sharing their new knowledge would indeed, as William Buchan (1729–1805) wrote, 'guard against the destructive influences of ignorance, superstition and quackery'.[45] Some of the authors wrote explicitly for rural populations, which presumably needed further enlightenment in health matters. Issues of diet, life-style, and health maintenance were just as important as remedies. Presumably, readers of these medical books, such as aristocrats, and even the clergy, would generously share the new medical advice with their servants and workers. Ministers and priests continued to participate in medicalized folk-healing schemes, a fact attested to by *Primitive Physick*, a widely circulated health manual by the Methodist John Wesley (1703–91).[46]

THE NINETEENTH CENTURY

A first step in the evolution towards medical supremacy came in post-revolutionary France with the rise of the Paris Medical School. At first, shortly after the Revolution, matters seemed unfavourable for medical professionals. Deprived of a privileged monopoly while their authority as experts was disparaged, physicians witnessed the brief rise of an ideology that emphasized citizens' self-government in health matters, individual autonomy, and domestic healing. Subsequently, however, a new plan for the promotion of 'the people's health' emerged, which sought to include professionals into a national policy of medical care. The new basis for this healing schema was the formal unification of medicine and surgery, a merger of momentous consequences. A second tier of less-trained medical practitioners, the *officiers de santé*, were to work in the countryside. Moreover, medicine was to be practised primarily in hospitals for the benefit of those who could not afford payments for individualized care. In view of dramatic urban population increases, Parisian hospitals became the workshops of a clinically oriented medicine that made great strides in the understanding of human disease.[47]

Systematic autopsies carried out on thousands of deceased French hospital patients allowed physicians to make further discoveries concerning the ravages that disease had wrought on individual organs and bodily systems. Through the use of physical methods of diagnosis, especially percussion and auscultation, numerous new clinical–pathological correlations were established. Such clincial knowledge and skills, obtained under conditions unavailable to lay people, allowed medical professionals to gain control over their relationship with the sick. Until this time, they had relied almost entirely on their patients' selective accounts to reach a verdict. Now, seasoned through the clinical and pathological examinations of indigent hospital patients, practitioners achieved new authority and status.[48]

Another tool, the 'numerical method', prompted comparisons between clinical findings and therapeutic outcome with the hope that medical understanding eventually could be improved through the employment of statistics. Initially, this approach generated fierce debate and faced rejection since it threatened the supremacy of knowledge culled from the individual clinical cases that were traditionally defended by most physicians. Despite such reservations, a new era in clinical investigation was launched. Some of the intuitive, impressionistic quality of medical practice, a customary symbol of professional healing subsumed under the term 'art of medicine', was overshadowed by novel methods of quantitative evaluation. The result was a gradual recognition that many articles of the traditional materia medica, as well as time-honoured practices such as bloodletting and blistering, were harmful to patients. Also eventually discredited was the heroic or aggressive therapeutic approach especially popular in America, featuring high doses of remedies and vigorous depleting practices aimed at impressing the sick through the achievement of palpable physiological changes.[49]

By mid-century, conventional forms of therapy such as bleeding and purging were discarded by sceptical practitioners, creating a significant void. That they had survived since classical antiquity pointed to the essential conservatism inherent in all healing activities, domestic and professional. Further assessment of remedies belonging to the traditional materia medica revealed that many agents were ineffective. In the past, substantive changes in medical treatment had always been potentially threatening to professional image and legitimacy. However, faced with scientific views of human functioning in health and disease, many physicians now sought to discover new drugs which could be experimentally proven to have specific pharmacological effects and therapeutic value.[50]

Cultural expectations based on humoralism and bodily constitution persisted, as did notions regarding the healing powers of the human body. Rejection of traditional medical practices shifted public support toward therapeutic strategies proposed by varieties of unlicensed practitioners and organized folk-healing practices, especially in America. Faced with a crucial gap in medical care, a series of sects emerged, eager to provide unorthodox alternatives to discredited professional schemes. Thomsonianism's herbal treatments, Grahamism's vegetarianism, and Priessnitz's hydropathy became therapeutic approaches attracting numerous followers, including members of the regular medical profession. Another domestic and folk tradition focusing on manipulative techniques and bone-setting eventually crystallized into two more systematic healing schemes: osteopathy, initially a drugless system of care featuring spinal manipulation, and its offspring, chiropractic, which went on to elaborate a concept of spinal displacement as the universal cause of disease.[51] (➤ Ch. 28 Unorthodox medical theories)

Europe, in turn, witnessed the birth of another healing scheme, homoeopathy, which had splintered from orthodox practices. Established in Germany during the late eighteenth century, this movement was originally designed as a therapeutic alternative to the depleting methods of the 'regulars', while later it promised to counteract the growing therapeutic scepticism exhibited by the hospital-based orthodoxy. Homoeopathic care was based on the principle of *similia similibus*, a postulated similarity between the actions of specific diseases and drugs that led to cancellation of the former and resulted in cures. At first, traditional remedies were progressively diluted to avoid iatrogenic effects, and ultimately prescribed in infinitesimal dosages. From its very inception, homoeopathy's growing popularity resided in its ability to pledge a holistic, individualized, and at least not harmful approach to healing, in stark contrast to contemporary depletions and the depersonalized care attributed to the professional mainstream.[52]

Early nineteenth-century attempts in German lands to establish a science of medicine using Kantian principles foundered, given the elementary state of the sciences considered basic for an understanding of the phenomena of health and disease in humans. By the 1830s, however, reliance on the theories, methods, and technologies of science finally began to bear fruit. A decentralized and competitive German university system steeped in research ideals fuelled a broad range of studies in the biological sciences. Initial discoveries in microscopic anatomy and embryology, physiology, chemistry, and pathology led to important advances in the knowledge of cellular structures, nerve electrophysiology, and the optics of human vision. As scientific research became an attractive career goal for medical professionals, especially in Germany, France, and Britain, it quickly provided a much more detailed understanding of bodily processes. After the 1860s, with the advent of microbiology, a new and invisible world of pathogenic agents was progressively revealed to researchers, physicians, and the public at large, opening up further possibilities for the control of disease.[53] (➤ Ch. 6 The microscopical tradition; Ch. 11 Clinical research; Ch. 16 Contagion/germ theory/specificity)

Thus, in a single generation, European medicine between 1840 and 1880 dramatically revised and expanded its knowledge base, providing practitioners with unprecedented precision in defining and explaining sickness. Physicians adopted comprehensive, scientific models of human physiology and pathology based on results obtained in countless experiments designed according to the methods of Claude Bernard (1813–78). 'Scientific medicine,' he wrote, 'like the other sciences, can be established only by experimental means, i.e. by direct and vigorous application of reasoning to the facts furnished us by observation and experiments.'[54] Later in the century, new diagnostic procedures came to rely on biochemical analyses and microscopic evaluations. (➤ Ch. 8 The biochemical tradition) The question was whether this more sophisticated scientific understanding of health and disease could be applied at the bedside, and whether such insights translated into better medical care.

The new scientific healing emphasized objectivity in the collection of data, largely dispensing with the patient's narrative in favour of specific measurements of biological activity. A new emphasis on empiricism established different criteria for therapeutic efficacy. The use of previously heralded panaceas (specifics) became a mark of ignorance, even quackery. Rejecting such cures, progressive medical circles adopted a marked therapeutic scepticism, even a nihilism, that witnessed the use of a few purified drugs with known pharmacological properties and a return to the healing power of nature. 'Medicine is after facts, it does not matter who is at the bedside, the sick person has become a thing', commented one German physician in 1870.[55] Patients were now viewed as disease material, objects for experimentation to further the gathering of new knowledge. In discarding its long-valued cures, medicine lost some of its most cherished symbols.

For several decades, therefore, 'scientific' practitioners were forced to rely mostly on the therapeutic qualities of their diagnostics and explanatory models, competing for patients loyal to entrenched folk-healing systems such as homoeopathy and 'natural therapy'.[56] Yet, even in the face of mounting costs and limited therapy, an increasingly better-educated public demanded medical services. This was mainly due to the activities of surgeons, who now achieved strikingly better results with their complex interventions employing anaesthesia as well as antiseptic and later aseptic methods. (➤ Ch. 42 Surgery (modern)) Before the end of the century, however, the first practical fruits of scientific medicine such as protective vaccines and effective sera emerged from the laboratories.[57]

Long before such impressive achievements, small groups of skilled workers, in a practice dating back to the sixteenth century, negotiated insurance coverage that included medical care. These plans were adopted on a larger scale to meet the needs of industrial workers, resulting in the establishment of compulsory insurance against sickness, first in Germany, and then in other parts of Europe. These state-sponsored programmes, such as the early German 'Krankenkassen', provided financial protection in the event of illness and for the payment of medical services.[58]

THE TWENTIETH CENTURY

In recent times, medicine has gained tremendous power and prestige through its increased ability to intervene directly in disease processes, often reversing them, and sometimes effecting cures. New generations of physicians have adopted scientific rationality and methodology to justify and carry out their healing tasks. Belief in the mind/body dualism, an ontological view of disease, as well as an emphasis on objective, numerical measurements and probabilistic reasoning, characterize what is now known as 'scientific' medicine. Aseptic surgery, chemotherapy, endocrinology, and scientific nutrition quickly dispelled previous notions of therapeutic impotence. This new spirit of confidence is reflected in the words of a prominent American scientist, Lawrence J. Henderson (1878–1942), who has been credited with the statement that in the early 1900s 'a random patient with a random disease, consulting a doctor chosen at random had, for the first time in the history of mankind, a better than fifty-fifty chance of profiting from the encounter.'[59]

The revolution in therapeutics accelerated after the Second World War with the advent of antibiotics and a new generation of synthetic drugs; their discovery was hailed as the greatest achievement in the history of medicine. These spectacular developments occurred in concert with advances in chemistry and pharmacology that produced a host of very effective agents for the treatment of many life-threatening diseases, thus decisively enhancing the prominence of biomedicine at the expense of other healing schemes. For the first time, physicians were able to arrest the natural history of most infectious diseases instead of helplessly witnessing or even actively hastening their course. Armed with a number of therapeutic options, practitioners could cure. The prognostic implications of such scientifically based healing were momentous.[60]

Tensions between the impersonality of universal medical science and the sick person's desire for emotional support and understanding in medical care were exacerbated. Professionals considered scientific competence more important than establishing a relationship with their patients. In fact, getting involved with the emotions of those seeking care was usually discouraged as an approach that was associated with sectarians and quacks. The physician's detached stance was the proper badge of scientific objectivity. By the 1930s, however, voices were heard in the medical profession contending that the science and art of medicine were complementary, not antagonistic. 'One of the essential qualities of the clinician is interest in humanity, for the secret of the care of the patient is in caring for the patient', wrote one medical authority.[61]

A key locus of medical care experienced a dramatic transformation: the hospital. From an institution exclusively devoted to the care of the poor, it gradually became an establishment where new diagnostic techniques and treatments could be provided to all classes of society. The success of that transformation can be seen, especially after 1900, in the explosive growth of hospitals in Europe and America. The 'new' hospital also provided an identity to scores of medical professionals training and working in it. Hospital affiliation became a hallmark of professional identity and status. An alliance between research, teaching, and delivery of care made hospital practice the very centre of professional medicine.[62]

While the concept of localized pathology had laid the groundwork for medical specialization in the preceding century, scientific advances and technological development now provided the decisive impetus. Medicine divided its labour and reorganized healing around particular areas of interest as its members struggled among themselves to control the market-place. The process brought new status, prestige, and income to the specialists, many of whom worked within institutional settings such as hospitals and clinics.[63]

In economically advanced countries without state-sponsored medical care plans such as America, professional healing remained a desirable commodity in the market-place, selected by choice or ability to pay. Physicians functioned as small entrepreneurs, and their practices were conducted like businesses. Yet, by the early 1900s, the ideologies of individualism and unfettered capitalism flagged, allowing for the establishment of more collectivist principles that sought to advance the public good. A social insurance movement began to provide medical-care coverage to workers of all classes and occupations. As the effectiveness of scientific medicine in developed countries reached new heights in the 1950s and 1960s, a new ideological framework emerged that argued for a right to health care guaranteed by the state. The result has been the creation of numerous national and local schemes that provide medical care to citizens.[64] (➤ Ch. 57 Health economics)

Driven by the industrial efficiency model, hospitals since the turn of the century have become repositories of the most advanced and prestigious medical technology. After the Second World War, hospital development accelerated in most developed and affluent countries, spurred by growing demands for more medical services. Since the early 1950s, additions such as neonatology and intensive-care units, cardiology and cardiac-catheterization laboratories, as well as transplantation services, have increased the range and complexity of care in such institutions. Staffed by specialists and equipped with sophisticated but expensive technology, hospitals have become formidable bureaucracies requiring resources to support ever greater numbers of staff and administrative personnel. These developments have had far-reaching effects by allowing state-of-the-art medical care to be provided to a broad spectrum of the eligible public under the various private and state-sponsored health plans. However, while highly beneficial in dealing with the physical effects of acute illness, most hospital routines continue to be detrimental to the rapport between physicians and their patients, a relationship already compromised by the impersonality of scientific medicine.[65] (➤ Ch. 36 The science of diagnosis: diagnostic technology; Ch. 68 Medical technologies: social contexts and consequences)

As in other fields of human endeavour, the technological fix in the health-care sector has been a particularly American addiction, one that has rapidly spread to other countries. 'Good' medicine is increasingly defined according to technical criteria that find their expression in charts, peer reviews, and insurance audits. In many parts of the world, hospitals compete fiercely to be the first in a given geographical area to obtain new and more-sophisticated medical equipment. As a result of changes in treatment, fragmentation in the medical market-place, and an economy of increasingly scarce resources, this premier but expensive medical institution is now under attack, in part a victim of its own success. Many American hospitals are now closing their doors, unable to survive in a competitive economic environment that is forcing a major restructuring of the entire delivery scheme. In countries with a national health-care system, decrepit physical plants and technological obsolescence compromise hospital treatment.[66]

In most regions of the world, the rapidly escalating cost of medical care has profound implications for the future.[67] Decisions often must be made on the basis of available economic resources rather than on medical need alone. Ethical and legal issues complicate therapeutic plans, and rationing care is now a fact of life. (➤ Ch. 37 History of medical ethics; Ch. 69 Medicine and the law) Because of differing objectives and priorities, health professionals are increasingly at odds with institutional managers and health planners. In corporate or governmental contexts, the power and professional status of salaried physicians is eroding, and their medical decisions are often overruled. As medical practice shifts from hospitals to ambulatory settings, even the venerable hospital becomes an 'endangered species'.[68]

Today, the biomedical establishment faces issues of medical-care availability, quantity, quality, and distribution. No other healing scheme in the domestic or folklore sector holds such a prominent position. Yet, both the status and income of medical practitioners is in danger. The needs of an ageing population in the developed countries of the world suggest a new structure of long-term care different from current complex and costly models. (➤ Ch. 46 Geriatrics) Historically, traditional indexes of the public's health such as mortality and morbidity rates have been used to define patterns of acute ill health. But should they be viewed as consequences of insufficient medical care? Must such demographic characteristics continue to determine a population's allotment of medical care?[69] (➤ Ch. 71 Demography and medicine; Ch. 72 Medicine, mortality, and morbidity)

If not, then future research must focus on the social, psychological, cultural, economic, and political factors that inhibit and facilitate access to and delivery of all types of medical care to individuals and communities. This must include contemporary domestic-healing networks as well as surviving fragments of folk medicine, especially in Third World countries with limited resources. With the application of systems theory to illness, concepts of causality are being broadened to include an array of forces located both within the human organism and the external environment. Social and psychological factors link up with biological elements, placing medical care within a much broader scaffolding. In the end, we face a paradoxical situation illustrated by recent reform movements such as 'holistic' or 'humanistic' medicine. These particular approaches seek to restore the focus of medical care, to encompass again the whole person within the social environment, and to transcend the conventional body/mind duality with its narrow scientific focus on localized dysfunction and pathology. At the centre of this broadened vision are notions of balance and harmony that hark back to traditional frameworks of explanation.[70]

Given the enormous cost of technically assisted care, many contemporary planners are promoting medically supervised domestic-healing practices, now termed by some the 'pre-primary health-care system', with medicine acting as the legitimate back-up alternative. Modern studies have demonstrated that as much as 90 per cent of basic care is still provided within the popular sector. Conversely, in an effort to decrease costs, reformers are now determined to shift the locus of medical care from the expensive hospital back to the home, to community health centres, and to outpatient clinics. Such care options will be placed in the hands of the consumers themselves, who will work with physicians and health-system managers to focus on health maintenance in addition to disease treatment. Practitioners and patients, in turn, are encouraged to forge more egalitarian relationships and establish a spectrum of co-operative interactions not unlike those hitherto employed in traditional domestic and folk-healing strategies.[71]

Today's modern medical care is centring the whole ill person within a societal context, while vigorously supporting self-care efforts. Modern goals aim to provide personal health information and training programmes for patients, intending to make them fully fledged partners in the healing enterprise. Indeed, in developed countries, 'patient power' is on the ascent, with Aesculapian supremacy eroding within anti-authoritarian cultural climates. In one formulation, medical care is now considered the authority of last, not first, resort to be consulted when the domestic system fails.

CONCLUSION

In the end, our historical tour of medical care can be said to have come full circle. From almost complete reliance on domestic healing practices in preliterate societies, social developments supported the gradual differentiation of folk-healing roles, especially the appearance of shamans and priests. The medical role was increasingly professionalized in early civilizations down to classical antiquity and the Middle Ages in Europe. Further evolution in more modern times eventually culminated in the establishment of a transcultural, scientifically informed type of medical care characterized by precise diagnostics, effective therapeutics, and enhanced prognostics that has also led to the empowerment of sub-specialist practitioners. While monopolistic in intent, the ascent of professionalism never implied the end of medical pluralism; the expansion of scientific medicine since the late nineteenth century has not replaced activities carried out in other healing spheres. Demographic, political, and above all economic forces now compel us to reconsider a familiar process in the delivery of medical care. Amply informed by the tenets of biomedicine, many curing efforts may, once again, be performed by the sick themselves. (➤ Ch. 70 Medical sociology)

NOTES

1 Cecil G. Helman, *Culture, Health and Illness*, 2nd edn, London, Wright, 1990; Corinne Shear Wood, *Human Sickness and Health: a Biocultural View*, Palo Alto, CA, Mayfield, 1979; Robert A. Hahn and D. Gaines Atwood (eds), *Physicians of Western Medicine: Anthropological Approaches to Theory and Practice*, Dordrecht, D. Reidel, 1985.

2 Peter Wright and Andrew Treacher (eds), *The Problem of Medical Knowledge. Examining the Social Construction of Medicine*, Edinburgh, Edinburgh University Press, 1982; T. J. Trenn, 'Ludwig Fleck's "On the question of the foundations of medical knowledge"', *Journal of Medicine and Philosophy*, 1981, 6: 237–56; C. Rosenberg, 'Woods or trees? Ideas and actors in the history of science', *Isis*, 1988, 79: 565–70.

3 Morris J. Vogel and Charles E. Rosenberg (eds), *The Therapeutic Revolution. Essays in the Social History of American Medicine*, Philadelphia, University of Pennsylvania Press, 1979; W. E. Mitchell, 'Changing others: the anthropological study of therapeutic systems', *Man*, 1977, 8: 15–20; G. B. Risse, 'The history of therapeutics', *Clio Medica*, 1991, 22: 3–11.

4 Howard Brody, *Placebos and the Philosophy of Medicine*, Chicago, IL, University of Chicago Press, 1980; Brody, *Stories of Sickness*, New Haven, CT, Yale University Press, 1988; Arthur Kleinman, *The Illness Narratives: Suffering, Healing, and the Human Condition*, New York, Basic Books, 1988; Byron Good and Mary-Jo Del Vecchio Good, 'The semantics of medical discourse', in E. Mendelsohn and Y. Elkana (eds), *Sciences and Cultures: Anthropological and Historical Studies of the Sciences*, Dordrecht, D. Reidel, 1981, pp. 177–212.

5 C. Leslie, 'Introduction'; A. Kleinman, 'Medical systems as cultural systems'; R. H. Elling, 'Medical systems as changing systems'; and J. M. Janzen, 'The comparative study of medical systems as changing social systems': all published in a special issue, 'Theoretical foundations for the comparative study of medical systems', *Social Science and Medicine*, 1978, 12B: 65–7, 85–93, 107–15, 121–9.

6 C. C. Hughes, 'Medical care: ethnomedicine', in M. H. Logan and E. E. Hunt Jr (eds), *Health and the Human Condition: Perspectives on Medical Anthropology*, North Scituate, MA, Duxbury Press, 1978, pp. 150–8; Arthur Kleinman, *Patients and Healers in the Context of Culture*, Berkeley, University of California Press, 1980: Wilbur H. Watson (ed.), *Black Folk Medicine: the Therapeutic Significance of Faith and Trust*, New Brunswick, NJ, Transaction Books, 1984.

7 Mircea Eliade, *Shamanism, Archaic Techniques of Ecstasy*, trans. by W. R. Trask, Princeton, NJ, Princeton University Press, 1964; Horacio Fabrega Jr and D. B. Silver, *Illness and Shamanistic Curing in Zinacantan: an Ethnomedical Analysis*, Stanford, CA, Stanford University Press, 1973; the Kwakiutl text 'I desired to learn the ways of the shaman', in Franz Boas (ed.), *The Religion of the Kwakiutl Indians*, part II, New York, Columbia University Press, 1930, pp. 1–41.

8 E. K. Ritter, 'Magical expert (asipu) and physician (asu). Notes on two complementary professions in Babylonian medicine', *Assyriological Studies*, 1965, 16: 299–321; G. B. Risse, 'Imhotep and medicine: a reevaluation', *Western Journal of Medicine*, 1986, 144: 622–4; J. Worth Estes, 'Egyptian healers', *The Medical Skills of Ancient Egypt*, Canton, MA, Science History Publications, 1989, pp. 13–26; A. L. Basham, 'The practice of medicine in ancient and medieval India', in C. Leslie (ed.), *Asian Medical Systems*, Berkeley, CA, University of California Press, 1977, pp. 18–43; Paul U. Unschuld, *Medicine in China: a History of Ideas*, Berkeley, CA, University of California Press, 1985.

9 'The Oath', in G. E. R. Lloyd (ed.), *Hippocratic Writings*, trans. by J. Chadwick, Harmondsworth, Penguin Books, 1978, p. 67.

10 L. Edelstein, 'The Hippocratic physician', in O. Temkin and C. L. Temkin (eds), *Ancient Medicine*, Baltimore, MD, Johns Hopkins University Press, 1967, pp. 87–110; I. M. Lonie, 'A structural pattern in Greek dietetics and the early history of Greek medicine', *Medical History*, 1977, 21: 235–60.

11 Ludwig Edelstein and Emma J. Edelstein, *Asclepius*, 2 vols, Baltimore, MD, Johns Hopkins University Press, 1945; Ralph Jackson, *Doctors and Diseases in the Roman Empire*, Norman, OK, and London, University of Oklahoma Press, 1988, ch. 6, pp. 139–69.

12 L. Edelstein, 'Empiricism and skepticism in the teaching of the Greek Empiricist School', in Temkin and Temkin, op. cit. (n. 10), pp. 195–203; Heinrich von Staden (ed. and trans.), *Herophilus: the Art of Medicine in Early Alexandria*, Cambridge and New York, Cambridge University Press, 1989: V. Nutton, 'Museums and medical schools in classical antiquity', *History of Education*, 1975, 4: 3–15.

13 J. H. Phillips, 'The emergence of the Greek medical profession in the Roman Republic', *Transactions and Studies of the College of Physicians of Philadelphia*, 1980, 2: 267–75.

14 A. Z. Iskandar, 'Galen and Rhazes on examining physicians', *Bulletin of the History of Medicine*, 1962, 36: 365.

15 R. W. Davies, 'The Roman military service', in D. Breeze, and V. A. Maxfield

(eds), *Service in the Roman Army*, Edinburgh, Edinburgh University Press, 1989, pp. 208–36.

16 D. W. Amundsen and G. B. Ferngren, 'The early Christian tradition', in R. L. Numbers and D. W. Amundsen (eds), *Caring and Curing. Health and Medicine in the Western Medical Traditions*, New York, Macmillan, 1986, pp. 40–64.

17 'The rule of St Benedict', in M. B. Strauss (ed.), *Familiar Medical Quotations*, Boston, MA, Little Brown, 1968, ch. 36, p. 372.

18 R. Greer, 'Hospitality in the first five centuries of the church', *Medieval Studies*, 1974, 10: 29–48.

19 T. S. Miller, 'Byzantine hospitals', in J. Scarborough (ed.), *Symposium on Byzantine Medicine*, Washington, DC, Dumbarton Oaks Library, 1983, pp. 53–63.

20 M. W. Dols, 'The origins of the Islamic hospital: myth and reality', *Bulletin of the History of Medicine*, 1987, 61: 367–90.

21 B. Rowland (trans.), *The Medieval Women's Guide to Health*, Kent, OH, Kent State University Press, 1981: J. Stannard, 'Medicinal herbals and their development', *Clio Medica*, 1974, 9: 23–33; M. Green, 'Women's medical practice and health care in medieval Europe', *Signs*, 1989, 14: 434–73.

22 T. S. Miller, 'The Knights of Saint John and the hospitals of the Latin West', *Speculum*, 1978, 53: 709–33.

23 J. H. Mundy, 'Hospitals and leprosaries in twelfth- and thirteenth-century Toulouse', in J. M. Mundy and R. W. Emery (eds), *Essays on Medieval Life and Thought Presented in Honor of Austin P. Evans*, New York, Columbia University Press, 1955, pp. 181–205.

24 Vern L. Bullough, *The Development of Medicine as a Profession*, Basle, Karger, 1966; Nancy G. Siraisi, *Medieval and Early Renaissance Medicine*, Chicago, IL, University of Chicago Press, 1990.

25 See, for example, Noel and Jose Parry, *The Rise of the Medical Profession: a Study of Collective Social Mobility*, London, Croom Helm, 1976; Andrew Abbott, *The System of Professions: an Essay on the Division of Expert Labor*, Chicago, IL, University of Chicago Press, 1988.

26 J. M. Riddle, 'Theory and practice in medieval medicine', *Viator*, 1974, 5: 157–84; Marie-Christine Pouchelle, *The Body and Surgery in the Middle Ages*, trans. by R. Morris, Cambridge, Polity Press, 1990.

27 Carlo M. Cipolla, *Public Health and the Medical Profession in the Renaissance*, Cambridge, Cambridge University Press, 1976.

28 R. Palmer, 'Physicians and the state in post-medieval Italy', in A. W. Russell (ed.), *The Town and State Physician in Europe from the Middle Ages to the Enlightenment*, Wolfenbüttel, Herzog August Bibliothek, 1981, pp. 47–61; Katharine Park, *Doctors and Medicine in Early Renaissance Florence*, Princeton, NJ, Princeton University Press, 1985.

29 J. J. Bylebyl, 'The school of Padua: humanistic medicine in the sixteenth century', in C. Webster (ed.), *Health, Medicine, and Mortality in the Sixteenth Century*, Cambridge, Cambridge University Press, 1979, pp. 335–70.

30 Paracelsus, 'Seven defensiones. The reply to certain calumniations of his enemies', trans. by C. L. Temkin, in *Four Treatises of Theophrastus von Hohenheim Called Paracelsus*, Baltimore, MD, Johns Hopkins University Press, 1941, p. 16.

31 Lester S. King, *The Growth of Medical Thought*, Chicago, IL, University of Chicago Press, 1963, ch. 3, pp. 86–138.

32 J. F. Malgaigne, *Surgery and Ambroise Paré*, trans. by W. B. Hamby, Norman, University of Oklahoma Press, 1965; M. Pelling, 'Appearance and reality: barber-surgeons, the body, and disease', in L. Beier and R. Finlay (eds), *London, 1500–1700: the Making of the Metropolis*, London, Longman, 1986, pp. 82–112; A. Wear, R. K. French and I. M. Lonie (eds), *The Medical Renaissance of the Sixteenth Century*, Cambridge, Cambridge University Press, 1985.

33 Charles Webster, *The Great Instauration: Science, Medicine, and Reform, 1626–1660*, London, Duckworth, 1975.

34 R. C. Sawyer, 'Strangely handled in all her lyms: witchcraft and healing in Jacobean England', *Journal of Social History*, 1989, 22: 461–85; Keith Thomas, *Religion and the Decline of Magic*, New York, Scribner's, 1971.

35 R. French and A. Wear (eds), *The Medical Revolution of the Seventeenth Century*, Cambridge, Cambridge University Press, 1989.

36 Thomas Sydenham, 'Medical observations concerning the history and cure of acute diseases' (1676), in *The Works of Thomas Sydenham, M.D.*, trans. by R. G. Latham, 2 vols, London, Sydenham Society, 1848, Vol. 1, p. 11.

37 J. G. L. Burnby, *A Study of the English Apothecary from 1660 to 1760*, London, Wellcome Institute for the History of Medicine, 1983.

38 G. B. Risse, 'Medicine in the age of enlightenment', in A. Wear (ed.), *Medicine in Society: Historical Essays*, Cambridge, Cambridge University Press, 1991, pp. 149–72.

39 Arnulfe d'Aumont, 'Santé', in D. Diderot (ed.), *Encyclopédie ou dictionnaire raisonné des sciences, des arts et des métiers*, Paris, 1751–65, Vol. XIV, p. 630 (quotation trans. by G. B. Risse); Matthew Ramsey, *Professional and Popular Medicine in France, 1770–1830: the Social World of Medical Practice*, Cambridge, Cambridge University Press, 1988.

40 A. Cunningham and R. French (eds), *The Medical Enlightenment of the Eighteenth Century*, Cambridge, Cambridge University Press, 1990.

41 George Rosen, *From Medical Police to Social Medicine*, New York, Science History Publications, 1974.

42 Dorothy and Roy Porter, *Patient's Progress: Doctors and Doctoring in Eighteenth-Century England*, Cambridge, Polity Press, 1989.

43 Irvine Loudon, *Medical Care and the General Practitioner, 1750–1850*, Oxford, Clarendon Press, 1986; W. F. Bynum and R. Porter (eds), *William Hunter and the Eighteenth-Century Medical World*, Cambridge, Cambridge University Press, 1985; Bynum and Porter (eds), *Medical Fringe and Medical Orthodoxy, 1750–1850*, London, Croom Helm, 1987; Roy Porter, *Health for Sale, Quackery in England, 1660–1850*, Manchester, Manchester University Press, 1989.

44 Michel Foucault, *The Birth of the Clinic, an Archeology of Medical Perception*, trans. by A. M. S. Smith, New York, Vintage Books, 1975; Guenter B. Risse, *Hospital Life in Enlightenment Scotland, Care and Teaching at the Royal Infirmary of Edinburgh*, Cambridge, Cambridge University Press, 1986; Toby Gelfand, *Professionalizing Modern Medicine*, Westport, CT, Greenwood Press, 1980.

45 William Buchan, *Domestic Medicine*, 14th edn, Philadelphia, 1795; C. J. Lawrence, 'William Buchan: medicine laid open', *Medical History*, 1975, 19: 20–35.

46 R. Porter (ed.), *Patients and Practitioners. Lay Perceptions of Medicine in Pre-industrial Society*, Cambridge, Cambridge University Press, 1985; S. J. Rogul, 'Pills for the poor: John Wesley's "Primitive Physick" ', *Yale Journal of Biology and Medicine*, 1978, 51: 81–90.

47 Foucault, op. cit. (n. 44); Erwin H. Ackerknecht, *Medicine at the Paris Hospital, 1794–1848*, Baltimore, MD, Johns Hopkins University Press, 1967.

48 Russell C. Maulitz, *Morbid Appearances, the Anatomy of Pathology in the Early Nineteenth Century*, Cambridge, Cambridge University Press, 1987; G. B. Risse, 'A shift in medical epistemology: clinical diagnosis, 1770–1828', *Proceedings of the 9th Symposium on the History of Medicine (East and West)*, Osaka, Japan, Tanaguchi Foundation, 1987, pp. 115–47.

49 T. D. Murphy, 'Medical knowledge and statistical methods in early nineteenth-century France', *Medical History*, 1981, 25: 301–19.

50 John H. Warner, *The Therapeutic Perspective: Medical Practice, Knowledge, and Identity in America, 1820–1885*, Cambridge, MA, Harvard University Press, 1986.

51 William G. Rothstein, *American Physicians in the Nineteenth Century*, Baltimore, MD, Johns Hopkins University Press, 1972; N. Gevitz (ed.), *Other Healers: Unorthodox Medicine in America*, Baltimore, MD, Johns Hopkins University Press, 1988.

52 R. Cooter (ed.), *Studies in the History of Alternative Medicine*, New York, St Martin's Press, 1988; Martin Kaufman, *Homeopathy in America; the Rise and Fall of a Medical Heresy*, Baltimore, MD, Johns Hopkins University Press, 1971.

53 W. Coleman and F. L. Holmes (eds), *The Investigative Enterprise, Experimental Physiology in Nineteenth-Century Medicine*, Berkeley, University of California Press, 1988; Bruno Latour, *The Pasteurization of France*, trans. by A. Sheridan and J. Law, Cambridge, MA, Harvard University Press, 1988.

54 Claude Bernard, *An Introduction to the Study of Experimental Medicine*, ed. H. C. Green, New York, Dover Publications, 1957, p. 2; orig. pub. 1927.

55 Robert Volz, *Der aerztliche Beruf*, Berlin, Lüderitz, 1870, p. 32–3.

56 I. Waddington, 'Professionalization and the development of medical autonomy', *The Medical Profession in the Industrial Revolution*, Dublin, Gill & Macmillan and Humanities Press, 1984; C. Huerkamp, 'The making of the modern medical profession, 1800–1914: Prussian doctors in the nineteenth century', in G. Cocks and K. H. Jarausch (eds), *German Professions, 1800–1950*, New York, Oxford University Press, 1990, pp. 66–84.

57 M. Vogel and C. Rosenberg (eds), *The Therapeutic Revolution*, Philadelphia, University of Pennsylvania Press, 1979; Owen H. Wangensteen and Sarah D. Wangensteen, *The Rise of Surgery: From Empiric Craft to Scientific Discipline*, Folkestone, Dawsons, 1978.

58 Gertrud Kroeger, *The Concept of Social Medicine as Presented by Physicians and Other Writers in Germany, 1779–1932*, Chicago, IL, Julius Rosenwald Fund, 1937; L. Machtan, 'Workers' insurance versus protection of the workers: state social policy in Imperial Germany', in P. Weindling (ed.), *The Social History of Occupational Health*, London, Croom Helm, 1985, pp. 209–22.

59 H. L. Blumgart, 'Caring for the patient', *New England Journal of Medicine*, 1964, 270: 449–56.

60 Jonathan Liebenau, *Medical Science and Medical Industry: the Formation of the*

American Pharmaceutical Industry, Baltimore, MD, Johns Hopkins University Press, 1987; Odin W. Anderson, *Health Services in the United States: a Growth Enterprise since 1875*, Ann Arbor, Michigan Health Administration Press, 1985.

61 F. W. Peabody, 'The care of the patient', *Journal of the American Medical Association*, 1927, 88: 882.

62 Charles E. Rosenberg, *The Care of Strangers*. The Rise of America's Hospital System, New York, Basic Books, 1987.

63 George Rosen, *The Structure of American Medical Practice, 1875–1941*, ed. C. Rosenberg, Philadelphia, University of Pennsylvania Press, 1983; Bradford H. Gray (ed.), *The New Health Care for Profit*, Washington, DC, National Academy Press, 1983.

64 R. L. Numbers (ed.), *Compulsory Health Insurance, the Continuing American Debate*, Westport, CT, Greenwood Press, 1982; A. Digby and N. Bosanquet, 'Doctors and patients in an era of national health insurance and private practice, 1913–1938', *Economic History Review*, 1988, 41: 74–94; Charles Webster, *Problems in Health Care: the National Health Service before 1957*, London, HMSO, 1988.

65 Eliot Friedson (ed.), *The Hospital in Modern Society*, New York, Free Press, 1963: Geoffrey Rivett, *The Development of the London Hospital System 1823–1982*, London, King Edward's Hospital Fund, 1986.

66 Louise Russell, *Technology in Hospitals: Medical Advances and their Diffusion*, Washington, DC, Brookings Institute, 1979; Rosemary Stevens, *In Sickness and in Wealth: American Hospitals in the Twentieth Century*, New York, Basic Books, 1989.

67 Rashi Fein, *Medical Care, Medical Costs, the Search for a Health Insurance Policy*, Cambridge, MA, Harvard University Press, 1986.

68 Everett A. Johnson and Richard L. Johnson, *Hospitals under Fire: Strategies for Survival*, Rockville, MD, Aspen Publishers, 1986.

69 J. R. Hollingsworth, *A Political Economy for Medicine: Great Britain and the United States*, Baltimore, MD, Johns Hopkins University Press, 1986; David Mechanic, *From Advocacy to Allocation: the Evolving American Health Care System*, New York, Free Press, 1986.

70 June A. English-Lueck, *Health in the New Age: a Study of California Holistic Practices*, Albuquerque, University of New Mexico Press, 1990; M. W. de Vries, R. L. Berg and M. Lipkin Jr (eds), *The Use and Abuse of Medicine*, New York, Praeger, 1982.

71 Paul Starr, *The Social Transformation of American Medicine*, New York, Basic Books, 1982; Eli Ginzberg (ed.), *From Physician Shortage to Patient Shortage, the Uncertain Future of Medical Practice*, Boulder, CO, and London, Westview Press, 1986.

FURTHER READING

Jackson, Ralph, *Doctors and Diseases in the Roman Empire*, Norman, OK, and London, University of Oklahoma Press, 1988.

Leslie, Charles (ed.), *Asian Medical Systems*, Berkeley, University of California Press, 1977.

Mechanic, David, *From Advocacy to Allocation: the Evolving American Health Care System*, New York, Free Press, 1986.

Porter, Roy (ed.), *Patients and Practitioners: Lay Perceptions of Medicine in Pre-industrial Society*, Cambridge, Cambridge University Press, 1985.

Ramsey, Matthew, *Professional and Popular Medicine in France, 1770–1830: the Social World of Medical Practice*, Cambridge, Cambridge University Press, 1988.

Reiser, Stanley J., *Medicine and the Reign of Technology*, Cambridge, Cambridge University Press, 1978.

Rosenberg, Charles E. *The Care of Strangers. The Rise of America's Hospital System*, New York, Basic Books, 1987.

Schipperges, Heinrich, Seidler, Eduard and Unschuld, Paul U. (eds), *Krankheit, Heilkunst, Heilung*, Munich, Karl Alber, 1978.

PART II

BODY SYSTEMS

5

THE ANATOMICAL TRADITION

Roger French

THE ORIGINS OF HUMAN DISSECTION

Systematic dissection of the human body began in Bologna, in the *studium* of arts and medicine, where surgery was taught alongside internal medicine. There are possible antecedents for medical dissection in the needs of the law *studium* to discover the causes of death when considering the lethality of wounds, poisoning, stillbirth and related cases. Legal support for dissection would naturally have been forthcoming in such circumstances; and provided that clerics were not involved, the church raised no objections.

The first systematic dissector we know of was Mondino de'Luzzi (*c.*1275–1326), whose *Anathomia* seems to have been complete by 1316. There are a number of features of the situation that must be noted if we are to understand the magnitude of the change that was happening in Western medicine. The first is that anatomy had little part to play in medical education before this time. It had no place in the medieval medical textbook, the *Articella*. The anatomy of the *Canon* of Avicenna was fragmented throughout the author's systematic presentation of the medical theory of each part of the body. The commentators' treatment of this anatomy was not complete by Mondino's time. Anatomy was not included in the medical statutes, some sets of which expressly exclude it. Gentile da Foligno (d. 1348) thought anatomy was 'the alphabet of medicine', but in practice, followed the 'usual error' and produced no commentary on it.[1] Of the ancient medicine available at the time, the most authoritative was the Hippocratic, which was not anatomical. The medical school of Salerno, where for more than a century anatomy of a sort had been learned by dissecting pigs, did not progress to human dissection and was being eclipsed by the rise of the medical faculties in the *studia*.

So in adopting the practice of teaching anatomy by the cutting-up of dead human bodies, the Bolognese doctors were doing something very unusual. In no other culture was dissection systematically performed, nor was medicine anatomical. Of course, anatomy looks to us a natural part of medicine, and we might be tempted to see the appearance of dissection as part of the development of medical education appropriate to a time when surgeons were being educated with physicians in a university. But there still remain to be answered the questions: why there? and why then? Moreover, there are some strange things about dissections on the model of Mondino, which slowly spread across Europe. They were based on the 'three venters' of the body, the abdomen, thorax, and cranium, and the organs each contained. The containing membranes of these cavities, however, were precisely the boundaries beyond which the surgeon could not proceed in his operations on the living body. The limbs, where the surgeon could indeed operate, were characteristically omitted from Mondinian anatomies.

The organs of the three venters were in fact the domain of the physician, who gave internal medicines and drew symptoms from internal pains. The three venters were dissected in a sequence (abdomen, thorax, head) which avoided the worst effects of putrefaction, but which was also the 'philosophical' sequence of the three fundamental faculties of the body: nutritive, vital, and animal. In dissecting and discussing each organ in the cavities, the Mondinian anatomist followed a rote of observables that had been first suggested by John of Alexandria (*fl.* seventh century AD) in commenting on Galen's *De Sectis*. Observables like 'position', 'size', and 'shape' had more to do with the categories of Aristotle (384–322 BC) than with medicine or surgery, and it was not until long after John of Alexandria that a seventh, medical observable was added: the disease to which each part was liable. Finally, in discussing their reasons for performing dissections, Mondinian anatomists rarely put medical or surgical purposes higher than third on their list. Mondino's own reasons for writing were, 'First to satisfy friends; second for intellectual exercise; third to overcome the forgetfulness of age.'[2]

In other words, something more was happening than the simple improvement of anatomical knowledge in the development of surgery and medicine. In fact, the physicians were manipulating anatomy for their own professional purposes. This is an extension of the story of how medicine came to be rational, that is, based on chains of reasoning (rather than, for example, purely on experiential knowledge). This reasoning was ultimately that of Aristotle, and the first people in the West to use Aristotle's physical works were the Salernitans. They found that these books were useful in explaining the summaries of Greek medicine with which they were familiar (this was largely because Galen had used the same works of Aristotle in rationalizing the apothegmatic medicine of Hippocrates). From the Salernitans, the medical commentators of the thirteenth century developed a huge apparatus of natural philosophy to underpin medicine. Part of the reason for doing so was to justify a view that saw medicine as a true *scientia*, a system of knowledge capable of demonstrative truth and appropriate for the new universities. Their enemies saw medicine as a manual trade, and tried to exclude it from the universities as ignoble and 'lucrative'. However, with the help of the old authors, the new doctors not only ensured the place of their subject in the universities as a higher discipline, but claimed, mostly with success, a monopoly of the practice of internal medicine, backed by the legal claims of the faculty. Their argument here was that the rationality of their medicine made it better than that of those who practised manual, craft, experiential medicine, which was now faced with suppression. In other words, the learned and rational physicians had separated themselves from the group earlier criticized by the enemies of medicine.

In the north, particularly in France and England, these moves resulted in the separation, in terms of education and practice, of the surgeons from the physicians. Those few, like Henri de Mondeville (*c.*1260–*c.*1320), who championed the cause of surgery, did so by urging surgeons to become as learned and as Latinate as physicians.

By Mondino's time, medical men had begun to discover the value of the texts of Galen (AD 129–*c.*200/210). This 'new Galenism', an effort to find and use the texts, produced a Latin version of Galen's complete work on the nature of the parts of the body shortly after Mondino had finished *his* anatomy book. Galen's book was sophisticated, philosophically and anatomically, in a way that was unknown in the early fourteenth century. Indeed, it was too sophisticated; in its place was generally preferred a curtailed and corrupt, but simpler, version of it that had come into Latin by way of Arabic. In other words, into a medicine that was partly Hippocratic, Byzantine and Arabic, aphoristic and authoritative, there came Galen's rational, philosophical and, above all, anatomical medicine. As a provincial but plausible Greek doctor in Rome, Galen had brought himself to the bedside of the emperor by convincing Romans of these three virtues of his medicine. In what amounted to a genius for self-advertisement, Galen performed vivisections on pigs in the middle of Rome, demonstrating his masterful knowledge of nerves and muscles as he silenced the squealing of the animal by compressing its recurrent laryngeal nerves.

It was the learned and rational physician who now saw that the rationality of medicine lay in its anatomical basis. It became an important part of his public image, on which his claim to superiority lay. This is why the physicians in the universities insisted on public displays of human dissection, wrote them into the statutes, and built theatres for them. It is also why natural philosophy was invariably put above medicine in their reasons for dissecting.

83

The first reason was generally concerned with demonstrating the wisdom and providence of the Creator; His skill often enough constituted a natural-philosophical reason, in second place. Surgery was rarely mentioned. Where the surgeons carried out their own dissections in their own organizations, the practical nature of the demonstration left few historical records: clear evidence of the social role of the physicians' anatomical knowledge and display.

The rational and learned fourteenth-century doctor, like Galen himself, wanted to show that the body was intelligible. Its intelligibility resided in the form and function of its parts. *Anatomia* remained the study of form and function jointly until the seventeenth century. Not only that, but the Galenic, medical 'function' was identified with the Aristotelian 'purpose' or cause. Both ancient authors seemed to agree that true knowledge could only be achieved from knowledge of purpose. In addition, Aristotelian philosophy included extensive discussion about what constituted true knowledge, how it could be acquired and how it could be tested. In the age of the universities, these matters were of the essence, for the student addressed them in the dialectic of the first part of the arts course. If he went on to become a master of arts, he tackled the question of the 'true knowledge' of the natural world, from the principles of natural change to the actions of animated beings.

The physician who stressed his rationality and learning was not only addressing learned colleagues in other disciplines in the university, but also potential students, who by deserting one master for another could have some influence on what they were taught. He was also addressing patients, many of whom would have been through a university and so would know what knowledge was. In all cases, Galen's rationality was accepted: real medicine was anatomical.

HELLENISM IN THE RENAISSANCE

Two movements of the early Renaissance were of great importance for later anatomy. The first was humanism, at first a way of teaching literary subjects from classical examples. Two of its principal features came to have an effect on medicine: the recovery, and the historical evaluation, of ancient texts. In anatomy, this meant primarily Galen's *On the Use of the Parts* and the *Anatomical Procedures*. Philological and historical studies now showed what Galen had said, and why he differed from other great authors, like Aristotle. A second stage in humanistic anatomy was the preparation of digests from wholly classical sources like the short teaching texts of Jacobus Sylvius (1478–1555) and Joannes Guinter (c.1510–74) in Paris. The huge anatomical texts of Gabriele Zerbi (1445–1505) in Padua, and Jacopo Berengario da Carpi (1470–1530) in Bologna, in the early sixteenth century were 'humane' anatomy in their philological and historical approach.[3] But both were also proud of being men of the schools, professional teachers whose business, as they saw it, was to acquaint their audience with the whole range of anatomical literature, including the distinctly non-humane Arabic authors. Both Berengario and Zerbi recognized the presence of another group of scholars interested in anatomy. They were part of the second movement mentioned above, Hellenism. The Hellenists were Greeks and their sympathizers who, before 1453, wanted to preserve Byzantium from collapse and who afterwards argued for the preservation and superiority of Greek over Latin culture. Their spokesman in anatomy was Alessandro Benedetti (c.1450–1512), whose little manual of anatomy used Greek sources only. By such processes the West chose to find its intellectual origins in Greece. Humanists and Hellenists agreed in finding Latin and Arabic anatomical terminology to be derived from the Greek, and much of the reduplication and confusion over terminology was reduced by the use of Greek terms by men like Sylvius. From Bologna, human dissection spread slowly to other European centres. For example, the Germans were dissecting by the early sixteenth century. Even though their linguistic and political history had been so different from that of the Latin humanists and Greek Hellenists, they joined in the claim for a Greek intellectual paternity. The German Johannes 'Eichmann' (1500–60) became 'Dryander' and dissected human heads in Marburg. But the German humanists suspected, with reason, that their humane studies were not at the Italian level. For their anatomy, they went back to Mondino, of whose text Dryander produced an edition in 1541. So did Martin Pollich of Mellerstadt (d. 1513), who sought help from real Italian humanists in his squabble over astrology with a Leipzig teacher of medicine, another man of the schools.

After Bologna, the greatest centre of human dissection was Padua. Padua was popular with foreign students, and no doubt the students were popular at least for economic reasons with the town. Here was another reason for the importance of anatomy: not only was it an identifying feature of the learned physician, it was of commercial benefit to his *studium* and town. This is reflected by the Paduan statutes at the time of Zerbi. They gave unusual emphasis to two points, the performance of the public dissections, and the suppression of unlicensed practice. To make sure no one misunderstood, it was directed that the statutes be read out publicly in the vernacular to the sound of trumpets. The two statutes are directly related. It was precisely on the grounds of being rational and learned that university doctors claimed that their subject was effective and that of empirics dangerous on the opposite grounds. Thus the university doctors persuaded the civil authorities that it was in the public interest that the faculty should have a monopoly of practice and power to prosecute practitioners without university training. Since the rationality of medicine was largely anatomical, the public display of human dissection underlined the learning, rationality, and political power of the physicians' medicine. Zerbi was a staunch ally of what was being defended in the Paduan statutes (in which he is mentioned). His anatomical textbook (published in 1501) is not, as some have thought, a tiresome piece of scholasticism, but a verbal display of rationality and learning designed to accompany the visual display of the public anatomies. His text on medical ethics could hardly be more explicit on the question of how the university physician should behave to preserve his reputation as learned and rational, and hence his monopoly. (➤ Ch. 37 History of medical ethics)

In Bologna, much the same can be said of Berengario da Carpi. Here, too, there were frequent dissections, and Berengario's book is devoted to showing that the practising anatomist, devoted to a study of anatomical parts actually perceptible, gives a special autonomy to his rationality and learning – it is an art not available to the philosopher or the medical man who is merely book-learned. Berengario called his anatomy '*anatomia sensibilis*', the anatomy of the perceptible. A similar claim for the autonomy of anatomy and for the validity of ocular demonstration was made by Niccolò Massa (1485–1569), who called it '*anatomia sensata*', that is, an anatomy of what had actually been seen.[4]

REFORMED ANATOMY

We need not suppose, of course, that Zerbi and Berengario were cynically exploiting the power of learned and rational medicine to impress, in order to promote the interests of their professional group. They quite naturally believed that anatomy as expressed by themselves was simply the best and so most useful. Berengario believed that his 'anatomy of sensibles' was better than the anatomy of Zerbi and his followers (the 'Zerbists'), which he saw as too literary and deferential to authority. Part of the very learning of the kind of anatomy they both studied was the authority of the great authors, but Berengario (more than Zerbi) contradicted them when he saw something else in the dissected body. (For instance he vigorously denied the existence of the Galenic *rete mirabile* in the brain.)

Even so, it was the eager young man from Brussels, Andreas Vesalius (1514–64), who made disagreement with the ancients a point of method in anatomy. Some time in 1539, while teaching the anatomy of the bones from Galen's books and from the skeletons of a man and of an ape, he made a guess that Galen had never dissected a human body. It was an outrageous guess, but one largely confirmed by later historians, and was made before Vesalius was experienced in anatomy. It meant, if taken seriously, that *all* of Galen's anatomical descriptions were potentially wrong, and that the business of anatomy was essentially to start all over again and check Galen's descriptions. Vesalius pursued his guess with the utmost vigour and with very little discretion. He attacked Galen (and 'his apes') with enthusiasm, sarcasm, and a zeal that very often misrepresents Galen's words or position.[5]

Vesalius's contemporaries were either horrified or fascinated. The only precedent for an attack on an ancient author in an age of humane and Hellenistic respect for antiquity had been half a century before, when Niccolò Leoniceno (1428–1524) had said that Pliny (AD c.23–79) made mistakes, a number of them anatomical. Leoniceno was a Hellenist by conviction and could indulge in the mutual suspicion of the Greek and Latin cultures on the Greek side. Pliny, after all, was a Roman and wrote in Latin, the language of the commentators that the Hellenists despised. Pliny thus looked like a hasty commentator upon or compiler of things Greek. Those who defended Pliny did so by championing the cause of Latin culture, the *res latina* in which Pliny was a great ornament to whom faith should still be given despite some of his factual errors.

Those who now, after Vesalius, sprang to Galen's defence used similar arguments. The case was different, however, for Galen (unlike Pliny) was Greek and his attacker (unlike Leoniceno) was a northener with no special pretensions to Greek scholarship. Moreover, while the battle for and against Galen was being fought, so was that for and against the Catholic Church. The defenders of Galen were most conspicuous among those who were also defending the church against Protestantism. The faith, they said, that had to be given to Galen (as to Pliny) was the same kind of faith that was given to the church fathers and the scriptures. The *res medica* and *res anatomica* were, like the *res latina* in the Pliny case, traditions of learning that must not be destroyed. Just as the church relied on its tradition of learning to find truth in the texts and reject the arguments of the Protestants, so the faith that ran through medical and anatomical learning ensured the reception and interpretation of the old texts and the transmission to future generations of modern discoveries. (➤ Ch. 61 Religion and medicine)

The zeal of Vesalius and the anger of Sylvius (in whose words are found most of the arguments above) show that what was at stake was more than intellectual enquiry or the development of a topic within medicine. Sylvius and Jean Riolan (the younger, 1580–1657) in Paris, Bartolomeo Eustachio (c.1500–74) in Rome, Gabriele Falloppio (c.1523–62) in Modena, and André du Laurens (1558–1609) in Montpellier all berated Vesalius for his impiety, lack of faith, and the damage he was doing to the medical tradition. None of these scholars had our distinction between anatomical and religious knowledge, because the church determined what was to be counted as knowledge; natural philosophy, of which anatomy was part, was still a religious business. What Vesalius seemed to be offering was 'knowledge' that was outside that control and therefore wrong. He was acting, it was said, with the language of religion 'in bad faith'.[6]

Some accommodation had to be made. Sylvius, Riolan, and William Harvey (1578–1657) saw that the body on the dissection table did not in every particular agree with what Galen had described. All three ascribed the difference to Nature, God's regent in the world, especially in the continual generation of human beings and animals. It seemed likely that the human body had changed over the centuries between Galen and the seventeenth century, a view that fitted in so well with Renaissance respect for the ancients, with the relationship between the non-naturals and the body in Greek medicine, and with contemporary despair of human morality, that it could hardly be denied.

By the end of the sixteenth century, anatomy had split up into groups over the Vesalius affair. Many Catholics wanted to defend Galen and the learned tradition in general. Archangelo Piccolomini (1525–86) in Rome attacked the description by Realdo Colombo (c.1510–59) of the passage of the blood through the lungs in this spirit, and constructed a highly Catholic vision of anatomy, centred on a view of God mediated by the church. A number of Protestants took the line that the individual's own duty to order his knowledge of God meant that authority had to be given to personal observation. A particularly Protestant development was the study of animals and plants in the natural world. Prompted by the words of St Paul that God is so present in the natural world that it is almost possible to reach out and touch him, many Protestants found it their duty to learn about the Creator from the structure of animals, His creatures. Many on both sides of the religious divide found it regrettable that there should be conflict. Conrad Gesner (1516–65) thought that there was available a philosophy common to both sides that should cut through their differences: it was Aristotle's natural philosophy, which in fact both sides did choose as the authority by which they hoped stability would be ensured in education. By the end of the sixteenth century in Padua, Hieronymus Fabricius of Aquapendente (1533–1619) was teaching aspects of the anatomy of animals, perhaps first prompted by Gesner's works, in an Aristotelian fashion in Padua.

Fabricius thought that Vesalius had begun the modern study of anatomy, but recognized that in refuting so much of Galen by dissection he had limited himself largely to morphology, the *historia* of the parts. With the renewed emphasis on Aristotle in the later sixteenth century, however, it was clear to Fabricius and others that true knowledge of a part rested on a knowledge of its function – its *purpose* – as much as on that of its structure. This was a significant part of Harvey's natural philosophy. We cannot discuss Harvey's discovery of the circulation here, but we should note two things about it. First, it was for him an anatomical business (as was generation). Second,

Harvey's declared reasons for anatomizing – and this was originally a surgical lecture course – were primarily the physicians' philosophical reasons: the 'action, function and purpose' of the parts.[7] (➤ Ch. 7 The physiological tradition)

This had been a notable trait: both Vesalius and Fabricius were appointed to teach anatomy and surgery. Both, in fact, concentrated on forms of anatomy that related more to the physicians than to the surgeons. Fabricius provoked the wrath of his German students by failing to give them human, surgical anatomy (and by mimicking their bad Latin accents). And when Harvey, Fabricius's pupil, returned to England as the seventeenth century began, it was to a country that shared a European notion of the nature of learned and rational medicine and the place of anatomy within that. But it was a country in which, on the northern pattern, surgeons were separate from and subject to the learned physicians. Harvey's professional body, the London College of Physicians, had had obligatory anatomy lectures since 1569, and in 1582–3 Lord Lumley (c.1534–1609) endowed another. It was originally surgical, with the express intention of bringing England up to the level of Italy, France, and Spain. Not surprisingly (given the argument of this chapter), it soon became a physician's, not a surgeon's business (for example, when Harvey was appointed). It should be noted that the surgeons were already making their own dissections. (➤ Ch. 41 Surgery (traditional))

We must note here one feature of the physicians' anatomy which was important for Harvey. The surgeons, learning their anatomy during apprenticeship, lectures or dissections, were acquiring directly useful knowledge. In contrast, the physicians were absorbing knowledge that was indirectly useful, as we have seen. It not only had to be highly visible knowledge, it had to be a true *scientia*, based on demonstration. But the only demonstrative method available to the dissecting physician was simple ocular demonstration. To strengthen this, the dissector took care to demonstrate his findings to as large an audience as possible, perhaps in the theatre. It was also helpful if the audience consisted of well-known people, whose probity and authority gave substance to the demonstration. And it helped, too, if the anatomist could contrive some form of experiment with clear-cut results. All three – ocular demonstration, distinguished 'jury', and experiment – had been used by Galen, and were well known to anatomists. They were used by Berengario, Massa, and particularly by Colombo, in demonstrating that vital spirits are generated in the lungs and transferred to the left ventricle of the heart by the 'venous artery' (historians call this the demonstration of the pulmonary transit of blood). It was in pursuing the same triple technique that Harvey discovered that the blood circulated.

While Harvey was bringing Fabrician anatomy to England, the champions of Galen in France were developing their vision of anatomy. Du Laurens petitioned Henri IV, who created a chair of anatomy and botany in Paris;

Riolan (in 1618) asked for an anatomy theatre. His argument rested largely on national pride, representing Paris as the modern Cos and Montpellier as the modern Cnidus; Sylvius had been the Herophilus of French medicine and Riolan himself was the modern Galen.

Bodies for dissection were not always in plentiful supply in the early seventeenth century. Sylvius, in the previous century, claimed that about fifteen or twenty bodies were available every year in Paris, but thought that most other centres made do with a single body every year. The authorities may have had scruples about the process of dissection, and Charles V consulted the university of Salamanca on the acceptability of dissection (he had a positive reply). By Du Laurens's time at the beginning of the seventeenth century, about four bodies were dissected every year. The teaching of anatomy to physicians did not utterly depend on dissection, and the French anatomists, including Du Laurens, developed a double mode of teaching, the analytic and synthetic. The analytic parallelled the actual dissection of the body in beginning with the whole and ending with the parts (ultimately the theoretically fundamental 'similar' parts). The method could also replace dissection. Synthetic teaching of anatomy was wholly theoretical and closely based in natural philosophy. Beginning with the elements, qualities, and humours, (➤ Ch. 14 Humoralism) it showed how the body had been constructed by nature by building up the similar parts into organic parts and these into the entire body. Such anatomy showed well the religious and philosophical (and professional) reasons for anatomy, but was of little use to the surgeon (who was anyway unlikely to hear it). Du Laurens also called the two methods 'descriptive' and '*scientificus*' (causal).[8]

NEW PHILOSOPHIES

We have seen above that the physicians' anatomy was closely linked in a number of ways to the natural philosophy that was the basis of theoretical medicine. Radically new natural philosophies were becoming available in the earlier seventeenth century, and their relationships to anatomy were necessarily different.

A general change in natural philosophy was that more people began to see that progress was possible. The controversy literature of the early seventeenth century (like that of Tobias Knobloch (1612) and of Du Laurens) partly reflects the needs of the schools for theses and disputations, generally found by apparent discord between the old writers. Such questions touched on topics like the 'origin' of the veins, the function of the spleen, the nobility of the heart, and the seat of the soul. Neoterical questions entered the literature with Vesalius's attacks on Galen and Colombo's demonstration that the 'venous artery' contains only blood. But with the discoveries of Gaspare

Aselli (1581–1625), Harvey, and Jean Pecquet (1627–74) it became clear that progress in anatomy was not limited to resolving the problems of the ancient literature. That is, the discovery of the lacteal vessels showed that there was another route, distinct from the liver, for the absorption of food. Clearly the first great 'concoction' of the body, the generation of blood in the liver from incoming food, was open to question. When Harvey showed that the blood circulated and did not therefore move unidirectionally from the liver, belief in sanguification in the liver was largely destroyed. It was completely destroyed when Pecquet demonstrated the passage of chyle directly into the subclavian vein. This destruction of the old made possible and necessary the construction of the new. The possibility of indefinite improvement was being opened up at the same time as people were listening to the similar message about natural philosophy as a whole from neoterics like Francis Bacon (1561–1626).

Another change in natural philosophy was in what constituted knowledge. For Harvey, the traditional relationship between structure, action, and use still generated knowledge of a part of the body, but it was the *purpose* that some of the new philosophers saw in this relationship that they objected to. Indeed, one of the objects of a natural philosophy of particles and local action-by-contact was to remove the purposeful nature currently attributed to motions involved in, for example, *horror vacui*. Although René Descartes (1596–1650) argued that the shape and disposition of the parts of a clock necessarily demonstrated its function, the old link between structure and function in the generation of knowledge was being broken. Descartes's friend, Cornelis ab Hogelande (1590–1662), expressed it clearly in explaining that there is no *purpose* in the valves of the heart shutting after the blood has been compelled to enter the arteries: it is simply the *mechanical* action of the blood pressing back to the heart that automatically closes the valve. Of course, this is evidence of God's original design, but that is all. To disregard purpose is 'to think mechanically'.[9]

What the mechanists objected to was not only Aristotle's teleological Nature, in which 'cause' (of motions and parts) is purposeful, but the immanent, provident and generative Nature that acted sometimes as God's regent in the day-to-day control of the body and sometimes as Galen's demiurge. When Harvey said that nature was sometimes slightly careless in piling the guts into the abdomen, the Galenic-theistic Nature was in his mind. Much more usual than Harvey's view was the belief that Nature does nothing in vain. It was implicit in this that all shape and action was purposeful. No mechanist or particulate philosopher would accept that action-use-utility was a precondition of knowledge of a part.

A philosophy based on particles, action by contact, and denial of purpose could not have the traditional interest in gross anatomy. If the basic bodily actions were the motions of particles through pores, as many thought, then fine structure, not gross, captured the interest. At the same time, microscopists like Antoni van Leeuwenhoek (1632–1723) were showing that gross structure did not vanish into homogeneity, but that diversity was continued, even multiplied, at great magnifications. This seemed entirely congruent with a functioning at the level of particles, and it reinforced the move away from the old teleology. (➤ Ch. 6 The microscopical tradition)

A third change pointed in the same direction – the decline of human dissection. Whether this was the effect of economic changes or of a philosophical loss of interest in gross anatomy, the result was the development of a number of techniques of teaching anatomy in the absence of a fresh cadaver. One of these was the attempted preservation of anatomical preparations or entire bodies. In the middle of the seventeenth century, Ludovicus Bilsius (de Bils) (1624–70) asked 25 florins to preserve four bodies, but he used brine, not the 'balsam' that was often sought as the agent of mummification; the subsequent decay is said to have caused his final illness and destroyed his entire collection. Another means of preserving flesh was brandy (which sometimes provided temptations for those handling the preparations). Some anatomists became skilled at making durable preparations by injecting vessels with a variety of substances. This had the advantage that it demonstrated fine structure in a way consistent with the new interests of philosophical anatomy. Lastly, artisans in Italy and elsewhere became skilled in making realistic wax models of parts of the body.

A fourth change discernible in anatomy in the seventeenth century also seems to be linked to those already mentioned. The woodcuts of Vesalius's *Fabrica* could hardly be improved upon, and a finer line could only be given by the use of metal. The copper plates of Giovan Battista Canano (1515–79) and later Guilio Casserius (c.1552–1616) had at least the potentiality of greater accuracy, but illustrations associated with the physicians' anatomy showed little improvement during the seventeenth century. The magnificent illustrations later used by Govert Bidloo (1649–1713) and William Hunter (1718–83) belong rather to the surgical tradition of anatomy, which is examined later (see pp. 96–99).

A last change we need to note is in the external circumstances of anatomy. The growing economic power of northern Europe eclipsed that of Italy where, compared with earlier centuries, something of a cultural decline became apparent. Human dissections ceased in Padua in the 1620s, apparently because of the cost. The last great Paduan anatomist was Adriaan van den Spiegel (1578–1625). Students from the north, who had traditionally travelled to Padua for part of their medical education, now began to feel that their needs could be met closer to home. Leiden, in particular, became known as a medical school. In London, comparatively recent lectureships in anatomy in the College of Physicians maintained some dissection. The shift to the north is illustrated by the Danish Bartholins, father and son: Caspar (1587–1629) was educated by Fabricius and Casserius in Padua, and published his 'institutes' of anatomy in 1611; his son Thomas (1616–80) was taught partly by Johan Vesling (1598–1649), (who left Padua when the anatomies stopped), and partly in Leiden. Thomas reissued his father's textbook with modern material, and produced a summary of recent 'controversies' on topics such as the lacteals: he was effectively addressing an audience whose centre of gravity was closer to Leiden than Padua.

In addition to economic changes, religious and political disturbances had their effects on anatomy. German-speaking countries suffered badly in the Thirty Years War, and Caspar Hofmann (1572–1648) was one of the few learned physicians to enter into contemporary controversies. Scholarly medicine itself came increasingly under pressure from the followers of Paracelsus (c.1494–1541), who thought in particular that corporeal anatomy was useless. In holding that a knowledge of medicine and drugs was God-given and not acquired, the Paracelsians were striking precisely at the learning on which the traditional doctor had based his public image. The rationality of this medicine, anatomy, was thus rejected on ideological grounds. In its place, they discussed a celestial anatomy in which the parts of the body corresponded with parts of the macrocosm. Many reformers considered, in a related way, that learned and traditional medicine was a monopoly protected and fostered by the physicians, much as priests fostered and defended a monopoly over the scriptures and their interpretation. English Puritans felt that traditional learned medicine had failed in the same way as the Roman church.

In England, indeed, the College of Physicians faced a double threat in the interregnum years. Its monopoly of internal practice was challenged, partly by sectarians opposed to monopoly and partly by 'chemical' physicians of Paracelsian lineage. In these circumstances, the public dissections as a social device to advertise the nature of the physicians' medicine came under pressure. Thomas Sydenham (1624–89), the most famous English doctor of that time, studiously avoided anatomical rationality in his practice of medicine.

THE ENLIGHTENMENT

The late seventeenth and early eighteenth centuries saw another group of related changes in anatomy. First, another natural philosophy became available, the Newtonian. It did not reach all medical centres of all countries with equal speed, but broadly had three effects of concern to anatomy. First, it reinforced the image of the body as a machine; second, it drew attention away from particle-to-particle contact and emphasized the hydraulic model of machinery; third, after the publication of the *Optics*, it encouraged medical practioners to use the notion of ether to explain how the body worked.

None of this gave any new interest to gross anatomy. In Italy, Marcello Malpighi (1628–94) was investigating small structures in big animals and big structures in small animals. His compatriot Giovanni Borelli (1608–79) was investigating animal movements in gross mechanical terms – levers, pulleys, centres of gravity, and so on. In Britain, and briefly in Leiden, Archibald Pitcairne (1652–1713) was working at the Newtonian hydraulic model. In Halle, Georg Ernst Stahl (1660–1734) dismissed anatomy as comprehensively as the Paracelsians by declaring that the soul acted as it pleased in the body and so function was unrelated to structure. His colleague, Friedrich Hoffmann (1660–1742), thought quite the opposite, and maintained, with the Prussian administration behind him, that anatomy was the basis of the rational and learned medicine that characterized the university doctor and gave him unassailable privileges over the surgeon and apothecary. In Leiden, Hermann Boerhaave (1668–1738) was working out a form of mechanism that centred on the fibre as the primary unit of the body. Action in the body still depended on solids, but their structure was fine, not gross.

This was essentially the end of the anatomy that the rational and learned doctor had used for so long to make a public statement about the kind of medicine that he, as distinct from all other kinds of practitioner, practised. This academic anatomy was now dealt with as part of the increasingly common 'institutes' of medicine, where it was taken as the first part of physiology, itself the first of Galen's five divisions of medicine (the others were pathology, semiotics, hygiene, and therapy). So for Boerhaave, Hoffmann, and (later) Albrecht von Haller (1708–77), anatomy was still in a sense fundamental to medicine, with the fine structure of what were traditionally the homogeneous, structureless, 'similar' parts housing somehow the moving powers of the body. Thus Hoffmann, relying partly on the recent periodical literature and anatomists like Frederik Ruysch (1638–1731) and Leeunwenhoek and his '*microscopium*',[10] began with the structure of the skin as a structured similar part. Upon such structures was built his physiology and pathology, in an 'institutes' format. He intended it also to be useful for surgery; however, as a state-backed learned physician in Prussia, this related more to his own belief that medical knowledge subsumes that of surgery, than to the surgeons' own search for anatomy, now so obvious elsewhere. Boerhaave's assimilation of anatomy into the first part of physiology was propagated by Haller in his edition of his teacher's lectures.[11] A similar format was adopted by Lazarus Riverius (1589–1655) in Montpellier.

A parallel change in the same period was that anatomists began to write histories of their subject. Daniel Leclerc (1652–1728) was followed by André Goelicke (1671–1744), James Douglas (1675–1742), Antoine Portal

(1742–1832), Thomas Lauth (1758–1826), Haller himself, and even Boer-haave, all of whom made greater or lesser attempts to trace out the history of gross anatomy. Clearly, there was some perceived change in anatomy that required legitimation; probably, it was the introduction of mechanism into anatomy and the consequent shift of attention to fine structure. For example, Bartholin's *Anatomia Renovata* of 1673 looks consciously new – he wrote of mathematics and mechanics in anatomy: bellows, syringes, pipes, bottles. Partly, too, it was that gross anatomy as a finite descriptive science was seen to have been left behind in an age of progress, in favour of fine anatomy. Simon Tissot (1728–97) certainly thought so: 'but in an age like the present, and upon a subject so much searched into as the human body, we do not flatter ourselves with discovering essential properties; all that we can naturally hope for, is to push farther those discoveries already made, which require no more than dexterity and patience to bring them to perfection.'[12]

With eighteenth-century improvement there was a place for 'research' in an almost modern sense. Progress like this must have been seen as possible since Harvey. Haller began the whole of the *Elementa Physiologiae* with a justification of the historical method of looking at the discovery of truth, which he maintained would improve the progress of anatomy.[13] It was indeed a method on which he claimed to be writing the book – clearly it involved also his extensive reference system.

We can summarize the history of academic anatomy with a glance at Haller's *anatomia animata*. Descartes's claim that the soul and the body belonged to mutually exclusive categories had cut right across current beliefs. These were that the soul, in addition to being the Christian vehicle of immortality, was the Form of the body in an Aristotelian sense. In seven-teenth-century terminology, the body was the instrument of the soul. In this way, the organs exercised faculties that were governed by the soul. From whatever source, particulate theories of matter made no use of the concept of faculty, and by the middle of the seventeenth century it was common to talk in terms of 'natural necessity', generally some kind of local mechanical and particulate cause, rather than of faculties. In anatomy, this meant that the shape of organs was no longer related to the instrumentality of the soul. The traditional function–form relationship was now hinged on the small, perhaps microscopically small, parts that seemed to illustrate the particularity of local natural necessity. The early-Enlightenment followers of Descartes equated 'soul' with 'conscious rationality' and found the body to be a machine. Such a view could assimilate Newtonian natural philosophy largely by making the machine one of tubes and moving liquids. Some such view was assembled by Boerhaave and became, as a result, very widespread in Europe at the beginning of the eighteenth century. It seemed to offer the hope that the actions of the body machine could be explored and explained on the basis of the laws of mechanics and mathematics. Ironically, it was precisely the detailed use of mathematics in the 1730s that showed that the body as a machine needed a source of motion to replace that lost by friction and to produce the apparently perpetual motions observed in the living body. Joseph Rosetti in Italy, François Boissier de Sauvages (1706–67) in Montpellier, Jerome Gaub (1705–80) in Leiden, and Robert Whytt (1714–66) in Scotland were part of an 'animist revival' in which the Hippocratic *impetum faciens* and 'healing power of nature' and the Christian soul were combined to supply a source of motion for the otherwise inert machine of the body. It no longer operated through faculties nor was it discernible through a structure–function relationship. Instead, it was investigated experimentally. In this way, Haller made his famous distinction between sensibility and irritability. The meaning of the phrase *anatomia animata* for Haller was that at the fundamental level mechanical explanations of the motion were inadequate. They explained what happened to motion once produced in the body, but could not account for the source of motion in an irritated and contracting muscle. The visible structure in which he saw mechanical laws being obeyed was still *anatomia*, but it was the structure of an essentially living body, *animata*, endowed with soul, if not in the traditional sense then at least the direct result of God's wisdom in designing the body. Something similar had been concluded in the case of the heartbeat late in the previous century by the arch-mechanist of Italy, Giovanni Borelli; and the ultimate appeal to the incorporeal was, in practice, not too dissimilar to that of some of the animists. The ultimate result was a widespread adoption of the notion that the living body has special, 'vital' forces which are ultimately not mechanical. And for the reasons just outlined, such vital functions no longer had a direct relationship to structure. The physicians' learned and rational medicine was lost from sight into an academic consideration of the 'Institutes' in parallel with the new vigorous growth of surgical gross anatomy.

SURGICAL ANATOMY

The growth of anatomy in the eighteenth century derived partly from a tradition distinct from the academic, the surgical. This is ultimately a reflection of basic changes taking place in learned society in the seventeenth century. The changes in natural philosophy occurred largely outside the universities. Harvey himself was demonstrating anatomy to the College of Physicians. The 'virtuosi' of the new natural philosophy did not work in a university context. Without a formal structure, they felt a need to communicate, and networks of correspondence were established. Formal structures like the Royal Society also played an important part in such communications. There were also less formal groupings, like the well-known '1645 group' and the 'invisible college'. There were attempts to formalize communication on a national and religious scale, with Protestant and Catholic 'corresponden-cies'. In anatomy, like-minded investigators set up 'clubs' or 'colleges', such as Bartholin's group in Copenhagen, and that in Amsterdam, which included Jan Blasius (1626–82), Jan Swammerdam (1637–80), and Ruysch among its members. Such groups periodically published their results, and periodicals rapidly became a major source of information for anatomical writers, such as Hoffmann in Halle.

These developments helped to break down the privileges of the old medical institutions. In England, the Royal College of Physicians did not grow as rapidly as the market for medical practice. Those taking medical degrees from Oxford and Cambridge were also small in number. In effect, the old monopolies could not be sustained and large numbers of physicians practised an all-round medicine – internal, surgical, and later obstetric. (➤ Ch. 47 History of the medical profession) It is evident that much of the demand for anatomical education in the early eighteenth century came from the students hoping to qualify for this kind of practice, although the anatomy they sought still dealt extensively with the interior organs on which they could not practise surgery. Yet, this was a knowledge that was useful for the practice of a medicine which was a mixture of the internal and manual. Moreover, on the European continent more than in Britain, the growing practice of forensic medicine and its post-mortem dissections made internal anatomy a useful accomplishment.

The upswing in human dissection began in the 1680s. By the early eight-eenth century, the medical students' Grand Tour took them to a number of centres in northern Europe, including if at all possible Leiden and Boerhaave, and probably Rheims for a cheap degree. The demand for anatomical training brought into existence a class of medical entrepreneurs ready to supply it. In Paris, private teaching of surgery offered an alternative to apprenticeship, and attracted foreign students. In London, a rapidly growing capital city without a university, William Cheselden (1688–1752) offered private instruc-tion in dissection and surgery at his house in Cheapside from 1713 to 1731, despite opposition from the United Company of Barbers and Surgeons, who claimed a monopoly. (➤ Ch. 48 Medical education)

The United Company illustrates many of these points. The *de facto* loss of monopoly by the old medical corporations not only made a mixed internal-surgical, general practice of medicine attractive to the student, but also encouraged the surgeons to aspire to internal medicine. They tried in 1689 and 1690 to secure an Act to allow them to practise internally, but were defeated by the physicians and apothecaries. Not only was economic and population growth increasing the market for a mixed, general practice of medicine, but the number of surgeons was growing rapidly. The first half of the eighteenth century saw the appearance of large numbers of ex-naval surgeons, who had already been licensed by the United Company. By 1713, after fighting France, the British fleet was the largest in the world, with 247 vessels. Each ship from the first to sixth rate carried a surgeon and mate. In meeting the needs of the navy, the United Company was licensing approximately two to three hundred surgeons a year. (There was a high turnover of surgeons in naval practice.) The naval surgeon in private practice could ignore guild restrictions of the Company, and it is arguable that the sheer numbers of such surgeons threatened the monopoly of the United Company. They had also been trained in internal medicine, so could claim a right to practise as physicians. Included among the naval surgeons were the Scottish surgeon-apothecaries, who had also been trained in internal medicine.

The United Company dissolved itself in 1745 in the interests of the surgeons' upward mobility. The new Surgeons' Company of London removed their objection to private anatomy teaching, which flourished. The most notable of the private London schools was that of the Hunters (William, 1718–83; and John, 1728–93). In practice, such schools offered much more than anatomy courses and went a long way to providing the qualifications for the kind of 'mixed' practice to be met in the growing urban centres. By mid-century, the London schools were offering more anatomy and surgery than those in Paris. In both centres, the hospitals too offered opportunities for the enterprising teacher to supply pupils with medical experience, sometimes including the provision of dissection material. In London, at Guy's Hospital in 1743, Drs William Bromfield (1713–92) and Frank Nicholls (1699–1778) gave courses of nearly forty lectures each, including anatomy, surgery, physiology, pathology, and midwifery. A 'surgeon' attending the private courses and the hospitals would, in fact, get a medical training. (➤ Ch. 49 The hospital) The Scottish universities took advantage of the new demand. In Edinburgh, Alexander Monro *primus* (1697–1767), a surgeon, excluded surgeons from the faculty, but taught surgical apprentices as well as medical students, in English.

The situation was somewhat different in France, where it was the surgeons rather than the apothecaries (as in England) who formed a class of general practitioner in civil life. The French surgeons became effectively organized in their profession. This reflected the centralized politics of the country as a whole, and drew its authority from the king's surgeon. This unity of profession was imposed from above on a hierarchy that included barbers and wig-makers: very different from the self-grouping of English surgeons based on common interest and (after 1745) on common vocation. The French surgical profession took over anatomy as a business as characteristic of them as it had been of the earlier learned physicians. The profession was well placed for the changes that took place at the time of the Revolution, for anatomy was seen as practical and useful to the civilian and soldier, while the theoretical physiology of the physician of the *ancien régime* was seen as speculative and imaginary. The new French surgical-anatomical medicine gave emphasis to diseased tissues, and the big hospitals provided the opportunity for systematic investigation of the relationship between symptoms in the living and physical lesions discovered after death by anatomical dissections. (➤ Ch. 9 The pathological tradition)

REFORM

In eighteenth-century Britain, market forces for medical education and practice led to a complex licensing situation. The private schools gave training but were not empowered to give licences. Of the universities, Oxford and Cambridge continued to produce small numbers of doctors, Aberdeen sold degrees and provided minimal instruction, while Glasgow prospered and Edinburgh flourished as a renowned school of training and qualification. There was the occasional bishop's licence. The Army and Navy Medical Boards continued to examine and license practitioners for military service, a licence that was valid in later civilian life. The Royal College of Physicians continued to produce the gentlemanly physician, able to command the highest fees.

This complex picture persisted until the reforming politics of the early nineteenth century. Central government in revolutionary France combined the roles of physician and surgeon for ideological and military reasons. In the new University of Berlin in 1810, the physicians and surgeons had equal standing, by order. In Scotland, the Universities Commission tried to construct a viable medical school from the fragmented teaching available in Aberdeen's Royal Infirmary, the rival colleges, each a university in its own right, and from private teaching. In England, too, it was ultimately central government that bowed to pressure from groups anxious for reform, largely those at the lower end of the scale of practitioners. Two results of these movements are of interest in the history of anatomy. First, the practical nature of the surgeons' concern with anatomy, combined perhaps with the concern of academic anatomy with fine structure, directed attention to the tissues of the body as the seats of diseases. This is evident with the Hunters and their colleague, Matthew Baillie (1761–1823), in London.

The second result of the reforming changes of the early nineteenth century was, in Britain, the passage of the Anatomy Act of 1832. Before this, the only legal supply of bodies for dissection was from the gallows, for the penalty for murder was not only hanging but subsequent dissection. But as a supply of dissection material, this was grossly inadequate for the rapidly growing demands of education. As the private schools continued to teach, the activities of the 'resurrection men' increased. So did public hostility, even to rioting and the destruction of dissection rooms. The suppliers of bodies found their task increasingly difficult and dangerous, and accordingly put up the price of their commodity. These things reached a peak in the late 1820s: while public outrage and vigilance were at a height, it was as cheap for a medical student to go abroad for his anatomy tuition as to stay at home. Disaster was imminent, partly in the collapse of the private teaching that furnished the bulk of students with their anatomical knowledge and which was profitable not only to the teachers but to other townsfolk.

When these students went abroad, it was to France; post-revolutionary legislation there had secured a supply of bodies from the destitute classes. It was clear to Jeremy Bentham (1748–1832) that some such system was needed to control the situation in England: with it, he could end the practice of grave-robbing. His first proposal for reform in 1826 was followed, coincidentally, by a legal judgement against two doctors whose dissection material had not come from the only strictly legal source, the gallows. This case made all anatomists liable to legal punishments. (➤ Ch. 69 Medicine and the law) A hastily convened parliamentary Select Committee reported in favour of Bentham's proposal. Some three months later, the activities of William Burke (1792–1829) and William Hare (fl.1829) were discovered after their sixteenth victim was found in the dissection rooms of Robert Knox (1791–1862). (Some indication of the scarcity of bodies is suggested by the £700 spent annually by Knox in securing a supply.) Held up briefly by the Reform Bill, the Anatomy Act became the law in August 1832. The Act established an Anatomy Inspectorate, the first of a number of centrally controlled Benthamite reforms which appeared in 1832. But the Act did not increase the number of bodies available for dissection. Its effect was to replace the supply of bodies from the resurrection men with a supply of unclaimed bodies of paupers dying in workhouses. The Inspectorate was, in practice, powerless to prevent arrangements between the parish authorities, who had responsibility for the sick poor as well as workhouse inmates, and the hospitals, which offered beds for the sick poor in exchange for bodies from the workhouse. What had been an additional punishment for murder – dissection – now became a gratuitous reward of poverty. The hospitals, in addition, could rely on their own mortuaries. It meant the end of the private schools, which had depended on equally 'private' supplies of bodies. This alone could be policed. (The Hunters' school had already closed, in 1831.)

NOTES

1   Gentile da Foligno, *Avicenne Medicorum Principis Canonum Liber Unum cum Lucidissima Gentilis Fulg. Expositione*, Venice, 1520.

2 Jacopo Berengario da Carpi, *Commentaria in Anatomia Muondini cum Amplissimis Additionibus*, Bologna, 1521.
3 Berengario, op. cit. (n. 3).
4 Niccolò Massa, *Anatomiae Liber Introductorius*, Venice, 1536.
5 A. Vesalius, *De Fabrica Corporis Humani*, Basle, 1543.
6 B. Eustachio, *Examen Ossium et de Motu Capitis in Opuscula Anatomica*, Venice, 1563.
7 G. Whitteridge (ed.), *The Anatomical Lectures of William Harvey. Praelectiones Anatomiae Universalis. De Musculis*, Edinburgh and London, Livingstone, 1964.
8 A. du Laurens, *Historia Anatomica*, Frankfurt, 1602.
9 C. ab Hogelande, *Cogitationes quibus Dei Existentia; item Animae Spiritalitas et Possibilis cum Corpore Unio Demonstrantur: necnon, brevis Historia Oeconomiae Corporis Animalis proponitur, atque Mechanice explicatur*, Leiden, 1676.
10 F. Hoffmann, *Operum Omnium Physico-Medicorum Supplementum Secundum in Tres Partes distributum . . . Pars Tertia*, Geneva, 1753.
11 H. Boerhaave, *Praelectiones Academicae in proprias Institutiones Rei Medicae*, ed. A. von Haller, 3 vols, Venice, 1743.
12 A. von Haller, *A Dissertation on the Sensible and Irritable Parts of Animals*, trans. and with a preface by M. Tissot, London, 1755.
13 A. von Haller, *Elementa Physiologiae Corporis Humani*, 8 vols, Lausanne and Berne, 1757–66.

FURTHER READING

Bynum, W. F. and Porter, Roy (eds), *William Hunter and the Eighteenth-Century Medical World*, Cambridge, Cambridge University Press, 1985.
Ceard, J., Fontaine, M.-M. and Margolin, J.-C., *Le Corps à la Renaissance. Actes de XXXe colloque de tours 1987*, Paris, Aux Amateurs de Livres, 1990.
French, R. K. and Wear, A. (eds), *British Medicine in the Age of Reform*, London, Routledge, 1991.
Gelfand, T., *Professionalizing Modern Medicine. Paris Surgeons and Medical Science and Institutions in the Eighteenth Century*, Westport, CT, and London, Greenwood Press, 1980.
Lind, J. R., *Studies in Pre-Vesalian Anatomy. Biography, Translations, Documents*, Philadelphia, PA, American Philosophical Society, 1975.
Maulitz, R., *Morbid Appearances. The Anatomy of Pathology in the Early Nineteenth Century*, Cambridge, Cambridge University Press, 1987.
Richardson, R., *Death, Dissection and the Destitute*, London, Routledge & Kegan Paul, 1987.
Siraisi, Nancy G., *Medieval and Early Renaissance Medicine*, Chicago, IL, University of Chicago Press, 1990.

6

THE MICROSCOPICAL
TRADITION

Brian Bracegirdle

Human beings are intensely visual animals, relying on their sense of sight
for most of their information about their individual worlds. This extraordinary
sense allows the unaided eye to gather data from objects millions of miles
away, to a close distance of about ten inches. Closer than that and some aid
to vision is needed. Simple lenses used as spectacles were introduced by
about 1350, and the microscope, providing higher magnifications, was introduced c.1600. This tool began to revolutionize science in 1830, was widely
used by 1870, and had become totally ubiquitous by about 1970. The microscope has provided scarcely credible results in the life sciences, and most of
all in medicine. I shall summarize work accomplished before 1830, and treat
in some detail what has been discovered since then.

EARLY HISTORY

Seventeenth-century microscopy provided a picture of an entirely new world,
being at once a stimulus and a difficulty. The stimulus was perfectly understandable – the illustrations in *Micrographia* (1665) by Robert Hooke
(1635–1703) are still a source of wonderment and pleasure to readers now
hardened by a plethora of sophisticated graphics; this book undoubtedly
established the microscope as an instrument. The difficulty was philosophical:
no framework existed for so startling a world picture as that revealed by
magnifications of about thirty times, and it would be slow to develop.
    True, sustained, scientific work was carried out in the later seventeenth
century by Antoni van Leeuwenhoek (1632–1723), who was the first to see
bacteria, for example. He worked with an idiosyncratic type of instrument
and was secretive as to his methods; therefore his results were largely unre-
peatable and did not exert the influence that might have been expected, in

spite of widespread dissemination by the Royal Society.[1] The results from the seventeenth century were very patchy: Hooke described cells for the first time, although without the dynamic understanding that is the true importance of the concept; and others described structures such as capillaries. (➤ Ch. 5 The anatomical tradition)

In the eighteenth century, the microscope was relatively little used. Of course, in a hundred years, some valuable results were obtained, but scientific work was sporadic and carried out by only a few individuals, who laboured in isolation. Large numbers of instruments were made, and designs were improved mechanically, making them much more convenient in use. Popular books were published in many editions, and a market in permanent preparations for inspection by the amateur was established. Such sliders require a certain dexterity for their manufacture, but had to be provided to allow purchasers of instruments to have something to view. The preparations followed original work in some cases: *The Construction of Timber* (1770) by John Hill (1716–75), for example, ensured that all slider sets would contain wood sections.

The historian of microscopy is fortunate in that large numbers of instruments (from about 1680 onwards) and preparations (from about 1750 onwards) have survived, allowing cross-checking between literature and the devices that allowed the literature to be produced. In spite of this, there are two main pitfalls for the historian: the one being the impossibility of adopting the mental attitude of earlier workers, with their relative lack of knowledge; the other, being the fact that truly scientific preparations do not survive except in very rare cases.

One special example must be quoted from the eighteenth century: the preparations made by William Hewson (1739–74) that still survive in the Hunterian Museum of the Royal College of Surgeons of England. Hewson worked in the school of anatomy run by William Hunter (1718–83), and between 1768 and 1771 made more than two hundred preparations, some dry and some wet. All were injected specimens and all still yield good-quality images with modern instruments. They are the most important surviving eighteenth-century scientific preparations. They are very typical of their age in that the highly developed technique of injecting blood and other vessels with various coloured media was used: this gives a stunning appearance on inspection, and (depending on the skill of the injector) a great deal of information about the course of the minute blood vessels, but nothing of the finer detail of most tissues. The techniques of preparing material to reveal cellular details were not to become established until a century later.

THE NINETEENTH CENTURY

By the beginning of the nineteenth century, interest in the finer structure of the body was increasing. M. F. X. Bichat (1771–1802) published his *Traité des membranes* in 1800, putting forward a science of anatomy and pathology based on a classification of tissues in the body, with their distribution in organs and their special diseases. (➤ Ch. 9 The pathological tradition) What is totally surprising to modern histologists about this monumental effort is that Bichat used only a hand-lens, as he actually mistrusted the compound microscope and its results. Neither did he use the word 'histology'. This name was introduced by A. F. J. C. Mayer (1787–1865) in 1819, in his small *Ueber Histologie*, which offered a division of tissues that differed only slightly from that of Bichat. This work was published at a time when Bichat's criticisms of the microscope were being amply justified. In the 1820s, a number of papers were published which described all tissues as being made up of globules of matter of a uniform diameter of about 1/300 mm. A good example of such a 'globulist' is Henri Milne-Edwards (1800–85) who could not, of course, realize that his results were due to what we would nowadays describe as diffraction effects resulting from the use of a microscope objective of far too small an aperture for its magnification.

And there the use of the microscope would have had to stop for the scientific study of histology and the later sciences of cytology and bacteriology, had it not been for a wine-merchant, J. J. Lister (1786–1869). He was the father of Lord Lister, the famous surgeon, and he was also the father of microscopical theory. In 1826, he had made for himself an instrument which had a far better high-magnification performance than any preceding it, based on experimental investigation of existing lenses. He published in 1827 with the physician Thomas Hodgkin (1798–1866) a paper that marks the beginning of modern histology, because it described the structure of tissues accurately as being composed of fibres and the like, rather than of 'globules'. By 1830, Lister had worked out the principle of aplanatic foci,[2] and provided opticians at last with the means to design objectives of good scientific performance. This was the breakthrough which would enable the microscope to be applied to medical training, diagnosis, and research on a grand scale.

By 1830, then, the instrument was waiting in the wings. At that time, most accepted that living matter arose spontaneously from non-living; it was not known that cells had nuclei nor how they reproduced; the normal structure of cells was a mystery and the abnormal not even contemplated; and the various causes of disease were merely conjectural. The microscope would alter all this.

During the 1830s, a scientific body of microscopical knowledge began to be established, in spite of the fact that the instruments used had no better performance than those of Leeuwenhoek, as Lister's work had not yet borne fruit very widely. However, the microscopes were a lot easier to use and were applied enthusiastically by a school led by Johannes Müller (1801–58) in Berlin, and others. The work was wide ranging, and papers on many tissues and organs were published, resulting in the formation of a corpus of knowledge and recognition of the importance of the microscope not only in medical research but also in medical teaching. It was this generalized application of the instrument to medicine which was the really important consequence of a decade of intense activity in microscopy.

CELL THEORY

It was in the 1830s also that interest in the cell as an entity began to develop apace, although it would be many years before the cell was widely accepted as the unit of life, and many more before its divisions were understood. It is, for example, remarkable that the classic by Charles Darwin (1809–82), *On the Origin of Species* (1859), has no entry for the word in its index. The names of M. J. Schleiden (1804–81) and T. Schwann (1810–82) are usually associated with the first establishment of cell theory, but in very different ways. In addition, the work on animal tissues by J. E. Purkinje (1787–1869) and others of the Müller school mentioned above was the basis that enabled Schwann to survey what was known of such tissues for comparison with his own work on plant cells, *Mikroskopische Untersuchungen* (1839).

Schwann accepted Schleiden's theory of the formation of plant cells by aggregation of granules into nuclei which then expanded into cells, and applied it to animal cells. The amorphous 'cytoblastema' was supposed to be the ground substance out of which cells were produced, and this was in perfect accord with the current ideas of the formation of cells out of the exudate of blood vessels. The concept of the cytoblastema was extended to include all that we now classify as intercellular material – varying only in viscosity: high in cartilage, medium in areolar tissue, low in blood! However, it was Schleiden who helped Schwann to see that the cell and its nucleus was the basic component of both plant and animal tissues. Although Schleiden was totally mistaken in his views on the development of cells, so powerfully did he argue and so resolutely defend an increasingly untenable position that he held back progress in understanding the nature of the cell for many years. He said that ways in which cells divide were either by exogeny, by formation of cells in a formless clump, or by endogeny, the development of one cell inside another. This in spite of several observations which showed cells dividing as we know them to do today. (➤ Ch. 7 The physiological tradition)

Schwann, then, established cell theory as early as 1839, but this considerable advance was totally overshadowed by Schleiden's waywardness. It was fortunate that Purkinje and Müller had described embryonic skeletal tissues because they, like plants, show a definite cell wall with minimal preparation. It was the sheer technical difficulty of demonstrating cell walls in a variety of other animal cells that held back wider acceptance of the cell theory. And it was Schleiden's unfortunate choice of specific plant material for investigation that led to error in describing as typical, cell divisions which are actually very unusual. He took as typical the development of the embryo-sac after fertilization, virtually in fact the only example where cells *are* formed without cell walls being laid down between them. However, as botanists described further examples of cell formation Schleiden's theories became less and less tenable. Several workers investigated the nature of the ground-substance of cells, especially in animals, in the 1830s and found it to be contractile and glutinous. Purkinje used the word 'protoplasm' to label it in 1839. This progress in cell theory was held up for years because it was not realized that only nuclei give rise to nuclei, so that the concept of nucleus and protoplasm forming a cell was some time in coming.

Work in embryology helped to overcome this difficulty. Good descriptive studies of cleavage had shown nuclei without their significance being understood, but slowly the concept became established that division of a cell into two equal daughter cells was the normal method by which cells increased in number during normal growth. Technical advances in both microscope and specimen preparation were required to visualize what went on when the nucleus divided.

By about 1850, the high power of a good instrument had the resolution of a modern 4 mm objective, and by about 1870, this had been given improved contrast also. With the introduction by Ernst Abbe (1840–1905) of homogeneous immersion by 1880, and of apochromatic objectives by 1890, the resolution (but not the contrast) of the microscope system had reached its theoretical maximum. Instruments were convenient in use and relatively cheaper than they had been, and their use in medicine was firmly established. Proper fixing of tissues, rendering them subsequently inalterable and simultaneously making more visible their component parts, was slowly established by about 1870. Colouring of specimens by applying various stains took off during the 1860s and was normal by about 1880. Sectioning of properly supported specimens was achieved in the 1880s, to give a battery of preparative techniques much as we still know them. However, it was not *until* the 1880s that all this was routine and widely followed. The difficulties faced by individual workers in the period 1830 to 1880, when so much was achieved but so much was misunderstood, cannot easily be overestimated.

It is in this context that understanding of the nature of the nucleus and its division must be seen. Nuclear details are at about the limit of visibility of the light microscope, and as those carrying out the work had no understanding of the significance of the processes, there was no conceptual framework to assist. In the 1840s, several workers had described a radiating appearance inside cells during cleavage. This kind of observation owed much to a fortunate choice of material, for it was to be many years before it was apparent that in some species the details of nuclear division are very clear, while in others they are just the opposite. It was thus not until the 1860s that the sequence of events started to become clear, and a great deal of work was published in the 1870s, when papers often included details of fertilization as well as subsequent nuclear divisions. By the end of the 1870s, Walther Flemming (1843–1905) emerged as a leading researcher in the field, and published in 1882 his famous *Zellsubstanz, Kern und Zelltheilung* synthesizing cytological research. He gave the name 'mitosis' to nuclear division, and set out the steps followed, noting that the chromosomes divided longitudinally: this was still not universally acknowledged. It was also recognized that, in some species at least, there was a constant number of chromosomes.

It was also late in the 1880s that a different type of division, in the germ cells, finally came to be understood, largely through the work of Theodor Boveri (1862–1915) and of W. A. O. Hertwig (1849–1922), although it was not until 1905 that J. B. Farmer (1865–1944) and J. E. Moore (b. 1892) introduced the word 'maiosis' (later altered to 'meiosis') to describe the special type of nuclear division that results in a halving of the number of chromosomes. It required an immense amount of work throughout both animal and plant kingdoms, to establish that meiotic division occurs in all sexually reproducing organisms. It is difficult to recall nowadays that the significance of the process was not to be understood for many more years. Although J. G. Mendel (1822–84) had carried out his work on what was later to be called inheritance (entirely without need of a microscope) in the 1860s, it had to be rediscovered in 1900 before the concept of the unit character of inheritance had a chance of becoming established.

It was in the United States that the significance of meiosis was revealed in 1902, in the fundamental work of W. B. Cannon (1871–1945) and others. The paper by W. S. Sutton (1877–1916) dated 1903 sets out the matter once and for all, and forecasts the nature of what we now call genes.[3]

More microscopical research was needed to establish the identity and behaviour of sex chromosomes, linkage, and other phenomena of inheritance. The real breakthrough occurred when T. H. Morgan (1866–1945) chose *Drosophila*, the fruit fly, as his experimental animal.[4] This breeds once every two weeks, has four readily observable chromosomes, and rapidly produces mutations which can be studied to enable maps of genes to be made: this had been done for fifty genes by 1915, a remarkable breakthrough. A vast amount of work was thus triggered and continues to the present day, including the discoveries leading to our understanding of nucleic acids. As part of this work, ultraviolet microscopy was applied. First developed by A. Köhler (1866–1948) in 1904, and requiring lenses made only from quartz (which alone transmits the short wavelengths), the technique provided greater resolution than visible wavelengths. In the 1930s, T. O. Caspersson (b. 1910) in Sweden used electronic means to record and amplify the images, allowing him to provide absorption curves for very small particles of material, giving information about the distribution of nucleic acids in the cell. In these various ways the functions of the nucleus and its various parts were slowly unravelled, to culminate in the discovery of the double-helix structure of DNA by J. D. Watson (b. 1928) and F. H. Crick (b. 1916) in 1953.

In the history of microscopical observations of cells, the nucleus attracted much attention because it was clearly visible – almost at the limit of resolution of the instrument. Other organelles were not so clearly visible, and their structure, and indeed their very existence, were questioned until the advent of the electron microscope. A fundamental difficulty with such complicated components is in their preparation for viewing. Until later in the nineteenth century, this was unsatisfactory, and much of the work published described essentially pathological structures. It is a fairly modern concept that to prepare and to observe tissues in a wide variety of ways will alone enable us to form a reasonably accurate picture of their true make-up. Such means were developed only slowly.

In the first explosion of work in microscopy of the 1840s and 1850s, the papers themselves describe pathological changes taking place as, for example, nerve fibres were excised and examined. The introduction of hardening agents arose from the need to allow easier excision: the fixing action was a happy by-product. Details of the introduction of reagents and techniques to carry through the exceptionally complicated series of events required to prepare a tissue mount can only be briefly summarized here, in the specific context of cytology. In 1833, chromic acid was first used as a hardening agent, but many workers still continued to use water or blood serum for mounting for another twenty years. Another important substance for fixing, osmic acid, was used from 1864, and this was to be very hepful in cytology later in the century. The now universally applied formaldehyde was not introduced until 1893. Unfortunately, to quote such a few bare dates may actually conceal truth rather than reveal it. The first mention in the literature of these substances is just that: it does not represent in any way their widespread use and thus any marked influence on microscopical research. In general this would be slow to develop, especially in the earlier years.

The same must be said of the introduction of staining techniques. A note of the mere first use of a dyestuff may be quite misleading: very often it is how it is used that is significant. Natural staining substances such as carmine and haematoxylin illustrate this very well. If carmine is not used at the right concentration for the right length of time, minute structures are simply not shown up, causing errors to be reported in the literature. If haematoxylin is not used with a mordant, it usually fails to stain, with similar results. For cytology, the use of metallic impregnation, as opposed to simple colouring, was the key to revealing minute details, and although the technique attracted attention in the 1860s it was 1880 before it was reliable and repeatable. It has already been said that infiltration and serial sectioning were techniques of the 1880s, and thus it is not surprising that it was during that decade that cytology began to yield impressive results.

The fibrous nature of cytoplasm was revealed as a net-like structure in fixed tissues, and it was not until the end of the century that W. B. Hardy (1864–1934) showed that the fixatives used profoundly affected the appearance of the cytoplasm. This meant that little had been achieved in elucidating its structure. Certain cytoplasmic inclusions had been described before then, and named 'mitochondria'. These structures attracted much attention in the early 1900s, and because it was possible to observe them in unfixed cells as well as in fixed ones, and to colour them while living with vital stains, their existence was not seriously contested. It required differential centrifugation to show that mitochondria are concerned with respiration, and the same technique also revealed a range of other particles from cytoplasm.

A major controversy arose concerning the very existence of another organelle, the Golgi bodies. This network shows up clearly in some cells treated with metallic impregnation, but many theories were put forward to explain them – for example, that they were merely vacuoles actually formed as a result of impregnation. Even in 1954 the dispute still raged, but since then, electron microscopy has shown that they do exist, along with many other minute and highly complicated structures in the cytoplasm.

MORBID ANATOMY

The above remarks apply to the normal, but it was in the context of the pathological that the concept that all cells arise only from cells was first stated. The microscope was applied to morbid anatomy only very slowly, although work on normal histology began in the mid-seventeenth century. This was due less to technical shortcomings in the instrument than to eighteenth-century theories and attitudes. As we have seen, Schwann realized the commonality of cellular structure between plants and animals, but was mistaken as to how cells arise. Pathology at that time relied on gross observations resting on purely hypothetical systematics. R. C. Virchow (1821–1902) first cut through these thickets, decisively rejecting both free cell formation and spontaneous generation: in 1855, he published a paper on cellular pathology in his own journal urging the wider use of the microscope by pathologists, and set out his famous aphorism '*omnis cellula e cellula*'. He later delivered a series of lectures on cell theory applied to understanding the phenomena of disease and healing: in 1858, these were published as his famous *Cellular-pathologie*. This seminal work came to revolutionize medical thought, but other views were widespread, and the English version of 1860 was received with some criticism in England. Lionel Beale (1828–1906), in London, was largely responsible for overcoming this entrenched opposition, but it took most of the 1860s. All of this was accomplished in the almost total absence of knowledge as to how diseases were spread. (➤ Ch. 16 Contagion/germ theory/ specificity)

A further interest that occupied many minds last century was an understanding of the process of inflammation, largely building on the theories of John Hunter (1728–93), as published in his *A Treatise on Blood, Inflammation and Gunshot Wounds* (1794). Pioneer experimental work was carried out by Dr Todd of Brighton, who punctured the web of frogs' feet, allowed them to heal for various periods, and then mounted the result for the microscope. On his death, the slides were sold to the Hunterian Museum at the Royal College of Surgeons, where the young John T. Quekett (1815–61) helped the eminent Benjamin Travers (1783–1858) to inspect them. Having decided that the actual living inflammation would have to be inspected, they then set up their own series of frogs, and the outcome was duly reported in Travers's *The Physiology of Inflammation and the Healing Process* (1844). Both of these endeavours represented long programmes of sustained scientific work, applying the microscope to the problem. The preparations survive in the museum.

Much of the preoccupation with injection of blood vessels seen in the nineteenth century may stem from studies of inflammation, the capillaries, and the origin of pus. This was of obvious practical concern in the surgery of the times, and it was Joseph Lister (1827–1912) who drew attention to the fact that vascular dilatation preceded tissue changes. J. Cohnheim (1839–84) proved in 1867 that white corpuscles migrate through capillary walls, thus forming pus, although why they should do so was unclear until E. Metchnikoff (1845–1916) demonstrated their phagocytic action. The local chemical control mechanisms of inflammation, the role of histamines and antibodies, took much longer to demonstrate, and the whole is a good example of many workers combining to solve a problem which at first looked very simple.

HISTOLOGICAL LITERATURE

The results already described were obtained by a relatively few dedicated research workers. What of the generality of medical practitioners, in their work and in their training? Clearly, the microscope figured little in medical courses before the 1830s, in which decade alone it became established as a research tool, as we have seen, to provide a basis of histological knowledge by the early 1840s. The books by F. G. J. Henle (1809–85) on the epithelia, *Symbolae ad Anatomiam* (1837), and on more general histology, *Allgemeine Anatomie* (1841), were key works. The first textbook in English was that of A. H. Hassall (1817–94), *The Microscopical Anatomy of the Human Body, in Health and Disease* (1846, 1849): this included the first description of the corpuscles of the thymus, and is very well illustrated, albeit largely with pictures derived from injected preparations. The first textbook in any language entirely devoted to preparative and manipulative techniques was Quekett's *Practical Treatise on the Use of the Microscope* (1848). It is thus no coincidence that courses in histology for medical practitioners took off in the 1840s. Guy's Hospital Medical School in London included such work from 1843, while J. H. Bennett (1812–75) in Edinburgh and H. W. Acland (1815–1900) in Oxford offered courses from 1845. Quekett had very comprehensive facilities at the Royal College of Surgeons shortly afterwards, and published his lectures in 1851, as well as producing many thousands of preparations (some of them from Hunter's earlier specimens). Many of these survive, and provide a most important scientific resource to the present day, supported as they are by published and manuscript material. (➤ Ch. 48 Medical education)

Some study of published textbooks of histology is most revealing of the progress of the science. The important 1842 booklet by J. Paget (1814–99) contains in its fifty-one pages a summary of virtually all contemporary knowledge, but includes nothing of retina or inner ear, nerve endings or nerve structure. Quekett's *Lectures on Histology* (1851) are a blend of plant and animal histology, omitting many of the usual tissues. Some works had appeared on the European continent, notably in Germany, but also by such as A. Donné (1801–78) in France, and it was from Germany that the first textbook of histology in the modern form was published by R. A. von Kölliker (1817–1905), a colleague of Virchow, in 1852. He was the first to apply the cell theory of Schwann to descriptive embryology, and a well-illustrated English version appeared the next year. It is worth quoting from the author's preface:

> Medicine has reached a point, at which Microscopical Anatomy appears to constitute its foundation, quite as much as the Anatomy of the Organs and systems; and when a profound study of Physiology and Pathological Anatomy is impossible, without an accurate acquaintance also, with the most minute structural conditions.

Further consideration of nerve and sense-organ entries in textbooks is enlightening, as these tissues are still among the most difficult to prepare and to interpret, and thus offer a useful guide to progress. Research on these topics went on apace in the 1850s and 1860s, with important papers published as a result of the application of new staining techniques. Kölliker's *Manual of Human Microscopic Anatomy* (1860) is a convenient starting-point, and there is a much better depiction of retina than in the version of only a few years earlier. The *Handbuch der Lehre* of 1869–72 (translated into English virtually as the volumes appeared) by S. Stricker (1834–98) contained an entry on retina written by Max Schultze (1825–74), and represents an enormous gain in knowledge compared with an edition of Stricker thirteen years earlier. The 1869 book included contributions from no fewer than ten histologists writing on the eye and its appendages alone – a remarkable group from one country. L. A. Ranvier's (1835–1922) ambitious *Leçons sur l'histologie du système nerveux* (1878) has excellent plates, and is another landmark text. C. Golgi (1844–1926), and S. Ramón y Cajal (1852–1934) later applied most powerfully techniques of metallic impregnation to the elucidation of nerve structure, and others had worked specifically on brain, culminating in the work by A. W. Campbell (1868–1937), *Histological Studies on the Localisation of Cerebral Function* (1905), impossible to conceive without the foregoing.

BACTERIOLOGY

During the fifty years immediately following J. J. Lister's announcement of his discovery of aplanatic foci in 1830, as we have seen, microscopy came of age. Its very complicated techniques were developed, in specimen preparation as in optical technique. Ernst Abbe formulated the theory of the instrument in such a way as to enable him to design homogeneous immersion systems that could yield high magnification coupled with appropriate resolution. He designed also the apochromatic objectives, using new kinds of glass, which gave better-quality images than ever before. More important still, his computations allowed manufacturers to begin to make objectives on a rational, rather than trial-and-error basis. This came to mean that a large number of instruments of good quality and smaller cost could become available, allowing the microscope a very wide use by the end of the nineteenth century. By then also an entirely new use for the instrument had developed, one that would require widespread effort and the use of instruments that performed at the theoretical limits. This was the science of bacteriology.

Microscopical progress had provided medicine with insights unimagined at the start of the century, giving a functional basis to knowledge both normal and pathological. The cell had become recognized as the unit of life, and a beginning had been made on understanding how it reproduced. For the patient at the receiving end, the advent of anaesthetics by mid-century had controlled pain and allowed surgery to proceed at a proper pace, but the risk of infection remained. However, the work by Louis Pasteur (1822–95), built on by Lister and others, enabled the germ theory of disease to take root in the 1870s, but it needed the genius of H. H. R. Koch (1843–1910) to establish it. We find it very difficult nowadays to put ourselves in the position of our predecessors, threatened quite frequently with death from epidemic disease, but having no knowledge of how it was transmitted, and faced also with death after sustaining a possibly quite simple injury when it was followed by fever and infection. The sheer difficulty of discovering and proving that one of a group of very similar minute parasitic plants was responsible in a particular case was enormous. (➤ Ch. 52 Epidemiology)

In 1840, F. G. J. Henle's chapter on miasmata and contagia was published in his *Pathologische Untersuchungen.* (➤ Ch. 15 Environment and miasmata) In this he set out his belief (he had no proof) that the cause of contagious disease was living material in the infected patient giving rise to the symptoms of the disease. He was unable to discover any such material, but did draw attention to the muscardine disease of silkworms already shown to be due to a fungus. He also laid down that such material must always be shown to be present with the disease, and be isolatable and able to reproduce the disease in a susceptible animal. This was a very important series of statements, but the microscopy of the time could not demonstrate the small organisms now known to be involved, nor could other techniques isolate them. The germ theory was thus unprovable, and fell into disrepute for a while.

By 1850, forms had been seen in the blood of cows with anthrax, independently by C. J. Davaine (1812–82) in France and F. A. A. Pollender (1800–79) in Germany. In the 1860s, Davaine continued his work, called the forms 'bacteria', and supposed that they were similar to those shown by Pasteur to cause butyric fermentations. Pasteur's famous work on flasks of broth opened in the pure air of mountains and in the air of cities, and left open with dust-trap tubes, attracted attention and brought back to the scientific mind the germ theory. However, it needed Koch, in 1876, to prove that Davaine's bacteria were indeed the cause of anthrax. It should not be supposed that the medical and scientific worlds at once accepted that bacteria might cause human diseases of various kinds. Under the microscope, most are so similar that the possibility of their being actually many different species was not entertained, and some influential workers still believed that they arose by spontaneous generation. H. Charlton Bastian (1837–1915), for example, believed this until the end of his life, as he could not conceive that there could exist forms of life capable of withstanding the temperature of boiling water – a not unreasonable belief for the time!

The real breakthrough was not microscopical as such, but the discovery of pure-culture techniques, based on cultivation on solid media. Originally using the fresh-cut surface on a potato, Koch soon solidified other media by using gelatine, so that by 1881, bacteriology was poised to develop as a science. Later, agar was used as the solidifying agent, and in 1887 R. J. Petri

(1852–1921) introduced his famous dish. A major microscopical difficulty is that bacteria are hardly visible under the microscope, unless they have been treated in a variety of ways. Different bacteria require very different techniques, and thus a long time was to elapse before it could be realized just how wide is the variety of organisms that display so narrow a range of form.

Koch himself was responsible for much progress. In 1882, largely unaided, he commenced the science of clinical bacteriology by staining smears from tuberculosis autopsy material with dilute alkaline methylene blue for twenty-four hours. This demonstrated bacteria in thin films, but he could not do so in sections. The difficulty here is that the bacteria are not numerous, and stain to resemble tissue components. He was successful in counterstaining with vesuvin, and this stimulated Paul Ehrlich (1854–1915) to work on the topic, using aniline oil in his mixture. The time taken was shorter, and proved repeatable and definite in its results. This was of first importance clinically at the time, for tuberculosis was a major scourge. Such direct microscopy was rapidly applied to other diseases and results came thick and fast. Fortunately, the many aniline dyes already available, and tested in general histology, proved capable of application also in bacteriology. The Gram stain was introduced in 1884, and later became virtually mandatory as part of the description of an organism. To the popular mind, however, it was the identification of the cholera organism which was a major triumph, for the disease was feared and widespread. (➤ Ch. 11 Clinical research) In 1883, Koch went to Egypt to investigate an outbreak, and concluded that comma-shaped germs in the gut were the cause. This was denied the next year by E. E. Klein (1844–1925) from England, as similar-looking organisms were found in the absence of the disease. It was, of course, part of Koch's additional technique to characterize the organism by its action in liquefying gelatine, and not alone by its simple stained appearance. This brought about the adoption of biochemical and nutritional as well as morphological techniques in bacteriology, and these would loom ever larger in the years that followed.

TWENTIETH-CENTURY DEVELOPMENTS

After 1900, the use of the microscope became ever wider, as improvements in manufacturing techniques were evolved. There was, at the one end of the spectrum of instruments, the very complete research outfit with its remarkable complement of accessories, largely the preserve of the wealthy English amateur. Although this was rarely used for serious scientific research, the requirement ever to produce improved optics stimulated the industry as a whole. At the other end of the spectrum was the, usually continental, model shorn of all but the basics, made and sold cheaply, and used very widely in training and research. This last rapidly became the subject of assembly-line manufacture by such as Leitz, making very large numbers of instruments available for use during and after the First World War. This was most timely, in view of the rise in systematic public-health work. (➤ Ch. 51 Public health)

From the beginning of the twentieth century, interest had developed in fresh material – that is, in material that was still living. Much of this was single-celled (Protozoa), sometimes stained intravitally to provide that contrast necessary for visualization. The difficulty with such work was that it was at the limits of resolution, and lacked visual contrast. Further biochemical work proceeded apace in the first half of the century, and was applied increasingly at the micro level, to stimulate the development of the science of histochemistry.

A scarcely credible amount of microscopical work was carried through before the Second World War. Scientific research started to become organized in much the same way as today, with larger laboratories and more staff than ever before. It was possible to organize a salaried career in medical research in hospital, university or even commercial laboratories, and many did so all over the world. The microscope coped very well indeed with stained material, for which preparation techniques were by now routine and rapid. Many scientific preparations survive from every decade of this century (although often largely forgotten in cupboards in medical schools), and it is possible to check the literature against the slide in a systematic manner. Also, many eminent scientists' preparations survive in archives and museums, and are of the greatest importance.

The microscope did not cope very well with living material, since it lacks the necessary contrast. This difficulty was not resolved until the 1950s, when the phase-contrast microscope was widely used. Invented by F. Zernike (1888–1966) in the 1930s but held up by the Second World War, this instrument allowed those working with individual living cells to see what they were doing at adequate resolution for the first time. The techniques of cytosurgery developed apace, for example, and have continued to do so with the formulation of long working distance optics, inverted instruments, and the like. This was a revolutionary achievement, and it was closely followed by an even more useful contrast technique – differential interference. Several workers developed systems that showed up minute differences in optical path as differences in colours to which the eye is very sensitive. Initially these were difficult to set up, but by the 1970s such systems as that of G. X. Nomarski were coming into widespread use for medical work, making it still easier to perform cytosurgery and to inject separate living cells.

A further development in light microscopy (which many had said was dead with the advent of electron microscopy) was to be of major significance in medical work: fluorescence techniques. Some cell components have the ability to absorb shorter wavelengths (invisible to the eye) and to re-emit them as longer wavelengths (visible as colours). Special fluorochromes were slowly discovered which were taken up by highly specialized parts of the cell, to reveal their exact whereabouts. By the later 1970s, this was a growth area of considerable potential in medical research. In the later 1980s, with the separately developed ability to make fluorochromes with immunological bindings, it became possible to target individual molecules for inspection in the living cell. This is a development which our predecessors could never have imagined, and one which holds the greatest potential for research into normal and especially abnormal cytology and inheritance. (➤ Ch. 36 The science of diagnosis: diagnostic technology; Ch. 68 Medical technologies: social contexts and consequences)

The modern ability to inspect living tissues and cells has brought about a resurgence in the use of frozen sections. These had a vogue in the 1870s and early 1880s, before infiltration and serial sectioning were established as the prime research means. Supporting the tissues by freezing them in an ice-salt mixture enabled them to be cut quite easily – for fixing and staining and examining in the conventional way, as few optical means of providing contrast were to hand. When it was discovered that ether could be used to provide the cooling (in the days before the refrigerator existed to give ice on demand), the use of what we now call cryosections was popular. In the early 1900s, a jet of carbon dioxide from a cylinder provided a more attractive means of cooling, and such sections were sporadically used in biopsy, as results were obtainable while an operation was in progress to help determine its course. In the 1930s and later, cryosections were needed for work in tissue culture, for example, and their use is now widespread (using microtomes built into efficient freezers) in research and in routine biopsy.

At the present time, the light microscope is used so very extensively throughout industry as well as research that it is difficult to imagine modern life without it. The results achieved are so widespread, often as part of a much wider effort involving a spectrum of techniques, that it is true to say that all medical progress now includes microscopical research, to the extent that it is impossible to list individual achievements. Science now relies on teamwork, the days of individual achievers at the bench being part of history.

The same is true of the other fundamental twentieth-century discovery – the electron microscope. From a shaky start in the 1930s, to the beginnings of wider commercial availability in the 1950s (when such an instrument was still regarded with awe even in advanced research establishments), the TEM (transmission electron microscope) is nowadays ubiquitous. Its brother the SEM (scanning electron microscope) had a slightly later start, but is now equally widespread in use. The attraction of the TEM is that it provides magnifications and resolutions up to one thousand times that of the light microscope, with all that that implies for the inspection of cellular components even down eventually to the molecular level. The SEM provides magnifications from about fifty times upwards, giving a 3-D effect with enormous depth of field – far greater than light optics manage. Between them, in the various modes in which they can be used, they have provided remarkable insights into medicine.

The fundamental knowledge of the electron beam had been established last century, but in 1924 it was shown that it could be regarded not only as a negatively charged particle but also as a wave. Hans Walter Busch (b. 1884), two years later, showed that focusing by magnetic coils was analogous to using lenses. Max Knoll (b. 1897) and E. Ruska (1906–88) used two such lenses to make, by 1931, the first electron microscope: it magnified only 17 times, soon increased to x400. This was very rapid development, outlined here to contrast with the very much slower evolution of the light microscope. In 1933, Ruska, persevering in face of many difficulties, built the instrument which is the ancestor of all existing electron microscopes. Commercial production models of TEMs were installed in Germany in 1939, in the USA in 1941, and in the UK in 1945. They were applied to life-science specimens somewhat slowly, as such material required very awkward preparative techniques.

The light microscope's basic image-forming mechanism is one of absorption, the specimen reducing the amplitude of the light passing through it to produce contrast. In the electron microscope, absorption plays virtually no part, the contrast being due to differential scattering of electrons by the atoms of the specimen; these electrons are off axis and blocked by the objective aperture. The amount of scattering increases with the amount of material in the specimen, and a heavy metal such as osmium was used to fix the material as a consequence – an interesting return to an important light-microscopy reagent but for a very different reason. The sections of material used had to be extremely thin, and it is also of interest that the Cambridge rocking microtome, developed by 1885, was of such quality as to be readily adaptable to cutting sections one-hundredth of the original design thickness. Other designs followed, all of them cutting extremely small pieces of tissue. This is an important matter, as the material which can be dealt with is only a very small sample of the whole, and much of the art of TEM work is in choosing the initial sample.

Apart from new designs of microtome, which advanced the specimen to the blade at a very slow and highly controlled rate, a major difficulty was that of the blade itself. Material for cutting came to be embedded in resins and from 1950, sections of high quality were cut by the edge of a fractured piece of plate glass. This apparently trivial discovery was of the very first importance.

In the 1960s, then, the use of the TEM spread apace in medical work and results accumulated that showed something of the true complexity of the fine structure of the cell. Better electronic control of the high-voltage power supply allowed higher magnifications to be achieved routinely in the research laboratory, and in the 1970s it became much easier to section material and to reconstruct the original. This development of the science of stereology has been of much importance in all life-science work.

In the 1970s also, the scanning electron microscope began to become important. This instrument relies on a different principle to produce its images, which are built up for presentation on a cathode ray tube. The images produced are of the surface of the specimen, providing great depth of field and complementing the TEM perfectly. During the 1980s, the TEM was very highly developed, to make routine the capture of more of the reflected energy for analysis with very sophisticated modules. Results from such work give a vast amount of information about organelles obtainable in no other way. More recent attention to observing fracture surfaces and the like with the SEM has shown ever more detail of cytological structure, so that virtually every medical problem nowadays is investigated by electron microscopy as part of a whole armoury of techniques, each applied by experts to provide a pool of results.

Such a pool, or rather torrent, of results creates its own difficulties as well as providing the means for progress. From the earliest days of Hooke in 1665, the intensely visual pursuit of microscopy in whatever form has positively required the production of illustrated reports of work accomplished. In the earlier days, these took the form of engravings made by an engraver from pictures drawn by an artist under the direction of the actual observer. Opportunity for mistake and misinterpretation was rife. The use of photomicrography from about the middle of the nineteenth century very slowly brought some greater degree of objectivity to the reporting, although it would be the turn of that century before photomechanical production of halftones was a possibility in the illustration of scientific papers. Even nowadays, the use of more than a limited number of halftone illustrations, especially in full colour, in a publication is strongly discouraged on grounds of expense. This is a major stumbling-block in communicating results, especially as very sophisticated methods of image manipulation have been evolved.

Image analysis relies on the ability of sophisticated electronic systems to capture the elements of an image, to store it, and to allow various of these elements to be manipulated at will. False colours can be added, and all manner of measurements made of the components. This bald statement conveys virtually nothing of the remarkable possibilities of the systems in use, but the ability to clean up an image by removing background 'noise', and then to analyse the picture systematically has already proved a very powerful tool in many different applications.

New methods of light microscopy have also been developed, an example being that of confocal scanning. This technique allows a light microscope to focus on a very thin layer of living tissue, perhaps below a surface, to observe actual life processes in action.

The first heyday of microscopy was a century ago, when light microscopes were applied widely and systematically for the first time, to the study of bacteriology. The second heyday of microscopy is now, when a remarkably sophisticated range of instruments is applied very much more widely and systematically to the study of all manner of normal and pathological medical problems, but as part only of an attack using a very wide range of techniques and equipment.

NOTES

1 The usual source on Leeuwenhoek is the somewhat uncritical C. Dobell, *Antony van Leeuwenhoek and his 'Little Animals'*, London, Bale, 1932; reprinted Dover Books, 1960. A more modern summary is B. Bracegirdle (ed.), *Beads of Glass: Leeuwenhoek and the Early Microscope*, London, Science Museum, 1983.

2 This complicated technical topic, and others, are discussed by B. Bracegirdle, 'Famous microscopists: Joseph Jackson Lister, 1786–1869', *Proceedings of the Royal Microscopical Society*, 1987, 22: 273–97.

3 W. S. Sutton, 'The chromosomes in heredity', *Biological Bulletin*, 1903, 4: 231–51.

4 T. H. Morgan, 'Sex-linked inheritance in *Drosophila*', *Science*, 1910, 32: 120–2.

FURTHER READING

Baker, J. R., 'The cell-theory: a restatement, history and critique', I: *Quarterly Journal of Medical Science*, 1948, 89: 103–25; II: ibid., 1950, 90: 87–108; III: ibid., 1952, 93: 157–90; IV: ibid., 1953, 94: 407–40; V: ibid., 1955, 96: 449–81.
Beale, L. S., *The Microscope in Medicine*, 4th edn, London, Churchill, 1878.
Bracegirdle, B., *A History of Microtechnique*, London, Heinemann, 1978.
——, 'Light microscopy, 1865–1985', J. Quekett Microscopical Club, 1989, 36: 193–209.
Bradbury, S., *The Evolution of the Microscope*, Oxford, Pergamon Press, 1967.
Carpenter, W. B., *The Microscope and its Revelations*, 8th edn, rev. by W. H. Dallinger, London, Churchill, 1901.
Foster, W. D., *A Short History of Clinical Pathology*, Edinburgh, Livingstone, 1961.
——, *A History of Medical Bacteriology and Immunology*, London, Heinemann, 1970.
Francon, M., *Progress in Microscopy*, Oxford, Pergamon Press, 1961.
Grainger, T. H., *A Guide to the History of Bacteriology*, New York, Ronald Press, 1958.
Hughes, A., *A History of Cytology*, London, Abelard-Schuman, 1959.
Hughes, S. S., *The Virus, a History of the Concept*, London, Heinemann, 1977.
Leeson, Leeson and Paparo, *Text/Atlas of Histology*, Philadelphia, PA, Saunders, 1988.
Russ, J. C., *Computer-Assisted Microscopy*, New York, Plenum, 1990.
Sharp, L. W., *Introduction to Cytology*, 3rd edn, New York, McGraw-Hill, 1934.
Slater, C. and Spitta, E. J., *An Atlas of Bacteriology*, London, Scientific Press, 1898.
Watt, I. M., *The Principles and Practice of Electron Microscopy*, Cambridge, Cambridge University Press, 1985.

7

THE PHYSIOLOGICAL TRADITION

E. M. Tansey

The word *physiologia* was first employed by Jean Fernel (*c*.1497–1558), who derived it from the Greek *physis*, a loose translation of which might be the somewhat ambiguous 'nature'. 'Physiology' was not in routine use until the nineteenth century; before then, both the subject matter and the term itself were subsumed in disciplines and words such as anatomy or the 'institutes of medicine'. Like much scientific thought, physiological ideas can be traced back to the ancient Greeks, to the Hippocratic Corpus, and to Aristotelian natural philosophy, although as an independent experimental science it is much more recent, emerging distinctly only around the middle of the nineteenth century. It did so from older traditions of theoretical medicine: from anatomy, and to a lesser extent from the natural sciences, and it became clearly identified as the study of the *function* of living matter. In turn, this definition narrowed as plant physiology was increasingly recognized as a specialization of botany, and the term 'physiology' became largely synonymous with 'animal physiology'. From the late nineteenth century onwards, the discipline matured, developed and diversified, and contributed to the further subdivision of modern biomedical sciences. Biochemistry, pharmacology, biophysics, endocrinology, and the neurosciences, to name but a few, all owe variable proportions of their intellectual heritages to physiology. Thus the boundaries of what constitutes physiology have been in constant flux, remain so to the present day and will, no doubt, continue. Whilst acknowledging these underlying dynamics, this account will assess the work of those who contributed to the growth of physiological thinking in a predominantly chronological framework, into which a necessarily brief consideration of factors such as institutionalization, funding, professionalization and technical advances will be integrated. Throughout, the word physiology will be used in the modern context of the functional study of the animal body unless otherwise indicated, and the topographical emphasis will be on western Europe and the United States of America.

PHYSIOLOGY IN THE ANCIENT WORLD[1]

The early observation that many living creatures were warm, but became cold when dead, was utilized in explaining the nature of living organisms and the constitution of life itself. The source and distribution of animal heat, the distinguishing feature that apparently conferred the property of living-ness, and its disruption and dissolution in disease and death, preoccupied medical philosophers and practitioners. Theories of life and living function in the ancient world were dominated by two traditions. Hippocratic writings (fifth to third centuries BC) emphasized the significance of the four bodily humours, each with different physical properties: warm, moist blood; the contrasting moist but cold phlegm; black bile which was cold and dry; and the warm but dry yellow bile. The fine balance between these, and the prevailing elements of fire, water, earth, and air, accounted for disposition towards health or disease. (➤ Ch. 14 Humoralism) Aristotelian natural philosophy identified the heart as the seat of the soul, the central nutritive organ, and the source of vital heat. Aristotle (384–322 BC) proposed that blood was produced in the heart, the mechanical action of which was caused by the contraction of warm cardiac blood after mixing with cold blood arriving in the left ventricle from the lungs. Within Greek culture such unifying concepts of form and function in living things merged comfortably with ideas of medicine and healing, which combined both body and soul in a coherent account of the nature of human beings. Almost five centuries later, Galen (AD 129–c.200) modified and codified these earlier accounts into a form that was to endure for over a thousand years. They can be briefly summarized: nutriment was absorbed by the liver, where it was transformed into blood; transported to the heart, the blood passed through invisible pores in the septum from the right to the left side, where it was mixed with the *pneuma*, or life spirit, drawn from the external world by the act of breathing; thus vitalized, the blood then ebbed and flowed in the major arteries and veins. These ideas persisted for many centuries. Preserved through the Dark Ages in the Arab world, and then recovered by the Western world in the late medieval period, they were easily incorporated into Christian traditions of creation, and became accepted, unquestioned, dogma. Challenges to these concepts, and the religious and medical authorities that maintained them, did not occur until the Renaissance. (➤ Ch. 61 Religion and medicine)

THE RENAISSANCE

Philosophical emphasis on reasoning from experiment, as advocated by Francis Bacon (1561–1626), and developments of new or improved instruments, like the astronomical telescope, with which to explore the natural world, encouraged bold enquiry about structure and function of living organisms, and in particular acknowledged humans as legitimate objects of scientific study. Concern with the working of the body in health and disease became recognized as the theoretical basis of practical medicine, and was taught under the auspices of the 'institutes of medicine', and closely associated with anatomy, pathology, and medical practice. Simultaneously, conceptual and technical advances in many other areas of Renaissance science, such as those in chemistry, mechanics, and architecture, emphasized shifts from more abstract accounts to the realization that new knowledge could have practical importance. (➤ Ch. 5 The anatomical tradition; Ch. 9 The pathological tradition)

An outstanding example is provided by William Harvey (1578–1657), who challenged the Galenic view of blood generation and distribution in his classic treatise on the movement of the heart and blood in animals, *Exercitatio anatomica de motu cordis et sanguinis* (1628). He postulated that the blood constantly circulated around the living body, having arrived at this radical conclusion by experimenting upon the circulatory systems of a wide range of animals; by reflecting on the significance of what he saw; and by demonstrating his results and explanations to his colleagues. Harvey established that blood was ejected from the right ventricle into the pulmonary circulation, returning to the left side of the heart, and then pumped around the rest of the body, being returned to the heart through a system of veins. Paradoxically, Harvey promoted the existence of components he was unable to see, most notably the presence of the capillary bed, whilst simultaneously dismissing the existence of the widely accepted, but never seen, cardiac septum pores. His work explained observed form – the multi-chambered heart, the distribution and gross morphology of the blood vessels (especially the pulmonary vessels), and the venous valves – in terms of proposed function derived from experimental manipulations. Conversely, the function ascribed to these parts was explained in terms of their structure – the muscular, multi-chambered heart was the pump of the system; the veins returned blood to the heart because they contained valves that prevented backwards flow. Harvey's influence continued most strikingly in Oxford, where a group of physiologists, including Robert Boyle (1627–91), Richard Lower (1631–91), Robert Hooke (1635–1703), and John Mayow (1641–79), using animal experiments and specially constructed equipment, studied the composition of the air, the process of respiration, attempted the first blood transfusion, and continued work on the circulation of the blood.[2]

The morphological advances made during the seventeenth century continued to promote new questions about the component parts of the animal body, and new scientific expertise in mechanics, thermodynamics, and optics – to say nothing of that in more apparently relevant subjects like chemistry, microscopy, and pathology – all contributed to further studies of physiological function.

Following Harvey, another Englishman, the clergyman Stephen Hales (1677–1761), confirmed the pulsatile nature of the circulation. Trained in mathematics and physics, he put these to use by attempting a quantitative assessment of the blood pressure, a precursor to the technique later developed into a routine diagnostic tool. Hales measured pressure by inserting brass tubes into the jugular vein and the carotid artery of a living horse, and observed that the arterial pressure, calibrated in feet and inches, was much greater than the venous pressure. He tried to determine several mechanical parameters of the circulatory system, and suggested that blood vessels could constrict or dilate under different conditions.

By this time, there was beginning to be more widespread, albeit still cautious, recognition that the *measurement* of biological parameters might be important in understanding the underlying physiological processes. One adherent of this view was Santorio Santorio (1561–1636), who examined fluctuations in normal human functions. To do this, he invented an instrument to count the pulse rate and also used a thermometer to assess the body's temperature. More startling, however, were his metabolic experiments, in which he charted his own body weight, food intake, and excreted output, using a specially constructed chair-balance. These revealed the regular loss, through 'insensible perspiration', of a small amount of body weight, and provided the theoretical basis of all modern metabolic investigations. (➤ Ch. 35 The art of diagnosis: medicine and the five senses)

THE ENLIGHTENMENT

By the beginning of the eighteenth century, the freshness of the Renaissance gave way to the more rational exploration of the Enlightenment. Modes of investigation were restricted, the principal approaches limited by technical prowess at blunt dissection with a knife, aided perhaps by a low-power hand-lens. From these developed diverse, but still anatomically based, enquiries such as those that involved the removal and grinding up or chemical dissociation of body tissues, to identify constituent parts. From such exercises emerged different and differing accounts of functional mechanisms.

Hermann Boerhaave (1668–1738), a professor of the institutes of medicine at Leiden University, attempted to provide a rational scientific foundation for medical practice. He proposed that integrated functional *systems* operated both independently, and to some extent synergistically, within the body, to form a coherent whole. In this, he was strongly influenced by the mechanistic philosophies of René Descartes (1596–1650), who in *De Homine* (1662) likened the body to a clockwork mechanism, functioning according to mechanical laws and principles. Boerhaave further considered the body to be composed of a series of vessels through which vital body fluids ebbed and flowed, and it was the movement, obstruction or stagnation of these fluids that subsequently accounted for health or disease. Such views were not without their critics, one of the most prominent being Georg Stahl (1657–1734), who was dissatisfied with such mechanist theories for the unique properties of living matter. He proposed an alternative 'animist' theory, which maintained that the human body was merely the temporary casing of a controlling *anima* or immortal soul created by God. John Hunter (1728–93) likewise proposed a 'life-principle' to account for the property that distinguished living organisms from non-living matter.

Boerhaave's interpretations and teachings, however, influenced generations of medical practitioners and theorists, one of whom was Albrecht von Haller (1708–77), an intriguing Swiss citizen who was a physician, poet, and government official. Haller closely annotated an edition of his teacher's writings and produced several major works of his own, including *Primae linea physiologicae* (1747) and *De partibus corporis humani sensibilibus et irritabilibus* (1752), critically developing Boerhaave's theories by further dividing animal organs and tissues according to their reactive properties, into 'sensible' and 'irritable' parts.

Haller's major extension of the Boerhaavian concept of vessels was to postulate that the solid parts of the body were composed of fibrous particles, the constituent fibres being of three main categories. Connective fibres formed the vasculature, membranes, and supportive tissues of the major organs. The other two categories, nerve fibres and muscle fibres, were endowed with particular vital properties, these being *sensibility*, or responsiveness to painful stimuli (nerve fibres); or *irritability*, the property of contractility in response to stimulation (muscle fibres). Haller's theories, based on experimental procedures and observations on animals and humans, thus not only typified organ structures according to their fibre composition, but also ascribed to those fibres *physiological* sensitivities which in turn accounted for their responses to specific stimulation.

These revolutionary new concepts of irritability and sensibility achieved widespread acceptance, and promoted further modification and interpretation. Johann Blumenbach (1752–1840) in Göttingen delineated several additional vital properties, including a 'moulding' quality responsible for regenerative actions, whilst William Cullen (1710–1790), a professor of medicine at the institutes of medicine at Edinburgh, concentrated his account on just one vital characteristic, that of the nervous system, which he considered as a reactive 'filter' between the organism and its environment. Haller's ideas were thus being reformulated, reworked, and amplified by many theorists, but they remained essentially qualitative. For example, Xavier Bichat (1771–1802), from Montpellier, performed dissections and examinations from which he proposed a theory of twenty-one different membranes or tissues as the fundamental units of living matter. Whilst not apparently employing a microscope himself, Bichat's proposals encouraged its more widespread use by others, and promoted histological investigations. (➤ Ch. 6 The microscopical tradition) This stimulated a wide range of new studies at a level below that of the whole organism and, in turn, these studies facilitated the formulation of new questions about function.

Towards the end of the eighteenth century, experimental, especially quantitative, approaches were becoming more routine and accepted. A particularly novel procedure had been adopted by the French naturalist René Réaumur (1683–1757), in his studies of digestive processes and their relationship to fermentation. He trained a pet kite to swallow and regurgitate small fenestrated tubes filled with food, and careful examination of these indicated that meat was more fully digested in the stomach than were starchy foods. Similarly, by using small pieces of sponge rather than tubes, Réaumur obtained samples of gastric juices. Lazzaro Spallanzani (1729–99), famous also for performing the first artificial fertilization, extended Réaumur's practice and observations. By swallowing and regurgitating linen pouches, he emphasized that gastric function was only one component of the digestive process. Like Réaumur, he was unable to analyse the chemical nature of the gastric secretions he obtained, but observed that outside the body they induced decomposition of foodstuffs, especially when warmed.

In the final decade of the eighteenth century, the accidental observation that a frog muscle contracted when a metal pin in the spinal cord was stimulated by contact with another metal led Luigi Galvani (1737–98) to postulate the existence of animal electricity, arguing that the muscle mass itself was a reservoir of electricity that caused the muscles to function. A lengthy and acrimonious debate developed with Allessandro Volta (1745–1827), as the latter maintained that electricity had to be applied to a muscle to make it contract. The debates continued long after Galvani's death and were not adequately resolved until Emil du Bois-Reymond (1818–96) (see p. 129) integrated Galvani's concept into a theory of the electrical nature of the nervous impulse.[3]

THE BEGINNING OF THE EXPERIMENTAL TRADITION

The nineteenth century brought an increasingly industrial society, and an air of pragmatism that gradually permeated scientific and medical studies. Paradoxically, as industry and technology encroached on daily life, there were movements away from mechanist explanations of living processes. In Germany in particular, Romantic ideas, encapsulated in the *Naturphilosophie* movement, provided a system of beliefs about, and reflections on, natural processes that reached a peak of acceptability and influence in the first half of the century. These changing perspectives and the spreading, although reluctant, embrasure of technology were accompanied by a growing acceptance of the power, both real and rhetorical, of scientific claims.

The flourishing of the hospital encouraged recognition of medicine as a specialized activity by professionally trained and regulated personnel, carried out in a designated building. (➤ Ch. 49 The hospital). Additionally, the growing awareness among medical practitioners that disease processes involved pathological changes emphasized dynamic *functional* aspects of health and illness. Both factors were important in the subsequent development of the ways in which physiological questions were in turn recognized and then addressed. Within European medicine, attention began to shift markedly away from the medical schools of universities such as those of Leiden and Edinburgh, with their learned Enlightenment values, to newer establishments which emphasized more practical approaches and consequent applications. These were often associated with key figures, such as Claude Bernard (1813–78) in Paris and Carl Ludwig (1816–95) in Germany (see pp. 127–30), and students from across Europe and even from North America began to travel the roads recently traversed by pathologists and chemists, to learn new attitudes and methods for the promotion of physiology. (➤ Ch. 48 Medical education)

During this period, physiology's ensuing growth and differentiation into an independent experimental science can be clearly identified. Although assorted influences operated at divergent periods in different countries throughout the nineteenth century, similar sequences and rhythms of development can be discerned: the creation of full-time research and teaching positions; the provision of adequately equipped institutions for research and teaching; the establishment of professional journals and societies; and wider opportunities for travel. These factors all contributed to integrated advances towards professional physiological studies, especially across western Europe and North America. As laboratories and technical expertise improved, other factors became associated with, and in turn influenced, this diversification, most notably the increasing use of experimental methods; that is, the deliberate and systematic manipulation of natural processes. Moves in this direction were facilitated in particular by the growing acceptability of the use of animals in experiments, an approach considerably accelerated towards the end of the century by the routine use of reliable anaesthetics. Instrumental techniques improved, especially as microscopes became increasingly available, powerful, and accurate. Additionally, sophisticated, specifically designed items of equipment were produced, and their employment became the accepted norm for those pursuing scientific activities, and also for later translation into diagnostic procedures. (➤ Ch. 36 The science of diagnosis: diagnostic technology) Some explicit examples will be given below (pp. 132 ff.). At the same time, both physicians and surgeons sought to enhance their professional status and recognized that claims to exclusivity demanded specialist training. Thus by the end of the nineteenth century, several significant components of the supporting structure for professional physiological study were in place. (➤ Ch. 47 History of the medical profession)

THE PLACE OF WORK: INSTITUTES AND LABORATORIES

The most consistent and successful of the early attempts to provide dedicated facilities for the pursuit of new scientific endeavours were taken in France and Germany, represented here by Claude Bernard and Carl Ludwig. The latter in particular provided a model for the development of physiology across the world.

In France, two distinct stimuli promoted physiology during the first half of the nineteenth century. Hospital medicine in Paris fostered a revolution in medical practice, which, with the concomitant creation of the clinic and the furtherance of bedside clincial teaching, had encouraged practitioners to formulate and then to test explanations of disease processes.[4] (➤ Ch. 11 Clinical research) From this inherently medical tradition arose several of France's most distinguished physiologists, including Bichat, François Magendie (1783–1855), and his pupil Claude Bernard. Recent literature has highlighted also the significance of the veterinary schools as cradles of physiology, because the mighty French war machine provided a regular supply of diseased and old army horses for experimental purposes.[5] Thus in both medical and veterinary contexts, experimental physiology was increasingly promoted because of its recognized utility.

In different German states, the rise of experimental techniques was accompanied by the ready recognition that this new approach required an infrastructure of support, of specialized rooms and even buildings, of equipment and instruments. Several states, for varying reasons, advocated and provided specialized institutes for the pursuit of experimental medical research, and Breslau, Heidelberg, Leipzig, and Munich all developed laboratories and institutes for the support and promotion of physiology. These specialized places of work, with full-time research staff, provided a physical base to which students could be recruited and from which, subsequently, acolytes could be dispatched.[6] In France, in contrast, the absence of such well-equipped institutes and laboratories hampered the development of physiology.

CLAUDE BERNARD (1813–78)[7]

Claude Bernard has a twofold importance in the history of physiology: first as an experimentalist in his own right; and second, and of substantial consequence for the advance and spread of new ideas and techniques, as a teacher. The two functions are clearly intertwined: as the investigator of metabolic function, the elucidator and promoter of the concept of the *milieu intérieur* – one of the fundamental principles of general physiology – and as the developer of new methods and techniques in animal surgery, his reputation spread and attracted to his laboratory students from across Europe and America. From Bernard's work came much physiological knowledge, including an elucidation of the digestive role of pancreatic juice in lipid metabolism and of the biosynthetic capabilities of the liver in carbohydrate catabolism. Also, by selective use of the poison curare, he followed his teacher Magendie in differentiating the sensory and motor properties of mixed nerves, and further determined that muscles, when their nerves had been poisoned, could still contract when directly stimulated – a practical demonstration of the 'irritability' suggested by Haller. Much of Bernard's experimental and philosophical approach to physiology and medicine was guided by the principle of coherence – that organs and tissues functioned in an integrated manner, and that organic functions followed a determined pattern to maintain an environmental constancy that he termed the '*milieu intérieur*', later developed into the theory of homeostasis by the American physiologist Walter B. Cannon (1871–1945).

For much of his career, Bernard worked in a cramped basement in the Collège de France, from which his students returned to their own countries to reproduce his methods, set up their own laboratories, and teach the next generation. Bernard's emphasis on practical experimental techniques and the use of living animals in research did, however, attract some opprobrium, especially in the days before anaesthesia. His advocacy of the new science of investigative physiology as the intellectual and practical basis of medical education and practice was an equally significant part of his career, his most momentous work being *Introduction to the Study of Experimental Medicine* (1865). In this, he developed experimental physico-chemical approaches to biological phenomena whilst emphasizing that the deterministic conditions of each experiment must be carefully noted. He elaborated further that disease states such as diabetes were malfunctions of these fundamental mechanisms, and stressed that expert knowledge of physiological systems should be recognized, supported, and incorporated into routine medical teaching.

CARL LUDWIG (1816–95)

Traditionally, a physiological 'Gang-of-Four' have been viewed as the founders of institutionalized, regularized physiological practice in the German states. These were Carl Ludwig, Emil du Bois-Reymond, Ernst von Brücke (1819–92), and Hermann von Helmholtz (1821–94).[8] All made several outstanding contributions to physiological science, and all were taught by Johannes Müller (1801–58). Müller is best remembered for his theory of specific nerve energies, which stipulated that stimulation of any given sense organ gave rise to its own peculiar sensation and no other. In 1843, du Bois-Reymond showed that a flow of electric current was involved not only in muscle contraction, as suggested by Galvani, but also in nerve conduction, and he proposed that the transmission of excitation between a nerve and muscle was due to this flow. Helmholtz delivered a vital blow to vitalism when, among others, he established a law of the conservation of energy – that energy was neither created nor destroyed. He measured the speed of conduction in a nerve fibre, recognized that a delay occurred at the neuro-muscular junction, and proposed a mechanism of colour vision involving retinal cones that were differentially sensitive to red, green, and violet (blue). Equally versatile, if less successfully so, was Brücke, who also studied sense-organ physiology, intestinal motility, salivary secretion, and fat metabolism.

Particularly important was Carl Ludwig, who occupies a similar niche in the hierarchy of physiological deities to that of Claude Bernard, although Ludwig, first in Zurich and later in Leipzig, was more influential than his French counterpart in training and inspiring visiting physiologists. Indeed, unlike Bernard, his own research career is often overshadowed by the deference afforded to his crucial role as mentor to the next generation of physiologists. But like Bernard, it was Ludwig's skills and talents in experimental methods that drew students: work on the blood and the innervation of blood vessels; and studies of renal and respiratory physiology, including the substantial proposal of a filtration-reabsorption mechanism for kidney function. In designing and implementing new pieces of equipment, such as the stromuhr for measuring the rate of blood flow, and the kymograph, the forerunner of all graphic recording instruments used in physiology, Ludwig made practical contributions to the conduct of physiology that survive to this day. The crux of his scientific belief was a determined anti-vitalist stand, a demand that physiological phenomena be explained only by reference to the known laws of physics and chemistry. Those views spread from Ludwig's laboratories during the final decades of the nineteenth century to most countries of continental Europe, including Imperial Russia, and to Scandinavia, across the English Channel to Britain, and beyond to North America. His intellectual 'family tree' includes practically every notable physiologist practising at the turn of the century, testimony to his outstanding success as an inspirer of the next generation. One later historian remarked that it was 'almost an obligation for every young and ambitious physiologist to spend at least a year studying with Ludwig'.[9]

BRITAIN IN THE 1870s

In Britain, the early promotion of physiology was directly stimulated by the developments epitomized by Bernard and Ludwig, and depended on the enthusiastic endeavours of a few highly committed men. William Sharpey (1802–80) followed his medical training in Edinburgh with a continental grand tour of European medical establishments before returning to become Professor of Anatomy and General Physiology at University College London. From that position, Sharpey's advocacy of new methods, approaches, and ways of thinking about functional organization was typified by his use of histology, and his teaching concentrated upon the use of the microscope. His pupils included Michael Foster (1836–1907) and Edward Schäfer (1850–1935), both of whom, in conjunction with their Edinburgh-trained colleague John Burdon Sanderson (1828–1905), provided the principal struts for the future support of British physiology. Foster left London in 1870 to become the first Praelector in Physiology at Trinity College, Cambridge: thirteen years later, he was translated into the first Professor of Physiology there, and from both positions did much to establish the prominent Cambridge Physiological Laboratory and to promote physiology in Britain. When Foster departed for Cambridge, Schäfer continued to develop the teaching of histology at University College London, whilst Burdon Sanderson, who succeeded Sharpey in 1874 as Jodrell Professor, organized courses in 'practical physiology' which included chemical, mechanical, and functional experiments. Ten years later, Sanderson became the first Waynflete Professor of Physiology in Oxford and was succeeded by Schäfer. Thus the three most influential positions in English physiology were filled by Sharpey's protégés, all united by a common aim to promote the subject, and with synergistic approaches.[10]

Physiology, especially for teaching purposes, was organized into three main areas that reflect the divisions of the subject at the end of the nineteenth century: *histology* was an integral part of physiology such that the need for natural light for microscope work was a significant consideration in the design and building of new physiological laboratories; *chemical physiology* was a natural extension of the physico-chemical approach promoted by Bernard and Ludwig and their adherents, and was concerned with the chemical analysis of body fluids and constituents; (➤ Ch. 8 The biochemical tradition) *practical physiology* most closely resembled what is thought of as physiology in the late 1900s – the experimental manipulation of organs and tissues, the investigation of their innervation and vascularization, and studies of integration, co-ordination, and regulation within the body as a whole. These latter approaches, to a limited extent for teaching, usually demonstration purposes, but more especially for research practices, required the use of living animals. In Britain, this more than anything else distinguished physiological approaches to experimental medicine, and brought physiology and its practitioners to the attention of a wider public. Briefly, concern about the use of animals in such work aroused suspicion and distrust which resulted in a Royal Commission in 1875, the recommendations of which were incorporated in legislation in the Cruelty to Animals Act of 1876. Thus in Britain, people and places involved in such work had to be registered with the Home Office: experimental procedures, except in special cases, had to be conducted entirely under terminal anaesthesia; and official reports of experiments had to be provided every year. This law and its implementation had an important unifying effect on physiologists, as will be discussed below (see p. 134).

THE TWENTIETH CENTURY

By the end of the nineteenth century, physiology was accepted in most quarters as an important component of medical teaching, although its integration was necessarily patchy and proceeded uncertainly in some medical schools and colleges.[11] Physiologists were poised to promote, develop and shape the discipline in unprecedented ways as the new century opened. Their attempts to understand the functional integration and control of living systems have proceeded, at varying paces and at several different levels of analysis, from that of the whole animal – via a physiological system – a specific organ or tissue, down to the cell, sub-cellular component, or molecule. Several factors have fuelled the exponential growth in physiological researches during the past century. These include the increasing availability and diversity of a professional workforce, and new intellectual approaches and fresh challenges from neighbouring and interdigitating disciplines. The design and production of specialized instruments have been crucial, and it is no accident that two major technical businesses, the Cambridge Scientific Instrument Company and the Harvard Scientific Company, both started in the physiological laboratories of, respectively, Cambridge and Harvard universities. Of necessity, therefore, the remainder of this chapter will be perfunctory, and will be divided into two complementary areas: before discussing some specific physiological subjects and themes of the past century, consideration will be given to additional significant factors in the promotion and development of the subject.

PUBLICATIONS: JOURNALS AND BOOKS

Journals, textbooks, societies, and meetings were all vital for the promotion of physiology. In Germany, Johann Reil (1759–1813) established the *Archiv für die Physiologie* in 1795, a tradition followed by many, such as Eduard Pflüger *Archiv für die gesamte Physiologie der Menschen und der Tiere* (established 1868: now the *European Journal of Physiology*).[12] In Britain, the *Proceedings* and *Philosophical Transactions* of the Royal Society, and from 1866 the *Journal of Anatomy and Physiology*, served the needs of the small physiological community. From the mid–1870s, Michael Foster began to collect the papers published from his laboratory, and the success of the bound copies of *Publications from the Cambridge Physiological Laboratory* encouraged him to found, in 1878, the *Journal of Physiology*, the early volumes of which contained original research papers and a bibliographic section summarizing the physiological literature of the period. From its inception, the *Journal* had an American editor and received regular contributions from American laboratories until the American Physiological Society organized the publication of the *American Journal of Physiology*, which first appeared in 1898 and was finally taken over by the Society just before the First World War. In Britain in 1909, increasing discontent with the authoritarian editorial attitude of the privately owned *Journal of Physiology* (the proprietor was John Newport Langley (1852–1925)) resulted in the establishment of the rival *Quarterly Journal of Experimental Physiology* (now *Experimental Physiology*); both titles are now owned by the Physiological Society. In America, the *Journal of General Physiology*, now associated with the Rockefeller University and the Society of General Physiologists, was started by Jacques Loeb (1859–1924) in 1918; and later, in 1948, the *Journal of Applied Physiology* was established by the American Physiological Society to reflect the needs of human physiologists. Inevitably, the pressures of more papers in a wider range of sub-disciplines using an increased diversity of physiological approaches have promoted the appearance of two rather different but complementary kinds of journals: first, specialized titles that provide a forum for the detailed research papers in contemporary physiology; and second, the appearance of broad-based review-style and news journals such as *Physiological Reviews* (established 1921); *Annual Reviews of Physiology* (1939); and, more recently, *News in the Physiological Sciences* (1986).

A significant tool in promoting physiology was the student textbook; regularly updated and revised editions reinforced the pace of progress, and the utilization of new methods of presentation – wood-cut illustrations, tables, diagrams, halftones, colours, and an increasing array of graphic techniques – have all been successfully incorporated over the past century. From nineteenth-century Germany, several influential volumes emerged, one of which, Müller's *Elements of Physiology*, was translated into English in 1838 by the London physician William Baly (1814–61) and metamorphosed into one of the most successful of English-language textbooks: the final, forty-third edition, appeared in 1960. During its publication lifetime, it had six editors, under whose names it was often known (W. S. Kirkes (1823–64), James Paget (1814–99), W. Morrant Baker (1839–96), W. D. Harris (1851–1931), W. H. Halliburton (1860–1931), and R. J. S. MacDowall (1892–1990)), and was finally terminated because it was considered too old-fashioned. Its first serious challenger had been the American *Textbook of Physiology* produced by W. H. Howell (1860–1945) in 1905, and attractively produced volumes such as those by Ganong, Samson Wright, Best and Taylor, and Guyton were more popular and successful by the 1960s.

Also in the final decades of the nineteenth century, books of practical exercises in physiology, with schedules of work in histology, and chemical and experimental physiology, and detailed laboratory manuals and handbooks started appearing. These were often produced by a teacher for a particular course, such as that by Burdon Sanderson at University College London, and then adopted and adapted by aspiring physiologists in other institutes as models for their own courses.

It is no coincidence that the leading figures in physiology emphasized the need to publish textbooks and monographs, not just for the broader band of medical students, but also for the small albeit growing population of students of physiology. The first major book in this category was Michael Foster's *Text Book of Physiology* (1877), which was followed by many others. The two-volume *Textbook of Physiology* (1898–1900), edited by Schäfer, contains contributions from many distinguished physiologists including Charles Scott Sherrington (1857–1952), Langley, and Leonard Hill (1866–1952), and provides an authoritative synopsis of turn-of-the-century physiology. Just before the First World War, Ernest Starling (1866–1927) produced the first edition of *Principles of Human Physiology* (1912), which had been preceded by his *Elements of Human Physiology* (eight editions, 1892–1907). *Elements* had been written to complement Schäfer's *Essentials of Histology* to provide a solid grounding in what then constituted physiology. *Principles* was much more comprehensive and aimed not only at undergraduates, but more explicitly at medical practitioners as a 'postgraduate' text. This classic, with its overt emphasis on human and mammalian physiology, went through many editions until the author's death in 1927, and continued under the editorship of Charles Lovatt Evans (1884–1968) until 1956.

Shortly after the first edition of Starling's *Principles* appeared, other major texts were produced: *Principles of General Physiology* (1915), by William Bayliss (1860–1924), was very different from contemporary volumes, emphasizing physico-chemical reactions and processes; *Applied Physiology* (1926), by Samson Wright (1899–1956) and based on his courses at the Middlesex Hospital, was specifically intended to give medical students an understanding of physiology with direct clinical relevance; Sherrington's *Mammalian Physiology* (1919) evolved during the First World War, when the few students still in classes at Oxford worked closely with their teacher to produce a major manual of surgical techniques and physiological experiments, one that was to have widespread influence in the teaching and practice of physiology. For well over half a century, generations of physiologists, in Britain and abroad, were trained in some or all of the laboratory methods advocated by Sherrington.

The production and updating of these authoritative textbooks and handbooks were necessary to educate new students, and also to promote postgraduate and specialist training and research. A particularly ambitious and successful scheme in this direction was launched by the American Physiological Society in 1959. Its multi-volume *Handbook of Physiology* was to provide 'the comprehensive but critical presentation of the state of knowledge in various fields of functional biology. It is intended to cover physiological sciences in their entirety once in about ten or twelve years and to supplement them thereafter.'[13]

The wide choice of books available, reflecting different perspectives and addressing several audiences, and the longevity and frequent revisions of some of the titles all attest to the rapid growth of the subject and the prime importance put on education and training by distinguished researchers. More recently, physiological sciences have been additionally promulgated in a variety of new media and study aids, including a battery of audio-visual material such as films, videos, and computer models. Many of these approaches have been adopted as an explicit response to disquiet at the use of animals in physiological teaching.

PROFESSIONAL SOCIETIES

By the end of the nineteenth century, there were medical societies at several universities or institutes across Europe and America at which physiological and other scientific papers could be read and discussed. Both the British Medical Association and the British Association for the Advancement of Science provided specialist 'physiological' sections, but in Britain the unusual circumstances of the 1876 Cruelty to Animals Act acted as a catalyst for the establishment of 'an Association of Physiologists for mutual benefit and protection', which became the Physiological Society. The society, from its beginnings, has always emphasized the importance of regular scientific and social meetings and has never had a permanent headquarters, preferring rather to hold its activities in members' laboratories, to promote a sense of coherent identity.[14]

An American Physiological Society had been founded as early as 1837, but the name is somewhat misleading, as it was principally a locally based society for hygiene and health, and seems not to have flourished. What survives today as the American Physiological Society was founded in 1887, modelled on the British society and sharing one founder-member, Henry Newell Martin (1848–96), in common. The structure of the American society has never been quite as intimate as its British counterpart, concentrating on fewer, larger meetings each year, although it responded earlier to the pressures of specialization by formally providing dedicated sections from the mid–1970s.[15]

The divisions, diversities, and increasing specialization of physiology can be illustrated in a small way by examining the formation of other biomedical societies from the Physiological Society. In 1911, the members who regularly met together within the framework of society meetings to discuss matters concerned with chemical physiology proposed the creation of a daughter 'Biochemical Club', the rules, regulations, and ethos of which were strongly influenced by its still vigorous parent. This became the Biochemical Society. Similarly, in 1931, the British Pharmacological Society budded-off from the Physiological Society – a further demonstration of the increasing diversity and specialization of 'physiology'. It was a British initiative that resulted in the International Congress of Physiological Societies in 1889 in Basle. Over one hundred physiologists from twelve European countries and the United States came together. Thereafter, the International Congress met regularly to hear papers, see demonstrations, and discuss work informally. The first temporary disruption was during the First World War, and a hastily convened meeting in 1920 in Paris was restricted to participants from allied and neutral countries; as such, it has been viewed by Congress historians with distaste and is included reluctantly in the official numerical sequence.[16] Conversely, the open invitation to Edinburgh in 1923 was refused by many French physiologists who objected to the inclusion of German and other 'enemy' physiologists. In 1929, the International Congress was held for the first time in the United States, and conference participation exceeded 1,000, with many physiologists travelling together across the Atlantic in a chartered vessel, the *Minnekahda*;[17] representatives of twenty-two nations, including China and Japan, were on board. Nine years later, the Congress met in Zurich and the idea of holding a separate pharmacological meeting was proposed. This, in time, became the International Pharmacological Congress. After the Second World War, the Physiological Congress developed rapidly; statutes for an International Union of Physiological Societies were approved in 1950, and a permanent Committee was established. Meetings were held in South America (Buenos Aires, 1950); in Asia (Tokyo, 1965); and in Australia (Sydney, 1983). Thus, an analysis of the first International Congress, held in 1889, emphasizes that physiology was then a small but growing activity practised in parts of western Europe and the United States. The subsequent congresses reveal physiology spreading across Europe and the English-speaking world, reaching across the globe, although African, Middle Eastern, and Asian involvement remains slight. (➤ Ch. 59 Internationalism in medicine and public health)

Much of the infrastructure to support physiology was developed in the decades around the turn of the century, at uneven, but broadly parallel, rates across much of Europe and North America. From then, the growing numbers of professional physiologists became engaged upon an increasing diversity of subjects and themes, using an equally expanding array of approaches and techniques, and it is clearly impossible to catalogue the discoveries and advances made in the past century. A telling illustration of the explosion of physiological sciences is provided in Table 1, which lists some of the winners of the Nobel Prize in Physiology and Medicine since its founding in 1901. Those whose achievements are clearly in fields distinct from the main principles and practices of physiology (that is, geneticists, virologists, clinicians, etc.) have been excluded, but those whose work has contributed to physiological understanding and progress, even if they did not consider themselves to be primarily physiologists, have been included. This table demonstrates eloquently the depth and breadth of recent historical developments, and the remainder of this chapter will be a distillation of some major advances, grouped within selected specialities. Asterisked dates in the text refer to the award of a Nobel Prize.

Broadly categorized, twentieth-century physiology has included detailed examinations, at several levels, of the functioning of particular organs or systems both *in vitro* and *in vivo*; investigations into the intrinsic and extrinsic control mechanisms of those systems by neural or blood-borne factors; broader studies, usually *in vivo*, of interaction and integration between different systems; and analyses of overall multi-organ, whole-body, integration and regulation. Some of these approaches will be exemplified by considering specific systems and physiological problems.

Table 1 Selected Nobel Laureates in Physiology or Medicine, 1901–91

Year of award	Name (dates)	Description of work
1904	I. P. Pavlov (1849–1936)	physiology of digestion
1906	C. Golgi (1843–1926); S. Ramón y Cajal (1852–1934)	structure of the nervous system
1908	P. Ehrlich (1854–1915)	mechanisms of immune system
1914	R. Bárány (1876–1936)	pathophysiology of the vestibular apparatus
1920	A. Krogh (1874–1949)	regulatory mechanisms of capillaries
1922	A. V. Hill (1886–1977); O. Meyerhof (1844–1951)	heat production in skeletal muscle; oxygen use and lactic acid production in skeletal muscle
1923	Sir Frederick Banting (1891–1941); J. R. Macleod (1876–1935)	insulin
1924	W. Einthoven (1860–1927)	mechanism of electrocardiogram
1929	Sir Frederick Gowland Hopkins (1861–1947); C. Eijkman (1858–1930)	anti-neuritic vitamins growth-stimulating vitamins
1931	O. Warburg (1893–1970)	nature and mode of action of respiratory enzymes
1932	Lord Adrian (1889–1977); Sir Charles Sherrington (1857–1952)	functioning of the nervous system
1936	Sir Henry Dale (1875–1968); Otto Leowi (1873–1961)	chemical transmission of nervous impulses
1937	A. Szent-Györgyi (1893–1986)	discoveries in cell metabolism, especially the role of vitamin C
1938	C. Heymans (1892–1968)	respiratory control mechanisms
1943	H. Dam (1895–1976); E. A. Doisy (1893–1986)	discovery of vitamin K chemical nature of vitamin K
1944	J. Erlanger (1874–1965); H. Gasser (1888–1963)	differentiated function of single nerve fibres
1947	B. Houssay (1887–1971); C. F. Cori (1896–1984); G. T. Cori (1896–1957)	anterior pituitary hormone in sugar metabolism; metabolism of glycogen
1949	W. Hess (1881–1973)	central control of autonomic function
1950	E. Kendall (1886–1972); P. S. Hench (1890–1965); T. Reichstein (b. 1897)	structure and biological effects of hormones from adrenal cortex
1953	Sir Hans Krebs (1900–81); F. A. Lipmann (1899–1986)	citric acid cycle coenzyme A
1955	A. Theorell (1903–82)	nature and mode of action of oxidative enzymes
1956	A. Cournand (1895–1959); W. Forssmann (1904–79); D. W. Richards (1895–1973)	cardiovascular pathology and cardiac catheterization
1957	D. Bovet (1907–92)	drug therapy, especially antihistamines
1961	G. von Békésy (1899–1972)	mechanics of inner ear
1963	Sir John Eccles (b. 1903); Sir Alan Hodgkin (b. 1914); Sir Andrew Huxley (b. 1917)	ionic mechanisms of inhibition and excitation of nerve cell membranes
1967	R. Granit (b. 1900); H. Hartline (1903–83); G. Wald (b. 1906)	primary physiological and chemical mechanisms in visual processes of the eye
1970	J. Axelrod (b. 1912); Sir Bernard Katz (b. 1911); Ulf von Euler (1905–83)	storage, release and inactivation of neurotransmitters in nerve terminals
1971	E. W. Sutherland (b. 1915)	cellular mechanisms of hormone actions

Table 1 Continued

Year of award	Name (dates)	Description of work
1974	A. Claude (1898–1983); C. R. de Duvé (b. 1917); G. Palade (b. 1912)	fine structure and function of the cell
1977	R. Guillemin (b. 1924); A. Schally (b. 1926)	hypothalamic-pituitary axis and role of protein hormones
1981	D. Hubel (b. 1926); T. Wiesel (b. 1924)	mechanisms of visual perception; functions of visual cortex
	R. Sperry (b. 1913)	functions of left and right cerebral hemispheres
1982	S. K. Bergström (b. 1916); B. Samuelsson (b. 1934); Sir John Vane (b. 1927)	prostaglandins
1986	R. Levi-Montalcini (b. 1909)	nerve-growth factor
1988	Sir James Black (b. 1924)	drug discoveries, e.g. beta-blockers
1991	E. Neher (b. 1944); B. Sakmann (b. 1942)	patch clamping of membranes

THE GASTRO-INTESTINAL SYSTEM: APPROACHES TO A PROBLEM

A major thrust of twentieth-century investigative techniques was the development of new ways to probe the major functional systems of the body. Largely assisted by advances in surgical techniques and chemical anaesthesia, experiments on animals revealed new levels of complexity in every system examined, and gastro-intestinal physiology demonstrates many of these features. The work of the Russian physiologist Ivan Pavlov (1849–1936; *1904) in the years around the turn of the century did much to elucidate functional mechanisms of different parts of the upper gastro-intestinal tract, and to understand the integrative controls of the system, especially the role of the vagus nerve. Pavlov was particularly expert in devising surgical approaches to the system, such as pouches and fistulae for the study of gastric and pancreatic function,[18] although his interests in the control mechanisms of the system eventually diverted almost completely into physiological psychology. Similar human studies were undertaken, necessarily rarely, by physicians. The first had been that by the American William Beaumont (1785–1853), whose patient, Alexis St Martin (c.1806-c.1884), had suffered a shotgun accident resulting in an anterior abdominable wall injury that rendered direct access to his stomach possible. From these studies, Beaumont made fundamental observations about the nature of gastric motility and the variations in flow of gastric juice in different conditions. Later examinations, again on an accident victim, 'Tom' (c.1886-c.1959), who as a child had sealed his oesophagus by eating hot clam chowder, thus needing surgical intervention, provided an extensive chronological account of gastric function.[19] An experimental refinement of this surgical method was by A. J. Carlson (1875–1956), who combined surgically induced fistulae in animals with the precise placement of balloons, from which he recorded movements of the stomach.

From the end of the nineteenth century, studies on the secretory functions of the gut, from the pioneering work of physiologists such as Bernard, Langley, Pavlov, and Bayliss and Starling on salivary, pancreatic, hepatic, and gastric secretion, expanded during the twentieth century into a wide range of complementary and synergistic examinations of gut histology, microbiology, biochemistry, endocrinology, and pharmacology.

A revolutionary new approach was adopted by the American physiologist Walter Cannon who devised a way, now in routine diagnostic use, of examining the internal workings of the body without recourse to surgery. To do this, he utilized newly discovered X-rays to examine the passage of radio-opaque food pellets along the gut. From an initial interest in the mechanisms of swallowing, and using a range of foods, he analysed the mechanical properties of every region of the gut, in humans and experimental animals. His famous 'J'-pictures of the shape of the stomach and pylorus during gastric emptying were originally traced on to lavatory paper held over the Roentgen screen, and are still the classic illustrations in many textbooks. Cannon's overwhelming concern with integrative physiology led him to consider the effects of varying food compositions on the rate of gastric emptying, and thereafter into an examination of emotional influences on gut function; from this came an extensive study of the control mechanisms of the autonomic nervous system. This work on neuro-effector systems and the ways in which different regulatory components interact and control each other resulted in a consideration of self-regulation, work encapsulated in Cannon's most famous work *The Wisdom of the Body*, first published in 1932. This was a detailed exposition of his theory of homeostasis, a direct but more sophisticated descendant of Claude Bernard's proposal of the constancy of the *milieu intérieur*.[20]

CARDIOVASCULAR PHYSIOLOGY: LABORATORY INTO THE CLINIC

To study the mechanisms of a rapidly beating heart, cold-blooded vertebrates and invertebrates were often used in preference to mammals. Much knowledge came from work on the heart's functions and its control, exemplified by the classical studies of W. H. Gaskell (1847–1914) of the muscles and the intrinsic and extrinsic regulation of frog and tortoise hearts. He showed that motor impulses from ganglia in the sinus venosus influenced heart rhythm but not the cardiac movements, which were due to muscle contraction. To extend such studies to the mammalian heart, several attempts were made to isolate it from neural control, and this was first successfully achieved by Michael Foster's student Henry Newell Martin in 1884, when he was Professor of Physiology at Johns Hopkins University. Martin maintained the heart by perfusion, a technique greatly facilitated by the development of suitable perfusion solutions by Sydney Ringer (1835–1910), amongst others. Martin's approach lasted well into the twentieth century until superseded by Starling's heart-lung preparation, used in the experimental studies from which Starling deduced his eponymous 'Law of the Heart', which related the contractile energy of a cardiac muscle fibre to its resting length. Later refinements in this area included more sophisticated perfusion pumps, the discovery and introduction of anti-clotting agents, and general improvements in perfusion and irrigation media. These developments all contributed to the creation of the apparatus for the first successful heart-bypass surgery in the early 1950s. (➤ Ch. 42 Surgery (modern)) In the same period, the technique devised by Adolf Fick (1829–1901) for calculating cardiac output was finally translated into a successful procedure for human diagnosis.

The heart's specialized conduction system was first investigated thoroughly by F. W. Stannius (1803–83), who demonstrated vagal inhibition and the intrinsic pacemaker. From embryological studies, Wilhelm His (1863–1934) discovered, in 1893, the auriculo-ventricular bundle of special conducting tissue that bears his name, often coupled with that of A. F. Stanley Kent (1863–1958), who discovered the bundle independently in the same year. Willem Einthoven (1860–1927; *1924) followed the British physiologist Augustus Waller (1856–1922), who provided the classic description of the electrocardiograph using a capillary electrometer, by developing the string-galvanometer that could accurately portray the electrical changes occurring in the human heart. This greatly facilitated laboratory and clinical examinations of the heart, such as investigations of the damage to the bundle of His that dissociated auricular and ventricular beats, and was a major development in the creation of modern electrodiagnostic techniques.

THE RESPIRATORY SYSTEM: APPLIED PHYSIOLOGY AND THE LABORATORY[21]

Two British physiologists in particular, John Scott Haldane (1860–1936) and Joseph Barcroft (1872–1947), made considerable contributions to understanding the mechanisms of respiration. Haldane, the nephew of John Burdon Sanderson, balanced interests in public health and respiratory physiology, and his early experiments on mine gases and physiological function in miners lead to a series of investigations in which he exploited physiological adaptive mechanisms in conditions of distress or disruption in a wide array of environmental conditions.[22] Like many physiologists, Haldane studied high-altitude responses. Claude Bernard's pupil Paul Bert (1833–86) had studied balloon-ists to discover that the respiratory gases dissolved in the blood exerted their effects not in proportion to their concentrations, but to their partial pressures; and the Italian, Angelo Mosso (1846–1910), determined that respiratory distress at high altitudes amongst mountaineers was occasioned by a lack of carbon dioxide. Haldane determined that oxygen tension in the blood was somewhat higher than in pulmonary air, and concluded, in a belief he held until his death, that the lungs secreted oxygen. In this he was strongly influenced by the theories of Christian Bohr (1855–1911) that pulmonary air exchange was predominantly the result of an active secretory process. This led to a protracted dispute with the Danish physiologist August Krogh (1874–1949; *1920), who believed that pulmonary gas exchange could be explained by diffusion processes, as did Barcroft.

Joseph Barcroft, a student of Michael Foster in Cambridge, became interested in the dissociation mechanism of the respiratory pigment, haemo-globin, examined the oxygen-carrying capacity of the blood, investigated the role of the spleen as the endogenous store of erythrocytes, and provided a major analysis of foetal respiration.[23]

As typified by many emerging physiological specialities, respiratory work needed new, increasingly sensitive and more portable analytical equipment. This resulted in the evolution of many eponymous pieces: for example, the 'Haldane' apparatus for gas analysis could measure oxygen and carbon dioxide very accurately, and was a cornerstone of respiratory physiology until super-seded by the 'Scholander' apparatus, which combined the same level of sensitivity but required a smaller-volume gas sample; the 'Van Slyke' for the manometric analysis of gases dissolved in blood and other fluids; and the 'Douglas' bag for the collection of gas samples for later analysis.

Concerns with respiratory physiology extended beyond investigation only of pulmonary gas exchange. One trend was to examine the airways themselves, an early contribution being made by K. E. R. Hering (1834–1918) and J. Breuer (1842–1925), who delineated two important neural reflexes, mediated via the vagus nerve. They showed that inflation of the lungs delayed the next inspiration, but that a maintained deflation increased the rate and depth of inspiration.[24]

Rather different approaches to respiratory function were developed primar-ily amongst members of what became identified as the biochemical com-munity, and will not therefore be assessed here, although insights into the cellular mechanisms of respiration and intermediate metabolism, by Otto Warburg (1892–1970; *1931), Otto Meyerhof (1884–1951; *1922), and Hans Krebs (1900–81; *1953), amongst others, contributed greatly to functional understandings of living organisms.

THE NERVOUS SYSTEM: INTEGRATIVE FUNCTIONS AND CHEMICAL MEDIATION[25]

The career of Charles Sherrington typifies the transition of physiology from the end of the nineteenth century to the middle of the twentieth century: from a medical interest to a defined, scientific speciality. Sherrington qualified in medicine in 1885, after studying with Michael Foster, and became Lecturer in Physiology at St Thomas's Hospital in London – the first specialist physiologist (that is, not a member of the medical staff) to hold such a post. He performed its poorly paid duties in conjunction with those as Superintendent of the Brown Animal Sanatory Institution, from where he studied rabies, visited Spain under the auspices of the Royal Society to investigate an outbreak of cholera, and was the first person in Britain to use diphtheria antitoxins successfully. (➤ Ch. 10 The immunological tradition) He moved to the Chair of Physiology in Liverpool in 1895, and thence to the Waynflete Chair at Oxford in 1913. During the First World War, he combined academic work with shifts in a munitions factory, studied fatigue, and devised his influential laboratory course in physiology, published as *Mammalian Physiology* (see p. 134). He was a distinguished bibliophile and published poet. As a research worker, it is for his careful analysis of the function of the nervous system that he is remembered, work that began in the late 1880s and occupied his entire career. The discrete anatomical unit of the nervous system was defined by S. Ramón y Cajal (1852–1934; *1906) as the neuron; Sherrington, utilizing the work of Magendie, who had clearly delineated the incoming and outgoing fibre paths of the nervous system, developed the theory of reflex integration, defining the functional unit of the nervous system as the reflex arc. Many complex activities and responses such as walking or breathing can be reduced analytically to a series of reflex arcs. Sherrington postulated that a reflex arc had to contain at least two neurons, necessitating intercellular conduction of the neural impulse at the space between neurons that he called the synapse. His studies, especially on primates, established the basis of modern physiological understanding of the nervous system: the nature of the reflex arc as studied in the flexion, extensor, and scratch reflexes; the reciprocal innervation of antagonistic muscles, from which he deduced that inhibitory mechanisms operated in the nervous system; the distribution and mechanisms of proprioceptors, especially the control of muscle tone and posture. All of these led to, and were subsumed in, two major concepts that emerge from his work: 'the final common pathway' and the 'integrative action' of the nervous system. The former referred to the convergence of reflex arcs originating from several sensory inputs on to one efferent neuron, the motor nerve of which thus forms a final pathway to the effector muscle. Sherrington considered the reflex to be a basic example of the integrative function of the nervous system, the principle of co-ordination and control that enabled the animal body to act as a whole.

In 1932, Sherrington shared the Nobel Prize with his compatriot and fellow neurophysiologist E. D. Adrian (1889–1977), who had also been trained in the Cambridge Physiological Laboratory. After the First World War, Adrian continued the work of his teacher Keith Lucas (1879–1916) on the nervous impulse, a critical factor in his success being his development of new techniques to record nervous activity. Of considerable interest to physiologists at this time was the problem of amplifying the very small electrical signals that they could record. Adrian used the capillary electrometer devised by Lucas, and constructed a system to amplify the neural signal, utilizing the thermionic valve amplifier, then in use in telegraphy and radio work. Simultaneously, the Americans H. S. Gasser (1888–1963; *1944) and J. Erlanger (1987–1965; *1944) incorporated valve amplification and also introduced the cathode ray tube, thus heralding the beginning of the electronic age in the physiological laboratory.

Adrian's sensitive recording apparatus allowed him to record afferent impulses from muscles, cutaneous nerves, and autonomic nerves, and enabled him to refine the technique so that he could record *in vitro* from a single nerve fibre stimulated by its end organ in an isolated frog muscle. This revealed that impulses carried in a sensory nerve varied in frequency dependent upon the intensity of stimulation, such frequency-coding being of fundamental importance in the understanding of the functioning of the nervous system. Adrian, alone or with collaborators, extended this work to the mammalian nervous system and confirmed that in the afferent fibres, and also in motor fibres, there was only one kind of nervous impulse, and that both sensory and motor information was produced by variation in the frequency of the impulse. His approach was broadly comparative and included investigations of several sense organs in several species. From this developed an understanding of the relationship between the initial sensory stimulus, the receptor response, the nature of the sensory nerve impulse, and the final integrated sensation recorded in the central nervous system. Adrian mapped out cortical projections from many sensory systems, revealing inter-species differences that reflected the mode of life of the animal, and studied human cerebral activity by using electroencephalography, a technique now used in the diagnosis and study of human neurological disease.

The work of David Hubel (b. 1926; *1981) and Torsten Wiesel (b. 1924; *1981) was a direct continuation of Adrian's sensory research. They analysed in finer detail the successive stages, or relays, along the visual pathway, providing a clear processing route from the receipt of the initial sensory stimulus by the retina to central perception, by single cell analysis of units of the mammalian visual system. They demonstrated that there was a marked increase in the specialization of neurons, which responded to increasingly complex visual stimuli at higher levels in the visual pathway.

When Sherrington published his first full paper in 1884 on neural degeneration, it was in collaboration with J. N. Langleya, a slightly senior Cambridge colleague. Langley, too, devoted his career to physiological research, although concentrating on the autonomic division of the nervous system. Especially with his colleague, W. H. Gaskell, Langley dissected the anatomical pathways taken by the two major component parts of the autonomic (a word he introduced) system, and his experimental work delineated much of the function of the sympathetic and parasympathetic branches. Particularly significant was his recognition of specialized sites of action at end-organs and ganglia, where the autonomic nerves exerted their effects. Strongly and mutually influential were the ideas that Paul Ehrlich (1854–1915; *1908) was evolving to explain the action of stains and dyes on living tissue and antibacterial drugs, from which arose two complementary and similar theories: Ehrlich proposed the 'side chain theory', Langley the 'receptive' theory, both of which were designed to account for functional interaction. From these theoretical accounts developed one of the most powerful concepts in twentieth-century biomedical sciences, the 'receptor' theory, which became utilized to account for cell–cell and cell–drug interactions in all manner of living tissues.

A student of Gaskell and Langley in Cambridge in the 1890s was Henry Dale (1875–1968; *1936), who became much interested in autonomic mechanisms. An early experiment revealed that the systematic administration of adrenaline to an anaesthetized animal closely mimicked the effects achieved by stimulating branches of the sympathetic nervous system. At the time, the relationship between the nervous system and the chemical stimulation was not clear, but Dale gradually discovered that the mechanism by which nerves communicate across the synaptic gap was due to the release of specific chemicals. He showed that autonomic ganglia, the end organs of the parasympathetic nervous system, and the neuromuscular junction could all be stimulated by a chemical called acetylcholine, which he also identified as a natural constituent of the animal body. Further analysis, using a particularly sensitive bio-assay system, the ventral muscle of the leech treated with the chemical eserine, revealed that acetylcholine was indeed released from the nerve endings at these sites. For this work on chemical neurotransmission, Dale shared the Nobel Prize with the Austrian pharmacologist Otto Loewi (1873–1961; *1936). Loewi's own experiments at the beginning of the 1920s had provided the first clear evidence that chemical substances were released by nerve terminals after stimulation, although he only hinted at their identities.

The concept of chemical neurotransmission was not uncontroversial, and for many years there was an active debate between those who supported it and those who believed that transmission across synapses was solely an electrical phenomenon. Much subsequent work, especially on isolated synapses of single nerve-muscle fibres, provided overwhelming proof of chemical neurotransmission at most synapses, and one of the principal proponents of the alternative view, J. C. Eccles (b. 1903; *1963), after formally announcing his 'conversion' to chemical mechanisms, formulated what became known as 'Dale's Law', which stipulated 'one neuron, one transmitter'.[26] As chemical neurotransmission achieved widespread acceptance it became the new orthodoxy, and it was widely assumed that only a few specific chemicals, including acetylcholine and noradrenaline, were involved in the process. This view was challenged, most notably by G. Burnstock (b. 1929), who suggested first that ATP (adenosine triphosphate, a compound known to be involved in metabolic pathways), might act as a neurotransmitter. He then expanded his ideas into a theory of co-transmission, that nerve terminals release not one substance, but a complex cocktail of two or more active chemicals. This, in turn, has developed into the concept of chemical coding, that nerves can be fully analysed, described, and manipulated by reference to the chemical mixture released at their terminals.

Dale's personal research during the first thirty years of the twentieth century was not confined to chemical neurotransmission: he first noted the oxytocic effects of extracts of the posterior pituitary gland (from which oxytocin was isolated in 1928), discovered histamine, and produced important work on anaphylactic shock, all of which illustrate his interest in broader questions about endogenous physiological regulatory mechanisms, especially chemical mechanisms; for this aspect of physiology he coined the term 'autopharmacology'. An unusual aspect of this concern was Dale's realization that as pharmaceutical and therapeutic dependence on natural substances developed, new analytical techniques and concords were necessary to provide a coherent framework in which medical research and practice could progress. Subsequently, Dale promoted national and international agreements on biological standards, based on reliable physiological responses, for a widespread of naturally occurring substances, as important a contribution to twentieth-century medical science as his experimental work.

THE ENDOCRINE SYSTEM[27]

When Dale began his research career on the autonomic nervous system in 1904, there was considerable interest in the use of chemicals in therapeutics. This had been accelerated by the evolution of the chemical and pharmaceutical industries, especially in Germany. Work such as that by Ehrlich encouraged scientific consideration of the effects and mechanisms of exogenously applied chemicals. Experiments like Dale's, emphasizing the role of endogenous chemicals, were also revealing chemical influences in an entirely different control system of the body, the endocrine system. (➤ Ch. 39 Drug therapies; Ch. 23 Endocrine diseases)

Ernest Starling and William Bayliss of University College London performed a crucial experiment in the history of endocrinology in 1902. They showed that the mucosa of the upper part of the intestine, on being stimulated by the presence of acid, released a chemical factor that induced pancreatic enzyme secretion. Careful experimental controls confirmed their finding and they named their new factor 'secretin'. Three years later, they had developed a generalized theory of this type of secretory process, and first used the word 'hormone' to describe such substances, replacing the previous phrase 'internal secretion'. Bayliss and Starling were not the first to observe the effects of such internal secretions. An earlier account from the same laboratory, by Schäfer and George Oliver (1841–1915) in 1894, had reported the pressor effects of extracts of the medulla of the adrenal gland. This substance, later identified as adrenaline, became the centrepiece of debate and discussion, then in new scientific research, as commercial interests represented by Parke, Davis & Co. became involved in physiological progress. Claims to have patented adrenaline and to exclusive commercial rights in it exacerbated worsening relationships between pharmaceutical manufacturers and scientists in America. Such tensions were still evident in 1921 when two Canadians, F. Banting (1891–1941; *1923) and C. H. Best (1899–1978), made perhaps the most famous endocrinological discovery, that of pancreatic insulin as the treatment for diabetes.

The history of endocrine research itself is too vast to incorporate into this account of physiological history, and only a brief but representative summary will be presented of one subdivision, that of the sex hormones.

The classic approach to endocrine research was established quite early: the removal of the suspected source of an internal secretion; and the charting of the consequent signs and symptoms of resultant disease, and their reversal by the injection of a crude extract prepared from the removed gland. The French physiologist and neurologist Charles Brown-Séquard (1817–94) followed a similar protocol in his controversial organotherapy, in which testicular extracts from animals were injected into male patients, including himself, with a claimed 'rejuvenating' effect. Properly controlled scientific studies on testicular extracts were reported in 1929 by the American L. C. McGee (b. 1904) and colleagues, who also introduced a bio-assay technique, the growth of the comb in castrated cockerels, to assess the potency of their extract, which contained androsterone. A few years later, testosterone was isolated, and during the same period, several ovarian hormones were isolated and named: oestrin (1923), progesterone (1929), oestriol (1930); oestrone (1930), and oestradiol (1936). Recognition of the fact that hormone levels altered significantly during pregnancy led to the development of a reliable pregnancy test by S. Aschheim (1878–1965) and B. Zondek (1891–1967) in 1928. By 1936, the plethora of work on endocrine mechanisms allowed the biochemist A. Doisy (1893–1986; *1943) to propose four firm scientific criteria for the identification of a hormone: confirmation that a gland produced the secretion; the availability of precise methods to detect the secretion; the production of an extract from which a purified hormone could be obtained; and finally, the chemical isolation, chemical identification, and synthesis of the hormone. A further major step was taken in 1938 by E. C. Dodds (1899–1973) when he announced the production of a synthetic oestrogen, stilboestrol.

Clinical observations that disease or damage to the pituitary gland some-times resulted in malfunction of the sex glands encouraged investigations into higher control mechanisms. Work by Aschheim and Zondek revealed the presence in the anterior pituitary of gonadotrophins, or hormones that in turn stimulated further glandular hormone release: for example, FSH (follicle stimulating hormone), which provoked the maturation of the ovarian Graafian follicles and the production of oestrone.

Yet a further stage in the control hierarchy was recognized by G. W. Harris (1913–72), who determined that the hypothalamus released 'factors' which either stimulated or inhibited pituitary function. This work has led to the discovery of many integrated control mechanisms, such as the hypothalamic–pituitary–gonadal axis. Understanding these stages in the control of sexual function has had widespread significance in the development of medical and social attitudes towards questions of fertility, infertility, contraception, and abortion.

From a functional viewpoint, the gradual elucidation of endocrine mechan-isms and the chemical nature of an increasing array of newly discovered hormones from organs not traditionally regarded as being endocrine, such as the gut and the heart, coincided with, and contributed to, the growing awareness of the role of chemicals in regulatory mechanisms of the body. In the mid-1950s, as the role of chemicals in neurotransmission (see p. 144) was increasingly accepted, a major distinction between neurotransmitters and hormones related to their site of action: a neurotransmitter had a clearly defined local action, a very short distance from its point of release; in contrast, a hormone exerted its effects at some distance from its site of production, being carried there in the bloodstream. From the 1970s onwards, fresh evidence and new concepts about the multitude of roles of endogenous chemicals in physiological regulation have blurred these distinctions.

Bayliss and Starling's original recognition of hormones as chemical messen-gers implied recognition of a target, a hormone receptor site. Analytical work in the 1970s and 1980s utilized membrane preparations to study receptor sites and revealed that most water-soluble polypeptide hormones bind to specific receptor sites on the surface of the cell membrane, in line with what had become the traditional view of cell–drug interactions. However, steroid hormones, soluble in lipid, could penetrate the membrane to act at specialized sites *inside* the cell, on either cytosol or nuclear receptors, and by interacting with DNA could evoke messenger RNA and consequently protein synthesis, a level of regulation that is a major conceptual leap from Bayliss and Starling's original experiments.

MEMBRANE PHYSIOLOGY

Investigations into membrane structure in the latter part of the nineteenth century were stimulated both by the cell theory and by the availability of increasingly sophisticated physical and chemical techniques. The studies of the botanist C. E. Overton (1865–1933) on osmotic pressure suggested to him the possibility of a specialized boundary mechanism, the cell membrane, that contained protein and lipid. This suggestion was further refined and developed by many others, and in 1935 J. Danielli (1911–84) and H. Davson (b. 1909) produced their theory of a permeable membrane, the dynamics and transport mechanisms of which have provided one of the most fruitful areas of modern physiological research.

Earlier physiologists knew from studies of injured nerve and muscle fibres that an electrical potential difference existed across their membranes, for which Helmholtz's pupil, Julius Bernstein (1839–1917), proposed a hypothesis in 1902. From chemical analysis, he knew that the interior of these fibres was rich in potassium but contained little sodium or chloride and suggested that this ionic imbalance resulted in a voltage across the membrane, as predicted by the equation devised by Walther Nernst (1865–1933). Nernst's work on the physics and chemistry of electrolytes showed that at the boundary between two different solutions of the same salt an electrical potential difference arises. Bernstein used the Nernst equation to devise a quantitative expression for the resting potential in muscle and nerve fibres and determined that the selective permeablility of the membrane to potassium ions established a negative resting potential inside, but that during excitation, that is, the passage of an action potential, the membrane permeability was transiently altered.

A major impetus to detailed work was the discovery in 1933 of the giant axon of the squid by the British zoologist J. Z. Young (b. 1907). The fibres were so large, up to 1 mm in diameter, that they had been mistaken for blood vessels until Young performed the simple experiment of electrically stimulating at one point and recording the generated impulse further along the fibre, thus confirming their conductile nature. Using the giant axon of the squid, A. L. Hodgkin (b. 1914; *1963), A. F. Huxley (b. 1917; *1963), and B. Katz (b. 1911; *1970) derived a mathematical hypothesis of the nerve action potential, which depended upon the external concentration of sodium ions.[28]

As in many fields, technical advances were critical. Membrane physiology was greatly facilitated by the availability of radioactive isotopes as tracers, just prior to the Second World War. The development of the flame photometer in the early 1950s eased the tedious analysis of precipitating and titrating sodium and potassium ions. In 1951, H. H. Ussing (b. 1911) proposed from his studies of membrane kinetics that there was a cyclical carrier mechanism of permeability, linking active sodium and potassium transport across the membrane. During the following decade, active transport of sodium ions was demonstrated across many membrane preparations – frog skin, skeletal muscle fibres, giant axons, and erythrocytes – and experiments on this mechanism led to the concept of the sodium pump, which maintains the ionic imbalance across the membrane. Further work recognized that the enzyme sodium-potassium adenosinetriphosphatase (sodium-potassium ATPase), a specific ion-transport enzyme, is embedded in the membrane of almost every animal cell and plays a vital part in the maintenance of the sodium pump.

Experimental manipulations have always been of considerable importance in the biophysical analysis of cell membranes, and two outstanding techniques have been developed since the Second World War. The voltage clamp, devised and refined during the 1940s and 1950s, allowed external control of the membrane potential, which could thus be maintained at desired levels, enabling subtle manipulations to be made to ionic currents. A substantial development, that of patch-clamping, was announced in 1976 by E. Neher (b. 1944; *1991) and B. Sakmann (b. 1942; *1991), which allowed minute portions, or patches, of membrane to be investigated in detail. They confirmed that when the membrane potential altered, it did so as ions crossed the cell membrane through specific ion-channels. This technique, which increased the sensitivity of previous methods by a factor of a million, allowed physiologists to study the discrete ion channels in more detail and to analyse the protein-molecule activities that regulate each channel.

CONCLUSION

Thus, as the twentieth century draws to a close, several shifts and developments in physiology can be discerned. Its close relationship to medical practice, heralded and promoted at the end of the last century, is no longer so apparent, although therapeutic utility is often proclaimed as a justification for experimental research. Levels of interest have progressively moved, from the whole animal to the integrated system; from the organ to the cell; from the cellular component to the ion. Associated with these movements has been the breakdown of 'traditional' departmental barriers (barely 150 years old) and the growth of new disciplines such as biophysics, neurosciences, etc. However, the physiological *approach* as the study of the function of living matter, has retained its identity, even if the boundaries of the subject itself are becoming increasingly indistinct.

NOTES

1 T. S. Hall, *Ideas of Life and Matter: Studies in the History of General Physiology 600 BC to AD 1900*, 2 vols, Chicago, IL, University of Chicago Press, 1969.
2 R. G. Frank, *Harvey and the Oxford Physiologists*, Berkeley, University of California Press, 1980.
3 M. A. B. Brazier, *Neurophysiology in the Seventeenth and Eighteenth Centuries*, New York, Raven Press, 1984.
4 J. E. Lesch, *Science and Medicine in France: the Emergence of Experimental Physiology 1790–1855*, Cambridge, MA, Harvard University Press, 1984.
5 P. Elliott, 'Vivisection and the emergence of experimental physiology in nine-teenth century France', in N. A. Rupke (ed.), *Vivisection in Historical Perspective*, London, Croom Helm, 1987, pp. 48–77.
6 See the essays in W. Coleman and F. L. Holmes (eds), *The Investigative Enterprise: Experimental Physiology in Nineteenth-Century Medicine*, Berkeley, University of California Press, 1988.
7 See, for example, F. L. Holmes, *Claude Bernard and Animal Chemistry: the Emergence of a Scientist*, Cambridge, MA, Harvard University Press, 1974.
8 P. F. Cranefield, 'The organic physics of 1847 and the biophysics of today', *Journal of the History of Medicine*, 1957, 12: 407–23; M. A. B. Brazier, *A History of Neurophysiology in the Nineteenth Century*, New York, Raven Press, 1988.
9 K. E. Rothschuh, *History of Physiology*, trans. by G. B. Risse, Huntingdon, New York, Robert E. Krieger, 1973, p. 207.
10 G. Geison, *Michael Foster and the Cambridge School of Physiology: the Scientific Enterprise in Late Victorian Society*, Princeton, NJ, Princeton University Press, 1978.
11 S. V. F. Butler, 'A transformation in training: the formation of university medical faculties in Manchester, Leeds, and Liverpool, 1879–84', *Medical History*, 1986, 30: 115–32; W. J. O'Connor, *Founders of British Physiology. A Biographical Diction-ary 1820–85*, Manchester, Manchester University Press, 1988; O'Connor, *British Physiologists 1885–1914: a Biographical Dictionary*, Manchester, Manchester Uni-versity Press, 1991.
12 T. H. Broman, 'J. C. Reil and the "journalization" of physiology', in P. Dear (ed.), *The Literary Structure of Scientific Arguments*, Philadelphia, University of Pennsylvania Press, 1991, pp. 13–42.
13 American Physiological Society, *Handbook of Physiology*, Baltimore, MD, Williams & Wilkins, 1959–78.
14 E. Sharpey-Schafer, *A History of the Physiological Society during its First Fifty Years 1876–1926*, Cambridge, Cambridge University Press, 1927; W. F. Bynum, 'A short history of the Physiological Society 1926–76', *Journal of Physiology*, 1976, 263: 23–72.

15 H. E. Hoff and J. F. Fulton, 'The centenary of the first American Physiological Society founded at Boston by William A. Alcott and Sylvester Graham', *Bulletin of the History of Medicine*, 1937, 5: 687–734; J. R. Brobeck, O. R. Reynolds and T. A. Appel (eds), *History of the American Physiological Society: the First Century 1887–1987*, Bethesda, MD, American Physiological Society, 1987; G. Geison (ed.), *Physiology in the American Context 1850–1940*, Bethesda, MD, American Physiological Society, 1987.

16 K. J. Franklin, 'A short history of the international congresses of physiology', *Annals of Science*, 1938, 3: 241–335; D. Whitteridge, *One Hundred Years of Congresses of Physiology*, Oulu, International Union of Physiologists, 1989.

17 Y. Zotterman, 'The Minnekahda voyage', in W. O. Fenn (ed.), *History of the International Congresses of Physiological Sciences 1889–1968*, Baltimore, MD, American Physiological Society, 1968, pp. 1–14.

18 I. P. Pavlov, *Lectures on the Work of the Digestive Glands*, trans. by W. H. Thompson, London, C. Griffin, 1910.

19 S. G. Wolf and M. G. Wolff, *Human Gastric Function: an Experimental Study of One Man and His Stomach*, 2nd edn, rev. and enl., Oxford, Oxford University Press, 1947.

20 S. Benison, A. C. Barger and E. L. Wolfe, *Walter B. Cannon: the Life and Times of a Young Scientist*, Cambridge, MA, Harvard University Press, 1987; W. B. Cannon, *The Way of an Investigator*, New York, Hafner, 1945.

21 See, for example, J. B. West (ed.), *Translations in Respiratory Physiology*, Stroudsburg, PA, Dowden, Hutchinson & Ross, 1975; P. Astrup and J. W. Severinghaus, *The History of Blood Gases, Acids and Bases*, Copenhagen, Munksgaard, 1986.

22 J. S. Haldane, *Respiration*, New Haven, CT, Yale University Press, 1922. See also Y. Henderson, *Adventures in Physiology*, Baltimore, MD, Williams & Wilkins, 1922.

23 J. Barcroft, *The Respiratory Function of the Blood*, Cambridge, Cambridge University Press, 1914; Barcroft, *Features in the Architecture of Physiological Function*, Cambridge, Cambridge University Press, 1934.

24 R. Porter (ed.), *Breathing: Hering–Breuer Centenary Symposium*, London, Churchill, 1970.

25 Useful histories of the nervous system include Brazier, op cit. (nn. 3 and 8); P. F. Cranefield, *The Way In and the Way Out: François Magendie, Charles Bell and the Roots of the Spinal Nerves*, Mount Kisco, NY, Futura, 1974; E. Clarke and L. S. Jacyna, *Nineteenth-Century Origins of Neuroscientific Concepts*, Berkeley, University of California Press, 1987. F. G. Worden, J. P. Swazey and G. Adelman (eds), *The Neurosciences: Paths of Discovery*, Cambridge, MA, MIT Press, 1975 offers accounts of twentieth-century neuroscience by neuroscientists.

26 Personal histories of work on chemical neurotransmission and the attendant debates are: Z. M. Bacq, *Chemical Transmission of Nerve Impulses: a Historical Sketch*, Oxford, Pergamon Press, 1974; W. S. Feldberg, 'The early history of synaptic and neuromuscular transmission by acetylcholine: reminiscences of an eye witness', *The Pursuit of Nature*, Cambridge, Cambridge University Press, 1977, pp. 65–83.

27 V. C. Medvei, *A History of Endocrinology*, Lancaster, MTP Press, 1987, includes twentieth-century work within the context of a broad historical survey. H. D.

Rolleston, *The Endocrine Organs in Health and Disease, with an Historical Review*, London, Oxford University Press, 1936, gives a broad review, especially strong on clinical matters, although necessarily restricted in its temporal range.

28 A. L. Hodgkin, 'Chance and design in electrophysiology: an informal account of certain experiments on nerve carried out between 1934 and 1952', *The Pursuit of Nature*, Cambridge, Cambridge University Press, 1977, pp. 1–21.

FURTHER READING

In addition to works listed in the notes, see:

Benchmark Papers in Human Physiology, a series of original papers and expert commentaries. Titles include: *Homeostasis; Cardiovascular Physiology; Hypertension; Contraception; Hypothalamic Neurons; Microcirculation; High-Altitude Physiology; The Heart and Circulation; Pulmonary and Respiratory Physiology; Cell Membrane Permeability and Transport; Electrophysiology;* Stroudsburg, PA, Dowden, Hutchinson & Ross.

The series *People and Ideas*, first published as *Men and Ideas*, includes *Circulation of the Blood; Renal Physiology; Endocrinology; Membrane Transport;* Bethesda, MD, American Physiological Society.

The Pursuit of Nature. Informal Essays on the History of Physiology is a collection of essays by several authors commemmorating the centenary of the Physiological Society, Cambridge, Cambridge University Press, 1977.

Essays in Biology, in Honor of H. M. Evans is a wide-ranging collection including several physiological entries, Berkeley, University of California Press, 1943.

Brooks, C. McC. and Cranefield, P. F., *The Historical Development of Physiological Thought*, New York, Hafner, 1959.

Foster, M., *Lectures on the History of Physiology during the Sixteenth, Seventeenth and Eighteenth Centuries*, Cambridge, Cambridge University Press, 1924.

Franklin, K. J., *A Short History of Physiology*, London, John Bale, Sons & Danielsson, 1933.

Fulton, J. F. (ed.), *Selected Readings in the History of Physiology*, 2nd edn, comp. by L. G. Wilson, Springfield, IL, Charles C. Thomas, 1966.

Fye, W. B., *The Development of American Physiology: Scientific Medicine in the Nineteenth Century*, Baltimore, MD, Johns Hopkins University Press, 1987.

Needham, D. M., *Machina Carnis: the Biochemistry of Muscular Contraction in its Historical Development*, Cambridge, Cambridge University Press, 1971.

8

THE BIOCHEMICAL TRADITION

W. H. Brock

As the science that deals with the chemical constitution of living systems and the dynamics of living chemical processes, biochemistry enjoys close connections with clinical medicine and the molecular biology which, since the 1950s, have formed the basis of our understanding of living processes. Although the term *biochemistry* was used by Felix Hoppe-Seyler (1825–95) in the first issue of *Zeitschrift für physiologischen Chemie* in 1877, the fully fledged autonomous discipline of biochemistry emerged only in the twentieth century. Essentially an interdisciplinary subject, biochemistry was formed from the chemists' 'vegetable' and 'animal' chemistry (which by the 1850s was identified as 'organic' chemistry and located within chemistry departments and institutes of chemistry), and the biologists', cytologists' and doctors' 'physiological', 'zoological' or 'clinical' chemistry (usually located within the physiology departments of medical schools). The subject also rapidly formed a meeting-ground for immunologists, nutritionists, and brewery chemists working on fermentation.

Like Darwinism and late-Victorian scientific naturalism, biochemistry was, in other words, fed by many streams, and only in the Edwardian period was the river broad enough to receive a geographical identity that separated it from its many tributaries and the land masses which had hitherto claimed its waters as their own. Despite its European headstart, the process of autonomy and professionalization was pioneered in the United States.

In Germany, despite its practitioners' influence on discipline-building abroad, physiological chemists tended to remain institutionally divided between chemistry and physiology. The result was that in the twentieth century Germany's greatest contributions to biochemistry tended to come from figures like Otto Meyerhof (1884–1951) and Otto Warburg (1883–1970), who worked in autocratically run research institutes rather than university schools of medicine or organic chemistry. Both British and American biochemistry benefited in decisive ways in the 1930s from the emigration of Jewish scientists such as Hans Krebs (1900–81) to Sheffield, England, E. Chargaff (b. 1905) to Columbia, M. Bergmann (1886–1944) to the Rockefeller Institute, R. Schoenheimer (1898–1941) to Columbia, and C. Neuberg (1877–1956 to New York and who founded the *Biochemische Zeitschrift* in 1906. On an international scale, encouraged by W. Weaver (1894–1978), the Rockefeller Foundation's decision in 1933 to encourage the application of physical and chemical techniques to the study of biological problems proved extremely significant in the opening up of new areas of biochemistry such as molecular biology, and in the training of post-war biochemists.

In Britain, the University of Liverpool gave academic recognition to the subject in 1902, when Benjamin Moore (1867–1922) was appointed to a chair of biochemistry within the School of Hygiene and Public Health. In 1906, after having a paper rejected by the *Journal of the Chemical Society* on the grounds that it was insufficiently chemical, and by the *Journal of Physiology* for being too chemical, Moore founded the *Biochemical Journal*. It was published at Cambridge where the physiologist Michael Foster (1836–1907) had brought the medically trained Frederick Gowland Hopkins (1861–1947) to a lectureship in chemical physiology in 1898. After years of gruelling teaching, Hopkins was appointed in 1914 to the then-unpaid Chair of Biochemistry. Three years earlier, in 1911, British biochemists founded a Biochemical Society which took over Moore's private *Biochemical Journal* as its official organ. With these encouragements, and above all by the endowment of Hopkins's research school at Cambridge by the Dunn benefaction in 1919 and by the publication of Moore's textbook (*Biochemistry*) in 1921, British chemists began to take an increasingly active interest in general biochemical problems. The term 'biochemistry' rather than 'physiological chemistry' was pressed by Hopkins in order to suggest the subject's biological generality and its separateness from medical physiology. Nevertheless, until after the Second World War most British biochemistry outside Cambridge remained an ancilliary sub-discipline to medical physiology and clinical medicine. (➤ Ch. 7 The physiological tradition)

In America, biochemistry developed within medical schools in its own right and not, as in Europe, as a sub-discipline of physiology. In 1882, after teaching medical students at the Sheffield Scientific School at Yale since 1874, R. H. Chittenden (1856–1943), a pupil of the German physiological chemist W. Kühne (1837–1900), was made a professor of physiological chemistry. This inspirational lead was copied by other medical schools in which, during the decade 1900 to 1910, a series of national changes in the medical curriculum brought 'biological chemistry' a favoured independent place. Although by the 1930s the expectation was that American biochemists would have received their primary training as chemists, their career opportunities remained focused on the medical school. On the communications front, outlets were to be found in the *Journal of Biological Chemistry*, which C. Herter (1865–1910) founded in 1905, and in the American Society of Biological Chemists founded in 1906.

PROTO-BIOCHEMISTRY

Ancient Greek 'biochemical' ideas were closely associated with the speculations of natural philosophers and physicians concerning the nature of matter and disease. Like other substances within the earthly sphere, the human body was usually conceived as a harmonious balance between four elements – earth, air, fire, and water – and four humours – blood, phlegm, and yellow and black bile. (➤ Ch. 14 Humoralism) Good health was a balance of these elements or humours; disease was an imbalance brought about by a faulty diet, an unsympathetic environment, or other factors such as the failure of the body's vital heat to blend (coction) food into the appropriate fluid or solid texture of the organism. Coction itself was not solely a mechanical process, but dependent upon an immaterial air-like *pneuma* which was the ultimate source of an organism's vitality. In the Aristotelian and Galenic systems of natural philosophy, the level of teleological and organizational sophistication of an organism was also explained in terms of vegetable, animal, and rational souls, which supervised nutrition, movement, and, in human beings, thought itself.

By the time of the so-called Scientific Revolution of the sixteenth and seventeenth centuries, developments in alchemy and chemistry, as well as a revival of interest in Gnosticism and Platonism, had encouraged new ideas concerning the processes of food assimilation, excretion, and breathing, as well as new practices in chemical drug therapy. In the light of the suggestions of Arabic alchemists of the previous centuries, emphasis was placed upon the principles of liquidity, metallicity, and solidity, or Mercury, Sulphur and Salt, in the understanding of chemical reactions. By the sixteenth century, alchemists had shown how to prepare mineral acids and to extract 'essences' or 'spirits' from plant and mineral substances by distillation.

Such empirical knowledge enabled the iconoclastic and eclectic Paracelsus (1493–1541) to reject humoral ideas of disease and replace them with the notion of infection by specific 'star-born' poisons. Deploying a literal version of the macrocosm–microcosm analogy, he argued that humans did not merely resemble the heavens and the earth, but were composed from them. Humans therefore consisted of mineral and astral components, of mortal and immortal elements, or spirits (*quintae essentiae*). Each spirit (whose 'signature' could be read by the expert, and perhaps a material useful as a medicine could be distilled from it) determined the form and function. This claim led Paracelsus to replace the traditional herbal remedies of Galenic medicine with chemical remedies. He saw these, and indeed all essences, as containing an 'internal alchemist' or *arcana* or *ferment* that had the power of separating the assimilable from waste. This reasoning was applied in detail to the processes of digestion and excretion, as well as fermentation. (➤ Ch. 12 Concepts of health, illness, and disease)

Paracelsus referred to the application of chemistry to medicine as *iatrochemistry* – an influential and revolutionary movement which insured that for the next several centuries medical practitioners received chemical training and/or took an interest in chemical science. In the hands of other Paracelsians, such as J. B. van Helmont (1579–1644) and Sylvius de la Boë (1614–72), the acidic nature of digestion, fermentation, the growth of plants, and the analogy between respiration and combustion all came under scrutiny. In the eighteenth century, however, Georg Stahl (1660–1734), an influential German physician and founder of the phlogiston theory of chemical composition, rejected iatrochemisty. He argued that chemistry could never lead to an understanding of vital functions, which were explicable only in terms of a vital principle or soul. This vitalists' charter did not, however, prevent chemists from continuing to explore living processes. For A. Lavoisier (1743–94), the oxygen gas which he detected in the atmosphere oxidized the carbon contained in food to release animal heat and the carbon dioxide exhaled in breath. Before his early death, he also laid the foundations for the analysis of organic compounds, while his contemporaries, J. Priestley (1733–1809), J. Ingenhousz (1730–99), and J. Senebier (1742–1809) began to explore the role of carbon dioxide in plant respiration and the nature of photosynthesis.

THE NINETEENTH CENTURY

The foundation of an 'assistant society' to the Royal Society, entitled the 'Society for the Improvement of Animal Chemistry', in 1808 is an early example of English chemists' and physicians' interest in biochemical phenomena. Despite the title 'Society', this was in practice a dining club consisting of, at the most, eleven members, including the chemist Humphry Davy (1778–1829), the pharmacist Charles Hatchett (1765?–1857) and his pupil, William Thomas Brande (1788–1866), the surgeons Everard Home (1756–1832) and Benjamin Brodie (1783–1862), and the physicians William Babington (1756–1833) and John Davy (1790–1868), Humphry's brother. As the Royal Society's Council noted, it was clear that 'this most useful pursuit [needs] the united talents of persons well-versed in chemistry, in anatomy and in physiology.'[1]

Between 1809 and its demise in 1825, the Animal Chemistry Society published sixteen papers on blood, urine, poisons, and the connection between nerves and animal heat. Its membership suggests that in the 1800s there was a core of London hospital consultants who saw chemistry as a useful tool in the elucidation of physiological processes. (➤ Ch. 11 Clincal research) Most of them looked to Jöns Berzelius (1779–1848), the Swedish doctor and chemist, for the analytical elucidation of the milk, blood, flesh, urine, and other solid and fluid components of living systems. Important contemporary British chemists such as W. H. Wollaston (1766–1828), J. Bostock (1773–1846), Thomas Thomson (1773–1852), and William Prout (1785–1850), as well as the surgeon Astley Cooper (1768–1841), were excluded from the Society. The Edinburgh-trained William Prout, for example, struggling to earn his living in London in 1812, was unable to obtain membership and he complained to Berzelius. Consequently, in order to further his career and gain attention and patronage, Prout gave public lectures on animal chemistry in 1813 and founded a journal in 1816, the *Annals of Medicine and Surgery*.

In an essay in this journal on the formation of blood, Prout noted that up until then (1816), physiology had reaped little benefit from chemistry. He blamed this situation on the fact that animal chemists were chiefly 'mere chemists'. 'Chemistry in the hands of the physiologist who knows how to avail himself of its means will', he predicted, 'prove one of the most powerful instruments he can possess.'[2] Prout is a good example of the physiological chemist. As a physiologist, he aimed to show through his work on respiration, analysis of milk, foodstuffs, blood, and urine how physiological chemisty could serve medicine in understanding the chemical basis of pathology and disease. (➤ Ch. 9 The pathological tradition)

Perhaps the best example of this approach is the analytical work which the British school of clinical chemists, A. Marcet (1770–1822), Prout, Golding Bird (1814–54) and H. Bence Jones (1814–73), did on urinary stones between 1812 and 1840. It was interest in the causes of the formation of kidney and bladder calculi that induced Prout to study digestion, on the principle which was to remain the hallmark of clinical chemistry up to the 1880s: that pathological chemistry could be comprehended only if the normal chemistry of the body was first understood. This assumption led Prout to the discovery of hydrochloric acid stomach secretion in 1824, to his analysis of milk in 1827, and to his nutritional observation that since milk was the universal pabulum and model diet, foodstuffs could be classifed according to the constituents of milk; namely, oleaginous materials (fats), saccharinous substances (carbohydrates), and albuminous or nitrogenous materials (proteins).

Prout, then, is a good illustration of the fact that long before Justus Liebig (1803–73) turned to the subject, animal and physiological chemists had not stayed content with the analysis of the fluids, secretions, and flesh of animal systems, but had begun to speculate about the chemical relationships between bodily substances and whether their *in vitro* synthesis would indicate anything concerning the *in vivo* transformations. For example, between 1827 and 1834, Prout developed a highly speculative physiological chemistry in which sugars, fats, and nitrogenous substances were transformed up, down, and across homologous chemical series by the addition and subtraction of the elements of water, electrolytic forces, and the addition of minute quantities of other elements. But how did the system work?

In common with the majority of chemists and physiologists in the first half of the nineteenth century, Prout believed that the chemistry of organized beings was intrinsically different from that of 'unorganized' materials. 'Their form is altogether different, and instead of being bounded by straight lines and angles, it is almost universally made up of some variety or combination of curves.'[3] Such differences were to be explained by a 'principle of organization' or a 'living' or 'vital' principle that was present in all organic materials. This governing power, which had been 'imbued by the Creator with a faculty little short of Intelligence', created (synthesized) organic substances from inorganic elements; such organic substances were in a state of combination different from those found in the mineral kingdom. There was a continuous struggle between the chemical forces and elementary substances of the inorganic kingdom and the organizing force of living organisms. The equilibrium of living systems could be maintained only by 'the constant and unremitting agency of the vital principle'. If this vital agency failed, either naturally through age or from sudden exhaustion, then death resulted and speedily restored the incarcerated atoms to their original inorganic state of existence. Such vitalistic notions, with variations, were common, though Prout more pragmatically went on in practice (like Liebig later) to discuss organization in terms of inorganic forces and substances. While accepting evidence of God's design in nature, Prout and other physiological chemists were prepared to subscribe to what has been described as a 'teleological mechanical' framework of explanations.[4]

Clearly, where today a biologist or biochemist attempts to explain the processes of life by appealing to the action of enzymes, electronic charges, or the programme of the genetic code, the early nineteenth-century scientist explained that a vital agency, or special powers, commanded, directed, and when necessary, modified the actions of subordinate inorganic powers of heat, electricity, and chemical affinities. These, in their turn, acted directly upon inert materials according to known laws of physics and chemistry. Inevitably, there were many different positions adopted over the role of vitalism in explanations of living processes. Some physiologists asserted, like Stahl the century before, that because life was such a completely different phenomenon from any inorganic one, the organized system could never be explained in terms of inorganic materials and forces; hence chemistry was a useless tool for the physiologist, whose discipline was to be concerned with 'biological laws' of a fundamentally different order from those of physics and chemistry. Such a viewpoint was strenuously opposed by A. F. de Fourcroy (1755–1809), Marcet, Bostock, Prout, J. B. A. Dumas (1800–84), and Liebig, who argued that since life depended upon inorganic elements such as carbon, the ordinary rules of chemical affinity were also developed by the vital force in living processes.

Although not all of Liebig's ideas were original, the essence of his work was its comprehensiveness and the apparent simplicity of an outlook that combined the concept of vital force in nature with that of a functional relationship between the inorganic world and plant and animal life. Following the demonstration by his friend F. Wöhler (1800–82) that the salts of organic acids are converted into carbonates when passed through an animal's system, just as they are oxidized to carbonates in air, and his discovery in 1828 of the isomerous nature of urea and ammonium cyanate, Liebig seems to have recognized that the barrier separating inorganic and organic chemistry was one of degree, not of kind. Like Lavoisier and P. S. Laplace (1749–1827) fifty years before him, Liebig was certain that animal heat could be explained in terms of the processes of combustion (oxidation) within the organism. Like Prout, this led Liebig to investigate the nature of foodstuffs – for which his elegant and simple copper oxide method of organic analysis had released the animal chemist from sweat, tears, and fearful expense in 1830 – and to distinguish 'plastic' (or structural) foods (nitrogenous substances) from 'respiratory' foods. Fats, which contained lots of carbon, could be likened to coal, while sugar and starches, being formed from fibrous plants, were like wood; both fats and sugars were fuels. Although these analogies did not stand up to detailed scrutiny in the 1860s, reference to plastic and respiratory foods were still to be found in British chemistry textbooks as late as 1888.

Liebig's reasoning as to how animal vitality could be understood within the framework of nature's laws was first revealed in his *Animal Chemistry* of 1842, the English translation of which, by William Gregory (1803–58), appeared simultaneously with the German edition. This extraordinary work was hailed in the *Lancet* as 'a book of sterling merit, of original thought, of transcendental merit' – extravagant praise from its editor Thomas Wakley (1795–1862). The publication of *Animal Chemistry* and its predecessor, *The Chemistry of Agriculture* (1840), aroused widespread discussion and enthusiasm among medical practitioners for whom Liebig's theory of continuous molecular action established a flexible concept of the cause of all contagious diseases, as well as fermentation and putrefaction. Much of the attraction of Liebig's *chemical* point of view was that it gave medical practitioners an advertisable public expertise against the non-medically qualified sanitarians, who advocated a miasmatic interpretation of disease.

Similarly, Liebig's 'black box' chemical equations, although speculative and erroneous and neatly satirized by Claude Bernard (1813–78), were nevertheless suggestive of how detailed chemical transmutations of foodstuffs, flesh and blood, and exhaust products might work at the cellular level. It must be emphasized, however, that Liebig was not the only animal chemist in the period 1840–50. He gave impetus to what was already well established. Indeed, Liebig's *Animal Chemistry*, whatever its influence, must be seen as the culmination of efforts extending over the previous fifty years to deduce chemical changes *in vivo* from the elementary quantitative analysis of milk, blood, flesh, and urine.

In *Animal Chemistry* Liebig argued that when an unstable or decomposing substance came into contact with another stable body, transmitted vibratory motion could cause the latter to decompose. This hypothesis at once explained disease (a form of putrefaction) and the fermentation of sugar to alcohol by yeast. Despite the recent microscopic observations of C. Cagniard-Latour (1777–1859) and Theodor Schwann (1810–82), and their interpretation that yeast fermentation was a biological (living) process (that is, yeast was a live organism), chemists tended to follow Liebig, who with Wöhler, published a notorious, slightly obscene skit on the biologists' claims.

After 1854, Louis Pasteur's (1822–95) work on fermentation, including the distinction between aerobic and anaerobic mechanisms, suggested that yeast fermentation was a by-product of cell metabolism; that it was something to do with the nature of life itself and its organization, and could not be reduced to the sort of biophysical-chemical mechanism that Liebig had advocated. Liebig challenged this view by asking Pasteur to explain the fermentative actions of cell-free pepsin and diastase, which A. Payen (1795–1871) and J.-F. Persoz (1805–68) had identified during the 1830s; the challenge was stimulated by Liebig's pupil, Moritz Traube (1826–94), who had speculated in 1858 that fermentations might be caused by soluble unorganized 'ferments'. The matter was not completely resolved until Eduard Buchner (1860–1917) prepared an extract of yeast, which he called zymase, in 1897. Some historians have argued strongly that this research at this late date, more than anything else, helped to separate biochemistry from general physiology by establishing a new chemical theory of metabolic action, the specific enzyme theory.[5]

Before then, under the influence of the cytologists' work of the 1860s, and of Liebig's and other physiological chemists' views that *organized* life must involve something beyond the purely physical and chemical, what historians have called the 'protoplasmic theory of life' held sway. In 1850, the chemist Thomas Graham (1805–69), while investigating the diffusion of liquids, distinguished gelatinous, or colloidal, materials from the freely diffusing crystalloids familiar to chemists and physicists. Graham, who made a fundamental study of this colloidal state, supposed that the particular form of aggregation that colloids assumed represented matter in a 'dynamical state', as opposed to the statical condition of ordinary liquids. Earlier, in 1835, during microscopical studies of foraminifera, Félix Dujardin (1801–60) had given the name *sarcode* (Greek, flesh) to the apparently structureless 'diaphanous, glutinous' substance from which these minute creatures were formed. For Max Schulze (1825–74), one of the many cytologists who developed Dujardin's sarcodic or protoplasmic theory of the cell, protoplasm was the most important substance in the cell in which were manifested all the chemical and morphological changes characteristic of cell life.[6] This homogeneous 'goo' was, for E. Haeckel (1834–1919), the active substrate of all vital motions and activities, whether of nutrition, growth, motion, or irritability. Although often conceived as a large molecule with side chains containing unstable groups which promoted analyses and syntheses, the theory tended to lead physiologists away from the specificity of chemical reactions within the cell and to adopt a biophysical explanation in terms of colloids and their properties. On the other hand, there were physicalist physiologists who borrowed notions from structural organic chemistry. For example, aware of the reactivity of cyano- and aldehyde groups and their use in synthetic organic chemistry, Eduard Pflüger (1829–1910) of Bonn (the originator of the concept of respiratory quotient) and others supposed that intracellular oxidations of these groups caused explosive ripples which constituted the phenomenon of vitality that Thomas Graham had posited of the colloidal state.

While recognizing that the protoplasm effected chemical changes *outside* the cell by secreting soluble ferments, there was no recognition that ferments played a role within the protoplasm. According to the botanist C. W. Naegeli (1817–91), the cell did not need them because it had available to it the molecular forces of the living matter, a much more energetic means of chemical action.

The new experimental botany of the 1880s, which is associated in Britain with the names of Sydney Vines (1849–1934) and Reynolds Green (1848–1914) and with Cambridge University and the Jodrell Laboratory at Kew Gardens in London, focused upon plant physiology. Influenced by German example and by evidence put forward by Charles Darwin (1809–82) that animal and vegetable protoplasm was similar, if not identical, the new school of botany tended to concentrate upon the chemical aspects of plant physiology. By asking what happened chemically during germination and plant 'digestion', these workers were inevitably led to the study of plant ferments and to their relationship with protoplasm. At the same time, a talented group of brewery chemists, Horace Brown (1848–1925) and Cornelius O'Sullivan (1841–1907)

of Burton-on-Trent, who had been inspired by Pasteur's industrially significant studies of wines and beers, also began to study the ferments associated
with plants and micro-organisms. It was O'Sullivan, for example, who began
kinetic studies of enzymes which revealed that they behaved like inorganic
catalysts.[7]

Close contacts were kept between the groups at Cambridge, Kew, and
Burton. They recognized the living cell as a veritable laboratory of enzymes.
Given the widespread distribution of enzymes in plants that the British groups
had uncovered by the mid-1890s, it is scarcely surprising that, like Traube
and Hoppe-Seyler before them, they decided that Pasteur's distinction
between organized and unorganized ferments was outmoded and that the
real difference between micro-organisms and higher plants (and by impli-
cation, animals) was one of degree and of division of labour.

Although such reflections were to be boosted by Buchner's discovery of
zymase, there remained difficulties with the enzyme theory, even after the
classically based synthetic organic chemistry of Emil Fischer (1852–1919)
had shown that their chemical structures could, in principle, be understood.

One other significant converging context arose from another new science
of the 1880s, bacteriology, which in the French context of microbiology had
also originally been concerned with Pasteur's work on fermentation. With the
establishment of the germ theory of disease in the 1880s, chemical pathologists and clinical chemists could begin to concentrate on the abnormal
rather than the normal: on the microbial infections and on the nitrogenous
compounds formed during the bacterial decomposition of cadaver proteins,
which Francesco Selmi (1817–81) called 'ptomaines'. The search for the
bacteriological toxins that ensued in Britain and on the European continent
was mirrored by the equally enthusiastic attempt to make antitoxins, or
chemicals which would stimulate the natural defence system that the vaccine
of E. Jenner (1749–1823) implied existed. (➤ Ch. 6 The microscopical tradition;
Ch. 10 The immunological tradition; Ch. 16 Contagion/germ theory/specificity)

The discovery c. 1900 of bacteriocidal 'alexines' within blood sera by Hans
Buchner and others, and the discovery in 1891 of the toxin–antitoxin reaction
by E. Behring (1854–1917) and S. Kitasato (1852–1931) offered a new
understanding of disease and immunity as an interaction between specific
chemical substances. Emile Roux (1853–1933) of the Pasteur Institute in
Paris, discoverer of the first bacterial protein toxin, could write in 1899, 'the
medicine of infectious disease has become microbial toxicology, and therapy,
the science of anti-toxins that Behring has revealed. The science of ferments
and of microbes both converge in the study of chemical reactions, which are
due to the most part to enzymes.'[8] Enzymes were, in other words, becoming
the subject, or common ground, of diverse research groups around 1900.

Of course, as Bernard Shaw pointed out later in *The Doctor's Dilemma*

(1906), (➤ Ch. 65 Medicine and literature) the bacteriologists and the immuno-chemists were overconfident in their claims that all disease could be eradicated once the relevant toxins were identified and destroyed either by naturally occurring alexines or by the chemical bullets introduced by P. Ehrlich (1854–1915). (➤ Ch. 39 Drug therapies) Hence the importance of the last converging stream, the study of nutrition to which Prout, Edward Smith (c.1818–74), and the public-health analytical chemists had already made significant contributions. The realization that certain exotic diseases (which were not insignificant in the days of European imperialism) or a mysterious impairment of health might be caused by unknown missing dietary factors, and that unknown accessory factors were also needed for the stimulation of maximum growth of animals, plants, and bacteria, had led by 1902 to the final stream which fed the river of biochemistry. (➤ Ch. 22 Nutritional diseases; Ch. 58 Medicine and colonialism)

THE TWENTIETH CENTURY

As classical organic chemistry in the hands of masters like Emil Fischer came to seem more and more routine, a game of repeated techniques as ritualized as the German Ph.D. system, chemists became increasingly attracted by the challenges of biology. That is, they returned to those areas of chemical physiology which had begun to seem important for the understanding of health and disease. Moreover, there was also the arresting challenge and insights offered by the new physical chemistry of F. W. Ostwald (1853–1932), H. J. van't Hoff (1852–1911), and S. A. Arrhenius (1859–1927), which promised fresh ways of studying the dynamics of metabolic processes. It was a Carlsberg brewery chemist who derived the fundamentally important pH scale of acidity in 1909.

In 1816, Prout had pleaded with physiologists to apply chemistry to their science. In the 1900s, it was the turn of organic and physical chemists to move into physiology and medicine and show that their hitherto poor ancillary relation, physiological chemistry, when rechristened biochemistry and given an enzyme research programme and a pH concept, could be regarded as the pivot of general physiology and medicine.

Twentieth-century biochemistry has been concerned with six main problems: the nature of proteins, nutrition, photosynthesis, metabolism, hormones, and molecular biology. Proteins had been first defined by Gerrit Jan Mulder (1801–80) in 1838 as a radical, $C_{40}H_{62}N_{10}O_{12}$, combined with variable amounts of oxygen, sulphur, and phosphorus, but after initial enthusiasm this definition was refuted by Liebig. Athough various useful chemical tests for proteins were devised, and several amino acids were identified as dehydration products, physiological chemists tended to view proteins as colloids which, by their nature, were not amenable to structural analysis. However, between 1899 and 1919, the German organic chemist Emil Fischer, using the classical techniques of analysis, esterification, and synthesis, produced suggestive evidence that proteins were strings of amino acids linked together by an amido group, $-CO-NH-CH=$. Although Fischer conceived these as chains (polymers) of larger peptide units, he worked within traditional ideas of molecular weights. During the 1920s, however, in an attempt to elucidate the colloidal state, T. Svedberg (1884–1971) developed the ultracentrifuge, which allowed H. Staudinger (1881–1965) to argue that proteins and enzymes were macromolecules rather than aggregates of simpler molecules in a colloidal state. In 1936 Linus Pauling (b. 1901) and A. Mirsky (b. 1900), arguing from the electronic theory of valency, suggested that protein stability arose from electron-sharing through hydrogen-bonding. Given the complexity of the experimental evidence and the uncertainty of the X-ray diffraction data on proteins pioneered by W. Astbury (1898–1961), several alternatives to the Pauling–Mirsky model were conceived during the 1930s. Decisive evidence for the linear, coiled-peptide theory was supplied in 1950 by the alpha-helix structure of the Pauling and R. B. Corey (1897–1971) and synthesis of insulin by F. Sanger (b. 1918) in 1955.

The surgically important and sustained investigations of agglutination and blood groupings by K. Landsteiner (1868–1943) between 1900 and 1940 attracted biochemists to immunology. Since the process whereby an antibody attacks an antigen appeared analogous to a chemical reaction in which bonds are broken and exchanged, it was natural for chemists to take an interest in the forces involved. In 1940, however, much influenced by his admiration for Landsteiner, Pauling invoked the mechanism of 'complementarity' whereby, like two pieces of a jigsaw, antigen and antibody surfaces fitted together stereochemically, allowing the antibody to destroy the invader. This speculation encouraged Pauling to take an interest in the structure of nucleic acids and the nature of gene replication. In 1948, extending his study of the structure and mechanism of haemoglobin oxidation in 1936, Pauling concluded that sickle-cell anaemia was a 'molecular disease' that originated in a deformity of the haemoglobin structure (haemoglobin S), which itself was caused by an inherited genetic fault. With the fuller understanding of molecular biology after 1953, molecular (or genetic) diseases became major areas of biochemical research with a bearing on both clinical and pharmacological treatment. (➤ Ch. 20 Constitutional and hereditary disorders)

Fischer's indominatable view that proteins, and therefore enzymes, had a definite chemical composition and that the mystery of life was amenable to chemical analysis, received strong support from F. G. Hopkins and the school of biochemistry at the University of Cambridge. In 1900, Hopkins isolated the amino acid tryptophane, which he showed was a necessary food factor in the growth and survival of mice. From this and other evidence concerning scurvy and 'imperial' diseases such as beri-beri, Hopkins argued that natural foods contained, over and above carbohydrates, fats, and proteins, 'accessory food substances' necessary for health. In 1912, convinced that all such substances were amines, C. Funk (1884–1967) named them 'vitamines'. Agricultural feeding experiments at the University of Wisconsin by E. V. McCollum (1879–1967) revealed that a fat-soluble principle (A) was important in diets, though it was left to medical practitioners to note its connection with xerophthalmia. Further Wisconsin experiments by H. Steenbock (1886–1967) made the chemical connection between vitamin A and carotene. The demonstration by Thomas Moore (b. 1900) in 1929 that carotene was a precursor of vitamin A enabled its structure to be determined by P. Karrer (1889–1971) in 1931, and the synthesis of A by R. Kuhn (1900–67) and C. Morris followed in 1937. Similar dietary and chemical studies in the 1920s by physiological and organic chemists led to the isolation, structural identification, synthesis, and commercial exploitation of a complete alphabet of fat- and water-soluble vitamins whose role as enzyme co-factors in metabolism was revealed during the same decades.

Although the study of the mechanism of photosynthesis in the 1920s had no bearing on medicine, it was important for the introduction of two further significant biochemical techniques: the use of bacteria (as opposed to the tissues of higher animals) and the introduction of radioactive isotopes by R. Schoenheimer in 1935. These together with the ultracentrifuge, the pressure manometer devised by Otto Warburg for studies of the rates of oxidation, his introduction of thinly sliced tissues in metabolic studies, and the introduction in 1941 of paper chromatography by A. J. P. Martin (b. 1910) and R. L. M. Synge (b. 1914) provided post-war biochemists with a powerful armoury of tools and techniques for the study of metabolism at cellular level.

Metabolic biochemistry began with successful attempts, such as those of A. Harden (1865–1940) and W. J. Young (1878–1942) on fermentation, to identify and isolate particular enzymes and to characterize their catalytic behaviour with specific substrates. From 1908 onwards, Warburg and Otto Meyerhof in Germany explored carbohydrate metabolism manometrically, and demonstrated how sugars were broken down by enzymes into pyruvic acid, acetaldehyde, and ethyl alcohol, while energy was released in the making and breaking of 'energy-rich bonds'. In 1946, building on this, as well as studies of liver glycogen synthesis by Gerty Cori (1896–1957), Hans Krebs unravelled the cyclic pathway whereby glucose and pyruvic acid undergo a complex metamorphosis into citric acid and oxalacetic acid involving several enzymes, co-factors and the adenosine triphosphate (ATP) discovered in muscle by K. Lohmann (1898–1978) in 1929. This elegant 'Krebs Cycle', which accounted for the intramuscular oxidation of carbohydrates, complemented Krebs's earlier work of 1932, in which he had established how ornithine is reduced to urea in the liver.

The existence of chemical secretions which regulate biochemical processes was first established by the physiologists W. M. Bayliss (1860–1924) and E. H. Starling (1866–1927) in 1902. Their isolation of the pancreatic hormone, secretin, was followed by the identification of pancreatic insulin by F. Banting (1891–1941) and C. H. Best (1899–1978) in 1922. These, and other hormones, were subjected to successful chemical analysis, and in many cases synthesis, by organic chemists and biochemists. Work on the steroids and the sex hormones proved especially important clinically and socially with the marketing of chemical contraceptives in the 1950s. (➤ Ch. 23 Endocrine diseases)

Nucleic acids, first detected in cell nuclei by F. Miescher (1844–95) in 1869, inspired little interest before the 1940s, when the advent of chromatography established that they, and not proteins, were responsible for genetic information. The analytical study by E. Chargaff (b. 1905) between 1946 and 1950 of the bases composing nucleic acids enabled F. Crick (b. 1918) and J. D. Watson (b. 1928), together with M. Wilkins (b. 1916) and Rosalind Franklin (1920–58), to exploit crystallographic modelling techniques, especially those of Pauling, to establish the double-helix structure of deoxyribose nucleic acid (DNA) in 1953. This model, which also suggested a process whereby genetic information was replicated, led to a heated international debate amongst traditional biochemists who viewed 'molecular biologists' (as Crick and Watson described themselves) as 'practising biochemistry without a licence'. Reconciliation came in the late 1960s when, through the good offices of Krebs and J. C. Kendrew (b. 1917), biochemistry was redefined as 'biology at the molecular level'.

Before Pauling's study of the chemistry of the haemoglobins in the 1930s and the establishment of molecular biology in the 1950s, 'inborn errors of metabolism', as A. E. Garrod (1857–1936) had termed them in 1909, had largely been confined to the clinical recognition of alkaptonuria, phenylketonuria, and several glycogen-related diseases. By the early 1980s, however, with the fuller understanding of the complexities of enzyme metabolism made possible by Krebs and others, well over a thousand clinical syndromes had been attributed to missing, or incorrect, enzymes. These, in turn, had been attributed to the effects of abnormal genes: to alterations in the base-pair sequences, or to the duplication or omission of gene sequences in the genetic code that were vital to the formation of specific enzymes and proteins.

Pauling, whose theoretical approach was representative of the new molecular biochemistry, concluded in 1968 that a great deal of mental illness could be attributed not just to possible genetic deficiencies but to a lower-than-optimum chemical concentration of nutrients vital to the brain's biochemistry. (➤ Ch. 21 Mental diseases) Although the medical community has proved unreceptive to his particular advocacy of vitamin C as a panacea for a gamut of illnesses, including the common cold, orthomolecular psychiatry and molecular medicine are proving to be fruitful areas of research. Together with the increasing possibilities offered by genetic engineering, clinical biochemistry holds the promise that a large number of enzyme-deficiency and related conditions may be slowly eliminated. Not surprisingly, therefore, biochemistry has come to replace anatomy as the basis of medical education in the twentieth century. It is now essential for the understanding of disease and diagnosis, and is the basis of pharmacology.

NOTES

1   See N. G. Coley, 'The animal chemistry club: assistant society to the Royal Society', *Notes and Records of the Royal Society*, 1967, 22: 173–85.
2   W. Prout, 'Inquiry into the origins and properties of the blood', *Annals of Medicine and Surgery*, 1816, 1: 10–26, 133–67, 277–89; see p. 12.
3   W. Prout, 'Observations on the application of chemistry to physiology, pathology and practice', *Medical Gazette*, 1831, 8: 257–65, 321–7, 358–91; see p. 261.
4   T. Lenoir, *The Strategy of Life: Teleology and Mechanism in Nineteenth Century German Biology*, Dordrecht, Reidel, 1982.
5   R. E. Kohler, 'The enzyme theory and the origins of biochemistry', *Isis*, 1973, 64: 161–96.
6   See J. S. Fruton, 'The emergence of biochemistry', *Science*, 1976, 192: 327–34.
7   See N. Morgan, 'The development of biochemistry in England through botany and the brewing industry 1870–90', *History and Philosophy of the Life Sciences*, 1980, 2: 141–66.
8   Quoted in Kohler, op. cit. (n. 5).

FURTHER READING

Allen, Garland, *Life Science in the Twentieth Century*, New York and London, John Wiley, 1975, ch. 6.
Brock, W. H., *From Protyle to Proton. William Prout and the Nature of Matter 1785–1985*, Bristol, Adam Hilger, 1985.
Buttner, J., *History of Clinical Chemistry*, Berlin and New York, Walter de Gruyter, 1983.
Coley, N. G., *From Animal Chemistry to Biochemistry*, Amersham, Hulton Educational, 1973.
Florkin, Marcel, *A History of Biochemistry*, 6 vols, Amsterdam, Elsevier, 1972–86 [= Vols 31–36 of M. Florkin and E. H. Stotz (eds), *Comprehensive Biochemistry*, 36 vols].
Fruton, Joseph S., *Molecules and Life: Essays in the History of Biochemistry*, New York, Wiley, 1973.
——, *A Skeptical Biochemist*, Cambridge, MA, Harvard University Press, 1992.

Holmes, F. L., Introduction to facsimile edition of J. Liebig, *Animal Chemistry* (1842), New York, Johnson Reprint Corporation, 1964.

——, *Claude Bernard and Animal Chemistry*, Cambridge, MA, Harvard University Press, 1972.

Kohler, R. E., 'The background to Eduard Buchner's discovery of cell-free fermentation', *Journal of the History of Biology*, 1971, 4: 35–61; 'The reception of Eduard Buchner's discovery of cell-free fermentation', ibid., 1972, 5: 327–53.

——, *From Medical Chemistry to Biochemistry. The Making of a Biomedical Discipline*, Cambridge, Cambridge University Press, 1982.

Leicester, H. M., *Development of Biochemical Concepts from Ancient to Modern Times*, Cambridge, MA, Harvard University Press, 1974.

Lieben, Fritz, *Geschichte der physiologischen Chemie*, Hildesheim, G. Olms Verlag, 1970; orig. pub. 1935.

Needham, J. (ed.), *The Chemistry of Life. Eight Lectures on the History of Biochemistry*, Cambridge, Cambridge University Press, 1970.

Olby, R. C., *The Path to the Double Helix*, London, Macmillan, and Seattle, University of Washington Press, 1974.

Teich, M., 'Ferment or enzyme. What's in a name?', *History and Philosophy of the Life Sciences*, 1981, 3: 193–215.

——, and Needham, Dorothy M., *A Documentary History of Biochemistry 1770–1940*, Leicester and London, Leicester University Press, 1992.

9

THE PATHOLOGICAL TRADITION

Russell C. Maulitz

'PATHOLOGY': ANCIENT AND MODERN

Pathology is ancient. 'Pathologists', specialists in anatomizing disease, are newcomers. Pathologists have worked at their craft (it has always been at least as much craft as science) for not much longer than a hundred years. Hence there is a first layer of meaning, namely the *professional* notion of pathology as a set of medical practices preoccupying a circumscribed set of medical actors. A second commonly acknowledged meaning of pathology lies, however, at the opposite pole: pathology without pathologists, pathology as a *biological* notion. It is no doubt a truism that the biological nature of 'pathology', in the guise of disease – the realist notion of the disruptive essence within the organism – is literally as old as life itself.

A third notion of pathology embodies its cognitive elements. Also dependent on human practice, this enterprise of inquiry into pathological change, at once *intellectual* and *craft-based*, is older than that reflected in the recent rise (and incipient fall) of pathology as an independent speciality. Though we shall need in this chapter to deal with both 'pathologies', professional and cognitive, the distinctions between them must be borne in mind, for this last sense of a pathological *tradition* is not only older, but also considerably less monolithic, than the recent emergence of 'the pathologist'.

In the earlier, craft–based enterprise, the 'pre-professional' tradition of pathology, physicians sought to fuse their everyday labours of hand, mind, and eye in understanding the loss of life. They sought to describe and understand disease not only through the exercise of schemes of disease classification, an impulse dating at least as far back as Greek antiquity. (➤ Ch. 17 Nosology) However, before the early modern period, medical thinkers often ignored the solid parts of the body and based their understanding largely on analysis of its fluids or 'humours'. In this framework, 'disease' entailed simply an imbalance of humours. (➤ Ch. 14 Humoralism) Hence we must look elsewhere for at least some of the early sources of impetus to anatomize disease.

One critical stimulus was medico-legal: post-mortem dissection performed to prove or disprove foul play. (➤ Ch. 69 Medicine and the law) Another was the sheer cachet of being cut up after one's death. Compilations of such autopsies began to appear during the Renaissance, most notably in the *Medicina* of Jean Fernel (1497–1558) and, a century later, the *Sepulchretum* of Théophile Bonet (1620–89). It was, in fact, Fernel who, in the second part of the work cited, introduced the term 'pathology' to denote the morbid appearances found in the subjects – usually royals and aristocrats – who fell to the anatomist's blade.

However, it was only around the mid- to late-eighteenth century, as we shall see, that physicians would add to these taxonomic and medico-legal designs through the critical and soon dominant motive of the pathological tradition: the impulse to localize the lesions of disease in their anatomical seats.

THE SEATS AND CAUSES OF DISEASE

'GENERAL' PATHOLOGY

As indicated in other chapters of this *Encyclopedia*, a remarkable change began to occur, perhaps as early as the seventeenth century, in the outlook of certain curious clinicians. Whereas pathology and anatomy had heretofore existed quite separately, and indeed had been reflected in ways of thinking about the body and its ills that had for centuries remained incommensurable one with the other, the two now converged. Within a few generations, by the early nineteenth century, the traditions of anatomy and of pathological theory had become tightly interwoven.

What did anatomy and pathology look like before the eighteenth century? The language itself becomes slippery and elusive. One may properly speak of pathological theory before, say, 1700, and one may properly speak of an anatomical tradition. But only with the advent of frequent and systematic dissection of the human body performed for the purposes of localizing disease can we find what counts as a meaningful pathological tradition. This phenomenon, though adumbrated by Bonet, Fernel, Thomas Willis (1621–75), and other seventeenth-century figures, was primarily an outgrowth of eighteenth- and nineteenth-century modernization.[1] I stress this point in order to draw a distinction marking a dramatic change in the medical world-view, a distinction between medicine preceding the era of pathological dissection and the practice of anatomical pathology that followed it.

Antedating the new tradition, perhaps by centuries, was what is now called general pathology. As every twentieth-century medical student learns, general pathology did not disappear or become displaced by anatomical pathology. General pathology was (and remains) essentially a collection of mental procedures for understanding disease through various theoretical systems devised to understand pathological change. An early outgrowth of classical Hippocratic and, more particularly, Galenic habits of thought in Western medicine, the impulse to rely on some system of general pathology in the medieval period became the badge of intellectual sophistication for the *physicus*, the educated physician. In the early modern period, this trend toward theoretical development in internal medicine and pathology, usually (but not always) based on the doctrine of humours, was focused increasingly in university settings. (➤ Ch. 48 Medical education)

By the Enlightenment, the notion of general pathology had become commonplace in medical parlance, discussed in standard works and the stock-in-trade of courses in the 'institutes of medicine'. In the eighteenth and nineteenth centuries, and indeed well into the twentieth, general pathology survived importantly to be taught in a number of formats and settings ranging from standard internal medicine to pathophysiology courses. Finally, woven into the larger tradition, general pathology, taxonomy, pathophysiology, and anatomy would become inextricable. (➤ Ch. 7 The physiological tradition)

MORBID ANATOMY

In the eighteenth century, the essential anatomical basis of pathology began to emerge, in a development that came to make morbid anatomy almost synonymous with the pathological tradition over the ensuing two centuries. The origins of this curious alchemy, by which pathology and morbid anatomy came to be superimposed, even now seem obscure. It is not possible to pinpoint all the factors that fostered this development; but it is at least possible, without attempting to assign relative weight or priority to them, to identify certain key elements, and in doing so, further to explore the world of the morbid anatomist in this critical seedtime for the pathological tradition.

In other words, among historians of medicine there is a growing consensus that over the course of the decades preceding the French and American revolutions, the course of the pathological tradition was redirected in a significant fashion, the first of two turning-points in the history of pathology. The determining steps in that change seem to have included the rise of an educated and socially well-placed surgical élite; an upsurge in medical practitioners' access to 'anatomical materials' – dead bodies – in large series of post-mortem dissections; an increase in hospital-based anatomical activity; and an upturn, at least among certain professional élites, in what one might term the internationalism of medical education and practice. We may review each of these determining factors *seriatim*.

It seems clear that in the latter half of the eighteenth century, a new configuration of relations developed between medical professionals and health institutions. A finely grained analysis of the economic and social conditions underlying this convergence lies beyond the scope of this chapter, but it is safe to say that in the European monarchies, surgeons gained in economic and political power during this period, a process that could only enhance the weight and consequence of their anatomical methods.[2] (➤ Ch. 41 Surgery (traditional))

Even when these surgeons lacked their internal-medicine counterparts' 'modern' model of university-prepared expertise, they still formed themselves into legitimate professional groups, bringing to bear highly particularized and well-shaped constellations of technical mastery based upon normal and morbid anatomy.[3] (➤ Ch. 47 History of the medical profession) This was certainly true in Britain and France. And in America, both before and after 1776, it was also true, if partly for a different reason: the levelling effect of the frontier. (In an important sense, even the settled American east coast remained a medical frontier until well into the nineteenth century.)

If the effect of changes in the sorting and classing of professional groups represented one key factor, another was the reciprocal relation between these changes and the classing of hospitals. To the extent that hospital care (and hospital-based medical and surgical education) became more prominent in the eighteenth century, it was primarily for the lower orders of society. Those whose entry to hospital ended in death became grist for the morbid anatomists' mill. In continental Europe, and to an extent in America as well, admission to hospital implied tacit permission for dissection of the body should the 'termination' of the patient's clinical course prove – as it so often did – to be his or her demise there. (➤ Ch. 49 The hospital)

As a result, the warehouse-like hospitals of some European capitals became centres, veritable assembly lines, for the practice, codification, and teaching of morbid anatomy. In Britain (and especially in Scotland), the supply of corpses was impeded by such legal niceties as permission from next-of-kin. This bottleneck, and in Britain the further barrier to the practice from a strong aversion among the laity, provided a booming business for the 'sack 'em up boys'. Such grave-robbing 'resurrectionists' perhaps saw themselves as offering an essential service. Only much later were they largely put out of business, after the Anatomy Act of 1832 finally provided for a regulated supply of bodies for dissection within a controlled market with clearly demarcated legal bounds.[4]

The quantitative argument, in which sheer numbers of patients led by a sort of 'mass action' to an upsurge in autopsy experience, can easily be pushed too far. It is difficult to assess the direct impact of eighteenth-century hospital growth on the pathological tradition. One suspects that the expansion of urban centres in Europe and America, with some attendant increase in disease, must have affected the store of available corpses, yet evidence on the issue is actually rather scant. Indeed, there is some evidence that, outside a few particularly squalid sites such as the Paris Hôtel-Dieu, physicians in voluntary hospitals in cities such as Edinburgh actually had relatively little opportunity to dissect: between their relatively less enfeebled population, and the weakest patients' families' reluctance to give consent for necropsy, many hospitals produced a paucity of dead bodies.[5]

It is also tempting to postulate a related impact from the eighteenth-century advance of warfare and military hospitals. As the lethality of weapons increased, wounds became ever more severe. Yet many of the major military hospitals, such as the Val de Grâce in Paris, were not founded until the end of the century, in response to a resurgence of warfare. And on military wards, such as there were, hospitalized soldiers and sailors were more likely to have been admitted for survivable conditions (venereal disease, enteritis, etc.) than for fatal battlefield injuries.

Nonetheless, the practice, and to a certain extent the theory, of morbid anatomy clearly grew apace before 1800, at least as a routinized teaching exercise based on materials 'as available' in hospitals. This qualification seems important in view of the misconception that has persisted since the influential work of the French historical philosopher Michel Foucault, to the effect that morbid anatomy was the crowning diadem created by the French school of medicine that flourished after 1800.[6] But in the second half of the eighteenth century, in many places – certainly, and to varying degrees, France, Germany, the Baltics, Russia, Italy, Britain, and America – surgeons and physicians were already keenly focused on morbid anatomy as a way of correlating post-mortem findings with ante-mortem diagnosis.

Such practitioners essentially saw the method of morbid anatomy as a way of 'proofing' their taxonomies of disease and improving their diagnostic acumen.[7] The second half of the eighteenth century, indeed, saw the development among physicians and surgeons of what virtually amounted to an internationally sanctioned effort to cut up every living thing that had stopped moving, including not just their own ordinary patients, but also their regents and royals, their families and colleagues.

No doubt there are good, if still partly conjectural, cultural reasons for this efflorescence of interest in picking apart the decayed human frame. The change may have stemmed partly from the decline of a religion-based repugnance to dissection among members of an increasingly secularized public. (➤ Ch. 61 Religion and medicine) There was also an intellectualized notion of the good of society. Hence in his magisterial survey of European public health and medicine in the 1770s, Johann Peter Frank (1745–1821), medical cosmopolite, Rousseau-apostle and inveterate traveller, could note that many 'sick commoners . . . in the last days of their suffering [had] instructed their heirs to have their corpses dissected . . . for the benefit of their fellow human beings who suffer from similar ills.'[8]

Frank singled out the traditional citadel of anatomical study, Italy, for special attention in connection with the salubrious new practice, carefully setting out the protocol whereby pathological specimens would be funnelled into institutionally supported morbid-anatomy museums.[9] In Italy and elsewhere on the Continent, such support tended to come from the university, hence indirectly the city-state. In Britain and America, it tended to come from guild structures such as the élite practitioner colleges. In every case, however, the efflorescence of pathological museums had the same three taproots: first, the clinical practice of medicine; second, the stimulus to attract more students (and hence fees) by means of the exhibition of rare diseases; and third, the impulse to classify not just disease, but also its material results.

EXPONENTS OF THE EIGHTEENTH-CENTURY TRADITION

This classificatory impulse, at once museological and clinical, spread quickly across international boundaries. In most major capitals, it resulted in major collections of oddities and organs: the pathological tradition for the first time writ large, for visual interrogation by one's peers. Many of these pathology collections survive to the present day. Perhaps the best known is that of John Hunter (1728–93), housed at the Royal College of Surgeons, London. It is no accident that Hunter, in part around his museological instincts, formed a reputation as a key British forerunner of the new nineteenth-century pathological anatomy (see pp. 176 ff.).[10]

Eclipsing even Hunter's reputation internationally was Giambattista Morgagni (1682–1771), successor at some remove to Andreas Vesalius (1514–64) in the anatomy chair at Padua. In 1761, Morgagni's *On the Seats and Causes of Disease* [*De Causis et Sedibus Morborum*], perhaps the most important pathological work before that of Rudolf Virchow (1821–1902) (see pp. 183–4), simultaneously capped both the grand Paduan tradition of general anatomy and the broader eighteenth-century European tradition of morbid anatomy.[11] (➤ Ch. 5 The anatomical tradition) With the *De Causis*, translated by the end of the decade into most consequential languages of Western medicine, Morgagni put the capstone on his own career as well.[12] He was almost 80 when he published this compendium of hundreds of cases, each correlating the pathology of individual bodily organs with the clinical courses exhibited by their former owners.

Given the limitations of inspection by the naked eye, Morgagni's work extended anatomists' scrutiny of individual body organs to body regions. He stressed the importance of the vascular system, and emphasized transmutations and sympathies between bodily regions. In one key case representation, for example, Morgagni introduced into medical discourse the peculiar yet powerful notion of pneumonia-induced 'hepatization' of the lung – the transmutation, by means of the instrumentality of disease, of lung into liver.[13] Morgagni is often portrayed as the architect of modern pathology, and in a way he was. But to see him as an 'early pathologist' is to miss how two other more salient features of his career epitomized the eighteenth-century phase, and largely the nineteenth-century phase, in the overall sweep of the pathological tradition. Recent studies re-emphasize Morgagni's 'connectedness' as a clinician, as a consultant to the Italian nobility, and consequently as an intimate of well-placed medical men, both established and aspiring, at home and abroad.[14]

Picture, then, John Morgan (1735–89), some-time Philadelphia institution-builder and in 1759 an ambitious young American student in Edinburgh. For a term that year, Morgan shared rooms with John Hunter. Four years later, as a newly fledged Edinburgh MD, Morgan set off on the obligatory Grand Tour of the European continent, alighting in Padua in July 1763. Repeated visits to Morgagni ensued, Morgan suing for the patronage of the older man and remarking on the similarity of their names: they must, Morgagni observed, be cousins.[15] But Morgan was interested in more than mere networks of contacts. He later wrote back to Morgagni that he was sending him, through commercial Venetian contacts, some wax-injected preparations illustrating the capillary circulation of the kidneys. In such a manner issued the language of morbid anatomy, as close as anyone could at that time come to a common discourse of international medicine, with the professional and intellectual benefits that attended such exchanges.[16]

Why did pathology become the first truly international medical tradition? One reason, as we have already seen, was the differential availability of pathological 'material' at different places and times. Another, perhaps less obvious, resided in the problems actually confronted by pathology-minded clinicians. Pathology was unlike, say, physiology, in which the elaboration of system was dependent in large measure on the concepts and especially the techniques brought to bear on particular problems. (Notions of nerve function, for example, depended, then as now, on matters such as whether whole-body or isolated nerve-muscle preparations were deployed.)

In contrast, the pathological tradition had by the late eighteenth century reached a point of convergence with mostly common elements, invariant across national boundaries. Whether in America, Britain, France, Germany, Russia, or Italy, clinicians faced certain repetitive problems at the post-mortem table. These were: when tissues grow and overgrow in exuberant fashion, how does one differentiate neoplastic from inflammatory change? How does one distinguish malignant from benign tumour? (➤ Ch. 25 Cancer) What is the nature of pus? How do wounds heal; and how does deranged wound healing kill? And finally, when blood ceases its free flow and, in various circumstances, forms clots, is such a process primarily a source of benefit or of mischief? These questions formed leitmotivs across all borders, a point to which I shall return.

Professionally, the late eighteenth-century impulse to investigate morbid-anatomy subjects can be portrayed as a project simultaneously embedded in three different social milieux. Men like Hunter and Morgagni got used to dissection – not only of the hospitalized poor, but equally their wealthy patients, their families, their fallen colleagues – as an extension of both their teaching and their practice. For them and others like them, in other words, this impulse to dissect at once advanced, first, the culture of professionalism, promoting clinical experience and career ascendancy; second, the culture of middle-class and aristocratic patient care, thereby promoting access to one perennial sort of paying customer; third, the culture of international medical education, thereby promoting access to the other major genre of paying customer: medical students.[17]

A NINETEENTH-CENTURY FLOWERING: PATHOLOGICAL ANATOMY

By the eighteenth century, medical authors commonly and increasingly spoke of 'pathological anatomy' when describing clinicians' practice of post-mortem dissection. In this chapter, I adopt the convention, however, of reserving this term to depict an array of dramatic innovations that were hammered out as part of the institutional changes following the French Revolution. Tempered in the crucible of the Paris Hospital in the Napoleonic and post-Napoleonic period, the innovations embodied in pathological anatomy essentially represented the practical implementation and the theoretical maturation of some well-established eighteenth-century pathological concepts.[18]

The group of early principals in this endeavour, most of them provincials drawn to Paris for medical advancement, included Xavier Bichat (1771–1802), Gaspard Laurent Bayle (1774–1816), and René Laënnec (1781–1826). Variously trained by Napoleon's some-time physician Jean Nicolas Corvisart (1755–1821) and by the Hôtel-Dieu chief surgeon Pierre Desault (1738–95) (the pairing of internist and surgeon is critical), Bichat and his colleagues combined the surgical notion of disease, localized at the level of particular organs and tissues, with medical notions of general, or systemic, pathological change. They did so largely without resort to microscopes, already in use by some experimentalists but still unable to supply crisp images, and chose instead to analyse disease in connection with its effects on individual tissue planes.

The notion of analysing pathological change in terms of bodily membranes and tissues was not wholly discordant with some similar ideas advanced by the French group's predecessors. Such ideas could be no more novel than was the disease substrate inviting their scrutiny: trauma, fever, enteritis, tuberculosis. In writing on gunshot wounds and inflammation, for example, John Hunter had adumbrated much of the work of Bichat and Bayle. The ubiquitous presence of inflamed tissues, in other words, invited precisely the sort of analysis that Hunter (and others) inaugurated, and that the early stewards of Paris medicine were soon to extend.

A generation later, Edinburgh surgeon John Thomson (1765–1846) could use the 'treatment of febrile and internal inflammatory diseases [considered to belong] exclusively to the province of the physician' as a prod for his colleagues to recognize that

> internal remedies [are] not only required in a large proportion of the diseases which are regarded as strictly chirurgical, but also that there are few diseases which come under the care of the physician, in which morbid affections, requiring the manual aid or practical skill of the surgeon, do not frequently occur.[19]

Thomson was hardly a professionally impartial observer. His plaint merely underscores the fact that, at least in Britain, the two branches, physic and surgery, remained too far apart, even in the 1810s and 1820s, systematically to assimilate a converging body of pathological theory. Hence it was in the French medical arena that these corresponding professional and conceptual changes took root in their earliest and most fully developed form.

Xavier Bichat, who was in many respects the veritable Mozart of eighteenth- and nineteenth-century medicine, first extended the medico-surgical analysis of tissue pathology in his 1799 *Treatise on Membranes*. In this and in his *General Anatomy*; in his projected subsequent *Pathological Anatomy*, published a generation later by his followers P. A. Béclard (1785–1825) and F.-G. Boisseau (1791–1836); and in the investigations of A. L. J. Bayle (1799–1858), Laënnec, and a number of their successors the human body in health and particularly in disease came to be conceived in a manner quite different from that visualized before the early nineteenth century. Bichat and Laënnec envisioned a sort of Russian-doll model of the body, a concentric affair in which tissue planes, enveloping and overlapping one another, invested the major organs of the thorax and abdomen.[20]

It was a surprisingly suggestive model, permitting its adherents both to understand and to predict pathological change in terms of 'sympathies' between the membranous tunics surrounding distant parts affected by unitary disease processes. At autopsy, serous membranes surrounding organs such as the heart, lungs, and abdomen were often inflamed in patients with, for example, disseminated tuberculosis. Mucous membranes of the gut were often affected by the bouts of enteritis that became, in turn, the central focus of a pathological system promulgated by perhaps the most influential Paris clinician-educator of the post-Waterloo period, namely François Broussais (1772–1838).[21]

And most of all, this was a model of pathological change that could only flourish, or at least only did flourish, under the system for educating medical practitioners that was introduced with the reopening of 'health schools' in France. These écoles de santé were established in 1794 in Paris, Strasbourg, and Montepellier. Medical teaching institutions such as these were clearly restored for local reasons, including the need to reverse some of the excesses of revolutionary corporate levelling; the need to provide practitioners to minister to an enlarging military corps; and, possibly, the opportunity to trade a little prime left-bank real estate. But the net result was as far-reaching as it was contingent: the amalgamation of surgeons' and physicians' outlooks into a coherent intellectual system.

Surgeons, used to extirpating the lesions of disease, and physicians, used to administering systemic medicaments, all suddenly now needed a blanket system that could unite heretofore disparate perspectives on the 'seats and causes of disease'. In its new aspect, pathological anatomy practically implemented that system. Philippe Pinel (1745–1826), like Corvisart a prominent figure in devising the newer approaches to medical education, said it as well as anyone in 1798: 'The art of healing is one and indivisible, and . . . as a consequence there is only one pathology.'[22] Here, for the first time, we see the emergence of a self-conscious new style of pathology.

Such a new, 'artificial', system of pathological anatomy was to have a number of interesting reciprocal effects on how the physician saw his own world. In particular, two rather different sorts of impact deserve comment. The first, at the professional level, was further to sustain the new internationalism of medicine, as trainees from everywhere in the old and new worlds arrived in Paris to imbibe the pathological tradition along with their clinical lessons. (Not surprisingly, such students, once back home, were successful in reimplanting the tradition in just the degree to which their indigenous systems supported the Gallic-style fusion of internal medicine and surgery.) (➤ Ch. 59 Internationalism in medicine and public health)

A second, cognitive consequence of the elaboration of pathological anatomy was its role in amplifying the importance of physical diagnosis. Diagnostic methods such as auscultation and percussion had multiple bases, but one of the most important was the impetus to correlate ante- and post-mortem findings. It comes as no surprise, then, to discover that the original French edition, quite unlike the English, of René Laënnec's benchmark 1819 *Treatise on Mediate Auscultation*, best known now for its early introduction of stethoscopy, fits squarely into the pathological tradition. In it, he explicitly fosters the new pathological anatomy: it is as much a work through which Laënnec could expound the principles of post-mortem dissection and tissue pathology as it was an encomium to the new, instrument-based techniques of physical examination. (➤ Ch. 35 The art of diagnosis: medicine and the five senses; Ch. 36 The science of diagnosis: diagnostic technology)

THE MID-NINETEENTH CENTURY: THE MICROSCOPE AS AUTHORITY

By the 1830s, pathological anatomists in Paris and elsewhere had begun to regularize, by means of elaborate methods for the classifying and teaching of morbid anatomy, ways of reaching consensus about macroscopic pathological anatomy.[23] Ironically, it was just then that they came to confront an instrument, the microscope, that challenged medical practitioners' accepted methods in pathology, their traditional ways of seeing the body in health and disease, and even the very means for attaining consensus. (➤ Ch. 6 The microscopical tradition)

Working microscopes had been available since the nineteenth century, but certain important optical characteristics limited their utility. Instruments relatively free of the most important forms of optical aberration, namely chromatic and spherical aberration, were introduced in most national settings around 1830. Among the earliest physician-investigators to use the new instruments were those who, like Thomas Hodgkin (1798–1866) in England and W. W. Gerhard (1809–72) in the United States, went to Paris and based their subsequent intellectual plans on the blueprint provided by pathological anatomy.

The effect of these new microscopes would be felt earlier in microscopical anatomy (soon to be called histology) than in pathology proper. That living tissues might be analysed into smaller constituents was a notion that for some decades had actually been gestating in various inchoate and fluid forms: those smallest functional elements had been variously dubbed fibres, globules, or even 'cells'. But the early concept of the cell lacked the microstructural specificity now imparted by the microscope. The critical level of specificity and a concrete notion, corresponding to the modern one, of living cells was communicated in 1838–9 by a pair of intriguing and rather mismatched German microscopists, the emotionally unstable lawyer-turned-botanist Matthias Schleiden (1804–81), and the soon to be self-exiled religious visionary physician Theodor Schwann (1810–82).[24] They did so by conjoining two specific ideas about the cell: its physiological primacy as a building block of living nature, either plant or animal; and a 'signature' sub-structural make-up, marked notably by the typical presence of a nucleus in each cell.

But the cellular model of microscopic anatomy, advanced by Schleiden and Schwann as well as by Robert Remak (1815–65) and others, made its way only slowly from biological theory into a form accessible to medical scientists. In part, it was not readily accepted; at first, it was quite unclear how cells reproduced. The romantic Schwann, seeking to unify all organic and inorganic nature, considered it likely that they crystallized from ambient tissue fluids or so-called blastema. But the intrinsic structural characteristics of living systems were such that embryologists and botanists had a better chance of working out these details than anatomists handling medical material. As a result, for a decade and a half the botanists and embryologists retained almost exclusive title to the use of the microscope for research in cellular structure and function.

It is interesting to note how much more pervasive microscopical investigation, both biological and, eventually, medical, was in the German states than in France, Britain, southern Europe, or the United States. To a certain extent, the imbalance in rates of activity may be more apparent than real. In Edinburgh, a prominent group of workers performed and taught histological experiments from the late 1830s.[25] In France, Alfred Donné (1801–78) and others actively pursued the fruits of microscopical research.[26] In America, J. B. S. Jackson (1806–79) and Alonzo Clark (1807–87) had both begun teaching pathological tradition in earnest in Boston and New York, respectively, by 1847, the year of the founding of the American Medical Association. Clark, at least, was charged by the Columbia trustees with the task of promulgating 'the recent application of improved microscopes to healthy and diseased structures'.[27]

But Jackson's and Clark's professorships were the only full-time American posts in pathology at that time, and for quite a while to come. That fact, and somewhat similar circumstances in Britain and France, underscores a stark distinction from the German position. There are various meanings one may attach to the expansion of Germany's system of higher education, spanning perhaps the latter two-thirds of the century, during Prussia's drive for hegemony. Although the subject lies outside the compass of this chapter, peculiar to this period in German history there clearly seems to have been a political and intellectual dynamic that fostered the emergence of hybrid disciplines in the medical sciences.

The emergence of one such field, histopathology, marked a new turning-point in the pathological tradition. Led by German investigators, clinician-pathologists between 1840 and 1860 launched a new phase of research, characterized by the fusion of histology and pathological anatomy. The German medical *paterfamilias*, Johannes Müller (1801–58), launched this new phase when, in a series of published scientific pieces and lectures in the late 1830s, he addressed the then (as now) hot issue of the 'finer structure . . . of morbid tumours'.[28]

Writing before the full elucidation of the cell theory itself, Müller was able nonetheless to introduce the microscope into the process of correlating bedside and organ- or tissue-based observations. The ability in some settings to move correlative diagnosis from the necropsy table to the microscope stage served another critical purpose. It allowed the physician to go beyond mere retrospective testing of diagnostic adequacy and hence therapeutic efficacy. He now had a way of providing prospective clues as to tissue diagnosis in a manner that could be expected, at least for some external tumours, actually to guide therapy. Thus the disclosure of a bone or breast tumour, for example, if shown to be of a certain histological type, might prompt an amputation operation considered to prolong survival. (➤ Ch. 11 Clinical research)

Partly because of the shift in the international epicentres of medical education from France and Britain to the German states – whence their forebears returned from formative *Wanderjahre* – historians of scientific medicine are used to depicting the critical single generation between 1840 and 1860 in the context of the triumph of Teutonic scientific and medical institutions. The truth is more complex and nuanced. The emergence of the particular form of histopathology that has lasted to the present day, its primogeniture properly credited to Müller's student, Rudolf Virchow, may be seen in part, but only in part, as a paradigm shift from the Schwannian notion of blastema to Virchow's concept of cellular continuity. But it may be traced as well to the convergence of information about the primacy of cellular life now flowing into international medicine from outside fields, notably botany, microscopy, and embryology, with inquiries coming directly from clinical medicine.

The same three clinical problems that had exercised Morgagni, Hunter, Bichat, and Laënnec remained sources of essential inquiry in the 1840s, 1850s, and 1860s; the formation of pus, the mechanism of thrombosis, and the origins of cancer. The intellectual lineaments of the pathological tradition can be traced through the use of any one of these problems as a marker of conceptual change. We may, for example, again use oncogenesis or cancer-cell formation as a useful probe. Twelve years before Virchow declared '*omnis cellula a cellula*', the French physician Hermann Lebert (1813–78) adumbrated the idea of the cancer cell as a specific, independent entity. But Lebert happened to adhere to the more humoralistic (and highly plausible) notion of the blastema, the ambient tissue substance from which the cancer cell was thought to derive.[29] In doing so, he followed in part the lead of his Viennese contemporary, Carl Rokitansky (1804–78), whose practical labours were absolutely prodigious. Rokitansky, however, probably undermined the impact and importance of his extraordinary experience at the post-mortem table by insistently embedding that experience within the older, humoralistic framework of general pathology.

When Virchow began a series of lectures on 'cellular pathology', in 1855, he fused one powerful set of ideas about cell specificity, culled from Lebert's and others' works, with another, drawn from biology and, in particular, the Berlin work of the unsung Jewish physician Robert Remak. But the fusion product, embodied in the concept that all cells originated from antecedent parent cell lines without the intervening participation of humoral elements, was perhaps less important intellectually than it may now at first seem. If one reads Müller, for example, on cancer formation, and one mentally 'substitutes' cell parentage for the chemico-humoral notions of cell origin to which he adheres, one finds little damage done to the clinical or scientific content, and great similarity to the later nineteenth-century cellular pathologists.

Politically, however, Virchow's move to fuse cell biology with tissue pathology was of signal importance: in 1855 when he lectured on the subject, and in 1858 when he promulgated a major text on the cellular basis of pathology.[30] Rejecting both his own teacher, Müller, and his Viennese counterpart, Rokitansky, Virchow's championship of the new *Cellularpathologie* was a political masterstroke. It was a conscious and highly successful attempt, undertaken by a tireless and intensely focused physician, to redirect the stream of the pathological tradition: not only did his new system secure Virchow's journey from Würzburg back to the key Berlin chair of pathology, but for half a century to come it cast Virchow himself in the role of both helmsman and lockmaster in that stream.[31]

Without the microscope, the cell could be considered in merely impressionistic terms. By emphasizing the role of the instrument, cellular pathology provided the focus for the development of pathology as a separate speciality. Virchow himself took advantage of this incipient possibility by developing his own, highly influential Pathological Institute in Berlin, and attracting a worldwide influx of students – much as Laënnec, Broussais, *et al.*, had done across the Rhine a half century earlier. Other Berlin luminaries, however, such as the surgeon Theodor Billroth (1829–94), saw this latest phase of the pathological tradition as more than a way of merely fostering another new, narrowly defined discipline or scientific career. Pathology was also a way of injecting both scientific culture and, perhaps even more important, clinical utility into the medical milieu of Bismarckian Germany.

Billroth, in particular, concerned to place surgery on solid scientific grounds, carefully tracked the work, performed in the 1860s by Virchow and his successors, on the origins of tumour cells. Billroth felt such work would be important in diagnosing and treating neoplastic disease. Indeed, it was in just that decade that pathological anatomy finally provided the tools by means of which inflammatory and malignant neoplasia could finally be differentiated. The new microscopical possibility, in reciprocal fashion, also now rendered the pathological tradition even more central in the physician's routine. It provided an additional layer of theoretical explanation, clarifying the differential origins of abnormal cells. It also added a layer of practical efficacy, enhancing the ability of the surgical pathologist to distinguish between disease processes that – while appearing similar to gross inspection – actually bore critically dissimilar prognostic and management implications.[32]

THE IMPORTANCE OF BEING VIRCHOW

To look at the phenomenon of an emerging research culture, and the centrality of the pathological tradition within that culture, is again to come back to the remarkable fashion in which Virchow's career operated as a syncytium, each element penetrating and reinforcing the next. Institutionally, as we have seen, he was able to 'jump start' the foundation of pathology as a separate discipline by newly re-emphasizing what was essentially an old technology, microscopy, and by insisting that the old role of prosector in pathological anatomy be expanded and elevated to the head of a separate institute. In such an expanded institute he was then able to operate at the personal and professional level by attracting a lively cadre of students, men such as Julius Cohnheim (1839–84) and Friedrich von Recklinghausen (1833–1910), who collectively went on to extend the pathological tradition in time, well into the twentieth century; in space, in an expanding Germany; and in conceptual scope.

Part of the very measure of Virchow's institutional and professional success was that his students at times contradicted and outstripped him. In old age he became rather depressed, partly because of the thwarting of his liberal civic beliefs – the political world, he felt, had passed him by – but perhaps in some measure because the scientific world had done the same. The notion of microbiology, the presence of alien bacterial organisms, as the basis of disease aetiology was, for example, an idea he could never fully accommodate to his image of the cell and its reactions as the bedrock of disease. Thus did the discipline of pathology give birth, however uneasily, to the discipline of bacteriology.

But even within pathology, Virchow's intensely localistic ideas about the role of the cell in pathological change were successfully challenged by his students. Most notably, Cohnheim, perhaps influenced by the more physiologically minded French school, demonstrated the phenomenon of inflammation to be the result of action at a distance from the point of anatomical injury. As white blood cells swarmed to a site of experimentally induced injury, Cohnheim showed their transmigration across vessel walls into injured tissue, forming pus and supporting the notion that the pus and circulating white cells were interchangeable entities.[33]

That Virchow's field of vision, in a biological and cognitive sense, was confined to the connective tissue cells disclosed on his microscope stage should not blind us to his larger disciplinary vision for pathology. It was his morphological method that constructed the edifice, both at the conceptual level of biological building-blocks as well as at the tangible level of institutional bricks and mortar. And it was in bricks and mortar that Germany led. In France, England, and the United States, individual investigators evinced interest, but only later, in the twentieth century, did their institutions begin to pull abreast of the German community.

PATHOLOGICAL PHYSIOLOGY AND CHEMISTRY

After Virchow, however, the pathological tradition became more complex, not just because pathologists went on to devise the methods of bacteriology, but also because they began quite early on to pay attention to the need to take their growing community beyond morphology: they sought to construct a science that would encompass not merely pathological anatomy, but also the subsidiary sciences of pathological physiology and pathological chemistry.

Such sciences, and the perception of a need to promote them, lagged behind pathological anatomy by no more than a decade or so, and ultimately came round to impact on the mainstream of the pathological tradition. While Cohnheim in gingerly fashion was opening up the anatomical dimension of pathology to those physiological procedures and modes of thought gaining currency in the mid-1860s, others took a distinctive approach to physiology and chemistry. Aware of new developments in pharmacy and organic chemistry, academic adminstrators in France, Germany, and elsewhere sought to yoke theoretical research concerns in fields such as physiological chemistry to traditional market-places that they saw represented in the clinical and scholarly communities.[34] (➤ Ch. 8 The biochemical tradition)

The clinic, and in particular the enterprise of training medical students, was seen to be particularly important in this regard. The patronage of clinical leaders, such as Carl Wunderlich (1815–77) and Billroth, hence played a key role in elaborating the several new interstitial sub-disciplines. Indeed, physiologists were learning about clinical and pedagogical utility what pathologists had already taken to heart: research is fine in a field as long as it carries a practical edge as well.

In the final quarter of the nineteenth century, both medical physiology and medical chemistry – the latter soon to be transmuted into biochemistry – developed both within and without pathology. Their evolution into independent disciplines are dealt with elsewhere in this volume (chs. 7, 8, 10, 11) and in the broader medical history literature. Their evolution within pathology, however, is just beginning to be understood.

Pathological chemistry probably began to emerge first, issuing from a long-standing nineteenth-century interest in the analysis of body fluids in disease.[35] By the 1870s and 1880s, it was further spurred, both by the independent development of medical, pharmaceutical, and industrial chemistry, and specifically by the rise of a sort of neo-humoralist strain of pathology in the French school. As early as 1859, Claude Bernard (1813–78), six years before he published his epochal *Introduction to the Study of Experimental Medicine*, was presenting a series of *Lessons on the Physiological Properties and Pathological Alterations of the Liquids of the Organism*.[36]

Simultaneously, and as part of his sinecure at the Collège de France, Bernard gave a course he dubbed 'experimental pathology', designed to demonstrate that 'the scientific study of pathology and physiology cannot really be separated, and that it is unnecessary to attempt to explain disease by means of forces or laws other than those governing ordinary living processes.'[37] Only in 1880 did he publish these lectures on the aberrations of body fluids in disease and the derangements imposed by poisons. Why did he wait so long? A clue lay in his conclusion to the volume's introduction: 'if today we may see the experimental impulse grow and develop abroad [read: Germany] by means of the creation and installation of magnificent laboratories, I cannot allow it to be forgotten that experimental medicine has its imperishable root, ancient and deep, in French soil.'[38]

In France, then, pathological physiology was wrapped up with pathological chemistry, in the Bernardian analysis of experimental changes in the morbid chemistry of vivisected animals. Both, in turn, were wrapped up with the teaching of classic late-nineteenth-century physiology. A generation later in Germany and in the English-speaking countries, pathological physiology, twisted into a somewhat more stunted and truncated branch of the pathological tradition, became a sort of pedagogical meeting-point between the basic medical scientific subjects and the clinic.

In research laboratories, a few investigators pursued another variant, experimental pathology, represented in Germany and America by the followers of Cohnheim, and in France by the disciples of Claude Bernard. Experimental pathology was especially important, through animal studies and the experimental extirpation of subjects' endocrine glands, in leading to the elucidation of mammalian hormonal mechanisms – a subject that had been near and dear to Bernard himself. (➤ Ch. 23 Endocrine diseases)

TWENTIETH-CENTURY OUTGROWTHS

From the 1890s on, investigators in Germany, America, and possibly Britain began to advocate a more formalized, physiologically oriented vision – actually no more than an attempt to revivify an early, under-developed Virchovian ideal – of this new experimental pathology. The purpose, as the American clinician George Dock (1860–1951) put it in 1904, was to reverse 'some of the errors and excesses of pathological anatomy'.[39] Around the time of the prior to the First World War reforms in medical education – in the United States the so-called 'Flexner reforms' – courses in 'patho-physiology' grew up in several medical schools. But these courses were never paralleled to an appreciable extent by the sort of concomitant research schools that characterized anatomical pathology or medical and pathological chemistry.

This functional or physiological strand of the pathological tradition, always in some uneasy equilibrium with the structural, exhibited its own rather peculiar and attenuated subsequent history. It more or less fell between the two stools of pedagogical utility and research methodology. Neither the physiologists nor the pathologists truly owned it, or owned up to it, from the research perspective. Fitfully, clinicians clamoured to fill the breach with a hodge-podge of facts about everything from cardiac electrophysiology to the hormonal relationships of endocrine organs. About once a generation, throughout the twentieth century, the utility of patho-physiology was seen to be an appropriate intellectual bridging mechanism between the pure, pre-clinical science subjects of the medical school curriculum and the practical subjects of the teaching clinic. And about once per generation this curious body of knowledge, never fully bounded by a discipline or research school, was trotted out to 'save' modern medical education from its own contradictions.

After the First World War, a new generation, probably the last greatly celebrated generation, of innovators in the pathological tradition grew up on both sides of the Atlantic. The importance of charismatic individuals and personal leadership continued unabated. Such a state of affairs was due partly to what remained, despite Virchow's over-arching theory of cellular pathology, the craft basis of the discipline: pathologists, in hospital-based residency programmes, were trained in what were essentially apprenticeships. It was due also to the peculiar combination of sheer driving energy and retentive intelligence that characterized the leaders upon whose patronage and direction younger generations depended.

Two examples must suffice, one illustrating the persistence of Old World influence and one the rise of the New. The disciples of Virchow collectively fanned out across greater Germany, von Recklinghausen to Strasbourg, for example, and Cohnheim to Breslau. By century's end, the fruits of the pathological tradition were finally finding their fullest impact in medical education throughout the industrial West and Japan. At that critical moment, the mantle of Virchow passed from the hands of his immediate intellectual progeny to the sons of the apostles, most conspicuously to the shoulders of Ludwig Aschoff (1866–1942) of Freiburg.

Trailed by his own international entourage, like Laënnec and Virchow before him, Aschoff produced both a school and a corresponding *œuvre* that could be seen as an expansive gloss on the nineteenth-century German school: further studies on the clotting of blood; appendicitis; the cellular pathology of rheumatism; vital staining; ageing; medical history. Passing around bits of tissue during long days of instruction for his pupils' inspection and research, Aschoff provided a sort of 'hands-on' experience for his polyglot group of followers (in 1912, several Americans, a Belgian, two Italians, a Russian, a Scot, several Japanese, and a bevy of Austro-Germans). By now, it was expected that the 'pathologist' – since the time of Virchow, increasingly a full-time specialist in anatomical (or to a lesser extent chemical) diagnosis – would spend most of his time in the autopsy and microscopy suites.[40]

But the worldly and well-travelled Aschoff was not above sending his assistants into the outback to pose as clinicians in the study of goitrous dogs or sideshow dwarfs. The clinical interest, as ever, remained strong in the pathological tradition, and this interest was more than simply a matter of pathologists' desire to correlate the morbid appearances of post-mortem or surgical tissues with the clinical course.

As late as the 1920s, indeed, it was still possible in most nations for the pathologist's billet to function as a way-station between one's early training and, as a young medical aspirant matured, a successful subsequent clinical career.[41] The reasons related to the utilitarian services the young pathologist-in-residence at a given hospital was called upon to supply: bacteriological diagnosis, perhaps, but above all, interpretation of surgical biopsy specimens. While accumulating experience simultaneously in the operating-room and the drawing-room, the enterprising surgeon-pathologist could, if trained by the likes of Aschoff, earn his keep at the microscope, differentiating between tumour and inflammation. (➤ Ch. 42 Surgery (modern))

But Aschoff and his students, clinically versed but steeped in pathology, clearly represented the specialized future. So, too, but with a slightly different twist, did the group of clinicians and pathologists at Harvard in the post-1900 generation. On the one hand, we can picture W. B. Cannon (1871–1945), eminent physiologist-pedagogue and quintessential discipline-builder, urging the creation of formal exercises in clinical-pathological correlation. Ten years later, patrician clinician Richard Cabot (1868–1939) founded the 'Case Records of the Massachusetts General Hospital', thus formalizing one of the oldest and most critical conventions of the pathological tradition. The 'CPC', or clinico-pathologic conference, was a set-piece consisting of mental and professional gymnastics pioneered by the Parisians three-quarters of a century earlier.[42] But by setting forth the canons of diagnostic proof in pathological terms, Cannon and Cabot, in the most formal manner possible, were also crystallizing the clear-cut, separate relations between the pathologist and the clinician. Those relations would persist throughout the ensuing century.[43]

But here, too, was Harvard pathologist William Councilman (1854–1933), surveying the modern hospital with its operating suites and laboratories and accounting for its increasing centrality and impact on medical thought, noting that 'laboratories have been erected . . . in which the investigation of disease could be more efficiently carried out . . . by means of the study of tissues or fluids from individual cases [as well as] the study of questions concerning disease.'[44] Councilman's view was prescient and ended up defining, even more than his colleagues' vision did, what the pathological tradition would look like by the end of the century.

In the decades following the generation of Aschoff, Cannon, Cabot, and Councilman, the laboratory became increasingly the locus of the pathological tradition, or what remained of it. It may or may not be mere semantic quarrelsomeness to state that pathology, at some ill-defined time around mid-century, underwent something like a mutation. Pathological anatomy finally yielded pride of place to pathological chemistry. Visitors to the 'pathology wings' of twentieth-century hospitals were much more likely to encounter vast banks of 'autoanalyser' equipment used to measure urea, glucose, and liver enzymes, than they were to espy organs in bottles. The new pathologists could look as much to Claude Bernard as to Rudolf Virchow for their intellectual roots.

As the importance of the laboratory, and specifically that of the so-called clinical chemistry laboratory, expanded, the prominence of the post-mortem suite waned. Hospitals were no longer required to maintain their rates of autopsies performed at a high percentage of inpatient deaths. In the most important medical journals, clinico-pathological conferences continued to be published, offering the elaborate puzzle-solving exercise pitting diagnostician against pathologist. But more often than not the denouement, the image of disease brought forth by the pathologist to etch the diagnosis into reality, was drawn from some vantage-point other than post-mortem dissection: perhaps a tell-tale biochemical test or an X-ray image. The image of the decaying cadaver had given way to that of the body as a chemical, micro-scopical, and radiological palimpsest.

Costs simultaneously escalated for the labour-intensive, ancient craft of pathological anatomy; no one found methods to automate the necropsy, a procedure that dragged for hours. Pathologists meanwhile became owners and operators of banks of radioisotopic imaging devices and the sort of automated chemical equipment just mentioned. Virchovian histology remained a subsidiary, if, especially for the surgeon in the operating-room, fitfully still-important, pursuit. But the biochemical autopsy and the immunochemical biopsy bade fair to supplant the pure morphologist's view. (➤ Ch. 57 Health economics)

At some level, however, the notion of clinico-pathological correlation, and with it the synergistic relationship of the pathologist to the clinician, remained intact. While craft had finally given way to Big Science, the caretakers of the pathological tradition survived and awaited still another turn of the lens-wheel, another, next method of picturing disease.

NOTES

1   On seventeenth-century beginnings see: Robert Martenson, 'Death into life: Thomas Willis and the constitution of medical knowledge in Restoration England', *Bulletin of the History of Medicine*.

2   Toby Gelfand, *Professionalizing Modern Medicine: Paris Surgeons and Medical Science and Institutions in the English Century*, Westport, CT, Greenwood Press, 1980.

3   Toby Gelfand, 'The surgical profession in the old regime', in Gerald Geison (ed.), *Professions and the French State, 1700–1900*, Philadelphia, University of Pennsylvania Press, 1984, pp. 149–80.

4   Ruth Richardson, *Death, Dissection and the Destitute*, London, Routledge & Kegan Paul, 1987.

5   Guenter Risse, *Hospital Life in Enlightenment Scotland: Care and Teaching at the Royal Infirmary of Edinburgh*, Cambridge, Cambridge University Press, 1986.

6   Michael Foucault, *The Birth of the Clinic: an Archeology of Medical Perception*, trans. by A. M. S. Smith, New York, Vintage, 1975.

7   Othmar Keel, 'The politics of health and the institutionalization of clinical practices in the second half of the eighteenth century', in W. F. Bynum and R. Porter (eds), *William Hunter and the Eighteenth-Century Medical World*, Cambridge, Cambridge University Press, 1985, pp. 207–56.

8   Erna Lesky (ed.), *Johann Peter Frank: a System of Complete Medical Police*, trans. by E. Vilim, Baltimore, MD, Johns Hopkins University Press, 1976, pp. 332–5.

9   Ibid.

10   Literature reviewed in text and notes of: Othmar Keel, 'Les rapports entre médecine et chirurgie dans la grande école anglaise de William et John Hunter', *Gesnerus*, 1988, 45: 323–41.

11   Giambattista Morgagni, *De Causis et Sedibus Morborum*, Venice, Remondini, 1761.

12   Benjamin Alexander (trans.), *Giambattista Morgagni: The Seats and Causes of Diseases*, London, Millar & Cadell, 1769.

13   Esmond Long, *A History of Pathology*, Baltimore, MD, Williams & Wilkins, 1928; reprinted New York, Dover, 1965.

14   Saul Jarcho (ed.), *The Clinical Consultations of Giambattista Morgagni: the Edition of Enrico Benassi (1935)*, Boston, MA, Francis A. Countway Library of Medicine, 1984.

15   Whitfield J. Bell, *John Morgan, Continental Doctor*, Philadelphia, University of Pennsylvania Press, 1965.

16   John Morgan, letter to Giambattista Morgagni, February 1765, quoted in Joseph

Carson, 'History of the Medical Department, University of Pennsylvania', MS Collections of the College of Physicians of Philadelphia (ZZ10c/4, Vol. 1).

17 The importance of the commercial aspect of teaching medical science subjects is stressed in L. S. Jacyna (ed.), *A Tale of Three Cities: the Correspondence of William Sharpey and Allen Thomson*, suppl. 9: *Medical History*, 1989, pp. ix-xxvii, see p. xv.

18 The classic study of the Paris Hospital remains Erwin H. Ackerknecht, *Medicine at the Paris Hospital, 1789–1848*, Baltimore, MD, Johns Hopkins University Press, 1967.

19 John Thomson, *Lectures on Inflammation, Exhibiting a View of the General Doctrines Pathological and Practical of Medical Surgery*, Philadelphia, PA, Carey & Lea, 1831; orig. pub. 1813.

20 Russell Maulitz, *Morbid Appearances: the Anatomy of Pathology in the Early Nineteenth Century*, Cambridge, Cambridge University Press, 1987.

21 Erwin H. Ackerknecht, 'Broussais or a forgotten medical revolution', *Bulletin of the History of Medicine*, 1948, 27: 320–43; Michel Valentin, *François Broussais, 1772–1838*, Dinard, Association des Amis du Musée du Pays du Dinard, 1988.

22 Quoted in Maulitz, op. cit. (n. 20), p. 51.

23 Russell Maulitz, 'In the clinic: framing disease at the Paris Hospital', *Annals of Science*, 1990, 47: 127–37.

24 Russell Maulitz, 'Schwann's way: cell and crystals', *Journal of the History of Medicine and Allied Sciences*, 1971, 26: 422–37.

25 Jacyna, op. cit. (n. 17).

26 Ann La Berge, 'Alfred Donné and early medical microscopy in France', *Bulletin of the History of Medicine*.

27 Russell Maulitz, 'Pathology', in Ronald Numbers (ed.), *The Education of American Physicians: Historical Essays*, Berkeley and Los Angeles, University of California Press, 1987.

28 L. J. Rather, P. Rather, and John B. Frerichs (trans.), *Johannes Müller and the Nineteenth-Century Origins of Tumor Cell Theory*, Canton, MA, Science History, 1986.

29 Erwin H. Ackerknecht, 'Le cancer dans l'oeuvre de l'École de Paris, 1800–1850', *Clio Medica*, 1985–6, 20: 125–34.

30 Rudolf Virchow, *Die Cellularpathologie in ihrer Begründung auf physiologische und pathologische Gewebelehre*, Berlin, Hirschwald, 1858.

31 Harold M. Malkin, 'Rudolf Virchow and the durability of cellular pathology', *Perspectives in Biology and Medicine*, 1990, 33: 431–43.

32 L. J. Rather, *The Genesis of Cancer: a Study in the History of Ideas*, Baltimore, MD, Johns Hopkins University Press, 1978, pp. 138–43.

33 Russell Maulitz, 'Rudolf Virchow, Julius Cohnheim, and the program of pathology', *Bulletin of the History of Medicine*, 1978, 52: 162–82.

34 Timothy Lenoir, 'Science for the clinic: science policy and the formation of Carl Ludwig's Institute in Leipzig', in William Coleman and Frederic L. Holmes (eds), *The Investigative Enterprise: Experimental Physiology in Nineteenth-Century Medicine*, Berkeley, University of California Press, 1988, pp. 139–78.

35 For example, A. B. Garrod, 'On the chemistry of pathology and therapeutics', *Lancet*, 1848, 1: 353 ff.; L. A. Becquerel and A. Rodier, *Traité de chimie pathologique appliquée à la médecine pratique*, Paris, 1854.

36 Claude Bernard, *Leçons sur les propriétés physiologiques et les altérations pathologiques des liquides de l'organisme*, Paris, Ballière, 1859.

37 Claude Bernard, *Leçons de pathologie experimentale et leçons sur les propriétés de la moelle épinière*, Paris, Baillière, 1880, p. vii.

38 Ibid., p. x.

39 Russell Maulitz, 'Pathologists, clinicians, and the role of pathophysiology', in Gerald Geison (ed.), *Physiology and the American Context, 1850–1940*, Bethesda, MD, American Physiological Society, 1987, pp. 209–35.

40 J. W. McNee, A. H. T. Robb-Smith and Robert Muir, 'Ludwig Aschoff: 1866–1942', *Journal of Pathology and Bacteriology*, 1943, 55: 229–36.

41 Russell Maulitz, ' "The whole company of pathology": pathology as idea and as work in American medical life', in Teizo Ogawa (ed.), *History of Pathology*, Tokyo, Taniguchi Foundation, 1985, pp. 139–61.

42 Russell Maulitz, 'In the clinic: framing disease at the Paris Hospital', *Annals of Science*, 1990, 47: 127–37.

43 Maulitz, op. cit. (n. 27).

44 Quoted in Maulitz, op. cit. (n. 41).

FURTHER READING

Ackerknecht, Erwin H., *Medicine at the Paris Hospital, 1789–1848*, Baltimore, MD, Johns Hopkins University Press, 1967.

Coleman, William and Holmes, Frederic L. (eds), *The Investigative Enterprise: Experimental Physiology in Nineteenth-Century Medicine*, Berkeley, University of California Press, 1988.

Foucault, Michel, *The Birth of the Clinic: an Archeology of Medical Perception*, trans. by A. M. S. Smith, New York, Vintage, 1975.

Gelfand, Toby, *Professionalizing Modern Medicine: Paris Surgeons and Medical Science and Institutions in the Eighteenth Century*, Westport, CT, Greenwood Press, 1980.

Long, Esmond, *A History of Pathology*, Baltimore, MD, Williams & Wilkins, 1928; reprinted New York, Dover, 1965.

——, *Selected Readings in Pathology*, Springfield, IL, Thomas, 1961.

Maulitz, Russell, *Morbid Appearances: the Anatomy of Pathology in the Early Nineteenth Century*, Cambridge, Cambridge University Press, 1987.

Morgagni, Giambattista, *The Seats and Causes of Diseases*, trans. by Benjamin Alexander, London, Millar & Cadell, 1769.

Rather, L. J., *Addison and the White Corpuscles: an Aspect of Nineteenth-Century Biology*, London, Wellcome Institute of the History of Medicine, 1972.

——, *The Genesis of Cancer: a Study in the History of Ideas*, Baltimore, MD, Johns Hopkins University Press, 1978.

Rather, L. J., Rather, Patricia and Frerichs, John B. (trans.), *Johannes Müller and the Nineteenth-Century Origins of Tumor Cell Theory*, Canton, MA, Science History, 1986.

Richardson, Ruth, *Death, Dissection and the Destitute*, London, Routledge & Kegan Paul, 1987.

Risse, Guenter B., *Hospital Life in Enlightenment Scotland: Care and Teaching at the Royal Infirmary of Edinburgh*, Cambridge, Cambridge University Press, 1986.

10

THE IMMUNOLOGICAL TRADITION

Paul Weindling

The origins of modern immunology are a matter of controversy. Some have attributed fundamental notions about contagion and resistance to ancient Greek medicine, particularly to the Hippocratic notion of a constitution; and Joseph Needham has seen ancient China as the progenitor of the science. More recent milestones have been the work of Lady Mary Wortley Montagu (1689–1762) and Edward Jenner (1749–1823) on smallpox inoculation and vaccination, respectively. A modern interpretation is that the 1880s marked a crucial turning-point with a stimulus coming from the bacteriological, cellular, and hereditary studies as related to pathology. (➤ Ch. 9 The Pathological tradition) Specialized journals were established in 1909 in Germany, and in 1915 in the United States, yet Peter Medawar (1915–87) has dismissed work prior to 1930 as 'composed from false empiricisms and confused terminology'. During the 1930s, immunology was modestly described as an 'applied science'.[1] The author of the definitive work on its history, Anne Marie Moulin, sees immunology emerging as a discrete science only with the concept of 'the immune system' in the 1960s, prompting the verdict that immunology has a very long prehistory going back to ancient medicine, but a very short history from the 1960s.[2] These divergencies suggest the need for caution in viewing immunology as a discrete science with clear origins and a readily identifiable subject matter.

Smallpox variolation and vaccination had made the concept of artificial immunity to disease familiar in the nineteenth century. Cholera raised the issue of differential responses. The rise of bacteriology and Pasteurian microbiology in the second half of the nineteenth century prompted discoveries and debates on the mechanisms of immunity. Studies of fermentation led Louis Pasteur (1822–95) in 1857 to the view that the culture medium of a ferment could accelerate or inhibit the growth of a micro-organism. By analogy, it could be possible to inhibit the spread of invasive organisms responsible for diseases. In the case of anthrax, Pasteur believed it was possible to attenuate the pathogenicity of the bacteria. Vaccines were synonymous with attenuated cultures. The notion that each disease had a specific causal microbe or bacterium triggered off experimental research and speculations on the body's responses to invasive pathogenic organisms. During the 1880s Pasteur became concerned with explanations for the virulence of fowl pest.

Robert Koch (1843–1910) developed technical methods like staining and culture techniques for the examination and culturation of bacteria. He enunciated principles suggesting that a disease was caused by a specific organism, which could be isolated, cultured, and experimentally reproduced by the inoculation of these cultures. Koch and his co-workers proved the bacterial causes of numerous infectious diseases (for example, anthrax, cholera, and tuberculosis) on the basis of these postulates. A specific disease also implied the possibility of a specific cure. (➤ Ch. 16 Contagion/germ theory/specificity)

The search for a therapy for diphtheria constituted a fruitful focus for disciples of Koch and Pasteur. Friedrich Loeffler (1852–1915) was able to separate the poison, which he characterized as an enzyme, from the disease. At this time, Loeffler thought of prevention in chemical terms of internal disinfectants rather than of specific immunity. Emile Roux (1853–1933) and Alexandre Yersin (1863–1943) established that the broth used as the culturing medium had poisonous properties. It was therefore the poison or 'toxin' that caused the disease rather than the actual diphtheria bacillus.

Emil Behring (1854–1917) became convinced that each pathogenic organism should have a specific opponent. A seminal paper of Behring and Shibasaburo Kitasato (1852–1931) dated 4 December 1890 described how they injected into healthy animals the poison or toxin produced by the culture of diphtheria and tetanus bacilli. They described the results as the formation of antibodies to a toxin. The bacteria or their products could thus be neutralized by sera from immunized animals. Clinical trials were undertaken, but only when Roux used increased dosages of serum obtained from horses was there any success in checking the infection. It was established that the earlier the treatment, the more likely the chances of recovery. (➤ Ch. 11 Clinical research)

These positive results seemed to open a general pathway to the control of infectious diseases. Such was the mood of optimism in the 1890s that Behring considered that sera could be produced for all diseases, including sexually transmitted diseases and cancers. (➤ Ch. 25 Cancer; Ch. 26 Sexually transmitted diseases) Subsequent research established the conceptual foundations of immunology. Behring used the term 'antitoxisch' in analogy to 'antiseptisch'. He did not have the concept of a specific substance or antitoxin, but referred to an activity or property. The term 'antitoxin' was coined by Guido Tizzoni (1853–1932) and Giusepponna Cattani (1859–1915) in 1891, when they spoke of '*antitossina*', which they believed might be a globulin. Paul Ehrlich (1854–1915) introduced the term '*Antikörper*' in 1891, and this was taken up by researchers working in association with Koch.[3] The term 'antigen' can be traced back to Ladislas Deutsch (Detre) (1874–1939) in 1899, and derived from the theory of Hans Buchner (1850–1902) that antibacterial substances were modified constituents of bacteria.[4] As Moulin has observed, language and terminology have taken crucial roles in immunological research.

The period 1890–1914 was an era of debate between advocates of cellular or humoral theories of immunity. (➤ Ch. 14 Humoralism) This is often naïvely characterized in terms of national and institutional rivalries with the cellularists predominantly at the Pasteur Institute and the humoralists at Koch's Institute for Infectious Diseases in Berlin. While it is certainly the case that Behring and Koch were leading advocates of the humoralist position, and Elie Metchnikoff (1845–1916) of the cellular case, divergences within their institutes and among researchers in others nearby should be appreciated. Moreover, despite the antagonism between Koch and Pasteur, there were many links between researchers attenuating the dichotomy, for example, between Behring and Roux, or between Metchnikoff and Rudolf Virchow (1821–1902). Although the Germans excelled in isolating specific causal organisms, and the French placed a greater emphasis on the body's responses to infection, all researchers were interested in the chemical processes of infection and of resistance to it. This is clearly shown by Ehrlich's deft probing of the chemistry of immune reactions, and his open admiration of Pasteur.

Koch insisted that there was no intercession from any cellular elements. The bactericidal properties of immune sera were open to challenge from cellular protagonists. Metchnikoff announced in 1884 a novel theory of the protective role of inflammation.[5] The founding of the Pasteur Institute in 1888 gave him a permanent base for pursuing research into this question. He linked immunity to survival and Darwinian selection.[6]

Ehrlich developed the analogy between immunity and nutrition. He calculated the 'immunity units' per gramme of dried serum, abandoning the use of living cultures as too unstable. He was convinced that toxins and antitoxins were chemical substances that attached themselves to the cell nucleus as 'side-chains'. He regarded these side-chains as groups of atoms capable of linkage and of receiving nutrients. He modified his theory in 1897, when he examined the chemical relations between toxin and antitoxin. He believed that antibodies were excess side-chains excreted by the cell protoplasm.[7] (➤ Ch. 8 The biochemical tradition)

Critics of the rigid causality of germ theory pointed out that bacilli of diseases like diphtheria could be present without causing any illness. Others, like Buchner, emphasized the role of spontaneous cure and the body's independent capacity to form antitoxins. There were naturally occurring bactericidal properties in body fluids. Buchner studied the bactericidal action of normal sera, which led to notions of natural resistance to infections and of the presence of natural antibodies and antibacterial antibodies. A priority was to stimulate the formation of natural antibodies by means of a healthy physical constitution and favourable physical environment. Dietary and social improvements were thus a means of promoting natural immunity to infections. Such social concerns were evident among French bacteriologists like Emile Duclaux (1840–1904) and Charles Richet (1850–1935), and among German public-health reformers. (➤ Ch. 51 Public health)

Breast-feeding was recognized as conferring natural immunity. Ehrlich in 1892 demonstrated the transference of anti-abrin and antiricin from female mice to their young by both the transplacental and mammary routes, and his work provided an immunological rationale for breast-feeding. In 1909, Paul Römer (1873–1937) introduced his guinea-pig intradermal method for the quantitative estimation of antitoxin in serum. This led to the development of the Schick test in 1913, providing a clinical method for determining immunity to diphtheria based on the antitoxin content of the blood. The test, named after Bela Schick (1877–1967) during the 1930s, was regarded as providing an indicator of the effect of the environment from Schick-positive to Schick-negative state under different conditions. This provided the foundations for the postulate of Frank Macfarlane Burnet (1899–1985) that in most animals around the time of birth, a state of immunological tolerance could be induced in order to suppress antibody production.

Behring had observed the phenomenon of hypersensitivity in 1893. Richet and Paul Portier (1866–1962) in 1902 introduced the concept of 'anaphylaxis' (as an antithesis to prophylaxis) after researches on toxins produced by marine organisms, which produced toxic reactions after a second injection. Anaphylaxis explained a condition of hypersensitive reaction by the body to sera. This changed views of asthma from being a 'nervous disease' to one associated with immunological factors. In 1903, Maurice Arthus (1862–1945) discovered local anaphylaxis as a response to intradermal injections of protein antigens. He established that Koch's injections of tubercle bacillus antigens elicited a local inflammatory response. Clemens von Pirquet (1874–1929) noted the lack of relationship to the circulating antibody, relating the tuberculin-type hypersensitivity to immunity and to pathological events at the site of infection.[8] Pirquet introduced the term 'allergy' in 1905 in the context of discussions of 'serum sickness', to which Schick also contributed. Links were made to hay fever in 1906, and asthma in 1910. These discoveries provided a basis for more recent work on immunopathological processes, in which the immune system can be seen as a cause of a disease. The research on allergy led to the discovery of Daniel Bovet (1907–92) concerning the benefits of antihistamines in treating asthma. (➤ Ch. 20 Constitutional and hereditary disorders)

Jules Bordet (1860–1961) and Octave Gengou (1875–1959) discovered the complement fixation test. They showed that antibody–antigen reactions could be measured. August von Wassermann (1866–1925) with Albert Neisser (1855–1916) and Carl Bruck (1879–1944) developed a diagnostic test for syphilis, as the recently discovered *Spirochaeta pallida* could not be cultured. They applied the complement test to syphilis, and showed this could be diagnosed by means of blood tests. In 1922, Gaston Ramon (1886–1983) introduced his flocculation test as a means of titrating toxin and antitoxin. In 1925, Reuben Kahn (1887–1979) gave details of a diagnostic flocculation test.

Almroth Wright (1861–1947) was a pioneer of prophylactic vaccination. He developed an antityphoid vaccine in 1897–8. His support for 'vaccine therapy' went with an attempt to reconcile Metchnikoff's cellular and Ehrlich's humoralist theories. He considered that the destruction of pathogenic bacteria by phagocytic cells was facilitated by specific antibodies in the serum.

Max von Gruber (1853–1927) studied the antigen–antibody reactions, claiming in 1896 that agglutinins were special types of antibodies. Agglutinins cause red blood cells to adhere together, and the method was later used to determine human blood groups. In 1901, Karl Landsteiner (1868–1943) distinguished the principal blood groups and showed that the grouping depends on the distribution of antigenic constituents. By determining the antigens present in any sample of blood, it was possible to assign the correct blood group. Injections of sera prompted analysis of the relations between the constituents of the blood and the mechanisms of immunity. In 1899 Bordet described immune haemolysis arising from the immunization of animals with foreign red blood cells. Ehrlich and Julius Morgenroth (1871–1924) failed to detect the formation of haemolytic auto-antibodies. Julius Donath (1870–1950) and Landsteiner studied the mechanism of haemolysis in 1904 in patients with paroxysmal cold haemoglobinuria. This work led to controversy over autotoxins. It was in this context that Svante Arrhenius (1857–1927) introduced the term 'immunochemistry' in 1904.

ANTITOXIC IMMUNITY

Although the emerging science of immunology enunciated certain general principles and techniques, how the pace of research has shaped utilization of vaccines has greatly varied. In the 1920s and 1930s, there was greater understanding of how viruses and rickettsia differed from bacteria. The following itemization of developments indicates how each disease presented distinctive problems. The outstanding successes achieved for diphtheria could not be replicated for cholera and syphilis, for example. Attempts to apply serotherapy to cancers were made during the 1890s. Thus prevention has continued to rely on such methods as the isolation of cases, disinfection, promotion of generally high levels of hygiene, and education; therapy with sera has had to compete with chemotherapy, surgery in the case of tuberculosis, insecticides like DDT (dichloro-diphenyl-trichloro-ethane), and oral rehydration therapy in the case of cholera. Antitoxic immunity was found to be of value in the following infections.

Diphtheria

In 1898, Ernst Salkowski (1844–1923) described a method of modifying toxin with formalin. Formalized toxin, or 'toxoid' was found to be non-toxic and harmless on injection, while retaining its antigenicity. In 1904, toxoid was used for the active immunization of horses and other animals by E. Loewenstein in Vienna and Alexander Glenny (1882–1965) in England. In 1909, Theobald Smith (1859–1934) suggested the use of toxin–antitoxin mixtures in children, a suggestion followed up by Behring in 1913. In 1923, Glenny, Allen, and B. E. Hopkins first suggested the use of toxoid for human immunization. Ramon used toxoid under the name 'anatoxine' in France; this was in widespread use in Canada from 1925, and in France from 1938 for all children aged one to fourteen.

Scarlet fever

In 1902, Moser used serum from horses immunized with whole-broth cultures of streptococci from scarlet fever cases. In 1907, Gabritchewsky immunized humans actively with a scarlet fever toxin. In 1925, George Dick (1881–1967) and Gladys Dick (1881–1963) produced a test for susceptibility to scarlet fever as well a scarlet fever antitoxin. The disease was ultimately controlled by chemotherapy.

Tetanus

After Behring and Kitasato showed that rabbits could be immunized by repeated small doses of tetanus toxin in 1890, it was found that the poison spread so rapidly that serum therapy had little preventive value. It was not until 1904 that antitoxin began to be used prophylactically on a wide scale in the United States. During the First World War, it was found that antitoxin reduced the incidence of tetanus amongst the wounded. (➤ Ch. 66 War and modern medicine) By 1933, Ramon and Christian Zoeller (b. 1888) were using toxoid for human immunization, which has become the routine method.

ANTIBACTERIAL IMMUNITY

Antibacterial sera have been used for treating the following: primary pneumo-coccal pneumonia, cerebrospinal meningitis, gonorrhoea, Weil's disease (lep-tospirosis), and anthrax. However, these sera have proved in many cases to be of doubtful value, and have been superseded by chemotherapy.

Bacterial vaccines have been found to produce antibacterial immunity in the following diseases:

Typhoid

In 1897, Wright and David Semple (1856–1937) used anti-typhoid vaccine for human vaccination. This was deployed successfully during the First World War. In 1934, Arthur Felix (1887–1956) and R. Margaret Pitt described the Vi antigen as a specially virulent component of typhoid bacilli. Attenuated strains containing this antigen were used in the preparation of vaccines.

Cholera

J. Férran (1852–1929) injected cultures during the Spanish cholera epidemic of 1884; Waldemar Haffkine (1860–1930) in 1892 prepared living vaccines; and in 1896, Wilhelm Kolle (1868–1935) introduced heat-killed phenolized vaccines. Leonard Rogers (1868–1962) used mass vaccination to prevent cholera among Islamic pilgrims. However, the results of large-scale vacci-nation campaigns remained inconclusive and, by the 1960s, vaccination was regarded as conferring only partial short-term immunity of two to three months.[9]

Whooping cough

In 1933, Thorvald Madsen (1870–1957) published the results of trials made in the Faroe Islands, showing that a vaccine made from a freshly isolated strain had only slight influence on prevention but decreased the severity of the disease. During the 1940s, there were experiments in the use of an antitoxin serum in prevention and treatment.

Plague

In 1895, Yersin obtained protection in animals with vaccines of *Pasteurella pestis*. In 1901, Haffkine published details of a heat-killed phenolized vaccine. Vaccines gave a useful degree of immunity for some months.

Tuberculosis

Koch's tuberculin vaccine aroused considerable controversy. So too did other vaccines, such as those produced by Friedrich Friedmann (1876–1952/3) in 1910 from turtle bacilli; by Henri Spallanger (b. 1882) from horses; and by Behring and Georges Dreyer (1873–1934). The diagnostic value of tuberculin was recognized and further diagnostic tests were develped by Pirquet in 1907, Ernst Moro (1874–1951), and Charles Mantoux (1877–1947) in 1908. Attention turned to the BCG vaccine developed by Albert Calmette (1863–1933) and Camille Guérin between 1906 and 1921 as a method for immunizing children. This consisted of a living culture from a bovine strain attenuated by growth in bile. There was only limited interest in BCG prior to 1945 in Britain, where curative methods were preferred. After 1943, the antibiotic streptomycin became available.

Meningitis, Haemophilus influenzae *b strain (Hib)*

Clinical studies of a vaccine for babies are currently underway in Britain. A vaccine is available in the USA for children over eighteen months of age.

ANTIVIRAL IMMUNITY

In 1897, Paul Frosch (1860–1928) and Friedrich Loeffler introduced the concept of diseases caused by agents that would pass through a bacteria-proof filter. It was not until the 1930s that understanding of the distinctive characteristics of viruses allowed for improvements in combating viral diseases. Martinus Willem Beijerinck (1851–1931) had in 1898 isolated by filtration the virus of the mosaic disease in the tobacco plant. The distinguishing characteristic of a virus is that it cannot multiply on anything less complex than a host cell. However, the variability of virus strains has posed a barrier to immunization in many diseases. Antiviral immunity has been found of value in the following:

Smallpox

Vaccination against smallpox has provided the classic instance of inoculation since the eighteenth century. By 1898, the inoculation with glycerinated calf-lymph had become standard in Great Britain. The disease has now been eradicated by the World Health Organization. (➤ Ch. 59 Internationalism in medicine and public health)

Rabies

In Great Britain, the preferred method of control has remained prevention by isolation and quarantine. While Pasteur used living vaccines, dead vaccines have also been introduced.

Measles

After Charles Nicolle (1866–1936) and Conseil showed in 1918 that specific protective antibodies were present in the blood of measles convalescents, sero-prevention and sero-attenuation was described by Degkwitz. During the 1930s, the use of placental extract rather than serum was recommended. In 1944, 'human immune serum globulin' was introduced by Cohn.

Typhus fever

Nicolle deduced in 1909 that epidemic typhus was spread by the body louse, and this was confirmed by studies during the First World War. The causal agent, *Rickettsia prowazekii* (named in commemoration of two researchers who died from typhus), was demonstrated by Henrique da Rocha-Lima (1879–1945) in 1916. Weigl prepared a vaccine from the intestines of infected lice in 1933, but its production was hazardous and labour intensive. In 1938–41, Herald Cox (b. 1907) grew rickettsiae in the yolk-sacs of developing chick embryos, constituting the basis of a vaccine. (➤ Ch. 19 Fevers)

Yellow fever

By 1910, extermination of mosquitoes meant the eradication of yellow fever from Cuba. Although experiments in preparing a vaccine from phenolized tissues dated from 1929, it was only in 1936 that an attenuated variant strain was cultivated by Max Theiler (1899–1972). The vaccine derived from this, cultured in chick embryos, was used with success by the United States Army during the Second World War. (➤ Ch. 24 Tropical diseases)

Canine distemper

In 1928, Patrick Playfair Laidlaw (1881–1940) and Dunkin devised a method of actively immunizing dogs and ferrets.

Poliomyelitis

During the 1930s, failed attempts to introduce a vaccine caused cases of paralysis and death in New York. After the virus was successfully cultivated in 1949, Jonas Salk (b. 1914) prepared a killed-virus vaccine. Following further refinements, this was successfully introduced during the 1950s.

Meningitis

Between 1905 and 1938, antisera were widely used in the treatment of cerebrospinal meningitis, but were found to be unsatisfactory. Vaccination is possible for certain forms of meningococcal meningitis, notably the cerebrospinal type prevalent in the tropics.

Other infections

Only partial or transitory immunity has been obtained with immunization against influenza, dysentery, botulism, and the common cold. Serum therapy was unsuccessful in cases of cancer and syphilis, including attempts to treat cancer by non-specific stimulation of the body's defence mechanisms. Chemotherapy was advanced by the introduction of sulpha drugs in the 1930s and penicillin in the 1940s: there was consequently less incentive to develop preventive immunization. (➤ Ch. 39 Drug therapies)

TRANSPLANTATION: THE ROLE OF THE IMMUNE SYSTEM

Skin-grafting gave a boost to immunological studies, in particular to the immunological basis of transplantation. By 1912, tumour-transplantation experiments had led to the finding that transplantation into another species and into unrelated members of the same species will generally fail, although autografts tend to succeed. (➤ Ch. 42 Surgery (modern)) During the 1920s, James Bumgardner Murphy (1884–1950) discovered the central role of lymphocytes in cell-mediated reactions, which included resistance to graft rejection, resistance to tuberculosis bacilli, and reactions against malignant tumours. Löwy has analysed conceptual, scientific, and professional differences to concerns with cellular immunity reactions from the 1950s.[10] Alexis Carrel (1873–1944) experimented on the transplantation of kidneys and the spleen. Although solving certain surgical problems and able to regraft a kidney back into a dog, he encountered the problem of rejection when an organ was transplanted.[11] In 1930, Leo Loeb (1869–1939) formulated the principle of biological individuality, which posed a barrier to the development of skin-grafting except when an individual's own skin was used. Medawar, a zoologist, began research on skin-grafting. His experience at the burns unit of the Glasgow Royal Infirmary confirmed in 1943 that skin-grafting from other species or from members of the same species could never be successful. Geneticists confirmed that among genetically heterogeneous individuals, it would be impossible to graft tissues or organs. Improved understanding of histocompatibility and immunosuppressive therapy led to attempts to find compatible donors and recipients for the transplantation of organs, a novel feature of modern surgery.

Macfarlane Burnet advocated that physiological approaches to the study of cellular immunity be combined with innovative biochemical and immunochemical research. The cell was of strategic importance in virology. Links were forged with protein chemistry, cellular physiology, and genetics. This is exemplified by his clonal-selection theory of antibody formation, and in the rediscovery of the role of lymphocytes in graft reaction. Lymphocyte studies became a key problem in a science that ceased to be a branch of bacteriology and took off as an expanding discipline in its own right. The term 'immune system' became current in the 1960s in the context of the elucidation of the key role of lymphocytes.[12] Understanding of immune deficiency diseases has led to the development of immunotherapy; for example, with regular doses of antibodies. The diverse disciplinary backgrounds of aforementioned researchers confirms that it is only in the 1960s that immunology as a separate scientific discipline became established. Its prestige, and public understanding of immunological concepts, have greatly increased as a result of the AIDS epidemic.

CONCLUSION

Advances in immunology and in vaccination have been accompanied by outbursts of public acclamation and hostility. The widespread hostility to compulsory smallpox vaccination re-emerged with opposition to many other vaccines. Enthusiasm for tuberculin in the 1890s rapidly evaporated. Antivivisectionists have taken a lead in opposing research on vaccines, and since at least the 1890s there has been much opposition to human experimentation. Certain reckless cases of experiments on disadvantaged social groups (for example, the poor, children, mentally ill and retarded, and prisoners) were publicized by opponents of the narrow scientific basis of vaccination. Tragic cases of serum sickness and anaphylactic reactions further increased public mistrust. Notable tragedies of defective vaccines being used (for example, BCG at Lübeck in 1931) have held up the introduction of potentially beneficial innovations. Nazi medical experiments were carried out in concentration camps to produce vaccines and sera (for example, against typhus and hepatitis), and these cases of human experimentation have become paradigmatic for unethical medical experimentation. (➤ Ch. 37 History of medical ethics)

Scientific concepts have also been challenged by those expert in immunology. In 1935, Ludwik Fleck (1896–1961), a Polish immunologist, examined the intellectual and social context of research into the Wassermann reaction, and formulated his sociological concept of an underlying '*Denkstyl*' or thought style arising among groups of researchers. Fleck's historical contributions on Wassermann merit comparison to the study produced for Nazi celebrations of Behring by Heinrich Zeiss (1888–1949) and Richard Bieling (1888–1967), deploying the concept of a Gestalt configuration in scientific discovery.[13] Fleck also had a holistic understanding of disease and a relativistic understanding of the sciences, which can be linked to his relativistic understanding of immunological concepts of species and of immune responses, for he considered that much of bacteriology and immunology failed to account for the complexity of observed phenomena. The history of immunology has therefore been a testing-ground for developments more broadly applicable to the history of science.[14]

NOTES

1   W. W. C. Topley and G. S. Wilson, *The Principles of Bacteriology and Immunity*, 2nd edn, London, Edward Arnold, 1938, p. 767.

2   Anne Marie Moulin, 'Immunology old and new: the beginning and the end', in Pauline M. H. Mazumdar (ed.), *Essays on the History of Immunology (1930–1980)*, Toronto, Wall & Thompson, 1989, pp. 292–8.

3   Paul Ehrlich, 'Experimentelle Untersuchungen über Immunität. II. Ueber Abrin', *Deutsche medizinische Wochenschrift*, 1891, 17: 1218; J. Lindenmann, 'Origin of the terms "antibody" and "antigen" ', *Scandinavian Journal of Immunology*, 1984, 19: 281–5.

4   Ibid.

5   E. Metchnikoff, *Virchows Archiv*, 1899, 96: 177.

6   E. Metchinikoff, *Leçons sur la pathologie de l'inflammation*, Paris, 1892.

7   E. Bäumler, *Paul Ehrlich. Scientist for Life*, New York, Holmes & Meier, 1984, pp. 61–7.

8   B. H. Waksman, 'Cell mediated immunity', in Mazumdar (ed.), op. cit. (n. 2), pp. 143–65.

9   W. E. van Heyningen and John R. Seal, *Cholera: the American Scientific Experience 1947–1980*, Boulder, CO, Westview Press, 1983, pp. 151–214.

10 I. Löwy, 'Biomedical research and the constraints of medical practice: James Bumgardner Murphy and the early discovery of the role of lymphocytes in immune reactions', *Bulletin of the History of Medicine*, 1989, 63: 356–91.

11 I. Löwy, 'The impact of medical practice in biomedical research: the case of human leucocyte antigens studies', *Minerva*, 1987, 25: 171–200.

12 Anne Marie Moulin, 'The immune system: a key concept for the history of immunology', *History and Philosophy of the Life Sciences*, 1989, 11: 13–28.

13 H. Zeiss and R. Bieling, *Behring. Gestalt und Werk*, Berlin, Bruno Schultz Verlag, 1941.
14 Ludwik Fleck, *Genesis and Development of a Scientific Fact*, Chicago, IL, and London, Chicago University Press, 1979; I. Löwy, 'The epistemology of the science of an epistemologist of the sciences: Ludwig Fleck's professional outlook and its relationship with his philosophical works', in R. S. Cohen and T. Schnelle (eds), *Cognition and Fact – Materials on Ludwik Fleck*, Dordrecht, D. Reidel, 1986, pp. 421–42.

FURTHER READING

Bibel, Deborah Jan, *Milestones in Immunology*, Berlin, Springer Verlag, 1988.
Mazumdar, Pauline M. H. (ed.), *Essays on the History of Immunology 1930–80*, Toronto, Wall & Thompson, 1989.
Moulin, Anne Marie, *Le dernier langage de la médecine, histoire de l'immunologie de Pasteur au Sida*, Paris, Presses Universitaires de France, 1991.
Parish, H. J., *Victory with Vaccines. The Story of Immunization*, Edinburgh, E. & S. Livingstone, 1968.
Silverstein, Arthur M., *A History of Immunology*, San Diego, CA, Academic Press, 1989.

11

CLINICAL RESEARCH

Christopher C. Booth

Clinical research is concerned with the study of human beings in health and disease. It may also require the use of experiments in animals, particularly if there are appropriate animal models of human disease. As with other types of research, it involves observation, experiment, and the development of new technology.

EARLY HISTORY

Through the centuries, physicians have carefully observed the diseases they have encountered. Smallpox, for example, was clearly described by the great Arabic physician, Rhazes, who worked in Baghdad and who died c.AD 960. During the seventeenth century, the outstanding observations of Thomas Sydenham (1624–84) did much to clarify the clinical appearance of many common infectious diseases. In the following century, the growth of medical societies and of medical publications produced a plethora of case reports, among which the first description of angina pectoris by William Heberden (1710–1801) remains pre-eminent. The correlation of clinical observation with pathological dissection after death was also a feature of the eighteenth century, exploited with particular success by G. B. Morgagni (1682–1771) in his classic work in Padua. (➤ Ch. 9 The pathological tradition)

The experimental method in clinical research was a product of the Renaissance. The great Italian artists and anatomists, who so vastly advanced knowledge of the structure of the human body, were contemporaries of Sanctorius Sanctorius (1561–1636) of Padua, who designed a number of ingenious instruments, in particular a highly sensitive weighing-machine in which he spent a considerable proportion of his life. His work established a long tradition of self-experimentation in clinical science. By the use of careful techniques of weighing, he was able to estimate the amount of 'insensible perspiration' that occurs in the human body.[1] But it is to William Harvey (1578–1657) that we owe not only the remarkable experiments, so simple and so timeless, which established the circulation of the blood, but also, in the words of the British clinical scientist, Sir Thomas Lewis (1881–1945), the bequest to us of

> Clinical Science, out of which physiology and pathology were afterwards born. Prompted and inspired by clinical observation and by dissections of the dead body, he proceeded farther by the method of experiment, using both man and animals, and harvesting and binding into one whole his abundant evidence.[2]

(➤ Ch. 7 The physiological tradition)

Although the Oxford physiologists were to extend the horizons of Harvey's discoveries during the latter half of the seventeenth century, it was not until more than a century later that his successors began to use his experimental method for the benefit of humankind. The studies of James Lind (1716–94) of the effect of different treatments in the cure of scurvy among seamen, for example, were not made until the 1750s; and the discovery of Edward Jenner (1749–1823), by experiment in humans, of the effectiveness of vaccination against smallpox was not published until 1798.

Technology in medicine has an older tradition than either clinical observation or physiological experiment. Since, as Benjamin Franklin (1706–90) so aptly remarked, human beings have always been tool-making animals, it was their capacity to make tools that led to the development of crafts such as carpentry, building, metal-smelting, weaponry, leather-tanning, weaving, and so on. From these crafts, there emerged through the ages the technology that has become one of the four environments within which humans live, the others being the cosmic, the natural, and the social. Medicine having first emerged as a craft, the technological environment has been of vital importance to its evolution in the modern era. For centuries, however, technology played little part in the practice of a physician, practical procedures being carried out by surgeons who were considered a lesser breed. The Hippocratic physician, for example, was bound by Oath not to undertake such technical procedures as cutting for the stone. (➤ Ch. 41 Surgery (traditional))

After the Industrial Revolution, however, science and technology came together. Technology became more firmly based in science and, conversely, science began to depend more and more on the pioneering of new technology. These developments have been increasingly reflected in medicine in the modern era. New discoveries have frequently depended on the creation of new techniques, new devices, and new methods of observation. The introduction of the stethoscope by R. T. H. Laënnec (1781–1826) made possible the examination of the heart and lungs. (➤ Ch. 36 The science of diagnosis: diagnostic technology) The pioneering work of Antoni van Leeuwenhoek (1632–1723) on the microscope in Delft at the end of the seventeenth century, belatedly taken up by pathologists more than a century later, made possible great advances in the nineteenth century. (➤ Ch. 6 The microscopical tradition) Techniques for examination of organs previously inaccessible to the clinical observer, for example the larynx, the optic fundus, stomach or lower bowel, not only extended the opportunities available to clinical investigators but also led to the development of new specialities. In the modern era, techniques such as computerized axial tomography and magnetic resonance imaging, which followed in the wake of the discovery by Wilhelm Conrad Roentgen (1845–1923) of the value of X-ray examination in 1895, have made the human body virtually transparent. (➤ Ch. 68 Medical technologies: social contexts and consequences)

THE NINETEENTH CENTURY

The emergence of clinical research as we know it today, however, had its origins in the nineteenth century. In France, the 'birth of the clinic' was a great stimulus to specialization in medicine.[3] Special clinics dealing with specific diseases encouraged the study of them. It was a development that was not confined to France. In England, Richard Bright (1789–1858) concentrated his research at Guy's Hospital on diseases of the kidney, pioneering the creation of nephrology as a speciality in medicine. Meanwhile, in Germany, the foundation of the University of Berlin by Wilhelm von Humboldt (1767–1835) in 1810 stimulated the growth of a university system which set out specifically to encourage research.[4] As the new sciences basic to medicine grew, strong university departments of physiology, pathology, and bacteriology were established, within which research was to be all-important.

So far as biomedical science is concerned, much was already known by the early years of the nineteenth century, for example, that life is maintained by chemical reactions of the same nature as those that occur in test-tubes. In 1847, Hermann von Helmholtz (1821–94) showed that the laws of conservation of energy applied as much to living tissues as to non-living things. The main ingredients of food – fat, carbohydrate, and proteins – were identified and their transformation in the body was studied. (➤ Ch. 8 The biochemical tradition) Mathematics, too, was found be an indispensable tool of medical science, physicians such as Pierre Louis (1787–1872) in Paris beginning to call statistical methods to their aid. Physics were also important: the induction coil, developed between 1830 and 1850, making it possible to make galvanometers of improved sensitivity; recording drums (kymographs) which could assist in the analysis of complex physiological phenomena; and even techniques for the study of the transmission of nerve impulses.[5]

It was also during the nineteenth century, particularly in Germany, that the microscope came into its own. Capitalizing on the improvements in microscopy that followed the production of good achromatic lenses by Joseph Jackson Lister (1786–1869), German histologists were able to show that all living organisms are made up of very small units or cells, not visible to the naked eye. In disease, there might be specific disorders of these cellular elements. By 1858, Rudolf Virchow (1821–1902) in his great work *Die Cellularpathologie* was able to demonstrate a whole new concept of human disease based on disturbances of the cellular structures of the human body.

The microscope was also of vital importance in the emergence of bacteriology as a new science. Leeuwenhoek and his successors had observed tiny organisms with their simple instruments, but the work of Louis Pasteur (1822–95) in France and of Robert Koch (1843–1910) in Germany, supported by many brilliant contemporaries, established the science of bacteriology. From 1875 onwards, a whole range of diseases was found to be due to infection by specific micro-organisms. (➤ Ch. 16 Contagion/germ theory/ specificity)

These scientific developments led to profound changes in the structure of universities and in attitudes to research. Departments in the new sciences of physiology, pathology, and bacteriology were created, particularly in Germany. Research institutes were also being set up. Popular subscription established a research institute for Pasteur in Paris, and in Germany the government supplied special laboratories for Koch and for the great pathologist Paul Ehrlich (1854–1915). In England, an institute was named after Joseph Lister (1827–1912), the pioneer of antiseptic surgery, and in Japan facilities were provided for Shibasaburo Kitisato (1852–1931), co-discoverer of diphtheria antitoxin with the German Emil von Behring (1854–1917). By the end of the nineteenth century, there had been a great burgeoning of the sciences basic to medicine. In the latter part of the century, young Americans flocked to the laboratories and clinics of the German medical schools and research institutes, just as earlier in the century they had visited the clinics of Paris. America soon began to emulate these new European traditions by establishing basic science laboratories in the universities and medical schools. The physiology laboratory of Henry P. Bowditch (1840–1911) at Harvard, the laboratory of physiological chemistry under Russell H. Chittenden (1856–1943) at Yale, and the physiology laboratory of Henry Newell Martin (1848–96) at Johns Hopkins were founded as early as the 1870s.[6]

Yet although there had been no hesitation in creating university departments in the basic sciences directed by full-time professors employed and paid by universities or research institutes, there had been by the end of the nineteenth century little comparable academic development in the world of clinical practice. The care of patients and the teaching of students in medicine occupied the time of the clinicians almost wholly, and they were remunerated partly from student fees as well as from their work as private practitioners. In Germany, however, clinical departments had their own laboratories and assistants, even though the professors often maintained large private practices. But the development of clinical science carried out in clinical departments by people devoted to research and working with patients in a clinical setting was to be a twentieth-century phenomenon. Stimulated by the German model, it was to begin and to reach its fruition in the United States.

THE AMERICAN EXPERIENCE

Although American medicine in the first half of the nineteenth century was very much dependent on European and particularly British medicine, specifically American contributions to medical research soon began to emerge. The classic observations of William Beaumont (1785–1853) on gastric secretion in an individual with a gastric fistula following a gunshot wound, which were carried out, as Walter B. Cannon (1871–1945) was to put it, 'in a backwoods army post, under the most unfavourable of conditions, without laboratory aid, with no journals or other literature to consult',[7] were a great stimulus to American physiology. Later in the century, Austin Flint (1812–86), remembered today for the cardiac murmur resulting from a relative narrowing of the mitral valve in the presence of left ventricular hypertrophy, was to be the most influential physician of his day. He had never studied in Europe, and as Sir William Osler (1849–1919) commented: 'He found his opportunities in country practice in Buffalo and Louisville, then frontier towns, and in New Orleans, and he had a national reputation before he reached New York'.[8] He was also one of the first to describe the gastric atrophy of pernicious anaemia, a condition to whose understanding and treatment future American clinical scientists were to make a major contribution. It must have seemed the end of an era to many when Flint died in August 1886. He was described by one his contemporaries as having had, as teacher, author, and investigator, more influence than anyone else on American medicine at that time.

But for American medicine, the year 1886 was, in fact, to be particularly propitious. In that year, the Association of American Physicians was founded, an organization that was to have a profound effect on the development of clinical research in the United States.[9] From the first, the Association determined that its membership should not be confined narrowly to those involved in the practice and teaching of internal medicine, but that it should include, even welcome, basic scientists – pathologists, bacteriologists, physiologists – as well as those who were doing exciting research in public health. This decision ensured that, for the future, clinical research workers and basic scientists would work together in creative multidisciplinary harmony. At the same time, universities were beginning to be involved in the teaching hospitals. (➤ Ch. 49 The hospital) As early as the 1880s, the University of Michigan had established that its clinical professors were on the university payroll and not dependent on income from practice or student fees. It remained, however, for some years a scientific rather than a practical or clinical institution. Of more importance to the newly developing world of academic medicine was the foundation of the Johns Hopkins Medical School and Hospital, which took in its first students in 1893. Its foundation professors were William Welch (1850–1934) in pathology, Osler in medicine, W. S. Halsted (1852–1922) in surgery, and Franklin Mall (1862–1917) in anatomy. They had all been deeply influenced by the clinics and laboratories in which they had trained in Germany, and the German model was followed in Baltimore.[10] Internships and residencies were set up following the German system, and at once a whole new generation of medical students was attracted to the new school. Many were to become leaders of their profession in cities throughout the United States.

A further important influence on clinical research was the emergence of specialization. As early as 1897, American physicians founded the American Gastroenterological Association. Other national societies, such as the National Association for the Study and Prevention of Tuberculosis, followed in the early years of the twentieth century, although the American Heart Association was not founded until the 1920s.

Meanwhile, there were two major developments that were to be vitally important for the encouragement of clinical research in the universities. The first was the introduction of a full-time system of clinical professorships within the medical schools throughout the country, with the provision of laboratories and assistants in the hospitals associated with them. The second was the establishment of a privately funded research institute with clinical facilities specifically set up for research: the Rockefeller Institute for Medical Research in New York City.

The individual who did most to encourage the development of the full-time system in clinical departments was William Welch, founder-member of the Association of American Physicians and foundation professor of pathology at Johns Hopkins. In an important presidential address to the Association in 1901, he argued cogently that there should be research opportunities for clinical staff in the universities comparable to those already available to the basic scientist. Whilst any young man who chose to make his career in basic science could find opportunities for the necessary training, Welch stressed that

with one or two exceptions, our hospitals do not offer the requisite opportunities

to young men who aim at the higher career in clinical medicine and surgery. . . .
It would seem that the training of physicians and surgeons has not kept pace
with the progress of medical science to the same degree as has that of the
specialties in the more purely scientific branches.[11]

Welch's views had undoubtedly been influenced by his experience in the
laboratory of Carl Ludwig (1816–95) in Germany. Ludwig, a physiologist,
trained many of the future generation of investigators who were to encourage
the new sciences in the Nordic countries and in Britain, as well as in
Germany and Austria.[12] He believed that the sort of change needed to
introduce effective clinical departments devoted to research would be more
likely to emerge in America than in Germany, where he deplored the rigidity
of the education system. Referring to the need for research-oriented clinical
departments, Max von Frey (1852–1932) wrote to Franklin Mall at Johns
Hopkins: 'You will remember that Ludwig often discussed this possibility'.[13]
Mall was an enthusiastic supporter of the idea that clinical departments
should be firmly based in the university and have similar research aims as
departments of basic science. He found in Lewellys Barker (1867–1943),
one of his young assistants who taught neuroanatomy, an able spokesman for
his views.

A year after Welch's presidential oration, Barker had the opportunity of
supporting his ideas in an influential address to the alumni of Johns Hopkins.
He argued powerfully that clinical professors should give their whole-time
commitment to teaching and investigation, so that students would obtain as
thorough a training in their clinical studies as they had received in the basic
sciences. He stressed that 'a modern university must be a centre of original
research, as well as a place of instruction'. It should be made up of 'scholars
who are not only familiar with the results of modern investigation, but who,
skilled in the methodology of their respective sciences, invade new territories,
searching diligently for new facts'.[14]

Barker succeeded Osler as Professor of Medicine at Johns Hopkins in
1905, when Osler accepted the post of Regius Professor at the University of
Oxford. There were, however, no funds then available at Johns Hopkins to
implement the full-time system. Nevertheless, Barker at once set up three
clinical research laboratories on the German model, the first in the United
States.[15] They were headed by young men who were full-time scientists
engaged in clinical investigation. The biological or bacteriological laboratory
was directed by Rufus I. Cole (1872–1966), the physiological laboratory was
headed by Arthur D. Hirschfelder (1879–1942), and the chemical laboratory
was under Carl Voegtlin (1879–1960), while a general clinical laboratory for
instruction was directed by Thomas R. Boggs (1875–1938). As Cole was to
describe the situation later, the opportunities for classical clinical observation
had never been better than under Osler, whose remarkable textbook of

medicine, first published in 1892 during his years at Johns Hopkins, provided the best clinical descriptions of human disease at that time. Barker, however, believed that the primary function of a university department of medicine should be something more. It should, he thought, be involved in the encouragement of experimental rather than purely observational research, and accordingly the professor of medicine should be free from the routine burdens of private practice and allowed to devote his time to his own investigations and to those of his staff. It was to be some years, however, before funds became available for the establishment of the first full-time professorships in the United States.

One of the most important initiatives in encouraging clinical research was undoubtedly the foundation in 1904 of the Rockefeller Institute for Medical Research.[16] Frederick T. Gates (1853–1929), one of the most influential advisers of John D. Rockefeller (1839–1937), had read Osler's textbook and concluded with good reason that at that time very little could effectively be done to treat the ailments of humankind. It was Gates who persuaded Rockefeller to invest in medical research. (➤ Ch. 63 Medical philanthropy after 1850) At first, the institute was entirely devoted to basic scientific studies, but right from the start there was an intention to set up a small hospital alongside the institute, which would be devoted to research in the clinic. This was finally opened in 1910. It had been intended that Christian Herter (1865–1910), a distinguished investigator of metabolic problems whose name was to be associated with the condition of coeliac disease, should direct the hospital, but he was unable to take up his position because he was suffering from myasthenia gravis. Rufus Cole, from Barker's department in Baltimore, was appointed in his place. It was to prove an inspired appointment. Cole at once recognized that the Rockefeller Hospital could play a major role in training the new generation of investigators who would be needed to fill full-time positions in clinical departments throughout the United States, and his early appointments were to include some of the most important investigators of the new era. It was also to provide an important training-ground for at least two clinicians who were to take up similar full-time positions in Britain in the years that followed the First World War. Cole and his colleagues fully understood the importance of recruiting basic scientists to work alongside clinicians. Donald D. Van Slyke (1883–1971) was appointed as the hospital's biochemist, and Oswald Avery (1877–1955), later to make the vital discovery that the genetic material in bacteria is DNA, joined in Cole's own programme of research in pneumonia, an often fatal disease in those pre-antibiotic days. Twenty years later, in 1930, Cole summarized his views on the work of the hospital. He considered that one of its most important features had been the stimulus it provided to other investigators in supplying them with new ideas, particularly because it encouraged the study of disease in the individual as well as in selected groups, both at the bedside and in the laboratory, to an extent that was hitherto unknown.[17]

Thus, by the end of the first decade of the twentieth century, there was beginning to emerge in the United States a significant body of young clinical investigators who were devoted to full-time research and teaching. The Association of American Physicians had now come of age, and S. J. Melzer (1851–1920) of New York proposed, with the support of other colleagues, that a new society was needed to provide younger investigators with a forum within which they could discuss their work. The American Society of Clinical Investigation was established in 1907, its membership being restricted to those under the age of forty-five years, so its early nickname of the 'Young Turks' was well deserved. It's journal, the *Journal of Clinical Investigation*, founded in 1924, has remained the leading journal of clinical research in the world, and the work of its vigorous and ambitious young members has provided the 'Old Turks' of the Association of American Physicians with just the stimulus that they needed.

A further highly significant influence on clinical research at that time was a report by Abraham Flexner (1866–1959) on medical education, which was published in 1910.[18] Flexner, educationalist brother of Simon Flexner (1863–1946), the first director of the Rockefeller Institute, drew attention to the lamentable situation in many of the medical schools that had sprung up throughout the land in the years following the ending of the Civil War. Frequently, such schools had no effective academic support and relied for their teaching on the activities of local practitioners. In many of them, research did not exist. Flexner considered that there were only five institutions that could properly be regarded as centres of medical research – Harvard and Johns Hopkins, and the universities of Pennsylvania, Chicago, and Michigan. He was an enthusiastic supporter of the full-time system, and he based many of his recommendations on the German model then developing at Johns Hopkins. Emphasizing the importance of internal medicine, he argued that academic internists should be able to 'devote their time and energy to painstaking study and experimentation, wide reading in many languages, discursive conversation and leisurely reflection . . . for the physician deals with the most complicated of mechanisms, the human body'. Soon afterwards, the Rockefeller Foundation, whose advisers now included Welch, made funds available to Johns Hopkins for the establishment of full-time chairs in clinical subjects, and with the stimulus provided by Flexner's report, this pattern spread throughout the United States in subsequent years. By the mid–1920s, there were as many as twenty institutions that could rival the best in Europe. Increasingly, clinical departments in the medical schools were staffed by full-time men and women, so that all specialities encouraged research and investigation in their chosen areas of practice. The full-time system received an even greater boost during the years that followed the Second World War, with the expansion after 1948 of the reorganized National Institutes of Health. For many years, research grants were liberally awarded to clinical departments, which grew enormously. P. B. Beeson (b. 1908) and Russell Maulitz have calculated that in 1947 there were perhaps six or twelve salaried faculty members on the staff of most departments of medicine. By 1974, in the University of Rochester, New York, to quote a typical example, the number of full-time staff in the department of medicine alone had risen to one hundred, and the number who were of professorial rank from one to twenty-three. (➤ Ch. 48 Medical education)

The question must be asked: how effective has the American organization of clinical research been and are its achievements unique? One cannot analyse the enormous output of American clinical departments, often published in the *Proceedings of the Association of American Physicians* or in the *Journal of Clinical Investigation*, but at the highest level it is possible to examine the record of American clinical investigators in winning Nobel prizes. In 1934, G. R. Minot (1885–1950) and W. P. Murphy (1892–1936) of Boston, together with the pathologist George Whipple (1878–1970), won the prize for their work demonstrating that pernicious anaemia, then a universally fatal disease, could be successfully treated with a liver diet. (➤ Ch. 22 Nutritional diseases) R. R. Cournand (1895–1988) and D. W. Richards (1895–1973) received the prize for their pioneering work on cardiac catheterization; C. B. Huggins (1901–89) for the treatment of prostatic cancer with hormones (➤ Ch. 23 Endocrine diseases); P. S. Hench (1896–1965), with his scientific colleague E. C. Kendall (1886–1972), for the introduction of steroid treatment; Rosalind Yalow (b. 1921) for the development of the technique of radioimmunassay; and M. S. Brown (b. 1934) and J. J. Goldstein (b. 1940) for their work on the molecular basis of lipid metabolsim. In 1966, Carlton Gajdusek (b. 1924) won the Nobel prize for his demonstration of the importance of slow viruses in chronic diseases of the central nervous system, particularly kuru, a disorder associated with cannibalism in New Guinea. More recently, J. E. Murray (b. 1919) and E. D. Thomas (b. 1920) have been rewarded for their introduction of transplantation of kidney and bone marrow. Of these, all but Huggins were members of the Association of American Physicians. By contrast, the only clinicians from other countries to have won Nobel Prizes have been the following: the Canadian surgeon Frederick G. Banting (1891–1941) won it for his contribution to the discovery of insulin; the German surgeon W. Forssman (1904–79), who first passed a catheter into his own heart, shared the prize with A. Cournand (1895–1959) and D.W. Richards; in 1903, Nils Finsen (1860–1904), a Dane, won the prize for suggesting that light was important in the treatment of lupus and smallpox, an avenue of research that has not fulfilled its early promise; and the Swiss surgeon Emil Theodor Kocher (1841–1917) was rewarded for his work on surgery of the thyroid gland. Egaz Moniz (1874–1955), a Portuguese physician, received the accolade for introducing cerebral angiography and, more dubiously, for the development of prefrontal leucotomy. Even more curious was the award to Julius Wagner-Jauregg (1857–1940) of Austria in 1927 for advising malaria inoculation for the treatment of dementia paralytica. With the exception of Sir Ronald Ross (1857–1932), who won the prize in 1902 for the discovery of mosquito transmission of malaria and whose work was carried out in India, no British clinical research worker has yet won a Nobel Prize.

GREAT BRITAIN

The development of clinical research within British medical schools and hospitals occurred more slowly than in the United States. By the end of the first decade of the twentieth century, there had been a number of outstanding British individuals whose contributions to clinical research had been internationally recognized. Sir James Mackenzie (1853–1925) had pioneered the use of the polygraph in the study of the heartbeat in health and disease. His follower, Sir Thomas Lewis (1881–1945), had begun his work on the electrocardiogram, invented by the Dutch physiologist and Nobel Laureate W. Einthoven (1860–1927), using the new technique for the analysis of cardiac arrhythmias. Sir Archibald Garrod (1857–1936) of St Bartholomew's Hospital in London had published his classic volume on *Inborn Errors of Metabolism*.[20] And surgeons such as Sir Victor Horsley (1857–1916) were making major contributions to neurosurgery and to the understanding of thyroid disease, the use of thyroid extract having been pioneered by G. R. Murray (1865–1939) in Newcastle in 1891.[21] In addition, Britain's role as a colonial power, particularly in Africa and the Orient, gave opportunities to men such as Sir Patrick Manson (1844–1922), Ross, and Sir David Bruce (1855–1931) in the newly developing disciplines of tropical disease. But, as in the United States, there were no clinical academic departments, headed by full-time professors, where young students could acquire the training necessary for clinical investigation. (➤ Ch. 24 Tropical diseases)

Sir William Osler was to be an important figure in Britain at this time. Translated from Baltimore to the Regius Chair of Medicine at the University of Oxford in 1905, he was dismayed at the medical educational desert that he encountered and which he repeatedly criticized in lectures at medical schools throughout the land. The current arrangements were so different from those he had enjoyed at Johns Hopkins. In 1907, with the twenty-year-old example of the Association of American Physicians to draw upon, he founded the Association of Physicians of Great Britain and Ireland, but there were to be important differences from the American model.[22] The British association did not include basic scientists, pathologists, physiologists, or bacteriologists, nor, at the beginning, those involved in public health. Furthermore, the British meetings, unlike those in the United States which welcomed all and sundry, were closed and were limited to those physicans who were members and their particular guests. The association has therefore remained an intimate club of mainly academic physicians and has had little contact with individuals in other scientific disciplines. Consequently, it has never had the same national impact on medical science as the American association. Furthermore its journal, the *Quarterly Journal of Medicine*, has continued through the years to publish descriptions of the natural history of disease rather than experimental work.

Before the First World War, the medical schools, particularly in London, were private institutions that for the most part had been founded before the University of London, with which they had little or no contact. There was very little encouragement of clinical research. The establishment of a Royal Commission on University Education in London, under the chairmanship of Lord Haldane (1856–1928), was to initiate the changes that led to the establishment of modern academic departments in clinical subjects, where there would be a proper emphasis on research, in British medical schools. The Commission's Report was published in 1913.[23] Haldane sought to introduce university education into practical subjects such as medicine, and the Commission was greatly influenced by the evidence of those with experience of both the German and the newly developing American medical scene. Professor Ludwig von Muller (1858–1941) came from Munich to outline the German system. Abraham Flexner extolled the virtues of German medical education as it had been developed in America and in particular at Johns Hopkins. Since there was no clinical departments in London with either laboratories or assistants, an American visitor, he told the Commission, would not wish to spend time in London but would learn far more from the schools on the European continent, particularly those in Germany. Osler, who gave evidence in 1911, the year he received his baronetcy, was scathing in his condemnation of the state of affairs in Britain. He had no hesitation in castigating the situation in the London medical schools, which had no clinical laboratory base, little or no link with the university, and no paid staff. In Oxford, he bewailed the fact that there was no clinical school whatsoever. He concluded that the only solution was 'an active invasion of the hospitals by the universities'.

It was the evidence of these individuals, together with that of the distinguished University College London physiologist E. H. Starling (1866–1927), that led to the Commission's recommendation that academic clinical units, led by full-time professors, should be developed in the London medical schools. Not unnaturally, there were immediate reactions from the senior and influential London consultants, who then controlled medical education there. Many opposed any change in the *status quo*. Their views were set out in the pages of the *British Medical Journal* by E. Graham Little (1867–1950) of St Mary's Hospital.[24] He adhered, as did many of his colleagues who were brought up in the Oxbridge system of medical education, to the idea that the opinion of the great universities of Oxford and Cambridge as to what constituted teaching of university rank was of prime importance. The London schools should therefore continue to teach Oxbridge graduates, who then returned to their native universities to be examined upon medical subjects, even though those universities took no interest in that form of education. As to research and teaching in Germany, he wrote that British doctors were 'sometimes shocked in Germany by what appears to the English-trained man as callous handling of the sick', a viewpoint no doubt influenced by European events in those years that led to the First World War.

The recommendations of the Haldane Commission were shelved during the war, which provided the reluctant London medical schools with an excuse for inactivity, but in 1919, St Bartholomew's Hospital appointed its first full-time professor of medicine, Sir Archibald Garrod, the great pioneer of biochemical genetics who had brought biochemistry to the bedside. Garrod, however, never took up the post, for he left St Bartholomew's the next year to succeed Osler, who had died in Oxford on the last day of 1919.

By 1925, there were five chairs of medicine established among the twelve medical schools in London, and Edward Mellanby (1884–1955), an influential investigator in the developing world of human nutrition, was a full-time teacher and research worker in a clinical department in Sheffield. Several of the London appointees had been greatly influenced by their experiences in the United States. Sir Arthur Ellis (1883–1966), a Canadian who became the first professor of medicine at the London Hospital Medical School and who was to make important contributions to knowledge of renal disease, was a contemporary at the Rockefeller Institute in 1910 with Sir Francis Fraser (1885–1964), who was to succeed to Garrod's chair at St Bartholomew's in 1920. Both men were therefore in the United States during the period when full-time chairs were being established and when the Flexner Report was the subject of widespread academic debate. They also had experience of the newly founded hospital of the Rockefeller Institute. Ellis wrote in the later years of that period of his life: 'I have often thought what a remarkable act of faith it was, that we should all have been consciously attempting to fit ourselves for full-time posts in medicine when no such posts existed anywhere'.[25] Fraser, more a remarkably successful administrator than research worker, was to play a major role in the developing world of clinical research in London, particularly in its association with postgraduate education.

The British professors, however, had very much less power and influence than their American counterparts. In America, the professor was not only head of a department that included all the sub-specialities in medicine or surgery, but was also chief of service of the clinical departments of the teaching hospitals which came increasingly under academic control. By contrast, the British academics simply controlled one unit among their clinical colleagues, who continued to spend much of their lives devoted to private practice. It is therefore not surprising that the battle between full-time academics and part-time consultants over who controlled medical education and clinical research in London was to rumble on for a full half-century. Nevertheless, by 1944, when a further report on medical education was published (the Goodenough Report),[26] the move towards academically controlled medical schools had made reasonable headway, and it now received enthusiastic support. Since that time, all medical schools have developed clinical departments in a wide range of subjects and the opportunities for clinical research in Britain have been greatly extended.

At the same time as the universities and medical schools were developing clinical academic departments at undergraduate level, with increasing facilities for clinical research, there were also important initiatives in postgraduate education that were to provide further opportunities for clinical investigation. There had been attempts to foster postgraduate education in London during the later years of the Victorian era but they had been based solely in the clinic. Sir Clifford Allbutt (1836–1925), from his Regius chair in Cambridge, had pointed out, however, that postgraduate education in medicine would fail unless it was based as much in the laboratory as in the hospital ward.[27] Osler, at the end of the First World War, played an important role in encouraging the emergence of postgraduate medical education. He considered that Britain was in a strong position to take over the status of Vienna and the German schools in postgraduate education in Europe. With H. C. Meakins (1882–1959) and the future Lord Dawson (1864–1945), he argued that doctors returning from war service urgently needed educational opportunities. There was also an imperial requirement. In those dying days of Empire, there was still an increasing flood of medical graduates from the dominions and colonies coming to London to seek specialist education.

In response to these needs, a committee was set up in 1921 under the chairmanship of the Earl of Athlone (1874–1957), recommending that there should be a specific school for postgraduate medical education attached to a hospital dedicated to this purpose.[28] In 1925, the existing London teaching hospitals were approached by a committee chaired by the then Minister of Health, Neville Chamberlain (1869–1940), to determine whether any would rise to the challenge. All refused, although St Bartholomew's Hospital, where Francis Fraser was now Professor of Medicine, declined only after very careful consideration. Finally, it was agreed that the school should be sited at Hammersmith Hospital in west London, where there was thought to be ample space for development. The hospital was a London County Council (LCC) institution which did not belong to the gilded élite represented by the independent London teaching hospitals, many of which were still reluctant to allow the establishment of academic clinical departments within their walls. The LCC, encouraged by their Chief Medical Officer, Sir Frederick Menzies (1875–1949), considered that the establishment of a medical school at one of their hospitals would play an important role in raising standards throughout the municipal non-teaching hospitals in London, many of which were regarded as low-grade institutions by the higher echelons of medical consultants.

Hammersmith was to prove an important development in British academic medicine. The new school was formally opened by King George V (1865–1936) in 1935, the year of his Silver Jubilee, nearly a quarter of a century after Osler had given his forthright evidence to the Haldane Commission. From the start, the hospital and medical school were planned to develop according to the Flexnerian pattern, which was proving so successful in the United States. The hospital consultant staff were to be provided from university funds administered by what became known as the British Postgraduate Medical School. The architect of this Flexnerian model, unique in Britain, was Francis Fraser, who came from his chair at St Bartholomew's to be head of the new Department of Medicine. The school was perhaps the only British equivalent to the Johns Hopkins Hospital, where the Foundation professors had had the opportunity, to use Osler's words, 'to blaze a perfectly new road, untramelled by tradition, vested interests or medical dead wood'.[29] It was to be at Hammersmith that clinical research workers such as E. G. L. Bywaters (b. 1910) carried out their classic studies of crush syndrome during the Second World War, where invasive techniques such as cardiac catheterization and liver biopsy were pioneered in Britain, and where open-heart surgery using cardiopulmonary bypass was first performed in this country. (➤ Ch. 42 Surgery (modern); Ch. 66 Medicine and modern war)) The clinical research at Hammersmith in that era was not greeted with unanimous enthusiasm by the traditional teaching hospitals in London, some of whose senior staff warned their students against going to work in an institution so deeply committed to experimental work in the human subject. Nevertheless, the school was to have a large number of research achievements to its credit and it played a major role, as did the hospital of the Rockefeller Institute in New York, in training a new generation of clinical research workers who became professional leaders elsewhere in Britain. In its early decades, the school was the most radical and nonconformist medical institution in the country. By the 1960s, it had become, in the words of the historian Noël Poynter:

the most advanced and successful in the British Commonwealth. It was an example of what can be achieved when the restrictions imposed by tradition and vested interests are loosened. This institution with its brilliant record has been of tremendous value in radically changing the attitudes of British doctors to medical education and the way it should be organized.[30]

At the same time, there were to be important developments in the University of Oxford, whose record in medical education had so disappointed Osler. The distinguished neurosurgeon Sir Hugh Cairns (1896–1952), who had studied with Harvey Cushing (1869–1939) in Boston, drew up a memorandum in the summer of 1935 arguing for the establishment of 'a complete school of medicine in Oxford'. Initially, it was to be a postgraduate school and as in the United States it was to be financed by private philanthropy, in this instance from the commercial success of the motor car. Lord Nuffield (1877–1963) contributed £2 million in 1936 for a new postgraduate school for clinical research in Oxford, which enabled the university to establish Nuffield chairs in clinical subjects.[31] Hugh Cairns was duly appointed to the Chair of Surgery, and L. J. Witts (1898–1982), after a brief sojourn at St Bartholomew's, where he had succeeded Fraser, became the first Nuffield Professor of Medicine. If the postgraduate initiatives in Oxford made perhaps a slower start than was the case at Hammersmith, recent years have witnessed a remarkable burgeoning of clinical research there. The American physician and infectious disease specialist Paul Beeson, who succeeded Witts, played a major role in encouraging these developments, and his successor, Sir David Weatherall (b. 1933), haematologist and pioneer of the application of the techniques of molecular biology to the study of human disease, has ensured that the Oxford school has become one of the world leaders in medical education and in clinical research in recent years. More recently, the University of Cambridge has founded an undergraduate school of medicine, which promises to provide important opportunities for clinical research in an environment where close links with the basic sciences, and particularly with molecular biology, are being established.

The development of opportunities for clinical research in academic clinical departments in Britain was, as in the United States, of great importance in encouraging an environment where clinical investigation could thrive. Yet the universities and medical schools provided little finance for medical research, concerned as they were with the problems of medical education. In the clinical arena, the financing of research has come from two main sources: a government-funded agency, the Medical Research Council (MRC); and the medical charities, such as the Imperial Cancer Research Fund, the British Heart Foundation, and the Wellcome Trust. The MRC also made other major contributions to clinical research: It not only gave its active support and encouragement to the newly developing clinical departments in the medical schools, but it also supported, throughout his career, the work of a remarkable individual, Sir Thomas Lewis, the architect of British clinical research in the years between the two world wars.

From the time of its foundation in 1913, the Medical Research Committee (which became the Medical Research Council in 1920) sought to encourage not only disinterested or 'pure' science, but also clinical research and experimental medicine.[32] In 1918, re-examining its role after the World War I, the Council acknowledged 'the urgent importance of using the resources of the Medical Research Fund to forward the science of experimental medicine and its study at the bedside, in close conjunction with all the resources of the modern laboratory'. The original members of the Medical Research Committee included two clinicians, the distinguished Regius Professor of Physic at the University of Cambridge, Sir Clifford Allbutt, and C. T. Bond (1856–1939), a Leicester surgeon of broad interests. As early as 1913, it was recognized that hospital beds might be required for research following the plan that had been adopted with such success at the Rockefeller Institute. It was then considered that they could be provided at Mount Vernon Hospital in Hampstead, London, which had been purchased by the Committee to house its Central Institute. With the outbreak of war in 1914, however, all plans had to be laid aside. After the war, the question of clinical research was reconsidered and the decision was taken not to develop a research hospital at Hampstead, partly on grounds of cost but also because 'it is undesirable . . . to divorce research work from higher teaching', a consideration which apparently did not apply to the MRC's determination to press ahead with a central institute, not linked with the university, devoted to the basic sciences. Instead it was decided to support a department of clinical research and experimental medicine at University College Hospital (UCH). Sir Thomas Lewis had been recruited by the MRC as their first full-time investigator in 1916, and he had carried out valuable work on cardiac neuroses. Now he was to have beds available at UCH for 'research work and higher teaching'. It was stressed, however, that although the clinical activities of the MRC were to take place away from the central institute at Hampstead, the National Institute for Medical Research (NIMR), Lewis's department was to be regarded as part of NIMR and its staff were expected to enjoy 'the fullest scientific intercourse with the others working there'. This ideal was not really to be fulfilled in future years, for Lewis always acted entirely independently.

At the same time, throughout the period between 1920 and 1930, the MRC gave active encouragement to the newly developing clinical academic departments in the London medical schools, providing research grants to talented individuals, as well as supporting Edward Mellanby's nutritional research in Sheffield and therapeutic research in Edinburgh. The first secretary to the MRC, Sir Walter Fletcher (1873–1933), a powerful figure who served from 1913 until his untimely death, was also influential in persuading both the Sir William Dunn trustees and the Rockefeller Foundation to provide financial support for building research laboratories at St Bartholomew's, St Thomas's and the London Hospitals as well as in Oxford, Cambridge, Edinburgh, and Cardiff.

By the early 1930s, Lewis had become the most influential figure in clinical research in Britain. He had now abandoned his research on electrocardiography, apparently fearful of being wedded to technology. But his department at UCH had become the Mecca for all aspiring clinical research workers. A Welshman, he was imbued with all the zeal of a nonconformist preacher in promoting the cause of clinical research. He continued to press the case for what he had come to term 'Clinical Science', arguing that 'Clinical Science has as good a claim to the name and rights of self-subsistence of a science as any other department of biology':[33] for example, physiology or pathology. To encourage the development of clinical science as a distinct entity, Lewis founded the Medical Research Society in 1930. Two years later, he changed the name of the journal *Heart*, which he had edited since 1907, to *Clinical Science*, a closer reflection of the more general approach that he now adopted. He did not always succeed in persuading others, however. The MRC, and particularly Fletcher, required convincing that there was truly a science of the clinic, and a president of the Royal Society, Sir Frederick Gowland Hopkins (1861–1947), had questioned the appropriateness of diverting funds to clinical research that might better be applied to the basic sciences.[34] This hesitancy to support clinical research in Britain in the 1930s was in marked contrast to the situation in the United States, where clinical investigators such as Minot and Murphy had already begun to win Nobel prizes.

Lewis, however, was not to be deterred. He believed that the MRC should do a great deal more for clinical research. In memoranda submitted in 1929 and again in 1942, he argued strongly for the creation of an institute of clinical research supported by the MRC[35]. It was not until 1970, long after Lewis's death in 1945, that the MRC opened its own Clinical Research Centre at Northwick Park Hospital, with no formal university affiliations. It was to be an ill-fated venture, in the 1990s it is scheduled for closure, on grounds that among others recall the MRC's comment in 1920 that 'it is undesirable . . . to divorce research work from higher teaching'.

Lewis's contribution to clinical research under the auspices of the MRC was undeniable. In the years between the two world wars, it was he who virtually alone convinced the Council of the need to 'forward the science of experimental medicine and its study at the bedside,' and he inspired a whole generation of research workers who were later to play major roles in the expansion of academic medicine in Britain after the end of the Second World War.

It may be argued that it was not his fault that some of his pupils, and later others, carried on a purely physiological approach to clinical research for too long, at a time when biochemistry, immunology, and cell biology were becoming more important. (➤ Ch. 10 The immunological tradition) There were, however, those who considered that by championing clinical science as a subject in its own right Lewis had caused a disastrous rift to develop between clinical research and the basic sciences, particularly at UCH. Sir Charles Lovatt-Evans (1884–1968), a professor of physiology, thought that Lewis had created an entirely artificial subject called 'Clinical Science', which was simply human physiology applied to the problems of clinical medicine. It is clear that Lewis ignored the importance of specialization. He was also suspicious of new technology, as is evidenced by his rejection of electrocardiography in his early years. Later, he was critical of the introduction of cardiac catheterization for physiological studies in England.[36] By the time of his death in 1945, it is clear that the developing world of clinical research, to which he had contributed so much, had moved on from the clinical physiology that Lewis had championed for so long.

In the immediate post-war era, the MRC was involved in two vitally important developments in clinical research. The first was the introduction of the randomized, controlled clinical trial. Advised by Sir Austin Bradford Hill (1897–1991), Professor of Medical Statistics and Epidemiology at the London School of Hygiene and Tropical Medicine, the Council set up in 1946 a trial of the efficacy of streptomycin in the treatment of pulmonary tuberculosis. The drug was in short supply in those lean post-war years and there was insufficient to treat all patients who might benefit. It was therefore considered ethically justifiable to carry out a trial in which one group of patients received streptomycin whereas a control group was treated with the then-accepted methods of treatment without the new drug. The design of the trial followed that adopted by R. A. Fisher (1890–1962) in his pioneering work in agriculture. Fisher had commented in *The Design of Experiments* in 1935 that randomization 'is necessary for the validity of using any test of significance', and the MRC trial emphasized the importance of randomization in selecting subjects for study. The results of the trial were startlingly successful: in the streptomycin-treated group, 7 per cent of the patients died, compared with 27 per cent in the control group, a difference that was highly significant statistically.[37] However, the results of the trial were infinitely more important and far-reaching than they were to be for the treatment of tuberculosis. As the *British Medical Journal* (*BMJ*) pointed out when reporting the trial in 1948, this was the first randomized, controlled trial of its kind to be reported in human subjects and it would serve as a model for other such studies.[38] The *BMJ* had not always been so perceptive. Since that time, the randomized, controlled clinical trial has provided the gold standard for all such studies. (➤ Ch. 39 Drug therapies)

The second important development was the application of epidemiology to the analysis of clinical problems, particularly those involved with the frailties of human behaviour. Once again, Bradford Hill was to be the key figure. In 1947, stimulated by the Chief Medical Officer at the General Register Office, the MRC had set up a conference to discuss the increased, and increasing, mortality from cancer of the lung. The MRC enlisted the aid of Bradford Hill, and with the aid of a grant from the Council, he was able to recruit the young Richard Doll (b. 1912), later Sir Richard and Regius Professor of Medicine in the University of Oxford, to join him in 1948 in analyzing possible causes of the disease. Their painstaking survey of patients from twenty London hospitals clearly showed that 'smoking is a factor, and an important factor, in the production of cancer of the lung'.[39] They went on to establish that the same conclusion applied nationally, and in an important study of members of the medical profession, they were able to show that mortality from the disease fell if individuals stopped smoking. These observations were not only important in showing the cause of a commonly occurring cancer in Britain, and subsequently in other countries such as the United States, but also in establishing the position of epidemiology in clinical research, at a time when laboratory scientists and many of those in traditional clinical academic departments considered subjects such as epidemiology to be 'soft science'. (➤ Ch. 25 Cancer; Ch. 52 Epidemiology)

In 1949, Sir Harold Himsworth (b. 1905) succeeded Mellanby as secretary to the MRC. A practising clinician, he had been Professor of Medicine at UCH in succession to T. R. Elliott (1877–1961). He was therefore concerned to encourage clinical research during his years as Secretary. He was to be Secretary during the years that followed the implementation of the National Health Service Acts of 1946, which resulted in the foundation of the National Health Service (NHS) in 1948. The Acts were to have important consequences for clinical research, for they gave ministers power not only to conduct research but also to assist others to do so. After due consultation between the Department of Health and the MRC, a Clinical Research Board, which included members from both bodies, was set up as part of the MRC. Extra funding was allocated at a later stage, and at the same time, facilities for decentralized research were to be provided by health authorities throughout the country.[40]

The years between 1950 and 1970, which coincided with Himsworth's tenure of the secretaryship, were to be a period of great expansion in the activities of the MRC throughout the country, particularly in clinical research. In that period, the Council founded eighty-two new research units. Of these, as many as forty-six were in the clinical field. Many of the units were set up in university departments and directed by university professors. It was during these years that the so-called dual-support system for medical research became established in Britain, the universities providing the core laboratory or clinical support and the MRC allocating research funds.

During the past two decades, the 1970s and 1980s, however, clinical research has faced increasing difficulties. The funding of medical research has not increased regularly every year as it did in previous decades, and research funds have therefore come under increasing strain. Basic scientists, their own funds under threat, have considered, as did Gowland Hopkins, that there was little justification for allocating scarce funds to research in the clinical disciplines. (➤ Ch. 57 Health economics) At the same time, there has been a great increase in the number of non-medical scientists who have been required for carrying out research in laboratories associated with clinical investigation. Clinical scientists have also faced an increasing problem with training. In a previous era, when the aspiring clinical scientist had undergone training in physiology as an undergraduate, it was relatively easy for him or her to undertake research in subjects such as cardiology and respiratory medicine whose research was often based on clinical physiology. Now, however, the clinician who would succeed in clincial research requires postgraduate training not only in his or her chosen clinical discipline, but also in biochemistry, immunology, cell biology, and particularly in molecular biology. It is for these reasons that distinguished clinical scientists have predicted the demise of the clinical investigator.[41, 42] Others have gone further in declaring that an 'age of optimism' is now over.[43] Nevertheless, for the future, if advances in basic biomedical science are to be applied in clinical practice and if new treatments are to be subjected to analysis before being introduced to the public at large, it continues to be imperative that a core of expert clinical investigators continues to play a major role in medical research in universities and research institutes.

ETHICAL CONSIDERATONS

In terms of its scientific base, clinical research differs in no way from the basic sciences. In ethical terms, however, clinical investigators are constantly faced with issues that constrain their freedom of action. It is clearly not possible to carry out experiments in the human subject that may be entirely acceptable in experimental animals. For centuries, the ethical standards of doctors, whether involved in treatment or in clinical investigation, were governed by the Hippocratic ethic. Doctors undertook to follow a system or regimen which would always be to the benefit of their patients, to give no deadly medicine to anyone even if asked, and never to induce an abortion in a woman. The Hippocratic tradition, amongst other undertakings, also enjoined doctors to respect the confidentiality of their patients. This ancient ethic was the guiding principle for doctors for more than two thousand years. (➤ Ch. 34 History of the doctor–patient relationship) During the present century, it has come under increasing strain. The old paternalistic certainties, under which the doctor knew best and decided what was right, are no longer acceptable. So far as ethics are concerned, Ian M. Kennedy (b. 1941) has rightly pointed out that: 'Medical ethics are not *separate from* but *part of* the general moral and ethical order by which we live. Decisions as to what the doctor ought to do must therefore be tested against the ethical principles of society.'[44] (➤ Ch. 37 History of medical ethics)

It was the participation of doctors in supporting the racial policies of Nazi Germany that most horrifyingly offended against all norms of medical ethics. After the Second World War, twenty-three Nazi doctors, many of whom had been involved in human experimentation, were tried at Nuremberg for war crimes, and several were executed. As one of the American prosecutors said at the tribunal, the atrocious experiments carried out in the Nazi concentration camps revealed nothing that civilized medicine could use. Nevertheless, they were medical experiments, carried out by qualified doctors, using scientific methods in however warped a cause. The Nuremberg Code, which emerged after the trials, was designed to ensure that never again would medical research be perverted in this way. The Code consisted of ten points giving ethical guidance to research workers. The first and most important reads: 'The voluntary consent of the subject is essential . . .' The principles embodied in the Code were further refined in the Declaration of Helsinki on medical research in 1964, which went on to define the difference between therapeutic experiments, in which clinical research is combined with professional care, and non-therapeutic experiments, in which there may be no benefit to the subject concerned but which may contribute to knowledge so that others may ultimately benefit. These guidelines, however, were only advisory to research workers, who continued to make their own decisions about the ethical propriety of their own experiments. At the same time, however, it became increasingly apparent that certain clinical experiments carried out in well-known medical schools or research institutes and published in respected medical journals did not conform to the Declaration of Helsinki. H. K. Beecher (1904–76) in the United States and M. H. Pappworth (b. 1910) in Britain were highly influential in criticizing experiments that were unethical because they had been carried out without the consent of the subject, with insufficient consideration of the risks involved, or on individuals such as prisoners who were in no position to refuse.[45, 46] (➤ Ch. 59 Internationalism in medicine and public health)

As a result of these developments, it became clear that a controlling structure was necessary to oversee the prosecution of clinical research. In all institutions where clinical research is carried out, there are now ethical committees, which include not only doctors and research workers, but also lay members, often a cleric or a lawyer, as well as nurses and medical administrators. One of the key issues facing these committees has been the question of informed consent. There are clearly problems when children or those with mental illness are involved, with the latter presenting a particularly difficult dilemma since psychiatric disorders most urgently require the application of the scientific method. In general, it is now agreed that no experimental procedure should be undertaken without the whole proposal being carefully explained to any potential subject, who should, if then agreeable, be asked to give signed consent. (➤ Ch. 69 Medicine and the law)

The evidence of the twentieth century shows clearly how important research, including human experimentation, has been in ensuring that scientific advances have been effectively applied to the ailments of humankind. The prevention of infective illnesses by immunization, the introduction of antibiotics, the discovery of new drugs to treat heart disease or ulcers of the stomach, and the remarkable advances in surgery that now permit the transplantation of organs as complex as the heart, lung, or pancreas, have all been the result of research based partly in the laboratory, partly in the clinic. For the future, clinical research will continue to require the active collaboration of scientists in the laboratory with caring doctors, working to agreed ethical principles, at the bedside.

NOTES

1 Sanctorius Sanctorius, *Medicina Statistica: Being the Aphorisms Translated into English by J. Quincy*, London, W. Newton, 1712.

2 Thomas Lewis, 'Clinical science', *British Medical Journal*, 1933, 2: 717–22.

3 Michel Foucault, *The Birth of the Clinic*, London, Tavistock, 1973.

4 H. H. Simmer, 'Principles and problems of medical undergraduate education in Germany during the nineteenth and early twentieth centuries', in C. D. O'Malley (ed.), *The History of Medical Education*, Los Angeles, University of California Press, 1970, pp. 173–200.

5 G. W. Corner, *A History of the Rockefeller Institute*, New York, Rockefeller Institute Press, 1964.

6 A. M. Harvey, *The Association of American Physicians, 1886–1986*, Baltimore, MD, Waverley Press, 1986, p. 2.

7 W. B. Cannon, 'Some modern extensions of Beaumont's studies in Alexis St Martin', *Journal of the Michigan State Medical Society*, 1933, 32: 125–64.

8 G. Thorn, 'Austin Flint: a biographical study of a founding member', *American Clinical and Climatological Association Journal*, 1959, 71: 51.

9 Harvey, op. cit. (n. 6).

10 Harvey, op. cit. (n. 6).

11 W. M. Welch, 'Presidential address to the Annual Meeting of the American Association of Physicians', cited by Harvey, op. cit. (n. 6), p. 188.

12 Karl E. Rothschuh, *History of Physiology*, Huntington, NY, Krieger, 1973.

13 Harvey, op. cit. (n. 6), p. 189.

14 Harvey, op. cit. (n. 6), p. 190.

15 Harvey, op. cit. (n. 6), p. 191.

16 Corner, op. cit. (n. 5), pp. 88–107, 249–83.

17 Corner, op. cit. (n. 5), p. 282.

18 Abraham Flexner, *Medical Education in the United States and Canada*, New York, Carnegie Foundation for the Advancement of Teaching, 1910.

19 P. B. Beeson and R. C. Maulitz, 'The inner history of internal medicine', *Grand Rounds: One Hundred Years of Internal Medicine*, Philadelphia, University of Pennsylvania Press, 1988, pp. 15–54.

20 Archibald Garrod, *Inborn Errors of Metabolism*, Oxford, Oxford Medical Publications, 1909.

21 G. R. Murray, 'Note on the treatment of myxoedema by hypodermic injections of an extract of the thyroid gland of a sheep', *British Medical Journal*, 1891, 2: 796–7.

22 Harvey, op. cit. (n. 6), pp. 173–7.

23 *Report of the Royal Commission on University Education in London* (Chairman: Viscount Haldane), London, HMSO, 1913.

24 E. G. Little, 'The University of London', *British Medical Journal*, 1913, 2: 1497.

25 Corner, op. cit. (n. 5), p. 106.

26 *Report of Interdepartmental Committee on Medical Schools.* (Chairman: Sir William Goodenough), London, HMSO, 1944.

27 C. E. Newman, 'A brief history of the Postgraduate Medical School', *Postgraduate Medical Journal*, 1985, 42: 738–40.

28 Ibid.

29 C. C. Booth, 'Half a century of science and technology at Hammersmith', *British Medical Journal*, 1985, 291: 1771–9.

30 F. N. L. Poynter, 'Medical education in England since 1600', in C. D. O'Malley (ed.), *The History of Medical Education*, Los Angeles, University of California Press, 1970, pp. 235–50.

31 C. C. Booth, 'Clinical research', in Austoker and Bryder (eds), *Historical Perspectives on the Role of the MRC*, pp. 205–41.

32 Ibid.

33 Thomas Lewis, 'The Huxley lecture on clinical science within the university', *British Medical Journal*, 1935, 1: 631–6.

34 F. G. Hopkins, 'Presidential address to the Royal Society', *Proceedings of the Royal Society, Series B*, 1934, 114: 181–205.

35 C. C. Booth, 'Clinical research and the Medical Research Council', *Quarterly Journal of Medicine*, 1986, 59: 435–447.

36 J. McMichael, foreword to D. Veral and R. G. Grainger (eds), *Cardiac Catheterisation and Angiocardiology*, Edinburgh, Churchill Livingstone, 1962.

37 Streptomycin in Tuberculosis Trials Committee, 'Streptomycin treatment of pulmonary tuberculosis. A Medical Research Council investigation', *British Medical Journal*, 1948, 2: 769–82.

38 Anon, 'Streptomycin in pulmonary tuberculosis', *British Medical Journal*, 1948, 2: 790–1.

39 R. Doll and A. Bradford Hill, 'Smoking and carcinoma of the lung', *British Medical Journal*, 1950, 2: 739–48.

40 A. Landsborough Thomson, *Half a Century of Medical Research*. Vol. II: *The Programmes of the Medical Research Council (UK)*, London, HMSO, 1975.

41 J. B. Wyngaarden, 'The clinical investigator as an endangered species', *New England Journal of Medicine*, 1979, 301: 1254–9.

42 M. Oliver, 'The shrinking face of clinical science', *European Journal of Clinical Investigation*, 1979, 7: 1–2.

43 C. T. Dollery, *The End of an Age of Optimism*, London, Nuffield Provincial Hospitals Trust, 1978.

44 Working Party Report, *Philosophy and Practice of Medical Ethics*, London, British Medical Association, 1988.

45 H. K. Beecher, 'Ethics and clinical research', *New England Journal of Medicine*, 1966, 274: 1354–60.

46 M. H. Pappworth, *Human Guinea Pigs*, London, Routledge & Kegan Paul, 1967.

FURTHER READING

Austoker, Joan and Bryder, Linda (eds), *Historical Perspectives on the Role of the MRC*, Oxford, Oxford University Press, 1989.

Corner, George W., *A History of the Rockefeller Institute 1901–1953. Origin and Growth*, New York City, Rockefeller Institute Press, 1964.

Drury, A. N. and Grant, R. T., 'Sir Thomas Lewis, 1881–1945', *Obituary Notices of Fellows*, London, Royal Society, Vol. 5, pp. 179–202.

Flexner, Abraham, *An Autobiography*, New York, Simon & Schuster, 1960.

Harvey, A. McGehee, *Adventures in Medical Research. A Century of Discovery at Johns Hopkins*, Baltimore, MD, Johns Hopkins University Press, 1974.

——, *The Association of American Physicians 1886–1986. A Century of Progress in Medical Science*, Baltimore, MD, Waverley Press, 1986.

——, *Science at the Bedside: Clinical Research in American Medicine 1905–1945*, Baltimore, MD, Johns Hopkins University Press, 1981.

Kennedy, Ian, *Treat Me Right. Essays in Medical Law and Ethics*, Oxford, Clarendon Press, 1988.

Lewis, Thomas, *Clinical Science Illustrated by Personal Experiences*, London, Shaw, 1934.

Maulitz, Russell C. and Long, Diana E. (eds), *Grand Rounds. One Hundred Years of Internal Medicine*, Philadelphia, University of Pennsylvania Press, 1988.

O'Malley, C. D. (ed.), *The History of Medical Education*, Los Angeles, University of California Press, 1970.

Phillips, Melanie and Dawson, John, *Doctors' Dilemmas. Medical Ethics and Contemporary Science*, Brighton, Harvester Press, 1985.

Rothstein, William G., *American Medical Schools and the Practice of Medicine*, Oxford, Oxford University Press, 1987.

Thomson, A. Landsborough, *Half a Century of Medical Research*, 2 vols, London, HMSO, 1975.

PART III

THEORIES OF LIFE, HEALTH, AND DISEASE

12

THE CONCEPTS OF HEALTH, ILLNESS, AND DISEASE

Arthur L. Caplan

WHY ARE HEALTH AND DISEASE SO IMPORTANT IN CONTEMPORARY SOCIETY?

Health and disease are concepts of importance in contemporary life. This is especially true if we happen to live in one of the nations of the industrialized world. Enormous sums of money, in America approaching nearly 12 per cent of the gross national product, more than $800 billion in 1992, are spent on health care. The nations of western Europe, Scandinavia, Canada, Australia, New Zealand, Korea, Singapore, and Japan spend large sums of money per person annually for medical care and other health-related activities. (➤ Ch. 57 Health economics) Many persons devote large amounts of their time to the pursuit of behaviours and life-styles that they believe will enhance their health and stave off disease.

The analysis of the concepts of health, illness, and disease is not a mere exercise in intellectual inquiry. Decisions about the meaning of these terms have direct and important consequences for daily life and the allocation of vast amounts of social resources.

The concepts of health and disease, and the persons and institutions concerned with them, did not always play such central roles in human affairs. As recently as the mid-nineteenth century, physicians and hospitals occupied minor, peripheral roles in nearly every society. Few persons actively pursued health by means of life-style, diet, or daily regimens of one sort or another. It is not clear that they could. The prevailing notions of health and wellness were not especially amenable to conscious pursuit by individuals.

During this same time, disease was feared and stigmatized, but was rarely the object of ministration by organized medicine, health care, or health-care institutions. The sick and the ill often turned to lay people – family as well as clerics. (➤ Ch. 30 Folk medicine) The situation today has changed radically. Why is this so and why do these concepts play such a central role in daily contemporary life?

The emergent concern with health and disease in this century is a function of many forces. The conquest of the pain associated with medical treatment, especially surgery, in the late nineteenth century by means of anaesthesia plus the demonstrable efficacy of twentieth-century medicine and public health in preventing or reversing many forms of infection, dysfunction, and nutritional deficiency surely constitute primary reasons for the prominence of concerns about health and disease. The demonstrable utility of various modes of conceiving disease, such as the germ theory, from the point of view of prophylaxis and cure compelled changes in the understanding of what disease and health mean. But, it was not simply the success enjoyed by medicine and its attendant conceptual models of health and disease over the past one hundred years that brought the concepts of health and disease to centre stage.

The historic connection in many theological writings, particularly Protestant, between health and moral character has played a key role in establishing the cultural importance of health and disease in Western societies. Disease and disability have been seen by many religious traditions as reflections of God's displeasure with sin and with the impure in mind if not in actual deed. The current interest in health and the prevention and avoidance of disease reflects the legacy of conceiving of disease and illness as instruments of divine displeasure. (➤ Ch. 61 Religion and medicine)

In a Western world grown far more secular in this century, at least in its public culture, disease, disability, and health have become transformed. Disease is no longer a sign of divine displeasure or a mark of sin. Disease is not seen as having instrumental value, it has taken on intrinsic importance. Health, in itself, is often interpreted as a sign of good moral character and individual worth, whereas disease is often equated with moral failure.

As the prospects for the control of illness and disease increased, the causal locus of the origins of disease began to shift toward the individual rather than outside forces or agents. This shift brought in its wake a shift toward the equation of health with good character and virtuous conduct. When those with cancer are told to use their mental powers to visualize cancerous cells in order to dampen their growth, when female workers are told they cannot hold jobs in a particular factory because the chemicals present pose risks to their reproductive well-being, when individuals are told they can use laughter or will-power to reverse the course of disease, when experts urge the control of diet, exercise, stress, or sexuality as the key to good health, then disease and health have taken a highly individualistic focus and, thus, are direct means for assessing the moral worth and value of human beings.

Technology also has had a role in the emergence of health and disease as central cultural concerns in the Western world. As nineteenth-century science, especially under the influence of Darwinism, began to diminish the boundaries that had made human beings seem special, unique, or distinctive, medicine became more willing to treat human beings as possible objects for scientific scrutiny and technologically based interventions.

Throughout this century and particularly since the Second World War, technology has come to play an increasingly important role in our health-care system. This is reflected in the emphasis in many modern health-care delivery-systems on the treatment of acute medical problems in hospital settings. The proliferation of neonatal units, CAT scanners, ultrasound, and organ and tissue transplants is a reflection of our collective faith in the power of technology and our belief that it can be used to identify and control the evils of disease and disability. Technology has reified health and disease, it has made it seem as if diseases are real entities in the world that can be observed, identified, manipulated, and eliminated. (➤ Ch. 36 The science of diagnosis: diagnostic technology; Ch. 68 Medical technologies: social contexts and consequences)

Prior to the First World War, there was relatively little that physicians or anyone else could do to combat the effects of acute disease and severe disability. The introduction of antibiotics, vaccines, transfusions, powerful diagnostic technologies, and technologically based therapies in the decades following the war transformed medicine from a profession focused on diagnosis and caring to one with at least a serious interest in curing. The expectations of physicians and patients have grown considerably and, as a result, the desire to be returned to a state of health after the onset of disease or injury seems more a matter of finding a competent professional than it does a matter for hopes, wishes, and prayers.

Particular political and social values place a special premium on health and the avoidance of disease. Health and the alleviation of disease and disability have key roles to play in highly competitive, capitalist societies. Societies committed to free-market economics can tolerate significant differences in the resources and status held by individual citizens, but such differences can only be accepted if there is a general acceptance of the means by which resources are acquired and held. A concern for equality of opportunity in economic life in many countries leads inevitably to the assignment of great weight to the preservation of health and the prevention of disease and disability.

The moral assessment of inequalities of power, possessions, and property is contingent upon the view that prevails of the opportunities that have preceded the creation of inequalities in the distribution of social goods. If some people are rich because they work hard and others are poor because they are lazy, then so be it. As long as a relative equality of opportunity exists, as long as the initial conditions for competing economically are seen as fair, then any differences that result are easier to accept on moral grounds.

If equality of opportunity is a critical moral component of the legal, political, and societal norms of free-market societies, then health and disease will be accorded special status. Those with congenital deformities or who suffer from disabling or chronic diseases, especially if they are infants or children, cannot be said to have an equal opportunity to compete with their peers for the goods and benefits that a competitive society makes available. The alleviation of disease and disability and the promotion of health are important political and cultural goals for the same reasons special priority is given to the provision of basic education, shelter, and food. All of these factors influence the extent to which equality can legitimately be said to exist with respect to opportunities and, therefore, to the extent to which the inequalities which result from a free-market approach to the distribution of social resources can be viewed as morally palatable.

Disease and disability become the object of concern in Western society because they are seen as a threat to equal opportunity, and in turn, to the moral foundation of economic life. The reductions in abilities and capacities that usually accompany diseases are threatening not only because they cause intrinsic harms to those beset by them, but also because they undermine the social commitment to the equity of competition and the fairness of the market as efficient methods for distributing social resources. Despite the fact that it may be expensive to redress the effects of disease or to prevent its occurrence, if fundamental inequities exist among people because of serious but remediable differences in their health and well-being, this is a state of affairs that is incompatible with the socio-economic orientation that seeks to reward striving, performance, and individual achievement. Economics plays a major role in thrusting the concepts of health and disease centre stage in developed nations that are organized around competitive markets. (➤ Ch. 70 Medical sociology)

HEALTH, DISEASE, AND THE SCOPE OF MEDICINE

If it is true that health and disease play powerful roles in filling important gaps left by the secularization of public culture and in legitimizing key presuppositions of prevailing socio-economic arrangements in Western societies, it is obvious why so much attention has centred in recent decades on their meaning and definition. The definitions accorded these concepts will play pivotal roles in establishing the boundaries of access to the health-care system, the limits of medical concern and professional control, and also of social obligation to share in the burden of alleviating disease, disability, and dysfunction. (➤ Ch. 4 Medical care)

Prima-facie obligations exist for government to correct the inequalities wrought by disease and illness. The answer to the question of what does or does not constitute a disease will determine not only how much authority and power is available to those responsible for alleviating the consequences of disease – physicians, nurses, public health officials, social workers, and other health-care professionals – but what government must do to shift resources toward those with special needs resulting from ill health in order to make economic and social life fair. (➤ Ch. 50 Medical institutions and the state; Ch. 51 Public health)

There has been much concern on the part of a variety of social commentators and ethicists from both ends of the political spectrum about the growing power and influence of medicine and other health-care professions in our society. Conservatives worry, for example, that physicians, nurses, and psychologists will introduce adolescent students to permissive attitudes toward sexual conduct in the guise of promoting 'health' education. Liberals fear, for instance, that the classification of homosexuality as a disease rather than a matter of personal behavioural preference or biological necessity will result in discriminatory treatment of homosexuals and the promotion of negative stereotypes. The definitions of health, disease, and illness are seen by many as political issues, requiring input from both professions and lay people.

Physicians are now able to control access to a wide variety of social and economic resources by the use of their authority as gate-keepers of eligibility for a wide spectrum of public and private programmes. Getting a job, receiving life insurance, permission to immigrate, admission to school, entry into and out of the armed services, access to legal compensation, exculpation from punishment, the ability to marry and to have and raise a family, are all controlled to some extent by doctors and other health-care professionals. Similarly, decisions about who will or will not be forced to receive medical care in hospital or institutional settings, who is or is not free to refuse medication or confinement, and what is or is not an acceptable form of medical treatment are controlled by physicians and other health-care personnel. (➤ Ch. 37 History of medical ethics; Ch. 69 Medicine and the law)

Health-care providers not only have the authority to enfranchise some members of society with social benefits or privileges, they also have the authority to excuse behaviour that, without medical exculpation, might be the object of police, judicial, or penal attention. Many groups have fought long and hard to have particular behavioural dispositions labelled as diseases; for example, alcoholics, gamblers, and those with chronic back pain. The disease label excuses certain behaviour that might otherwise be viewed as criminal, sinful, or lazy, and thus be subject to various forms of sanction.

Conversely, many groups, such as homosexuals and the disabled, have struggled to free themselves from being categorized as ill or diseased. Disease labels, while often exculpatory in terms of liability or responsibility, carry other burdens such as the stigma attached to illness and the assumption that those who are ill or diseased require treatment and cure from legitimate experts.

If the scope and domain of medicine and the related healing arts are to be accurately delineated, a clear understanding of the concepts of health and disease is a necessity. The definitions that are given to these concepts are critical both for understanding the possibilities and limits of health care as well as for understanding the moral obligations, rights, and responsibilities that ought to prevail between patients and providers in health-care contexts. ((➤ Ch. 34 History of the doctor–patient relationship)

THE RELATIONSHIP BETWEEN THE CONCEPTS OF HEALTH AND DISEASE

What is the nature of the logical relationship between health, illness, and disease? Many health-care professionals and a large percentage of the general public appear to view health and disease as logical opposites, while illness and disease are often used as synonyms. When asked if they are healthy or feel well, most people will answer affirmatively if they are not suffering from any particular disease or disorder at the time the question is asked. Looked at uncritically, health would seem to be no more than the absence of disease and illness. Disease and illness appear to connote any impairment in a person's sense of well-being or fitness.

But there are powerful reasons for questioning the appropriateness of viewing health and disease merely as conceptual opposites, and disease and illness as synonyms. Even if no particular disease is present, it is still possible to say that a person seems healthier or is healthier in certain ways than others. The average marathon runner or professional athlete is probably healthier, with respect to overall physical well-being, than the average philosophy professor, even if neither happens to be afflicted with a specific disease at the time the comparison is made. Health does seem to require the absence of disease or illness as a necessary condition, but it is not clear that this absence is by itself sufficient to define the nature of health.

The possibility that health is not simply the absence of disease or illness, but refers to something more, is reinforced by the activities of some contemporary health-care practitioners. Some see their job as more than simply the alleviation of disease. Psychoanalysts, plastic surgeons, nutritionists, and sports physiologists are interested not only in the prevention or alleviation of disease, but also, and perhaps sometimes only, the promotion of health. If health and disease were logically related to one another as contradictory concepts, it would be impossible to make any sense of the ideas expressed by such terms as 'maximize health' or 'positive mental health'. These ideas, as well as the notion that relative degrees of health can exist even in the absence of disease or illness, do appear to be meaningful and coherent.

Not only is the absence of disease not sufficient to establish the existence of health, diseases do not always impair or threaten health. Some diseases are unpleasant and disabling but do not compromise the health of the individual who has them. For example, enduring a short bout of measles or mumps during childhood, either through infection or inoculation, may actually be conducive to health. A person can be riddled with cancer, delusional, or suffer from hypertension, and yet remain entirely unaware of any symptoms of dysfunction. A person who is the carrier of the sickle-cell trait, while prone to certain problems under certain rare circumstances, is better protected against malaria than someone lacking this genetic endowment. The fact that one can be functioning well and feel healthy while suffering from a disease also hints that the concepts of illness and disease may actually refer to different states or conditions. Feeling sick is not the same as having a disease, since one can be ill but not diseased and diseased but not feel ill.

Some behaviours that are viewed as diseases in at least some circles – gambling, homosexuality, hyperactivity, or drug-addiction – have tenuous logical connections to the concept of health. Certainly, it is much less difficult to obtain agreement across social classes and different cultures about those states of the mind and body that constitute diseases than it is to secure agreement about which states are to be viewed as healthy. The use of addictive narcotic drugs and their relationship to health is viewed quite differently in Jamaica, Holland, Bolivia, and Peru than it is in the United States or Saudi Arabia.

While the view of health and disease as conceptual opposites may be widely accepted, there are reasons for calling this presumption into question. A strong case can be made for the view that the logical relationship between health and disease is not one of contradiction. The conceptual opposite of health might more reasonably be seen as unhealthy ; and the logical contradictory of diseased as non-diseased. Health and disease may exist as parallel concepts rather than as concepts defined only in terms of one another. While disease may be among the criteria that are used to define health, other measures or states may be necessary in order to attribute this state to an individual.

NORMATIVISM VERSUS NON-NORMATIVISM IN THE DEFINITION OF DISEASE

Perhaps the major point of contention among philosophers, doctors, and other health-care experts who have examined the meaning of health and disease is the extent to which value judgements are requisite for or are implicit in the definitions of these concepts. Many physicians and not a few philosophers believe that there is no need to resort to considerations of value in general or morality in particular to identify, understand, or analyse the concepts of health, illness, and disease. Those who subscribe to non-normativism believe that determinations of health and disease are matters of empirical fact and nothing more.

One of the ways in which the case for assigning a key role to values in the definition of health and disease is made by those who espouse the contrary view, normativism, is to observe that categories of disease vary from culture to culture and historical period to historical period. Moreover, what is supposed to be the same disease or the same state of health can produce very different experiences in different people.

Granted, not everyone has the same experience in conjunction with disease. One common way of responding to this fact is to use the term 'illness' to refer to the subjective perception or the phenomenological experience of disease. If anxiety causes some individuals to hyperventilate but causes a tightening sensation in the chest of others and a headache in still other persons, this wide range of symptoms, responses, and experiences can be captured by the term 'illness'.

Illness is by definition subjective and thus specific to time, place, and culture. Variations in illness are to be expected. It seems beyond dispute that illness, defined only as the experience of health or disease, is heavily influenced by the prevailing values and norms of a given society. Indeed, those who wish to defend the view that health and disease can be defined in purely objective terms without reference to values are more than willing to concede the historical and sociological findings of those such as Michel Foucault, Thomas Szasz, Peter Sedgwick, and G. Canguilhem that disease is irremediably a product of culture, economics, and ideology. But, by segregating the perception of disease and the response a disease elicits in a particular individual living in a particular society under the rubric of illness, those who seek a non-normative definition hope to be able to find univocal meanings for disease (and sometimes for health) which transcend the specifics of time, place, and person.

What is at stake in the battle over the role played by values is the objectivity of claims about disease and health. If values play crucial roles in shaping the meanings of not only illness but also health and disease, then it appears as if the prospects for objectivity in medicine and health care, which depend upon these concepts, are imperilled. If values infuse the analysis of disease, then diseases seem to be a product of human invention. Diseases would be categories imposed by human beings upon human beings, not states that they possess and which can be discovered by anyone who has learned the criteria and evidence requisite to make a diagnosis. The greater the role of values in the definition of health and disease, the worse the prognosis appears to be for both their objectivity and reality. Ideology and politics loom especially large in the classification of human behaviours and states as indicative of health or disease to the extent to which values appear, since values, unlike empirical facts, are seen as very much a product of social forces. And if disease and health are matters of ideology and politics, then the prospects for an objective, verifiable science of medicine seem diminished if not simply hopeless.

The clearest contemporary expression of the view that health and disease can be defined without explicit reference to moral values or ethical norms has been offered by the American philosopher Christopher Boorse. He argues that while it is true that different social, ethnic, and economic groups do not agree on the reference class of the terms health and disease, and while it is also true that professionals often disagree about the disease status of a particular condition or behaviour, it would be wrong to conclude from such facts that an objective definition of health or disease that does not rely on values is impossible to attain. Boorse contends that while different people or groups do disagree about the specific application of a disease definition to particular cases, this does nothing to disprove the possibility of locating an objective, value-free definition of disease. Illness is often subjective and variable. Disease need not be.

All organisms, including human beings, are the product of a long course of biological evolution. Human evolution has been driven by a wide variety of environmental demands which have conferred advantages on those creatures possessing certain phenotypic and genotypic traits. Since our minds and bodies have evolved in response to our evolutionary past, health consists in our functioning in conformity with our natural design, as determined by natural selection.

If kidneys exist as a result of evolving in response to the contingent forces of natural selection so that their function is to remove impurities from the body, if hearts evolved to pump blood to organs and tissues, if external ears evolved in order to allow the localization of sound, then in any human being (or any other organism, for that matter) possessing kidneys, heart, or ears, health consists, in part, in having a kidney that removes impurities from the blood, a heart that pumps blood to organs and tissues, and ears that can localize sounds. These organs were designed by evolution to perform such functions and when they do so, the organism that possesses them can be said to be healthy. If they do them especially well, regardless of why that is so, the person who owns them can be said to have a very healthy heart or an especially sound pair of kidneys.

If there is some failure in an organ system, if it loses the capacity to perform the function for which it was designed by evolution to perform, this is indicative of disease, whether it is perceived as illness or not. Natural design permits an analysis of health or disease independent of the experience of the person. Illness, but not disease, is in the mind of the beholder. Values need not enter into the definition of the concepts of health and disease at all. This is because the goals which drive evolution have nothing to do with ethics, morals, ideology, sociology, or values.

Evolution places a premium on survival and reproduction. Survival and reproduction are the only goals that matter for evolution. In order to attain these goals, all organisms, including humans, have evolved traits that increase their probability of survival and the transmission of genes into the next generation. Organisms that lacked the genotypes and phenotypes requisite for survival and reproduction become extinct. Only those with traits adequate for survival and reproduction are here today.

Disease can be defined as any impairment of the functions typical of a particular biological species, functions required to achieve the natural goals set, not by politics or culture, but by the twin demands of survival and reproduction. Are concepts such as survival and reproduction themselves value-laden? Neither of these terms is used in any moralistic or evaluative sense – survival and reproduction are merely the contingent by-products of a Darwinian system responding to a specific set of historical circumstances. There is nothing good or bad about them – they merely exist.

If one accepts the view that the goals of survival and reproduction have guided the evolution of every living organism on this planet, then health and disease can be understood solely in terms of the causal contributions various states, conditions, and behaviours make to the achievement of these ends. No resort to ethics or any other sort of value judgement is necessary. All that must be done is to determine whether the causal contribution of a particular trait or behaviour is positive or negative in terms of the overall capacity of a particular organism to achieve its biologically designed ends. The extent to which this is so determines whether or not the trait or behaviour is to be classified as healthy or diseased.

An especially persuasive argument that values need play no role in the definitions of health and disease is that a non-normative analysis works as well for assessing the health status of plants and animals as it does for humans. Veterinarians know what it means for a cat or a pig to be sick. Few would want to argue that, before they could say that an animal was sick or dying, they must resort to an examination of the animal's mores or understand the animal's values!

HEALTH AS NORMALITY, DISEASE AS ABNORMALITY

Non-normativism, the position that disease can be defined without reference to anything other than the empirical assessment of functions based solely upon the understanding of the purposes the functions were designed to serve, is closely related to the definitions of health and disease used in contemporary medical texts. Many physicians, if pressed to define health and disease, will respond that disease is anything that is abnormal and health is what is normal.

Normal and abnormal refer to statistical normalcy, not any sort of value judgement about a particular state or behaviour. The unusual, the uncommon, and the extreme become candidates for classification as disease. Those states and behaviours that cluster around the mean or for which there is relatively small variance become the reference class of health.

The statistical conception of health and disease has prevailed in Western medicine for many, many decades. It is a legacy of the ancient theory of humours and the more modern conceptions of 'balance' or homeostasis, which grounded thinking about health and disease for many centuries. Health for thinkers as diverse as Galen (AD 129-*c*.200/210), William Cullen (1710–90), and W. B. Cannon (1871–1945) consisted of the attainment of a balance or harmony in the workings of the body. Deviations or abnormalities in the composition of bodily fluids, or, in later times, organ systems, connoted disease. (➤ Ch. 14 Humoralism)

Physicians often do equate abnormal measures of blood pressure, blood chemistry, or body weight with disease, regardless of whether dysfunction or pain is present. But, the primary problem with the attempt to establish a value-free definition of both health and disease is that anything 'unusual' is considered a disease state even when it is not at all clear why it is unhealthy to be abnormal. It seems conceptually bizarre to say that the unusually tall, intelligent, strong, fast, or agile are diseased simply by dint of their abnormality or deviance. Those at the tail ends of the distribution of any state, trait, or behaviour would by definition be diseased, an analysis that seems too inclusive and at the same time indifferent to historical attempts to connect difference with dysfunction.

The problem raised by the advantages conferred by some forms of statistical deviancy for the statistical approach to the definition of health and disease is serious. Abnormality is a sign or indication that something may be wrong, but it does not seem, in and of itself, to constitute disease. If a value-free conception of these concepts is to be found, it would seem that the attempt to root disease and health in a functional analysis, perhaps based upon the recognition that human beings are biological organisms which have evolved to meet the challenges of a shifting set of environmental demands, has the best chance of succeeding.

THE PROPONENTS OF NORMATIVISM

Normativists believe that health and disease are concepts that are inherently value laden. They believe that to understand exactly what it is that these concepts mean or refer to, it is necessary to realize that decisions have to be made about states of the body or mind that must involve considerations of what is desirable or undesirable, useful or useless, good or bad. Normativists argue that no matter how many descriptive facts are known about the body or about the functions of a particular cell or organ system, it is impossible to decide whether or not a particular state of affairs represents health or disease without some reference to values.

Historically, the primary focus of philosophical attention on the part of physicians and others interested in health care has been the concept of disease. If disease could be adequately defined and interpreted, then it was believed that all other questions about the aims, goals, and purposes of health care would be resolved.

Normativism is sometimes confused with alternative forms of healing. While there are some exponents of normativism in the ranks of those who espouse holistic health or alternative forms of medical intervention such as spiritual or psychic healing, most normativists are only concerned to defend the position that values form an irreducible element in the definition of disease.

Perhaps the clearest illustrations of the ways in which values influence the definition of health and disease emerge from the realm of mental health and mental illness. A cursory glance at nineteenth-century American medical texts reveals that some physicians asserted with all of the authority at their disposal that women who enjoyed sexual intercourse or engaged in masturbation were certainly afflicted with various forms of mental illness and often a variety of corresponding physical ailments as well. Textbooks of the era were replete with diseases of the mind that seemed to afflict only black men and women in astounding numbers. One of the most important disorders was a condition labelled 'drapetomania', a horrible plague that denoted an obsessive desire on the part of a slave to run away from his or her owner. (➤ Ch. 21 Mental diseases)

Normativists are much impressed with illustrations of the ways in which values and cultural prejudices tacitly or even overtly influence medical determinations of health and disease. They point to contemporary disputes about the disease status of such conditions as homosexuality, premenstrual syndrome, and infertility, and ask how anyone could possibly conclude that labelling some particular physical or mental state as diseased or healthy involves nothing more than an empirical assessment of biological functioning.

Both historical and contemporary cases of shifts in beliefs or uncertainties as to the proper classification of various conditions make it clear that values play an inextricable, but entirely appropriate, role in defining health and disease. Moreover, as normativists point out, a key element of the definition of disease is that the states of the body and mind that are seen as diseases in various cultures are so viewed only as a result of the fact that people disvalue them. In a society burdened with overpopulation, infertility might be viewed as a healthy state. In a society wealthy enough to provide financial support for all newborns and a bias towards large families, infertility might be seen as a disease state meriting serious attempts at amelioration through surgical or pharmacological intervention.

One of the boldest attempts to formulate a normative definition of disease, which highlights the valuational dimension of this concept, is that of the psychiatrist Charles Culver and the philosopher Bernard Gert. Culver and Gert argue that the core meaning of disease involves the recognition that something is wrong with a person. They argue that diseases are actually a subcategory of a more general category labelled 'maladies'. The members of this class include not only diseases but also injuries, disabilities, and death itself. They argue that what is common to all these conditions is that human beings universally view them as evils. Other things being equal, people disvalue these states and try to avoid them if they can. (➤ Ch. 13 Ideas of life and death)

Unlike most non-normative analyses of health and disease, which view disease and health in terms of deviations from statistical normalcy or from various norms of species-typical functioning, Culver and Gert's position is that it is not dysfunction, but the perceived evil associated with dysfunction, that is at the heart of understanding the meaning of disease. In the case of a myocardial infarction, it is not the deviation from normal functioning which makes us classify this event as a disease. Rather, it is the loss of capacities, the onset of pain, and the risk to life itself, the evils associated with this dysfunction, which lead to the disvaluation of this particular deviation from functional normality.

While the members of different cultural groups or societies may not always agree on what constitutes an evil, every society recognizes certain states of the mind or body as evils to be avoided. While people may not always agree as to the identity of those mental or physical states that represent evils, they all recognize that a loss of abilities, a loss of freedom, pain, the loss of pleasure, or death are evils. Malady thus has the apparent advantage of unifying what may initially appear to be disparate states such as pain, injury, and death by allowing them to be grouped under the common criterion of states of the body or mind that people disvalue as evils. (➤ Ch. 67 Pain and suffering)

A weakness in this approach to the normative analysis of disease is that it makes the status of disease dependent upon the willingness of the members of society to recognize a particular state of affairs as evil. Those with hypertension may not feel any loss of capacity, but the physician operating with a non-normative sense of proper physiological functioning can say that disease is present even if the patient would not agree. Similarly, a culture that has no written traditions may be unaware and unconcerned about the presence of dyslexia in some of its members. But a psychologist studying the group may be aware that a non-disvalued abnormal condition is present and may wish to try and intervene to modify the problem in order to allow such persons to learn to read should they move into another society.

NORMATIVISM VERSUS NON-NORMATIVISM – WHAT IS REALLY AT ISSUE?

The debate about the role played by values in the definition of health and disease may appear to be nothing more than an abstract philosophical controversy having few if any consequences for either the clinical practice of health care or the formulation of health policy. However, once the underlying concerns motivating the debate are made clear, it can readily be seen that what is at issue are understandings about the aims of medicine and the scientific status of its practices.

Normativists and non-normativists are equally concerned with supplying a definition of health and disease that is capable of roughly capturing our intuitions about what ought to be classified as a disease and who ought to be viewed as healthy. But those offering definitions are also concerned with providing a definition that can help classify ambiguous states of the body or mind or resolve uncertainty where disagreements exist as to the proper classification of a condition as a matter of health or disease.

Aside from the aesthetic appeal of living in a world where conceptual matters admit of neat and tidy resolutions, there are important reasons for undertaking these definitional efforts. Unless medicine and the other health-care professions use definitions of disease and health that are clear and unequivocal, there is a grave danger that uncertainties will exist on the part of both health-care providers and patients as to the aims, goals, expectations, and hopes they bring to medical encounters. If health and disease are nothing more than socially determined, culturally mediated, and individually subjective concepts, then there is some fear that there will be little possibility of either placing medicine on a firm scientific footing or of finding consensus among experts and patients as to the proper limits of medical concern.

If one doubts that judgements of value are in any way objective, then the presence of values in the definition of health and disease will make it impossible for health care and medical science to rest upon an objective and universal foundation. If, on the other hand, value judgements are seen as amenable to objective reasoned argument, then their presence in the definitions of health and disease will do nothing to undermine the objectivity or scientific prospects of medicine and health care.

Why should it be presumed that values and objectivity or even consensus are incompatible? If it is possible to obtain agreement among rational human beings that some states of the body or mind are valuable and desirable while others are not, then it ought to be possible to accord an explicit role to values in the definition of disease and health without sacrificing objectivity, precision, or universality. Since there would seem to be no lack of agreement among both patients and health-care providers that under ordinary circumstances life is preferable to death, ability is preferable to disability, pleasure more desirable than pain, then those committed to normativism would appear to have at least some grounds for optimism that an objective foundation can be found upon which to rest value-laden definitions of both health and disease. While this may be harder to do for some conditions or states than others – for example, is it better to be born with large or small breasts? – it seems that the goods and evils that bring people into the health-care system, and motivate others to want to practise the art and science of health care, form at least a rough area within which consensus can be reached about what is good and what is bad and therefore what is health and what is disease.

The controversy over normativism and non-normativism which has occupied centre stage in recent thinking about health, illness and disease may be more illusory than real. If the motivation for the controversy is the fear over the subjective nature of values, then it may be possible to defuse the debate by noting that it is possible to achieve agreement and consensus about values as well as facts. If this position is acceptable, then it may be possible to define disease as disvalued dysfunction, where dysfunction is defined in terms of both human goals and the design of the human body (and mind, to the extent to which this can be known). Health would become valued forms of functioning, optimal or maximum, in certain systems or tissues. The extent to which values are seen as a source of difficulty for objectivity in the definition of health and disease will determine the degree to which one's sympathies lie in the normativist or non-normativist camps.

FURTHER READING

Useful discussions of the way in which values have shaped the understanding of disease can be found in Ronald Bayer's *Homosexuality and American Psychology: the Politics of Diagnosis*, New York, Basic Books, 1981. Two other especially illuminating sources as to the interaction of values and the concepts of health and disease are: Thomas Szasz, *The Myth of Mental Illness*, New York, Harper-Hoeber, 1961; and Michel Foucault, *Madness and Civilization*, London, Tavistock, 1965.

A historical overview of debates about the definition of health and disease is presented in the anthology edited by Arthur Caplan, H. Tristram Engelhardt and James McCartney, *The Concepts of Health and Disease*, Reading, MA, Addison-Wesley, 1981. The clearest exposition of the view that values play no role in the definition of disease can be found in two papers by Christopher Boorse, 'On the distinction between disease and illness', *Philosophy and Public Affairs*, 1975, 5: 49–68; and 'What a theory of mental health should be', *Philosophy of Science*, 1976, 44: 542–73. Arguments for the value-laden character of these concepts are presented in Henry E. Sigerist's classic work, *Civilization and Disease*, Chicago, IL, University of Chicago Press, 1943; and in Edmund D. Pellegrino and David C. Thomasma, *For the Patient's Good*, Oxford, Oxford University Press, 1988.

A useful analysis of the role played by the concepts of health and disease in explanations in medicine and of the ontological status of these concepts can be found in Edmond A. Murphy, *The Logic of Medicine*, Baltimore, MD, Johns Hopkins University Press, 1976; and Charles M. Culver and Bernard Gert, *Philosophy in Medicine*, Oxford, Oxford University Press, 1982. Lawrie Resnek gives an especially insightful analysis of the ontological status of disease in *The Nature of Disease*, London, Routledge & Kegan Paul, 1987.

13

IDEAS OF LIFE AND DEATH

W. R. Albury

THE OPPOSITION OF LIFE AND DEATH

Throughout the history of European medical thought, life and death have been regarded as opposites. This seemingly banal statement, however, requires two important qualifications. The first is that, prior to about 1800, there was no general conception of 'life' that could be used to separate plants and animals from the rest of nature. The three kingdoms of nature – animal, vegetable, and mineral – were seen rather as a continuum, in which minerals shared to a certain extent the growth, reproduction, and other characteristics later identified exclusively with 'life'.[1] Insofar as medical thinkers concerned themselves with plants and non-human animals, they did so largely in order to discover useful medicinal properties in the former and informative analogies to human anatomy and physiology in the latter. Thus it was specifically the living human being rather than life itself that formed the prime focus of medical interest in life and death prior to the nineteenth century.

The second important qualification that the initial statement above requires is that although life and death may always have been seen as opposites, nevertheless the nature of this opposition was, and still is, capable of being understood in different senses. Aristotle (384–322 BC), in his logical writings, identified four senses of opposition, three of which are of central importance for grasping the changes that occurred in medical conceptions of life and death from antiquity to the twentieth century. In Aristotle's characterization of the three relevant senses, 'things are said to be opposed . . . (i) as correlatives to one another, (ii) as contraries to one another, [or] (iii) as privatives to positives'.[2] And of these three types of opposition, it is the third one which was to serve as the fundamental organizing principle of medical discourses on life and death until the end of the eighteenth century; that is, until approximately the same time as the concept of 'life' in general began to be formed.

LIFE AND DEATH AS POSSESSION AND PRIVATION

Aristotle did not explicitly relate his discussion of 'positives' and 'privatives' to life and death, but all his examples of 'positives' were capacities that naturally develop at their appropriate time in humans:

> We say that that which is capable of some particular faculty or possession has suffered privation when the faculty or possession in question is in no way present in that in which, and *at the time at which, it should naturally be present.* We do not call that toothless which has not teeth, or that blind which has not sight, but rather that which has not teeth or sight *at the time when by nature it should.*[3]

And all his examples of 'privatives' were phenomena typically associated with human senescence and thus by extension with the end of life:

> 'There may be a change from possession to privation, but not from privation to possession. The man who has become blind does not regain his sight; the man who has become bald does not regain his hair; the man who has lost his teeth does not grow a new set.'[4]

The natural life-cycle of development and decay seems therefore to have served Aristotle as the underlying model of possession and privation in his logical works, so it is not surprising that his treatment of the relationship between life and death in other works took the form of an opposition of this type. And as we shall see, this same type of opposition continued to structure the view of life and death held by medical thinkers for many centuries thereafter.

So long as life and death were related to each other as 'possession' and 'privation', life was thought of not as a unitary concept but as a collection of faculties or properties, and death had to remain a theoretical nullity. In Aristotle's view, for example, 'it is the presence of the soul that enables matter to constitute the animal nature, much more than it is the presence of matter which so enables the soul.'[5] So notwithstanding the importance accorded by Aristotle and many other ancient writers to 'innate heat' as a material cause of life,[6] the soul was conceptually prior as an explanation of living phenomena. But the soul was a complex entity for Aristotle, with distinct parts responsible for such capacities as growth, sensation, change of quality, locomotion, and intellect.[7] Thus he held that 'it is not the whole soul that constitutes the animal nature, but only some part or parts of it',[8] and the life of the animal consists in the collection of faculties with which these various 'parts' of the soul endow it.[9] Indeed, it can consist in any of these faculties alone, for the word life

> has more than one sense, and provided any one alone of these is found in a thing we say that thing is living. Living, that is, may mean thinking or perception or local movement and rest, or movement in the sense of nutrition, decay and growth.[10]

The death of the animal, on the other hand, consists in the withdrawal of these faculties: 'when the soul departs, what is left is no longer a living animal, and . . . none of the parts [of the body] remain what they were before, excepting in mere configuration.'[11] Life is a plurality and death an absence.

The same pattern of opposition can be found in the Hippocratic Corpus. A late text on *The Heart*, usually dated around or after 260 BC, identified the left chamber of the heart as the source of the living body's 'innate heat'.[12] But it also held that 'man's intelligence, the principle which rules over the rest of the soul, is situated in the left chamber' of this organ.[13] This picture again involves a pluralistic concept of the soul, although one less developed than Aristotle's, together with heat as a material cause or condition of other life phenomena. The orifices of the heart 'are the springs of man's existence; from them spread throughout his body those rivers with which his mortal habitation is irrigated, those rivers which bring life to man as well, for if they ever dry up, then man dies.'[14] The author did not specify what it is in the blood that is essential for life: perhaps it is heat which the blood acquires in the heart, 'for the blood is in fact not a hot thing by nature . . . though it may be made hot';[15] perhaps it is nutritive matter, 'for the great artery feeds from the belly and intestines and is laden with food';[16] or perhaps, again, it is moisture, as suggested by the metaphor of rivers and irrigation;[17] or finally, perhaps it is all of these together. But when the flow ceases, death ensues.

The plurality involved in Aristotle's conception of the soul is underlined by the criticism made by Galen (AD 129-*c*.200/210) of the distinction between a vegetative part and a sensory part of the soul, and his own replacement of this terminology with a division of the faculties of living things into one class that are caused by nature (growth and nutrition), and another class caused by soul (feeling and voluntary motion). Hence animal life is composite: 'animals are governed at once by their soul and by their nature'.[18] And having regard to the natural faculties alone, without taking into account those of the soul, Galen argued that growth and nutrition – to which he added 'genesis' – are only the primary faculties and that these faculties in turn 'need the service both of each other, and of yet different faculties' such as attraction, retention, assimilation, and expulsion.[19] The result of this proliferation of faculties was that many individual phenomena of life were explained although life itself was not. From the point of view of the opposition between life and death, Galen's account added little to Aristotle's: life continued to consist in the possession of a pluralistic collection of properties, and death consisted only in their removal; that is, in nothing at all, '*ipsaque mors nihil*'.[20]

From the time of Galen to the middle of the eighteenth century, the properties of living things were attributed by various authors to the actions of numerous underlying causes, but death remained nothing more in medical theory than the outer limit of life. The concept of death functioned as a boundary designating the pure absence of vitality, involving no positive content of its own. As the principal medical contributor to the *Encyclopédie*, Ménuret de Chambaud (1733–1815), expressed it, 'One knows death only by its opposition to life, in the same way that rest is manifested by its direct contrast with motion'.[21] It has been suggested that the concept of life in the *Encyclopédie* was equally vacuous,[22] since the chevalier de Jaucourt (1704–79) defined life there as 'the opposite of death'.[23] But Jaucourt, who had once studied under Hermann Boerhaave (1668–1738),[24] followed Ménuret in giving life, 'in its common meaning', the positive characteristic of motion: of 'a continual movement of the solids and fluids of all animated bodies', and in opposing death to this organic motion as 'the absolute destruction of the vital organs, without them being able to restore themselves'.[25]

Physicians, of course, expressed views on the moral significance of death, as they did on that of life itself. Christian thinkers, for example, had added an immortal, personal soul (or part of the soul) to the other souls (or parts of the soul) that classical antiquity had regarded as active in human life. Thus the instant of death became a moment of immense theological consequence, since the dying person's immortal soul was irrevocably consigned at this moment to eternal damnation or bliss. But ethical and religious reflections on life and death, while accepted as a legitimate part of medical discourse in Christian Europe, were drawn from sources other than medicine. They affected medical practice by making the priest a more important figure at the deathbed than the physician, but they did not illuminate medical theory. (➤ Ch. 61 Religion and medicine)

Physicians also devoted much attention to investigating the effects of death upon the body: changes in its surface appearance, the onset of rigor mortis, and the dissolution of its parts through putrefaction. But by the middle of the eighteenth century, learned medicine, following the views introduced earlier by Georg Ernst Stahl (1660–1734), understood such effects as purely physico-chemical phenomena, as evidence that a special vital power had ceased to operate and that the inherently unstable compounds that made up the body had fallen once more under the sway of the ordinary laws of matter.[26] Thus Albrecht von Haller (1708–77) described the fate of the body's solid parts after death in the following terms: 'the earth, deprived of its bonds of union, insensibly moulders away and mixes itself with dust'.[27]

Life was now understood, both in medical thought and in popular culture, as being in some sense 'an exception to nature'[28] rather than as the actualization of nature's highest potential, as it had been for Aristotle.

Although it was not clearly conceptualized in a unified way, life was nevertheless something positive for eighteenth-century medical theory: it was a collection of properties that produced the vital movements and bound together the chemical constituents of the body. Death, on the other hand, was for medicine merely the withdrawal of this positive force, a discontinuous transition from the sphere of the vital to the sphere of the physico-chemical. As Edmund Goodwyn (1755–1829) put it: 'Of animal bodies there are only two general conditions, Life and Death; and since by *death* we understand the privation of life, there can be no intermediate state between them.'[29]

It is true that 'in the eighteenth century, medical interest in death grew all of a sudden to unique and extraordinary proportions, far beyond the continuous routine concern' of previous ages.[30] This interest, however, was oriented not toward giving the idea of death a conceptual content of its own, but toward defining ever more precisely the moment of transition separating vitality from its absence. The chief objects of this medical concern, then, were the problems of apparent death, of resuscitation, and of premature burial. The organism, it was found, dies in stages, from its exterior inwards; so diagnostic precision was required to determine the exact moment when 'absolute' death had succeeded apparent or 'imperfect' death and when resuscitation efforts could be abandoned.[31]

The view that the organism dies from its exterior inwards, together with the opposition between vital processes and physico-chemical phenomena, fell within an essentially defensive conception that regarded the power of life as the power to resist the encroachments of a hostile world. The classical idea of 'the healing power of nature', which was so central to the medical revival of Hippocratic thought during the eighteenth century, had reference to the nature of the living body, not to nature in general. In Boerhaave's words, 'The conjunct Power of all these Actions of the Body for preserving its own Health, which arises from the wonderful Structure of its Parts, is what *Hippocrates* calls NATURE '.[32]

Organisms, then, were conceptualized as little islands of vitality in a sea of physico-chemical materiality always threatening to engulf them.[33] Life was the collection of properties working to forestall this engulfment; hence the definition of Xavier Bichat (1771–1802) at the end of the century: 'Life is the totality of functions which resist death.'[34] (➤ Ch. 7 The physiological tradition)

In all cases, however, this resistance could only be temporary. At best, it would lead the organism to a 'natural death' which eventuates, according to Haller, 'from mere old age'.[35] Such a death, occurring 'through mere weakness, rather than through the oppression of any disease', results from the rarely of the body's parts with age and use.[36] But this natural limit is rarely attained, because 'very many people are carried off before this time by disease'.[37] Apart from diseases, other acknowledged causes of 'premature' or 'accidental' death were physical violence (wounds, injuries) and violent passions (sudden death caused by joy, terror, anger, etc.).[38]

The melancholy theme of the inevitable termination of life did seem to offer some salutary lessons for eighteenth-century thought, however. First, at the ethical and religious level, medical writers such as Johann Peter Frank (1745–1821) reminded their readers that 'contemplation of our natural end has a certain usefulness in improving the moral state of man'.[39] Second, at the level of social policy, it was argued by Frank and others that 'this contemplation can even help promote our physical well-being', by stimulating philanthropic legal reform in order to assure the humane treatment of the dying and the protection of the apparently dead from premature burial.[40] And finally, at the theoretical level, consideration of the role of death in the natural world produced, in the work of naturalists such as Carl Linnaeus (1707–78) and Georges-Louis Buffon (1707–88), the concept of the 'balance of nature': death, by limiting the population size of each species and therefore the numerical relations between species, serves to maintain the harmonious natural order.[41] But even this conception of balance, which was sufficiently optimistic to serve Linnaeus as a theodicy justifying predation in nature, still regarded death as pure negativity, as the purely quantitative subtraction of what was actually or potentially in excess.

For moral discourse, then, the eighteenth-century medical conception of death could contribute to a contemplative tradition begun 'long ago by non-Christian philosophers'.[42] For social reform, it could provide a focus for 'one of the numerous activities triggered by the dominant philosophical trend of the 18th century, the philosophy of Enlightenment'.[43] And for natural history, it could provide a new theory of the order of nature; but for medical theory itself, death remained simply the disappearance of life in nullity.

LIFE AND DEATH AS CORRELATIVES

Around the beginning of the nineteenth century, the medical conception of life and death began to undergo a series of important changes. From this point forward, death would increasingly acquire substantive characteristics of its own, while its theoretical locus was shifted from the exterior to the interior of life. And this new theoretical prominence of the concept of death made it possible for the first time for a science of 'life' to develop; it was only from this period that biology, as a unitary scientific discourse, could exist.[44]

Rather than standing in mute opposition to life, then, death became its most revealing mirror. First of all, in the new medical school of Paris, established by the Revolutionary government in 1794, the reunification of surgery with internal medicine and the reorganization of the hospital system led to the routine practice of autopsies for the first time. (➤ Ch. 49 The hospital) The discipline of pathological anatomy which arose out of this practice redefined the nature of disease in medical theory, with the organic lesions of the cadaver replacing the symptoms of the living patient as the privileged source of medical truth about disease.[45] The same Bichat who, as a physiologist, defined life by its ability to resist death, was able, as a pathological anatomist, to exhort his medical colleagues to 'open up a few corpses' as a way of dispelling 'that obscurity which [the] observation [of symptoms] alone could not dissipate'.[46] (➤ Ch. 9 The pathological tradition)

If the medical discipline of pathological anatomy made death theoretically informative for the first time, the zoological discipline of comparative anatomy – appropriating some of medicine's conceptual and procedural tools[47] – made death itself central to the definition of life. In the early years of the nineteenth century, Georges Cuvier (1769–1832), working at the Museum of Natural History in Paris, replaced the classical approach to zoological taxonomy, based on the external characters of species, with a new system based on their forms of internal organization.[48] And these forms of organization, in Cuvier's treatment, could only be understood as different ways of meeting the threat of death. Only when the animal was radically redefined as being capable of dying, could the necessity of its organic coherence become intelligible.

This new understanding of the relationship between life and death, which would make it possible for Cuvier to establish the correlation of anatomical parts as a fundamental principle of zoology, or for pathological anatomists to establish the correlation of symptoms and lesions as a fundamental principle of medicine, was itself a correlative concept. Life and death were no longer opposed as 'positive' to 'privative', but as correlatives in the logical sense of the term described by Aristotle: 'Such things, then, as are opposite the one to the other in the sense of being correlatives are explained by a reference of the one to the other.'[49] Indeed, in the strictest use of the term, correlatives must not only be explained by one another, but each must serve as a 'necessary condition of existence' of the other.[50] Moreover, since 'it belongs in all cases to one and the same science to deal with correlated subjects',[51] the new science of life would also of necessity be the science of death.

Cuvier gave theoretical expression to this correlative relationship in his formulation of the 'conditions of existence' which any species had to meet in order to survive: internal conditions that required that all the organs of a species constitute a harmonious unity (sharp teeth and claws accompanying carnivorous digestive systems, flat teeth and hooves accompanying herbivorous digestive systems); and external conditions that required that the organism as a whole be suited to its surroundings (fishes in water, rabbits on land).[52]

Thus death, which for Linnaeus and Buffon operated only quantitatively to limit the numbers in each species, became a force operating qualitatively to limit their very forms of organization. Or, to put the matter another way, for eighteenth-century naturalists, the conception of death functioned only a posteriori to cull the numerical excesses of already-existing species, whereas for Cuvier, death functioned a priori to determine the conditions of existence for any species whatsoever, actual or possible, living or extinct.[53]

As noted above, the Cuvierian conception of life emphasized not only the (internal) interdependence of the organs, but also the (external) dependence of the organism as a whole on its surroundings – on what Auguste Comte (1798–1857) would soon afterward call its milieu, or environment, using that term for the first time in its biological sense.[54] So life was no longer characterized by its resistance to the environment, but by its dependence upon it. Among many leading medical thinkers, the view was accepted that life was a state provoked or incited by the environment. François Broussais (1772–1838), whose system dominated medical thought in France early in the nineteenth century, asserted that 'the life of the animal is maintained only by external stimulations',[55] thus reviving in a new form the principle earlier enunciated by John Brown (1735–88).[56] Elsewhere in Europe, chiefly in the German and Italian states, Brown's own system, which had achieved only limited success before his death, became widely adopted.

Furthermore, life was no longer characterized for medicine by its resistance to death and disease; on the contrary, life itself became the principal source of its own destruction. Eighteenth-century medical writers had recognized excesses or irregularities in human activity as a cause of disease: Boerhaave, for example, cited the case of 'a Man that was order'd to carry Letters in haste to *Utrecht*, who, by excessive running, so forced the grosser Parts of his Fluids into the smaller Vessels, so to render the Obstructions incorrigible by any Art'.[57] And toward the end of the century, Brown had brought life and death closer together by insisting that the same external powers of nature that produced life and health in the organism also produced sickness and death.[58] But for Jean-Nicolas Corvisart (1755–1821), writing in 1806, and for Broussais after him, the normal functioning of the organism itself was to become intrinsically pathogenic.

According to Corvisart, the parts of the body, 'by the very fact of their action',[59] are pathologically altered, producing 'derangements which . . . are veritable organic diseases'.[60] In addition, the Cuvierian internal 'conditions of existence' are never fully satisfied: 'Each one of us comes into the world more or less vitiated, from which there follows some kind of defect in the equilibrium of our functions.'[61] The pathogenic effects of this imbalance follow even if no individual organ is defective at birth, because 'each organ in itself can be good and nevertheless be too strong or too weak relative to the other organs.'[62] Similarly, for Broussais, the excitation that maintains life 'is never uniform in the animal economy; it is always stronger in certain parts and weaker in several others, and predominates successively in different regions. This inequality often ends up deranging the equilibrium of the functions.'[63] And such derangements are pathogenic because 'health supposes the regular exercise of the functions; disease results from their irregularity.'[64] Far from resisting death then, life was represented here as producing it: as Corvisart put it, 'the very fact of life is the cause of death'.[65]

In the eighteenth century, medical texts had recognized a sense in which 'the Action of Life destroys itself'[66] by attrition or the wearing away of its parts. Boerhaave and Haller, for example, both noted these quantitative losses, and Haller pointed out that 'there would be no great distance between the end of our life and its beginning, unless these losses were repaired' continually by nutrition.[67] Brown, too, saw the decline of the organism in quantitative terms, as a loss of excitability: 'Under normal physiological conditions the excitability decreases slowly in quantity everywhere in the body from childhood to old age.'[68] For Corvisart and Broussais, however, the action of the bodily parts gave rise qualitatively to organic lesions. Thus while eighteenth-century medicine saw disease as an event interrupting life's inevitable progression towards natural death, nineteenth-century medicine began to see death as an event interrupting life's inevitable production of organic diseases.

The first decades of the nineteenth century, then, were attended by changes in medical thought which significantly altered the conceptual relations between life and death. In place of the image of life as a collection of properties resisting death from the onslaughts of the external world, one found a series of relays whereby the environment provoked life, life provoked disease, and disease provoked death. Instead of existing only as a 'privative' into which life would vanish in its final defeat, death now became the correlative of life: both an integral constituent and a necessary product of the vital process. But this transformation was only roughly sketched out at the beginning of the nineteenth century, although that period clearly marked the crucial turning-point. To appreciate the full extent of this development one must move to the latter part of the century.

Here, in the 1860s and 1870s, the scene abounds in paradoxes, for what was taken in the previous century for death has now become life, and what was taken for life has now become death. This reversal arose out of two important biological developments, one in bacteriology and the other in physiology.

First of all, the classic criterion of the death of the organism, putrefaction, was shown by Louis Pasteur (1822–95) and others to result, not from the privation of life, but from its microscopic profusion. In a condition of the total absence of life, the corpse would not undergo decay. As Pasteur wrote, 'the destruction of organic materials is chiefly due to the multiplication of microscopic living creatures.... In short, life appears in a new form after death, and with new properties'.[69] At the end of the eighteenth-century, the diagnostic certainty of putrefaction as a sign of death had come under question by physicians investigating the related problems of apparent death, resuscitation, and premature burial.[70] But notwithstanding the earlier iatro-chemical doctrine of fermentation, classically stated by Johannes Baptista van Helmont (1577–1644), it was only after Pasteur that medical thought regarded putrefaction as a uniquely and thoroughly vital process.[71]

Moreover, acceptance of the cell theory meant that the microbial process of putrefaction could not be regarded only as a special phenomenon of predation upon macroscopic organisms; for, as Rudolf Virchow (1821–1902) pointed out, each cell in the body, like each microbe, was 'an organism in miniature'.[72] Thus microbial action became the prototype of the activities of the living cells composing all organic bodies. It was from this perspective, then, that biologists could accept the assertion of the chemist Eilhard Mitscherlich (1794–1863) that 'life is nothing but a putrefaction', or Felix Hoppe-Seyler's (1825–95) slightly more cautious proposition that 'the vital phenomena of plants and animals have no more perfect analogy in all of nature than the putrefactions.'[73] (➤ Ch. 8 The Biochemical Tradition)

While it was the bacteriologist Pasteur who showed most clearly how life had been mistaken for death, it was the physiologist Claude Bernard (1813–78) who showed, correlatively, how death had been mistaken for life. 'It is worth noting', Bernard wrote, 'that... we are the victims of a habitual illusion, and when we wish to designate phenomena of *life*, we refer in reality to phenomena of *death*.'[74] This illusion he explained, elaborating on the views expressed earlier in the century by the chemist, Justus von Liebig (1803–73),[75] as follows:

> the phenomena of destruction or of vital death are those which capture the eyes and by which we are led to characterize life. The signs are evident and obvious: when movement is produced, when a muscle contracts, when volition and sensibility are manifest, when thinking takes place, when a gland secretes, the substance of the muscle, the nerves, the brain, the glandular tissue disorganizes itself, destroys itself and consumes itself. In this way every manifestation of a phenomenon in the living being is necessarily linked to an organic destruction; it is this that I intended to express when in a paradoxical form I said ...: *life is death*.[76]

Of course, Bernard also held that '*Life is creation*', the creative synthesis being expressed primarily in embryological development and the phenomena of growth and nutrition.[77] But he clearly subordinated this aspect of life to the previous one: 'Creative life exhibits itself only secondarily; it manifests itself only in the presence of death, or of the products of destruction.'[78]

Bernard's formulation would make the real presence of death, rather than the a priori threat of death, the condition of existence for life. But in this Bernard was only expressing at the level of the individual organism what Charles Darwin (1809–82) had put forward at the level of the species. For death in Darwin's theory was not, as in Cuvier's, a point of reference for the definition of possible organic forms, but rather an agent of natural selection whose effect was to mould and shape the forms of actually existing species. Through death, Darwin held, nature

> can act on every internal organ, on every shade of constitutional difference, on the whole machinery of life. . . . It may be said that natural selection is daily and hourly scrutinising, throughout the world, every variation, even the slightest; rejecting that which is bad, preserving and adding up all that is good. . . .[79]

It would seem, then, that the system of relays constructed earlier in the century, running from the environment through life to disease and death, was being broken down by the time of Bernard and Darwin. Not only did a line now run from death to life, but another one ran from life to the environment. Darwin pointed to the extreme complexity of the relations between species within the same environment, since the presence of each species modifies the environment for the others.[80] And Bernard emphasized this relationship even more strongly at the cellular level, for in higher animals the living elements of the body – the cells – are never exposed to the external environment, but exist within a fluid internal environment which they not only modify but also create.[81] Thus, while Bernard could agree with Broussais that for any of the phenomena of life 'there are always external agents, outside stimulants, that provoke the manifestations of the properties of a material that is always inert by itself', he also insisted that 'in the higher creatures these stimulants in reality reside within what we call an internal environment [which] . . . although deeply situated, is still external to the elementary organized particle which is the only part that is really living.'[82]

The new situation just described was not, however, one of a simple linear reversal, whereby the earlier series of relays was replaced by one in which death causes life and life causes its own environment. In fact, the picture was far more complicated, because the putrefactions and related phenomena – such as fermentations – which were understood as specific to life, were precisely the processes of destruction that had led to Bernard's paradoxical expression that life is death. 'When a part functions', wrote Bernard, '. . . the organ destroys itself. This destruction is a physico-chemical phenomenon, most always the result of a combustion, a fermentation or a putrefaction. Basically, it is the true death of the organism.'[83] Life and death, then, were understood as inextricably bound together, as correlatives, in every vital process: 'There is no life without death; there is no death without life.'[84] Every action of the organism became suffused with death, but rather than being the mechanical, inert, essentially alien death of eighteenth-century medical thought, it was now a peculiarly vital, organic, and intimate death since it involved a form of destruction unique to, and indeed constitutive of, living bodies. Theoretically, at least, death had been domesticated.

THERAPEUTICS AND CORRELATIVE DEATH

It might be expected that the internalization of death within life would have been associated with a pessimistic attitude toward disease and therapeutics in medicine. At the beginning of the nineteenth century, at least, this association can be found, in the work of Corvisart for example. Writing on heart disease in 1806, Corvisart stated that 'it is sometimes possible, I think, to prevent the disease, but never to cure it.'[85] Thus, he noted, 'one finds almost everywhere the fatal prognosis of death'.[86] Other medical figures, chiefly associated with the Vienna Medical School, were not so much pessimistic as sceptical about the state of medical knowledge, and advocated a programme of therapeutic nihilism.[87] But this sporadic 'academic movement' was vigorously opposed by most practitioners and did not represent the predominant approach to the therapeutics as it developed during the century.[88]

Shortly after Corvisart published his treatise on diseases of the heart, Broussais would begin to insist that most diseases were curable if treated early enough. 'The art of curing chronic inflammations' – which, according to Broussais, were the underlying cause of all serious disease – 'consists therefore in knowing how to prevent them or at least stop them before they reach the stage of *disorganization*', which irreversibly alters the tissues.[89] But 'from the moment when this disorganization is consummated, all hope of cure is lost'.[90] Broussais's therapeutic regime called for vigorous and repeated bleedings, principally by means of leeches, at the first sign of inflammation in order to diminish the over-stimulated irritability of the inflamed part: 'It is always dangerous not to halt an inflammation at its start.'[91] (➤ Ch. 40 Physical methods)

For Corvisart's resigned pessimism in the face of disease and death, Broussais substituted an aggressive therapeutic activism. But his object was not, like that of the neo-Hippocratic physicians of the eighteenth century, to strengthen the spontaneous healing power of nature by removing an excess of blood that was thought to stifle its action. Nor was it, like that of the aggressive therapeutics of Brown, to strengthen the debilitated excitability of the organism – a condition that Brown saw underlying all diseases. On the contrary, for Broussais it was excessive stimulation rather than exhaustion which resulted in disease, so that the withdrawal of blood from a part of the body had the effect, in his view, of lessening the vitality of that part and thus its susceptibility to over-stimulation. In basing his therapeutics on this local 'deadening' effect, Broussais made death an ally of medicine against disease. During the rest of the nineteenth century, this alliance was to be deepened and extended.

One element of the extension of this alliance was a change of attitude toward the subject of apparent death, which had so exercised earlier medical reformers. Some eighteenth-century writers had suggested that apparent death might have a spontaneous therapeutic function, since persons who recovered from this condition seemed to enjoy particularly long and healthy lives thereafter.[92] Early in the following century, the therapeutic focus was shifted in the direction of human intervention, and the suggestion was advanced that if a person requiring surgery accidentally fell into the condition of apparent death, or suspended animation, then the surgical procedure ought to be performed before the patient was resuscitated.[93]

As resuscitation techniques were improved, so that recovery was 'no longer unexpected', experimental trials were conducted which attempted actively 'to induce, for the needs of surgery, a state of suspended animation' – chiefly by means of asphyxiation.[94] Early investigations of the anaesthetic properties of such substances as nitrous oxide were thus interpreted according to the assumption that these gases also produced their characteristic effects by asphyxiation; finally, when general anaesthesia was introduced by American practitioners in the 1840s, 'there were many who took their discoveries to be new methods of inducing asphyxia, the type, but by no means the only type of suspended animation.'[95] (➤ Ch. 42 Surgery (modern))

The growing use of general anaesthesia from the 1840s onwards, and its association with asphyxiation and suspended animation, may help to explain why both 'the epidemic fear of apparent death and scepticism concerning the signa [by which death could be diagnosed] seem to have disappeared almost simultaneously around the middle of the 19th century.'[96] It was at just this period that 'the anaesthetists rapidly became ... the great resuscitators'[97] and that apparent death became a handmaiden of surgery rather than a harbinger of premature burial. Thus was the controlled death of suspended animation allied to the controlled destruction of the surgeon's knife.

Although the initial confusion of anaesthesia with asphyxia was soon dispelled, its association with death was unaffected by this change. According to Bernard's researches, anaesthesia was not just the metaphorical death of sleep, in which one becomes 'dead to the world',[98] but a process of suppression that 'extends to all vital manifestations, of whatever kind they may be'.[99] When a surgical patient is anaesthetized, 'it is on the more delicate protoplasm of the nervous centres that the anaesthesia first exerts its action and [thus] it is . . . the phenomena of consciousness and sensory perception that are the first to disappear.'[100] If the process of anaesthesia was not restricted to this first stage, however 'if the protoplasms of all the anatomical elements in all the tissues were affected at the same moment by the anaesthesia, all functions would stop simultaneously, and death would be instantaneous.'[101] Surgical anaesthesia remained, therefore, a form of controlled death.

Another form of controlled death also made its first therapeutic appearance in surgery, but soon spread to other medical fields as well. The association between putrefaction, fermentation, and wound infection – soon to be generalized to the germ theory of disease – led to the application of poisonous substances to the body with the specific aim of killing micro-organisms. (➤ Ch. 16 Contagion/germ theory/specificity) At first, as in the antiseptic surgery of Joseph Lister (1827–1912) these poisons were restricted to the surface of the body or localized in wounds caused by surgical incision or accidental trauma.[102] By the end of the century, however, the objective was to introduce such poisons systemically, by injection into the bloodstream, so that they could operate throughout the entire fabric of the body.

Of course, poisonous substances had been used as remedies long before this time. Mercury, for example, had been used against syphilis since the appearance of that disease in Europe during the Renaissance. (➤ Ch. 26 Sexually transmitted diseases) It was not, however, the poisonous quality of mercury that was originally held to lie behind its therapeutic usefulness, but its ability to produce copious salivation in the patient. A later age would look upon this as a symptom of mercury poisoning, but before the nineteenth century it was understood as an expulsion of the corrupt matter underlying the disease.[103] In other circumstances, where substances had been employed specifically because they were poisonous, as in the case of remedies for parasitic worms, both the host and the parasites were poisoned together; the success of the therapy depended on the host having a greater tolerance for the poison than did the parasite. Death here was not so much controlled as withstood.

By contrast to these traditional remedies, however, the chemotherapeutic compounds developed by Paul Ehrlich (1854–1915) in the decades before the First World War were specifically designed to be poisonous to a particular micro-organism without being toxic to its host.[104] Ehrlich illustrated his conception by referring to the German folktale of the Magic Bullet, which could be fired blindly but which unerringly found its way to the intended target. The most famous of Ehrlich's magic bullets, the arsenical compound salvarsan, introduced for use against syphilis in 1910, represented a significant improvement over mercury in both safety and effectiveness. Controlled death had passed from the surgical theatre, via the chemical laboratory, into the general practitioner's consulting rooms. (➤ Ch. 39 Drug therapies)

The nineteenth century's conceptual internalization of death within life was far from being an inducement to a passive or pessimistic attitude toward disease. Death itself was actively harnessed as a therapeutic agent. Although bloodletting, so favoured by Broussais, did not survive much past mid-century as a mainstream therapy, in spite of occasional revivals,[105] other means were found to control the vitality of the organism. Bernard, developing Broussais's conception of disease as a pathological intensification of a normal physiological process (or in other words, a quantitative rather than a qualitative variation from the normal state), laid the foundations for an experimental medicine oriented toward the control and 'normalization' of functional distrubances.[106] It was not through the depletion of the internal environment by bloodletting, but through its physico-chemical manipulation that Bernard proposed to master the phenomena of life, both normal and pathological.

> The general cosmic environment is common to living and to inorganic bodies; but the inner environment created by an organism is special to each living being. Now, here is the true physiological environment; this it is which physiologists and physicians should study and know, for by its means they can act on the histological units which are the only effective agents in vital phenomena.[107]

The nature of the organic or histological units – the cells – could not in Bernard's view be altered, since it results from the creative, synthetic aspect of life which defies control; nevertheless, 'because the plastic or synthetic phenomenon is subordinated to the functional or destructive phenomenon . . . we have an indirect means of influencing it experimentally by acting on the latter'.[108] If the organism keeps itself alive by constantly dying, one could control the way it lives by manipulating the forms of death it undergoes. This manipulation would thus constitute the 'conquest', 'domination', 'mastery', or 'subjugation' of life – all four terms (or their cognates) being used by Bernard in the brief compass of two paragraphs.[109] It was through the death within life that life itself was to be forced into submission.

The approach to therapeutics that developed throughout the nineteenth century interposed the physician between the dying patient and the priest in a number of ways. First, every patient was in some sense a dying patient; the moment of final death, which concerned the priest, was for the physician only the last point on a continuum of death extending from the moment of birth. Second, the immortal soul, which had fitted easily within a conception of life and death as possession and privation, was a discordant element within the nineteenth-century conception of life and death as correlatives. At the deathbed, the physician as believer might respect the soul, but there was no longer a place for it within medical discourse or a reason to defer to the priest on its behalf.

LIFE AND DEATH AS CONTRARIES

In 1903 Albert Dastre (1844–1917), Bernard's former student and his successor in the Chair of Physiology at the Sorbonne, criticized his master's description of the relationship between life and death. To say that 'life is death', or that the activities of the living organism destroy life itself, was for Dastre both 'hazardous' and 'obscure'.[110] The organism does not consume itself in the course of its normal activity, but burns reserve materials taken from the bloodstream, just as a steam-engine does not consume the iron and steel of which it is made but burns the coal that is shovelled into it.[111] The steam-engine analogy, which replaced Liebig's picture of the self-destructive effects of muscular activity, had in fact been put forward earlier by Liebig himself in order to 'furnish no unapt image' of the organism's metabolic self-regulation.[112] But to later critics of Liebig's theory, such as Edward Frankland (1825–99), the significance of this image lay in another direction. For Frankland, writing in 1866, held that his own studies of metabolism, and those of other researchers, were sufficient to 'prove conclusively' that, 'like the piston and cylinder of a steam-engine, the muscle is only a machine for the transformation of heat into motion'.[113]

Although what Virchow called 'the mechanistic interpretation of life'[114] had been advocated in various forms by medical thinkers since the seventeenth century, it had not previously intruded upon the relationship between life and death. Like other explanations postulating the effectivity of 'soul' or 'nature' or 'vital properties' in the body, the mechanical explanation of life was quite compatible with the concept of life and death as possession and privation. And for a long time it was also compatible with the concept of life and death as correlatives. But with the development of thermodynamics and the successful application of the principle of the conservation of energy to the study of living phenomena, both the science of life and the science of machines became subordinated to the same theoretical requirements. The machine was no longer a model for the living organism, as it had been since the seventeenth century. Or rather, it was no more, and no less, a model for the organism than the organism was for it, since both the machine and the organism were now to be understood as instances of a single general theory of the transformations of energy.[115]

This new view was elaborated over a considerable period of time, for 'while the principle of the conservation of energy had been discovered and experimentally confirmed by the middle of the 19th century, the introduction of this idea into biological thought and its application to metabolism still required a number of decades.'[116] By the end of the century, however, the thermodynamic outlook was so well entrenched in biology that when Max Rubner (1854–1932) 'finally produced incontrovertible experimental proof that the principle of the conservation of energy held for living systems',[117] his work was threatened with trivialization and 'he had to defend the importance of proving something which seemed so self-evident as to be accepted without proof.'[118] Thus we may say that around the turn of the century, the energetic principle was firmly established in biological thought.

The consequences of this development for the medical conception of life and death were far-reaching, for death became a contingent occurrence rather than an organic necessity. In principle, a machine can be kept functioning indefinitely, given adequate maintenance; the only limitation in practice is the one that arises from economic considerations when the cost of the required maintenance becomes prohibitive. There is no place within this vision for an intimate involvement of death in every living process: perfect health is maximal functional efficiency; disease is a maintenance problem; and death comes at that contingently determined moment when medical maintenance either reaches the limit of its technical capacity, or else is abandoned as no longer cost effective. Strictly speaking, then, the opposition of life and death is assimilated to that of health and disease an opposition not of correlatives but of contraries. (➤ Ch. 12 Concepts of health, illness, and disease)

Aristotle specifically identified one type of contrary opposition as applying to health and disease.

> Those contraries which are such that the subjects in which they are naturally present ... must necessarily contain either the one or the other of them, have no intermediate. ... Thus disease and health are naturally present in the body of an animal, and it is necessary that either the one or the other should be present in the body of an animal.[119]

Without accepting the metaphysical premises inherent in Aristotle's concept of a 'subject', twentieth-century medicine nevertheless has treated both health and disease, and life and death, as contraries.

A distinctive feature of contraries in Aristotle's sense is that 'it is possible that there should be changes from either into the other, while the subject retains its identity ... [f]or it is possible that that which is healthy should become diseased' and vice versa.[120] In twentieth-century terms, no machine functions at peak efficiency for long without a further input of energy from an external source in the form of maintenance work. The state of perfect health is achieved transiently, if at all, and then changes into disease; medical maintenance effects a change in the contrary direction and this process can in principle be prolonged without limit.

From at least the period of the Renaissance, visionaries had set for medicine the goal of prolonging life indefinitely, but it was only in the twentieth century that medicine acquired the technical means to convert this goal from a theoretical horizon to a guiding principle of practice. Indicative of the new agenda for twentieth-century medicine was an address on 'experimental therapeutics' given in 1900 by Ivan Pavlov (1849–1936) at the International Congress of Medicine in Paris.[121] Discussing his experimental work on dogs whose vagus nerves had been surgically cut at the neck, Pavlov described the series of steps he and his colleagues had taken to keep the animals alive after this injury, which had always been considered fatal.

In previous work on other species, it had been found that a tracheotomy was necessary to keep the animal from suffocating as a result of paralysis of the soft laryngeal tissues, but Pavlov's use of adult dogs, with their differently structured larynx, had overcome this problem. Next, it was necessary to establish a gastric fistula and close off the oesophagus, to prevent the frequent vomiting and regurgitation experienced by vagotomized animals from either obstructing their breathing and causing them to suffocate, or else introducing foreign matter into their lungs and causing them to die from chronic pulmonary inflammation. This being done, it was found that the animals were unable to digest their food properly, so Pavlov had to stimulate gastric secretion with a chemical agent before introducing food into the stomach through the fistula, and then rinse out the contents of the stomach with warm water after digestion was completed. Finally, apart from these direct interventions, the experimenters had to control the animals' environment in order to keep them alive: the vagotomized dogs could not survive doses of various medications that normal dogs tolerated without distress; their internal temperature was abnormally affected by exercise and by external heating or cooling; and their heartbeat, once accelerated, would not return to normal for several hours.[122]

Pavlov apologized to his learned audience 'for devoting so much time to this secondary question of physiology', but excused himself on the ground that 'there seems to be concentrated in it the fundamental idea' that he wished to convey to them. This fundamental point was that 'the survival of vagotomized animals, like an incalculable number of physiological and particularly medical facts, is a continuing triumph for the conception of the animal organism as a physical-chemical and mechanical entity.'[123] Thus far, Pavlov spoke in the common idiom of late nineteenth-century scientific medicine, but as he continued, he shifted to an engineering idiom more characteristic of medicine in the twentieth-century. 'In effect, in all the stages of the elaboration of our question is not the animal organism revealed uniquely as a machine – extremely complicated, undoubtedly, but all the same manageable and obedient as any other machine?'[124]

Pavlov shared with Bernard the vision of 'power over the animal organism',[125] but that power was not conceptualized as the domination or conquest of life and death; rather it was portrayed as 'a technology of living substance' in the sense of this phrase used by Jacques Loeb (1859–1924).[126] However, whereas Loeb's work concentrated on the manipulation of embryological development, Pavlov's aim was to 'salvage the machine' which would otherwise fall into 'complete ruin':

> As soon as possible, a broken part was replaced with another, equally necessary; but since, as a result of injury, it had lost some of its energy and regularity, external methods were used for supplementation. . . . The animal machine, thus repaired, continued to function with complete success. Is this not the step-by-step procedure of any mechanic to whom one entrusts the restoration of one or another complicated machine?[127]

In the nineteenth century, vivisectional experiments had been developed 'which depended for their success not upon the death of the animal but rather upon its survival for as long as possible'.[128] But according to Pavlov's conception of 'experimental therapeutics as a new and exceedingly fruitful method of physiological investigation',[129] keeping the animal alive after its vital functioning had been severely disrupted was now the principal object of the experiment and not just a means of studying one or another physiological process. And lest it be thought that this procedure, which Pavlov called 'physiological synthesis', was appropriate only for laboratory research, he stressed that 'physiological synthesis coincides with medicine and is identified with it.'[130] The physician who 'treats myxedema by preparations from the thyroid gland . . . does exactly the same as the physiologist who . . . gives an injection of thyroid extract to an animal deprived of this organ'.[131]

Pavlov's vision heralded the trajectory of medical development leading to hormone-replacement regimes, bionic prostheses, organ transplants, *in vitro* fertilization and gene therapy – all designed to maintain the human machine in efficient running order.[132] The only 'natural limit to the power of the aforesaid synthesis' for Pavlov was not really natural at all: it was contingently set by our 'insufficient knowledge of cellular life',[133] a problem that further research could be expected to dispel. And if there was no limit to the potential power of physiological synthesis, there was equally no limit to medicine's potential involvement in the patient's life: witness Pavlov's description of his animals as having been 'repaired' and as continuing 'to function with complete success',[134] even though they could 'no longer eat by themselves and digest their food adequately', and their health could be maintained 'only on condition of a life artificially simplified, with a bland and tranquil regime'[135] perpetually controlled by the experimenters.

In addition to the remedial maintenance which consists in the repair of damaged or defective organs, twentieth-century medicine has also embarked on a programme of preventive maintenance of the human machine. In earlier centuries, the mechanical image of the organism had made it possible to question 'whether the body was a good or bad machine'.[136] In the light of Darwin's evolutionary theory Ernst Haeckel (1834–1919) introduced, in 1866, the term 'dysteleology' to characterize the study of organs which were 'useless or inoperative . . . [or] indeed, hurtful and dangerous' such as the vermiform appendix, which was described as 'extremely dangerous, and . . . responsible for a number of deaths every year'.[137] This nineteenth-century concept of dysteleology, which Haeckel saw as a way of attacking speculative theories of 'purpose' in nature,[138] was transformed by twentieth-century medicine into a programme of surgical prophylaxis.

At the beginning of this century, for example, Elie Metchnikoff (1845–1916) of the Pasteur Institute argued that the human species no longer had any use for the large intestine, an organ which had first evolved in mammals very different from humans, and that its bacterial flora contributed 'nothing to the well-being of man',[139] but on the contrary were 'the source of many poisons harmful to the body'.[140] In view of these dangers, Metchnikoff held that it was 'impossible' to wait for evolution to bring about 'the suppression of an organ which has become useless'. Instead, he called upon science 'to accelerate or anticipate such a result', foreseeing the day, unfortunately 'perhaps in the distant future', when surgical excision of the large intestine would 'become normal'.[141] Although surgical prophylaxis on this scale did not become a routine procedure in the twentieth century, the programmatic outlook represented by Metchnikoff nevertheless ensured that Haeckel's dysteleology 'found its practical culmination in the removal of the healthy appendix' – or, one might add, the healthy tonsil or the healthy postmenopausal uterus – 'as an altogether useless and dangerous part'.[142]

In a world in which medicine is expected to provide a perpetual maintenance service for the human machine, disease can be 'frequent', 'constant', and even 'inevitable', yet at the same time be something 'outside the natural order' and 'clearly accidental'.[143] One might say that illness is only contingently inevitable, because 'science will conquer disease'; it will achieve 'the impossible' by allowing humans 'to remain forever in the fullness of health and protected from diseases'.[144] In similar fashion, death also is only contingently inevitable; it seems to have intruded into the natural order in some way that requires special explanation rather than existing there of necessity. As Metchnikoff put it, 'If natural death does exist, it must have appeared on the face of the earth long after the appearance of life.'[145]

August Weismann (1834–1914) had argued in the nineteenth century that unicellular organisms were not susceptible to natural death: as long as 'those conditions which are necessary for their life are fulfilled, they continue to live, and they thus carry the potentiality of unending life in themselves'.[146]

Multicellular organisms, on the other hand, were subject to natural death as a matter of evolutionary advantage to the species.

> I consider that death is not a primary necessity, but that it has been secondarily acquired as an adaptation. I believe that life is endowed with a fixed duration, not because it is contrary to its nature to be unlimited, but because the unlimited existence of individuals would be a luxury without any corresponding advantage.[147]

As a result of the differentiation of somatic cells and reproductive cells in multicellular organisms, these organisms need only live long enough to reproduce.

> Normal death could not take place among unicellular organisms, because the individual and the reproductive cell are one and the same: on the other hand, normal death is possible, and as we see, has made its appearance, among multicellular organisms in which the somatic and reproductive cells are distinct.[148]

Metchnikoff objected to Weismann's argument on the basis that '[i]t is impossible to regard natural death, if indeed it actually exists, as the product of natural selection for the benefit of the species,[149] a position that is shared, although on somewhat different grounds, by late twentieth-century biologists.[150] He did not, however, offer an alternative to Weismann's explanation of the origin of death, but referred instead to Loeb's recent work on natural death, which he believed showed that 'there is no good evidence for its existence'; the only potential exceptions were dismissed by Metchnikoff as 'purely accidental'.[151]

Dastre also invoked the work of Loeb, and used it together with Bernard's concept of the internal environment to explain, or rather explain away, natural death. He suggested that the life of any cell depended on 'the perfect constancy of its appropriate environment'. If this constancy is not maintained, then 'solely as a result of the imperfections of the extrinsic conditions of the environment, the living being is dragged down into deterioration and death.' In the multicellular organism, this environment, which is internal to the organism as a whole but extrinsic to the individual component cells, 'is depleted and poisoned around each cell as a result of accidents which happen to the other cells. Each one experiences therefore a progressive deterioration and finally a destruction which is in fact the rule, although in principle it is an accident.'[152] Dastre thus reinterpreted Bernard's concept of the internal environment in two significant ways: first, by insisting on the need for 'perfect constancy' in the cellular environment, whereas Bernard had at most required a dynamic constancy 'such that external variations are at every instant compensated and brought into balance';[153] and second, by locating the origin of death within the environment rather than within the living cell itself.

Although each cell suffers an accumulation of deleterious effects arising from 'the insufficiency or imperfection of the nutritive absorption or excretion', the work of Loeb and others showed that this decline could be reversed by an appropriate adjustment of the cell's environment.[154] Unfortunately, the multicellular organism is incapable of maintaining its internal environment in exactly the right balance needed to bring about this repair, and ultimately death ensues. Even so, for Dastre, the fact remains, that this sequence of events leading toward death is by no means 'a rigorous consequence of life itself'; on the contrary, 'it retains an accidental character', having nothing truly 'natural, inexorable and inescapable' about it.[155] Death may thus be 'the rule' and yet remain purely accidental to life itself, or, in the terminology used earlier, death is only contingently inevitable.

Neither Metchnikoff nor Dastre went so far as to suggest that the contingent inevitability of death could be abolished. Both men, however, envisaged the scientific possibility of postponing death indefinitely by redefining old age as a disease. Metchnikoff, for example, referred to 'the existing pathological character of old age', which he said was 'not a true physiological process'.[156] Dastre, too, held that 'old age, such as we know it, is a chronic illness and not by any means a normal phase of the vital cycle.'[157] Both agreed that old age could therefore be conquered by science and that the present experience of ageing gave no evidence of the natural term of human life. Death, when it came, would be painless, peaceful, and welcome, even, as it were, instinctive: 'If the cycle of human life followed its ideal course according to physiological function, then the instinct of death would appear in its time, after a normal life and an old age healthy and prolonged.'[158] (➤ Ch. 46 Geriatrics)

Late twentieth-century medicine still accepts as its ultimate aim the ideal set for it by such figures as Pavlov, Dastre, and Metchnikoff in the first years of the century: the perpetual maintenance of the human organism as a maximally efficient machine, and the indefinite postponement of the 'accident' of death. Given this aim, it is clear that 'the medical ideal, ever more closely to be approximated, must be bodily immortality.'[159] Such an ideal is not normally expressed in explicit terms, however. Rather than calling for the prevention of all deaths, one speaks, for example, of seeking to achieve 'further reductions in *premature* deaths'; but this more cautious formulation only thinly disguises the demand for immortality, since 'it often seems doubtful from our words and deeds that we ever regard any particular death as other than premature, as a failure of today's medicine, hopefully avoidable by tomorrow's.'[160]

The twentieth-century medical opposition between life and death, then, is one that reduces death once again to a kind of nullity, but not the nullity resulting from the privation of something positive. Death is now a nullity not because it is the loss of something internal to life, but because it is the failure of something external to life, the perpetual maintenance service of modern medicine. The consequences of this outlook can be seen in medical judgements about death and dying, for in practice '[d]ying is defined ... in terms of the actions – or failed actions – of the physicians. In keeping with the predominant technical bias of biomedicine, "dying" becomes a cultural metaphor which symbolizes treatment failure.'[161] Already, at the beginning of the century, Dastre had argued that when the physician 'declares that any particular person is dead, it is less a judgement of fact that he utters than a prognostication' that nothing he could do would restore the dying person to life.[162] Observations of medical residents in a contemporary hospital have shown a similar attitude:

> Patients were generally considered by residents to be dying when the residents determined that there was nothing they could do to reverse the course of the disease and the patient would not recover no matter what they did. In medical parlance, patients came to be seen as dying when 'all therapeutic options were exhausted,' 'there is nothing more we can do,' or 'we have nothing more to offer.' ... The words of these residents illustrate how the context of dying becomes defined in terms of the physicians' own treatment agenda.[163]

If the modern hospital permits the priest once again to assume a degree of pre-eminence over the physician at the side of the dying patient, it is only because a hospital bed cannot become a deathbed in medical terms until the physician has to some extent withdrawn from it. (➤ Ch. 37 History of medical ethics; Ch. 69 Medicine and the law)

In the late 1960s, when improvements in resuscitation techniques and the increasing feasibility of major organ transplants provided new ways for medicine to 'salvage the machine', as Pavlov put it, the definition of dying in terms of the end point of therapeutic activity found its natural counterpart in a new definition of death as irreversible coma rather than as the cessation of heart and lung functions.[164] The notion of irreversibility inherent in this redefinition of death was simply the prognosis, as Dastre had suggested at the beginning of the century, that 'the life of the brain, extinguished at this moment, will not be revived' by any therapeutic effort, even though 'there are many elements in this organism which are still living.'[165] Such a prognosis must be determined by the limits of therapeutic efficacy, a point nicely captured in a 1977 ruling of the Supreme Judicial Court of Massachusetts:

> Brain death occurs when, in the opinion of a licenced physician, based on ordinary and accepted standards of medical practice, there has been a total and irreversible cessation of spontaneous brain functions *and further attempts at resuscitation or continued supportive maintenance would not be successful in restoring such functions.*[166]

In earlier times, anxiety over the diagnosis of death was motivated by the fear of premature burial. In an age of organ transplants, concern was to become focused instead on the fear of premature dismemberment. To introduce cessation of brain functions as the criterion of death, in place of the traditional reliance upon cessation of heart and lung functions, conjured up visions of the comatose but still breathing, albeit mechanically supported,patient being vivisected by overzealous surgeons in their haste to obtain transplantable spare parts. That such a patient could be regarded by opponents of the brain death criterion as 'alive' despite being totally dependent upon artificial support systems for heart, lung, and other vital functions, did not merely reflect lingering nostalgia for the traditional heart–lung definition of death. It also reflected, more importantly, widespread acceptance of the living human body's dependence upon medical technology as a perfectly natural and indeed intrinsic feature of 'life' itself. (➤ Ch. 68 Medical technologies: social contexts and consequences)

As the definition of the brain-death criterion makes clear, in contemporary medicine dying and death are neither a part of life as in the nineteenth century nor the absence of life as in earlier ages. Today, a comatose patient today whose loss of spontaneous brain functions is irreversible by existing resuscitation techniques is 'dead'. Another comatose patient tomorrow, *in exactly the same physiological state* as the first one was today, is 'not dead' if in the meantime a new resuscitation technique has been introduced that can be used to reverse the coma. The criterion of death is technological rather than biological.

For modern medicine, then, life is not the opposite of death as the active is the opposite of the inert, for the same level of organic activity/inactivity can count as death at one time and life at another, according to the state of medical technology. Nor is life the opposite of death as the natural is the opposite of the artificial, for the greater the capacity medicine has to intervene technologically in the production and maintenance of life, the less sense it makes to characterize either life or death as natural.[167] In the twentieth century, both life and death fall under the aegis of a perpetual maintenance programme; their relationship must now be understood as the opposition between the self-declared successes and the 'accidental' failures of a single technological project.

NOTES

1   Arthur O. Lovejoy, *The Great Chain of Being*, New York, Harper & Row, 1960; Michel Foucault, *The Order of Things*, New York, Pantheon, 1970, pp. 157–62.
2   Aristotle, *Categories*, 11 b 15 ff. The fourth sense of opposition, 'as affirmatives to negatives', is not directly applicable to the problem of life and death, since it concerns linguistic propositions rather than natural objects.

3 Ibid., 12 a 29 ff (emphasis added).

4 Aristotle, 13 a 30 op. cit. (n.2), ff. Cf. Shakespeare's description of the end of human life: 'Last scene of all,/That ends this strange eventful history,/Is second childishness and mere oblivion,/Sans teeth, sans eyes, sans taste, sans everything.' *As You Like It*, II. vii. 163–6.

5 Aristotle, *On the Parts of Animals*, 641 a 26 ff.

6 Everett Mendelsohn, *Heat and Life: the Development of the Theory of Animal Heat*, Cambridge, MA, Harvard University Press, 1964, ch. 2.

7 Aristotle, op. cit. (n. 5), 641 b 5 ff, and *On the Soul, passim*, e.g. 411 a 25 ff.

8 Aristotle, op. cit. (n. 5), 641 b 9 ff.

9 Aristotle argued that the soul must be a unity (5, 411 b 5 ff) *On the Soul* but that the sense of unity in question seems to be spatial. At the very least, he admitted that the parts of the soul are 'distinguishable by definition' and distinct in nature in that they are found in various combinations in different species of living things (ibid., 413 a 31–b 24).

10 Aristotle, op. cit. (n. 9), 413 a 20 ff.

11 Aristotle, op. cit. (n. 5), 641 a 19 ff; cf. op. cit. (n. 9), 411 b 5 ff.

12 G. E. R. Lloyd (ed.), *Hippocratic Writings*, Harmondsworth, Penguin, 1978, p. 349. The heart was identified with the two ventricles, the auricles, and atria being regarded as appendages (ibid., pp. 349 n and 353).

13 Ibid., p. 351.

14 Lloyd, op. cit. (n. 12), p. 349.

15 Lloyd, op. cit. (n. 12), p. 351.

16 Lloyd, op. cit. (n. 12), p. 351.

17 The importance of moisture for the maintenance of life is discussed by Aristotle in his treatise *On Longevity and Shortness of Life*, ch. 5, 466 a 17 ff. For later developments of this concept, see Thomas S. Hall, 'Life, death and the radical moisture: a study of thematic patterns in medieval medical theory', *Clio Medica*, 1971, 6: 3–23.

18 Galen, *On the Natural Faculties*, Cambridge, MA, and London, Loeb Classical Library, 1916, p. 3.

19 Ibid., p. 33; cf. pp. 223–5.

20 Seneca, *Troades*, II; quoted in Albert Dastre, *La Vie et la mort*, Paris, Flammarion, 1918, p. 299; orig. pub. 1903.

21 Jean Joseph Ménuret de Chambaud, 'Mort (*Médecine*)', in Denis Diderot and Jean Le Rond D'Alembert (eds), *Encyclopédie, ou dictionnaire raisonée*, Paris, 1751–65, Vol. X, p. 718. Cf. Paola Vecchi, 'La mort dans *l'Encyclopédie*', *Studies on Voltaire and the Eighteenth Century*, 1981, 191: 986–94.

22 François Jacob, *The Logic of Life: a history of heredity*, New York, Pantheon, 1973, p. 89.

23 Louis, Chevalier de Jaucourt, 'Vie (*Physiolog.*)' in Diderot and D'Alembert, op. cit. (n. 21), Vol. XVII, p. 249.

24 John Lough, *The Encyclopédie*, London, Longman, 1971, p. 73.

25 Jaucourt, op. cit. (n. 23), p. 249. Cf. the nearly identical definition of death in Jaucourt's entry, 'Mort (*Hist. nat. de l'homme*)', ibid., Vol. X, p. 716.

26 On Stahl, see Thomas S. Hall, *Ideas of life and matter*, Vol. I, Chicago IL, University of Chicago Press, 1969, ch. 25, pp. 351–66, esp. p. 359; François

Duchesneau, *La Physiologie des lumières*, The Hague, Martinus Nijhoff, 1982, ch. 1.

27 Albrecht von Haller, *First Lines of Physiology*, New York and London, Johnson Reprint Corporation, 1966, Vol. II, p. 248; orig. pub. 1786.

28 Philippe Ariès, *The Hour of Our Death*, Harmondsworth, Penguin, 1983, p. 355.

29 Edmund Goodwyn, *The Connexion of Life with Respiration*, London, J. Johnson, 1788, p. 99 (emphasis in original).

30 Erwin H. Ackerknecht, 'Death in the history of medicine', *Bulletin of the History of Medicine*, 1968, 42: 19.

31 Ibid., pp. 19–23; Ménuret, op. cit. (n. 21), pp. 718–21, 726–7; Goodwyn, op. cit. (n. 29), p. 100; Johann Peter Frank, *A System of Complete Medical Police: Selections*, Baltimore, MD, Johns Hopkins University Press, 1976, pp. 265–7 (orig. pub. 1786); and Vecchi, 'Mort apparente et procédés de "ressuscitation" dans la littérature médicale du XVIIIᵉ siècle', *Revue de synthèse*, 1984, 105: 143–60.

32 Hermann Boerhaave, *Academical Lectures on the Theory of Physic*, London, 1742–47, Vol. I, p. 8 (emphasis in original). Cf. Max Neuburger, *The Doctrine of the Healing Power of Nature*, New York, 1932; Neuburger 'An historical survey of the concept of nature from a medical viewpoint', *Isis*, 1944, 35: 16–28.

33 Cf. Elizabeth Haigh, 'The roots of the vitalism of Xavier Bichat', *Bulletin of the History of Medicine*, 1975, 49: 77.

34 Marie-François-Xavier Bichat, *Recherches physiologiques sur la vie et la mort*, Paris, 1800, p. 1; cf. Jacob, op. cit. (n. 22), pp. 90–1, for similar formulations by non-medical writers.

35 Haller, op. cit. (n. 27), p. 247.

36 Haller, op. cit. (n. 27), p. 247, cf. Ménuret, op. cit. (n. 21), pp. 721–2.

37 Haller, op. cit. (n. 27), p. 246.

38 Ménuret, op. cit. (n. 21), pp. 722–3.

39 Frank, op. cit. (n. 31), p. 262; cf. Haller, op. cit. (n. 27), p. 248.

40 Frank, op. cit. (n. 31), p. 262; cf. Ackerknecht, op. cit. (n. 30), pp. 19–23.

41 Carolus Linnaeus, *Oeconomia Naturae* (1749) and *Politia Naturae* (1760), in [C. Linné], *L'Équilibre de la nature*, Paris, Vrin, 1972; Georges-Louis Leclerc de Buffon, 'Le lièvre' (1765), in Jean Piveteau (ed.), *Oeuvres philosophiques de Buffon*, Paris, Presses Universitaires de France, 1954, p. 365.

42 Frank, op. cit. (n. 31), p. 262.

43 Ackerknecht, op. cit. (n. 30), p. 20.

44 M. Foucault, *The Birth of the Clinic*, New York, Pantheon, 1973, chs 8–9; Foucault, op. cit. (n. 1), pp. 263–79; Jacob, op. cit. (n. 22), pp. 89–91.

45 Foucault, op. cit. (n. 44), chs 8–9; Ackerknecht, *Medicine at the Paris Hospital, 1794–1848*, Baltimore, MD, Johns Hopkins University Press, 1967, ch. 2; Alain Rousseau, 'Une révolution dans la sémiologie médicale: le concept de spécificité lesionnelle', *Clio Medica*, 1970, 5: 123–31; David M. Vess, *Medical Revolution in France, 1789–1796*, Gainesville, Florida State University Press, 1975, ch. 9; Toby Gelfand, *Professionalizing Modern Medicine*, Westport, CT, Greenwood Press, 1980, ch. 10.

46 Xavier Bichat, *Anatomie générale, appliquée à la physiologie et à la médecine*, Paris, 1801, Vol. I, p. xcix.

47 W. R. Albury, 'Appendix', in W. R. Albury and D. R. Oldroyd, From 'Renaissance mineral studies to historical geology in the light of Michel Foucault's *The order of things*', *British Journal of the History of Science*, 1977, 10: 209–11.

48 William Coleman, *Georges Cuvier, Zoologist*, Cambridge, MA, Harvard University Press, 1964, chs 2–3; Foucault, op. cit. (n. 1), pp. 263–79; Jacob, op. cit. (n. 22), pp. 100–11.

49 Aristotle, op. cit. (n. 2), 11 b 30 ff.

50 Aristotle, op. cit. (n. 2), 8 a 30 ff.

51 Aristotle, op. cit. (n. 5), 641 b 1 ff.

52 Georges Cuvier, *The Animal Kingdom*, London, Bohn, 1863, pp. 2–3; orig. pub. 1817.

53 Ibid., p. 4.

54 Georges Canguilhem, 'Le vivant et son milieu', in Canguilhem, *La Connaissance de la vie*, Paris, Vrin, 1971, pp. 132–4.

55 François-Joseph-Victor Broussais, *Examen des doctrines médicales et des systèmes de nosologie*, 3rd edn, Paris, 1829–34, Vol. I, p. 1.

56 Guenter B. Risse, 'The Brownian system of medicine: its theoretical and practical implications', *Clio Medica*, 1970, 5: 45–51; Risse, 'The quest for certainty in medicine: John Brown's system of medicine in France', *Bulletin of the History of Medicine*, 1971, 45: 1–12; Georges Canguilhem, 'Une idéologie médicale exemplaire, le système de Brown', in Canguilhem, *Idéologie et rationalité dans l'histoire des sciences de la vie*, Paris, Vrin, 1977, pp. 48–54; W. F. Bynum and Roy Porter (eds), *Brunonianism in Britain and Europe*, Medical History suppl. 8, London, Wellcome Institute for the History of Medicine, 1988.

57 Boerhaave, op. cit. (n. 32), p. 6 (emphasis in original).

58 John Brown, *Elementa Medicinae* (1780), para. 328, quoted in Canguilhem, op. cit. (n. 56), p. 51.

59 Jean-Nicolas Corvisart, *Essai sur les maladies et les lesions du coeur et des gros vaisseaux*, 3rd edn, Paris, 1818, p. xvii; orig. pub. 1806.

60 Ibid., p. xx.

61 Corvisart, op. cit. (n. 59), p. 371.

62 Corvisart, op. cit. (n. 59), p. 375.

63 Broussais, op. cit. (n. 55), p. xvi.

64 Broussais, op. cit. (n. 55), p. xvii.

65 Corvisart, op. cit. (n. 59), p. 381; cf. W. R. Albury, 'Heart of darkness: J. N. Corvisart and the medicalization of life', *Historical Reflections*, 1982, 9: 17–31; reprinted in Jean-Pierre Goubert (ed.), *La Médicalisation de la société française, 1770–1830*, Waterloo, Historical Reflections Press, 1982, pp. 17–31.

66 Boerhaave, op. cit. (n. 32), p. 6; cf. Haller, op. cit. (n. 27), p. 241.

67 Haller, op. cit. (n. 27), p. 242.

68 Risse, op. cit. (n. 56), 1970, p. 45.

69 Louis Pasteur, 'Report on fermentation addressed to the Minister of Education, April, 1862', in Hilaire Cuny, *Louis Pasteur*, London, Souvenir Press, 1965, pp. 158–9.

70 Ackerknecht, op. cit. (n. 30), p. 21.

71 On van Helmont, see Hall, op. cit. (n. 26), Vol. I, ch. 14, pp. 206–17; Henry M. Leicester, *Development of Biochemical Concepts from Ancient to Modern Times*,

Cambridge, MA, Harvard University Press, 1974, pp. 93–8; Walter Pagel, *The Religious and Philosophical Aspects of van Helmont's Science and Medicine, Bulletin of the History of Medicine*, suppl. 2, Baltimore, MD, Johns Hopkins Press, 1944. It is clear from all these accounts that Helmontian 'ferments' (1) were not identified in all cases with putrefaction and (2) were not uniquely associated with living beings.

72 Rudolf Virchow, 'The mechanistic interpretation of life' (1858), in Lelland J. Rather (ed.), *Disease, Life, and Man: Selected Essays by Rudolf Virchow*, Stanford, CA, Stanford University Press, 1958, p. 105. Cf. John R. Baker, 'The cell-theory: a restatement, history, and critique – part 1', *Quarterly Journal of Microscopical Science*, 1948, 80: 104–6.

73 Eilhard Mitscherlich and Felix Hoppe-Seyler, quoted in Claude Bernard, *Lectures on the Phenomena of Life common to Plants and Animals*, Springfield, IL, C. C. Thomas, 1974, p. 127; orig. pub. 1878.

74 Ibid., p. 29 (emphasis in original).

75 Justus Liebig, *Animal Chemistry, or Organic Chemistry in its Application to Physiology and Pathology*, New York and London, Johnson Reprint Corporation, 1964, pp. 209–231; orig. pub. 1842.

76 Bernard, op. cit. (n. 73), p. 30 (emphasis in original); cf. Virchow, op. cit. (n. 72), p. 107.

77 Bernard, op. cit. (n. 73), p. 29 (emphasis in original).

78 Bernard, op. cit. (n. 73), p. 252.

79 Charles Darwin, *On the Origin of Species by Means of Natural Selection*, Harmondsworth, Penguin, 1968, pp. 132–3; orig. pub. 1859.

80 Ibid., pp. 124–9.

81 Bernard, op. cit. (n. 73), p. 259.

82 Bernard, op. cit. (n. 73), p. 20.

83 Bernard, op. cit. (n. 73), p. 252.

84 Bernard, op. cit. (n. 73), p. 94.

85 Corvisart, op. cit. (n. 59), p. xxxiv.

86 Corvisart, op. cit. (n. 59), p. xxxiii.

87 See, for example, Erna Lesky, *The Vienna Medical School of the Nineteenth Century*, Baltimore, MD, and London, Johns Hopkins University Press, 1976, p. 122.

88 Owsei Temkin, 'The meaning of medicine in historical perspective', in Temkin, *The Double Face of Janus and Other Essays in the History of Medicine*, Baltimore, MD, and London, Johns Hopkins University Press, 1977, p. 46; Lesky, op. cit. (n. 87), p. 122.

89 François Broussais, *Histoire des phlegmasies ou inflammations chroniques*, 4th edn, Paris, 1826, Vol. III, p. 459 (emphasis in original); orig. pub. 1808.

90 Broussais, op. cit. (n. 89), p. 458.

91 Broussais, op. cit. (n. 55), p. lix; cf. Jean-François Braunstein, *Broussais et le matérialisme: médecine et philosophie au XIXe siècle*, Paris, Meridiens Klincksieck, 1986, pp. 77–81. On similar therapeutic developments in Britain and North America, see Peter H. Niebyl, 'The English bloodletting revolution, or modern medicine before 1850', *Bulletin of the History of Medicine*, 1977, 51: 464–83.

92 Vecchi, op. cit. (n. 31), pp. 146 ff.

93 Lloyd G. Stevenson, 'Suspended animation and the history of anaesthesia', *Bulletin of the History of Medicine*, 1975, 49: 508.

94 Ibid., pp. 484–7.

95 Stevenson, op. cit. (n. 93), p. 510; cf. Martin S. Pernick, *A Calculus of Suffering: Pain, Professionalization and Anaesthesia in Nineteenth-Century America*, New York, Columbia University Press, 1985, p. 43, for further evidence of the association of anaesthesia with death in the first half of the nineteenth century.

96 Ackerknecht, op. cit. (n. 30), p. 21; cf. Ariès, op. cit. (n. 28), pp. 402–4. Reflecting on this change, Ariès has argued that it was late nineteenth-century doctors who first introduced the concept of death as 'pure negativity' (ibid., p. 404), but the material he cites is concerned with questions of the exact moment of death and the status of the cadaver, rather than with the relationship between life and death in medical theory.

97 Stevenson, op. cit. (n. 93), p. 482.

98 Stevenson, op. cit. (n. 93), p. 482.

99 Bernard, op. cit. (n. 73), p. 182.

100 Bernard, op. cit. (n. 73), p. 182.

101 Bernard, op. cit. (n. 73), p. 182.

102 Joseph Lister, 'On a new method of treating compound fracture' (1867), and 'On the antiseptic principle in the practice of surgery' (1867), in Logan Clendening (ed.), *Source Book of Medical History*, New York, Schuman, 1942, pp. 610–21.

103 Girolamo Fracastoro, *Syphilis, or the French Disease* (1530), in Clendening, op. cit. (n. 102), p. 120.

104 John Parascandola, 'The theoretical basis of Paul Ehrlich's chemotherapy', *Journal of the History of Medicine*, 1981, 36: 19–43; cf. Erwin H. Ackerknecht, 'Cellular theory and therapeutics', *Clio Medica*, 1970, 5: 1–5.

105 Guenter B. Risse, 'The renaissance of bloodletting: a chapter in modern therapeutics', *Journal of the History of Medicine*, 1979, 34: 3–22.

106 Cf. Georges Canguilhem, *On the Normal and the Pathological*, Dordrecht, D. Reidel, 1978, pp. 17–46.

107 Bernard, *An Introduction to the Study of Experimental Medicine* (1865), New York, Dover, 1957, p. 76.

108 Bernard, op. cit. (n. 73), p. 253.

109 Bernard, op. cit. (n. 73), p. 273.

110 Dastre, op. cit. (n. 20), p. 212; cf. p. 220.

111 Dastre, op. cit. (n. 20), p. 223.

112 Liebig, op. cit. (n. 75), pp. 250–1.

113 Edward Frankland, 'On the origin of muscular power', *Philosophical Magazine*, 1866 (4th series), 32: 193–4; cf. Adolf Fick and Johannes Wislicensus, 'On the origin of muscular power', *Philosophical Magazine*, 1866 (4th series), 31: 501–2.

114 Virchow, op. cit. (n. 72).

115 Jacob, op. cit. (n. 22), p. 194; cf. p. 253.

116 George Rosen, 'The conservation of energy and the study of metabolism', in C. McC. Brooks and P. F. Cranefield (eds), *The Historical Development of Physiological Thought*, New York, Hafner, 1959, pp. 254–5.

117 Rosen, op. cit. (n. 116), p. 260.

118 Frederic L. Holmes, 'Introduction', in Liebig, op. cit. (n. 75), p. cxiii, with citation to Max Rubner, *Z. Biol.*, 1894, 30: 85.

119 Aristotle, op. cit. (n. 2), 12 a 1 ff.

120 Aristotle, op. cit. (n. 2), 13 a 16 ff.

121 Ivan Petrovich Pavlov, 'Experimental therapeutics as a new and exceedingly fruitful method of physiological investigation', *Bulletin of the New York Academy of Medicine*, 1974, 50: 1018–30; orig. pub. 1900.

122 Ibid., pp. 1021–5.

123 Pavlov, op. cit. (n. 121), pp. 1025–6.

124 Pavlov, op. cit. (n. 121), p. 1026.

125 Pavlov, op. cit. (n. 121), p. 1026.

126 Jacques Loeb, letter to Ernst Mach, 1890, quoted in Philip J. Pauly, *Controlling Life: Jacques Loeb and the Engineering Ideal in Biology*, Berkeley, University of California Press, 1990, p. 51.

127 Pavlov, op. cit. (n. 121), p. 1026.

128 W. R. Albury, 'Experiment and explanation in the physiology of Bichat and Magendie', *Studies in History of Biology*, 1977, 1: 88.

129 Pavlov, op. cit. (n. 121).

130 Pavlov, op. cit. (n. 121), p. 1028.

131 Pavlov, op. cit. (n. 121), p. 1028.

132 Cf. Michael D. Bayles, 'Physicians as body mechanics', in A. L. Caplan *et al.* (eds), *Concepts of Health and Disease: Interdisciplinary Perspectives*, Reading, MA, Addison-Wesley, 1981, pp. 665–75.

133 Pavlov, op. cit. (n. 121), p. 1028.

134 Pavlov, op. cit. (n. 121), p. 1026.

135 Pavlov, op. cit. (n. 121), p. 1024.

136 Owsei Temkin, 'Metaphors of human biology', in op. cit. (n. 88), p. 277.

137 Ernst Haeckel, *The Riddle of the Universe at the Close of the Nineteenth Century*, London, Watts, 1900, pp. 270–1 (orig. pub. 1899); with citation to Haeckel, *General Morphology*, Vol. II [*Generelle morphologie der organismen*, 1866], and *The Natural History of Creation* [*Natürliche Schöpfungsgeschichte*, 1868].

138 Ibid., p. 272.

139 Elie Metchnikoff, *The Nature of Man: Studies in Optimistic Philosophy*, London, Heinemann, 1903, p. 249.

140 Ibid., p. 252.

141 Metchinikoff, op. cit. (n. 139), p. 254.

142 Temkin, op. cit. (n. 136).

143 Dastre, op. cit. (n. 20), pp. 335–6.

144 Dastre, op. cit. (n. 20), pp. 336–7.

145 Metchnikoff, op. cit. (n. 139), p. 266.

146 August Weismann, 'The duration of life' (1881), in Weismann, *Essays upon Heredity and Kindred Biological Problems*, Oxford, Clarendon Press, 1889, p. 25.

147 Ibid., p. 24; cf. Weismann, 'Life and death' (1883), in Weismann, op. cit. (n. 146), pp. 136, 159.

148 Weismann, op. cit. (n. 146), p. 28.

149 Metchnikoff, op. cit. (n. 139), p. 267.

150 F. Jacob, *The Possible and the Actual*, Seattle and London, University of Washington Press, 1982, pp. 50–1.

151 Metchnikoff, op. cit. (n. 139), p. 266; with citation to J. Loeb, *Archiv für die gesammte Physiologie*, 1902, 93: 59. Cf. Pauly, op. cit. (n. 126), pp. 111–12.

152 Dastre, op. cit. (n. 20), p. 333.

153 Bernard, op. cit. (n. 73), p. 84.

154 Dastre, op. cit. (n. 20), p. 332. Cf. Pauly, op. cit. (n. 126), pp. 86–9; and Jacques Loeb, 'The role of salts in the preservation of life', in Loeb, *The Mechanistic Conception of Life*, Cambridge, MA, Harvard University Press, 1964, pp. 154–77 (orig. pub. 1912).

155 Dastre, op. cit. (n. 20), p. 332.

156 Metchnikoff, op. cit. (n. 139), pp. 278, 277.

157 Dastre, op. cit. (n. 20), p. 339. Cf. A. L. Caplan, 'The "unnaturalness" of aging – a sickness unto death?', in Caplan, op. cit. (n. 132), pp. 725–37.

158 Metchnikoff, op. cit. (n. 139), p. 283; cf. Dastre, op. cit. (n. 20), pp. 346–7. For a version of this scenario by a contemporary medical researcher, see Lewis Thomas, 'The deacon's masterpiece', in Thomas, *The Medusa and the Snail*, Toronto, New York and London, Bantam Books, 1980, pp. 107–12.

159 Leon R. Kass, 'Regarding the end of medicine and the pursuit of health', in Caplan, op. cit. (n. 132), p. 8. Kass treats the pursuit of health and the prevention of death as alternative goals for medicine, but the thrust of the present argument is that these two goals are continuous with one another in the context of the twentieth-century conception of life and death.

160 Ibid. (emphasis in original).

161 Jessica H. Muller and Barbara A. Koenig, 'On the boundary of life and death: the definition of dying by medical residents', in Margaret Lock and Deborah R. Gordon (eds), *Biomedicine Examined*, Dordrecht, Kluwer, 1988, p. 369.

162 Dastre, op. cit. (n. 20), p. 302; cf. p. 311.

163 Muller and Koenig, op. cit. (n. 161), p. 369.

164 Ad Hoc Committee of the Harvard Medical School, 'A definition of irreversible coma: report of the Ad Hoc Committee of the Harvard Medical School to examine the definition of brain death', *Journal of the American Medical Association*, 1968, 205: 337–40; reprinted in Stanley Joel Reiser *et al.* (eds), *Ethics in Medicine: Historical Perspectives and Contemporary Concerns*, Cambridge, MA, and London, MIT Press, 1977, pp. 504–7.

165 Dastre, op. cit. (n. 20), p. 302.

166 Quoted in William H. Sweet, 'Brain death', *New England Journal of Medicine*, 1978, 299: 410–1; reprinted in Edward S. Shneidman (ed.), *Death: Current Perspectives*, 2nd edn, Palo Alto, CA, Mayfield, p. 145 (emphasis added).

167 Cf. Pauly, op. cit. (n. 126), pp. 199–200.

FURTHER READING

Ackerknecht, Erwin H., 'Death in the history of medicine', *Bulletin of the History of Medicine*, 1968, 42: 19–23.

Ariès, Philippe, *The Hour of Our Death*, Harmondsworth, Penguin, 1983.

Canguilhem, Georges, *La Connaissance de la vie*, Paris, Vrin, 1971.

Dastre, Albert, *La Vie et la mort*, Paris, Flammarion, 1903.

Gervais, Karen Grandstrand, *Redefining Death*, New Haven, CT, and London, Yale University Press, 1986.

Hall, Thomas S. *Ideas of Life and Matter*, Chicago, IL, University of Chicago Press, 1969.

Jacob, François, *The Logic of Life: a History of Heredity*, New York, Pantheon, 1973.

Mendelsohn, Everett, *Heat and Life: the Development of the Theory of Animal Heat*, Cambridge, MA, Harvard University Press, 1964.

Shneidman, Edwin S. (ed.), *Death: Current Perspectives*, 2nd edn, Palo Alto, CA, Mayfield, 1980.

14

HUMORALISM

Vivian Nutton

Humoralism is a system of medicine that considers illness to be the result of some disturbance in the natural balance of the humours, within the body as a whole or within one particular part. It stresses the unity of the body, and the strong interaction between mental and physical processes. It is at one and the same time highly individualistic, for each person and each bodily part has their own natural humoral compositon (also known as *krasis*, mixture, or temperament), and universal, for the range of variation is limited and the same patterns of illness (diseases) can be seen to occur in many individuals. The natural balance of health is always precarious, for it is constantly subject to potentially harmful influences from one's diet, life-style and environment. Hence an appropriate diagnosis of the cause or causes of illness is far from simple, since it must involve an almost limitless range of factors both inside and outside the body. None the less, provided one can discover the proper healthy humoral balance within an individual, one cannot only restore the body to health (traditionally by allopathic means, but homeopathic remedies are not excluded), but can also devise means of maintaining that health for as long as possible. In humoralism, prophylaxis plays as great a role as therapy.

Historically, humoralism formed the basis for the Western tradition of medicine down to the nineteenth century. In its earliest manifestations, in sixth- and fifth-century BC Greece, it reveals no links with any of the medical systems elsewhere in the eastern Mediterranean, and the few apparent parallels with Indian or Far Eastern medical systems may well be fortuitous. By the second century AD, it had become dominant throughout the Roman Empire. The Arab conquests of the seventh century, and the subsequent translation of Galenic and Hippocratic texts into Arabic in the ninth century, ensured its primacy in Muslim lands, where, particularly in Pakistan, it continues to play a major role in the twentieth century, with certain aspects of modern Western therapeutics and clinical discoveries being incorporated within an overall traditional humoral framework. In the Middle Ages, the introduction of translated Arabic medical texts into the Latin West, from the eleventh century onwards, confirmed the importance of humoralism. In learned medicine as taught at the newly founded universities, it formed the basis for all medical understanding, and diagnosis and treatment were structured according to the pattern of the so-called six non-naturals. Although from the sixteenth century onwards many of the anatomical and physiological theories of its greatest Greek exponent, Galen of Pergamum (AD 129-c.200/210), were overthrown, the apparent therapeutic advantages of a humoralist explanation ensured its continuation, albeit in an attenuated form. The discovery of the circulation of the blood by William Harvey (1578-1657) only transferred to the blood many of the properties ascribed by Galen to the other humours, and many eighteenth-century theories of health and disease, for example those of Friedrich Hoffmann (1660-1742), William Cullen (1710-90), and John Brown (1735-88), maintained the idea of health as a form of equilibrium. Gabriel Andral (1797-1876) revived a stricter humoralism when, as a result of his researches in haemopathology, he attributed disease to changes in the constituents of blood, fibrin, albumins, alkalis, etc. Possibly under his influence, the Viennese Carl Rokitansky (1804-78) ascribed the creation of all pathological cells to specific *dyscrases* (bad mixtures) in the blood, an opinion he later retracted after strong criticism from Rudolf Virchow (1821-1902). (➤ Ch. 9 The pathological tradition)

A combination of the new cellular pathology, which concentrated on tissues rather than on bodily fluids, and chemistry might seem to have put an end to humoralism as a scientifically acceptable theory, although the lay person still continues to think of the processes of disease and therapy in terms that would have been familiar to Galen and Hippocrates of Cos (c.450-370 BC). Yet the isolation and identification of hormones and neurosecretions in the body as responsible for the maintenance of a natural balance, homeostasis, both physical and behavioural, can be taken as a rough confirmation of some aspects of humoralism. However, unlike their ancestors, these modern 'humours' are not the sources of all pathological conditions, and their interactions are far more complex than the mixtures of the Greeks. At the same time, modern epidemiologists have begun to focus again on the receptivity of the individual as a factor in certain diseases, and to isolate types, both physical and psychological, who are most at risk. This, however, may best be seen as a return to holism, rather than specifically to humoralism, for, although within the same general framework of unitary explanation, there is no recourse to what is the distinctive characteristic of humoralism, the humours themselves.

The word 'humour' goes back directly to the Greek word 'χυμός', which designates any fluid or juice. Sap in plants, blood in animals, and ichor in the gods are all humours, and on a purely empirical basis it would not be hard to attribute responsibility for life, at least in part, to these fluids. At the same time, there are other clearly natural bodily fluids in human beings that make their appearance only when sickness is present (for example, the mucus of a runny nose or the liquid stools of diarrhoea) and which may disappear again apparently spontaneously when the patient recovers. Hence, even before our earliest written medical records in Greek, it is possible to conceive of theories and therapies that involved these fluids, and that posited health as some form of equilibrium between them. It is an idea that finds close parallels among the so-called Presocratic philosophers, who in the sixth century BC were speculating on the ultimate make-up of the universe. By 450 BC, the weakness of arguments that focused on one single initial substance, or element (for example earth or water) had become clear, not least because of their failure to explain change and differentiation. Two alternative types of explanation took their place. One, favoured by the Ionian philosopher Heraclitus of Ephesus (c.540–475 BC), assumed a perpetual strife between two basic principles, fire and water. Although apparently stable, all matter was held in a precarious balance between the two as they flowed to and fro. Change was the only true constant, and stability could only be achieved by confining the flux within certain limits. By contrast, the Sicilian healer-philosopher Empedocles of Acragas (c.492–432 BC) posited an equally self-conflicting universe, but one created out of four elements, earth, air, fire, and water, which had become separated out from a primeval mixture. Each thing was made out of these elements in a particular proportion: bone consisted of two parts earth, two parts water, and four parts fire; blood of equal parts of each element. The stability of each object resided in the maintenance of the proper proportional balance between the four elements. The balance, once achieved, might remain steady, unlike in the Heraclitean theory of perpetual change, for its existence was guaranteed by the continuation of its due proportion. Processes like breathing could be explained by a regular alteration in the proportions of the elements within a particular organ.

It is against this wider, cosmological background that one should set the earliest surviving Greek medical writings in the Hippocratic Corpus. This is a body of medical treatises in the Ionic dialect of Greek, mostly written between 410 and 360 BC, although some may be several centuries later in date, and associated with the name of Hippocrates of Cos. Contemporaries talk of him as a great physician and teacher at Athens, but there is, as yet, no conclusive proof of his authorship of any specific treatise in the Corpus. Indeed, although certain tracts were clearly written by the same person, the diversity of opinions within the Corpus is at least as striking as their coincidences. It in no way represents a consensus within early Greek medicine, but rather the reverse.

Yet, even where there is a disagreement over details, substantial similarities may be detected in general outlook. Most authors in the Hippocratic Corpus saw health and disease as dependent on a balance or imbalance, although they might disagree among themselves over what it was that was or was not in balance. The author of *On Ancient Medicine* was openly scathing about philosophers like Empedocles and about those who talked about the body in terms of the hot, the cold, the wet, and the dry (an interpretation of the elements in qualitative terms). In their place, he posited a multiplicity of contending powers or properties, including hot and cold, sweet and sour, and astringent and insipid, increases or decreases in any of which might bring about disease. Other authors, like that of *Affections*, stressed the presence of harmful fluxes within the body, whose migrations determined the seat of the disease. By contrast, the author of *Regimen* adopted a view very close to that of Heraclitus, whereby it was argued that humans are made from fire and water, in continual flux, and that it required only a slight change towards an excess or deficiency of either for the body's balance to be disturbed and for illness to result.

In these, and in many other tracts, two bodily fluids, phlegm and bile, take on a major role as causes or as indicators of diseases. Phlegm is associated with water, bile with fire, and, in the two treatises *On the Sacred Disease* and *On Airs, Waters and Places*, the two are linked with an appropriate season, winter and summer, and with an appropriate geographical area, South Russia and Libya. They are used to explain racial characteristics, including cowardice and effeminacy, as well as more obvious mental disorders. (➤ Ch. 15 Environment and miasmata) In *On the Sacred Disease*, phlegm blocks the flow of air to and from the brain, which results in epileptic convulsions as the air tries to force its way through; bile, on the other hand, heats and dries the brain, thereby causing frenzied madness. The doctor's knowledge of these causes will not only enable the rejection of the simplistic explanation of divine intervention, but will lead to the correct allopathic treatment and, in some cases, appropriate prophylaxis.

By contrast with bile and phlegm, which, although naturally and necessarily present in the body, are usually mentioned only in negative contexts, blood is an extremely ambiguous humour. The most important fluid in the body for life, it also is a symptom and, according to some authors, a cause of illness. Haemorrhoids, nose-bleeds, and menstruation all indicate a harmful excess of blood, although whether it is the excess (or plethora), the blood itself, or one of its constituents that is responsible is a matter for open debate. According to the author of *On Humours* (which include urine, sweat, pus, and nasal discharges), the changing seasons can bring about a harmful excess of blood, which is to be relieved by bleeding, but the same condition can be equally caused by pleurisy and by bile. (➤ Ch. 40 Physical methods)

When and why the doctrine of *four* humours came to be is far from clear. In *On Diseases, I* and *On Affections*, the writer talks of the four qualities, hot, cold, wet, and dry, while at the same time relying on the bipolarity of bile and phlegm as the main explanation. The author of *On the Sacred Disease* shows a similar equivocation. Only in the texts *On Diseases, IV* and *On the Nature of Man* is there given a description of the human body in terms of four humours, seen in some way as the equivalent of Empedocles's four elements. Although careful clinical observation may well have suggested the existence, and importance, of particular humours, of itself this does not entail the idea that humans are *composed* of humours, and that these are four in number. The theories are the product of the interaction between the Greek doctor, who provides the observational data, and the Greek philosopher, who provides the categories by which these clinical experiences can be ordered.

At first, there was no general agreement as to which humours were the four. The author of *On Diseases, IV* suggests that they are blood, phlegm, bile, and water, which, like the sap in plants, provide nutriment to the body. They have their seats respectively in the heart, head, liver, and spleen, organs that were already supposed in early Greek medicine to be of immense significance for the proper working of the body. Indeed, it may be that it was from this pre-existing importance of the spleen as a reservoir of fluid and from its association with water that the author took water as the fourth humour in the schema.

The author's opinion was not followed, except in *On Generation*, a treatise which, in fact, may come from the same pen. Instead, there came to dominance a theory, first expressed in the Hippocratic Corpus in the treatise *On the Nature of Man*, which gave the fourth place to black bile or melancholy. This author's model is avowedly the four elements, but the description of the four humours avoids any correlation with elements, and uses instead one with the four qualities, hot, cold, wet, and dry. Exactly what the fourth humour, black bile, was, is still a matter for controversy. It may be identified with a clotting agent, or with the dark blood sometimes vomited as a result of a stomach ulcer, but according to some later Greek authors it also bubbled and fizzed when it hit the ground, and was likely to destroy whatever came into direct contact with it. In its destructive potential, and in its normal invisibility, it stood at the opposite pole from the generally beneficial and easily perceived blood. However, at least as influential in the adoption of black bile as the fourth humour was the fact that, according to the author of *On the Nature of Man*, the diseases that it caused could be fitted into a seasonal pattern. The idea that there was a cycle of diseases corresponding to that of the seasons was by no means unique, for the prevalence of phlegm in winter and bile in summer is found in many other texts in the Corpus. Nonetheless, the linkage of the four seasons with the four humours marks a major step. Each humour predominates in turn in a particular season of the year, and at a particular time in one's life: blood in spring and childhood; bile in summer and youth; black bile in autumn and adulthood; and phlegm in winter and old age. Such a schema had more than the virtue of conceptual neatness to commend it. It gave the doctor the opportunity to regulate the balance of the body by knowing in advance just what humour was likely to be excessive or deficient at a particular time, and by then taking appropriate action, either through removing the offending humour directly, for example through bloodletting or drugs, or through changing the body's overall mixture through diet and life-style. The neatness of its correlations gave this theory added explanatory force, and it appears to have been adopted by many other physicians in the fourth century BC. Its author was identified with Hippocrates, or, at the least, with his son-in-law Polybus (*fl.* 370 BC), an attribution that gave it added authority. It corresponded to some obvious phenomena. Even Erasistratus (*fl.* 270 BC), who vigorously attacked explanations for disease in terms of humours, seems at times to have spoken of humours as existing within the body, although he regarded them as in no way possessing the dominant powers ascribed to them by the Hippocratics.

Another of the attractions of this four-humour theory was its inclusiveness, for it could easily be combined with a theory like that of Philistion of Locris (*fl.* 380 BC) and of his pupil Plato (427–347 BC), which linked the four elements with the four primary qualities. Plato's cosmological myth, the *Timaeus*, opened up further possibilities, for, as well as ascribing diseases to changes in the four elements, and to excess or deficiency of air, phlegm, and bile, he also posited that differences between fevers arose through the influence of different elements. The author of *On the Nature of Man* believed all fevers to be caused by bile, but Plato differentiated between them and attributed the variations to the presence of other elements. (➤ Ch. 19 Fevers) Furthermore, in the *Timaeus*, he expressly linked physical and mental diseases together, giving a physical explanation for mental or moral conditions, a link that can be found, albeit less fully developed, in some Hippocratic texts.

It was Galen of Pergamum, philosopher as well as physician, who provided the first major synthesis of all these opinions. Convinced that Hippocrates was the author of *On the Nature of Man*, and that Plato in the *Timaeus* was drawing directly on the teachings of the great physician from Cos, he combined the two strands into an imposing system. He aligned the four humours with the four elements – although, for the most part, his clinical writings talk in terms of qualities, not elements – which in human beings could be combined into any one of nine natural mixtures or temperaments: one a perfect mixture of all humours, the rest having one or a pair of humours in slight predominance. Because these predominances were natural, they were not morbid, except in the sense that they created a predisposition to certain diseases. Galen also avoided relating the qualities of the humours exactly and in all particulars to the relevant visible bodily fluids by treating his elemental humours as invisible entities, recognizable only by logic. The blood in the arteries thus was formed from all four humours, but with a preponderance of elemental blood; a failure to identify black bile in similar quantity in the visible body thus was no objection to the presumed existence of black bile as a pure, elemental humour. The idea of the body built up from humours was easily extendable. Although, in theory, agnostic about the workings of the soul (or mind), in practice Galen was a strong somaticist, even eager to explain mental disease in terms of physical disorder (and vice versa). (➤ Ch. 21 Mental diseases) Temperament now affected the mind as much as the body, an idea that Galen found confirmed in Plato and also in the *Problems* ascribed to Aristotle, where the melancholic (or atrabilious) genius made a distinguished appearance.

Whether or not we believe Galen's claims that in his own day Hippocratism was out of fashion, his own combination of logic and experience, of theoretical sophistication and bedside practice, of massive book-learning and avowedly successful therapies, and, not least, his overpowering wordiness, proved irresistible. Famous already in his lifetime, his books became even more potent after his death. First in the Greek-speaking East of the Roman Empire, and then in the Latin West, Hippocratism, as viewed through Galenic eyes, became the dominant medical philosophy. The words of Galen gradually ousted from medical encyclopedias those of others in the Hippocratic tradition, and Galen's vision of Hippocrates as the author of *On the Nature of Man*, the creator of the theory of the four humours, and a believer in psychosomaticism became accepted as gospel. Such divergencies as later became apparent could be easily explained away or reconciled either medically or philologically. Hence, the disagreement over the fourth humour between the authors of *On the Nature of Man* and *On Diseases, IV* could be reduced by declaring that the fluid produced in the spleen was at one and the same time watery and black bile, and hence that both authors were in fact referring to the same substance, though by different names.

The attractiveness of the Galenic theory of humours lay also in the ease with which it could adapt to other disciplines, not least those of physiognomy and astrology. Physiognomical tables connecting physical and moral characteristics were thus given a convincing theoretical framework, and the truths of astrology could be seen to complement those of medicine. The fourfold scheme of the astrologer Antiochus of Ascalon (*fl.* AD 180) joined the four humours to the four cardinal points in the heavens, and gave to each three of the constellations; for example, phlegm was associated with Capricorn,

Aquarius, and Pisces. These connections, from fields peripheral to medicine, only confirmed the ability of Galen as a great astrologer as well as a great physician. Christians might also associate his humours with the saints, Peter, Paul, Mark, and John, and with musical modes. The sheer variety of the system and its ability to explain almost anything made it both convincing and unfalsifiable, for behind its apparent certainty lurked the possibility of error on the part of either practitioner or patient. If the patient failed to recover under the suggested therapy, the system itself offered many ways to explain why.

It comes as no surprise to find the Galenic theory of the four humours becoming so dominant, in Europe and in the Islamic world. It offered an apparently convincing explanation that linked together both man and macrocosm. The regularity of a divinely created universe, with the procession of the stars in their seasons, had its parallel in the regularity of the humours in the divinely created human body. Medieval illustrations of the body frequently draw on corrrespondence between the humours, the planets, seasons, and the like, and the belief in an occult (or hidden) cosmic sympathy, which became increasingly common in the Renaissance, provided further proof of the validity of such links. As a logical system, too, humoralism was impressive; for Galen's logic in proceeding to his conclusions is almost impeccable, and his Arabic interpreters, not least Avicenna (AD 980–1037), had refined his arguments still further. Provided that one accepted his premises, which he claimed were 'common notions', 'what everybody knew', his results were very hard to deny.

The advantages of this logical scheme can be best seen in the development within humoralism of the theory of the six non-naturals. Galen himself had spoken often of the natural constituents of the body, its elements, humours, mixtures, organs, bones, spirits, and faculties, and had contrasted the health of the body in its natural state with unnatural ill health, disease, its causes, and its symptoms. He also in several passages talked of the things that were, in his phrase, 'neutral', being neither necessarily good nor bad: food and drink, environment, rest and wakefulness, exercise, evacuation of bodily residues, and the emotions. Each of these had an impact on the humoral balance of the body, but it could be for better or worse, depending on the individual and his or her condition at the time. Nowhere, however, did Galen draw these scattered observations together into a coherent whole.

We have too little information to decide whether this was done first in late-antique Alexandria or by his Arabic interpreters. Certainly when Hunain Ibn Ishāq (AD 809–73) composed his treatise *Medical Questions and Answers*, he adopted the threefold scheme of talking first about the natural organization of the body, then about these neutral factors, and finally about unnatural (or anti-natural) disease. This summary of Galenic learning was repeated by all

Arabic writers in the Galenic tradition, who thereby shared a coherence of doctrine and a coherence of technical terms. From at least the time of Haly Abbas (d. AD 944), these six factors became identified as the crucial elements in the causation and cure of most diseases. (➤ Ch. 31 Arab-Islamic medicine)

Hunain's treatise was translated into Latin, probably in the eleventh century, as the *Isagoge* or *Introduction* of Johannitius. The translator introduced two significant changes: the question-and-answer form was replaced by a straightforward didactic account, and the six neutral factors were given a new name. Alongside the 'naturals' and the 'contra-naturals' were now the six 'non-naturals' ('*sex res non-naturales*'), a somewhat confusing title since they were indeed found in nature. The *Isagoge* in its Latin form is a model of concise exposition of complicated information, and it became the primary text for medical study in the medical schools that, from the twelfth century on, sprang up in Italy, France, and the rest of Europe. Every aspiring doctor learned the basic concepts from the *Isagoge*, and took cues from it. Hence, not only academic treatises, but also prescriptions and medical advice were structured according to the categories of the six non-naturals, since it was by regulating these that one could restore the body to health or, more importantly, prevent the natural balance of a body from tipping over into imbalance. Drugs as well as diet fell into this category of food and drink, bleeding as well as sexual intercourse and purgatives into that of evacuation, and great attention was paid to a proper environment or air. Nor was one's emotional state neglected, and a walk to a picnic in pleasant countryside with agreeable company might prove as effective a remedy as any elixir. By its stress on proper regimen, in the very broadest sense of the word, the schema of the six non-naturals offered an alternative to drastic intervention, as well as a hopeful explanation for mental disorder, and for the physical consequences of mental illness.

The non-naturals were but one component in the fully developed theory of humours, albeit one that at times enjoyed an independent existence. Similar ideas on the need to site people within their environment, and on hygiene and diet as crucial determinants of health and disease, were approved well into the nineteenth century by physicians who would have rejected contemptuously the humoral theories from which they sprang. (➤ Ch. 53 History of personal hygiene) At the same time, their patients maintained – and, at least in Clerkenwell, according to Vicky Rippere, continue today to maintain – opinions on the determinants of illness and recovery that would not have been out of place in the sixteenth century.

However, it was not only the doctrine of the six non-naturals that commended the theory of humours. Taken as a whole, it did provide a coherent rationale for treatment, and, in particular, for prophylaxis, that at least in part corresponded to what the patient also might observe. Many diseases, for example, do have a seasonal pattern, attack certain age groups and not others, and appear to resolve following treatment. Congenital and chronic conditions, as the humoralists rightly declared, are harder to treat successfully than acute; equally, they are less obviously fatal. It might also be argued that by forcing the physician to consider the patient as a unity, mind as well as body, the theory of humours brought within one explanation a whole range of phenomena that are today frequently treated as discrete. It could embrace a psychosomatic explanation of illness as much, or as little, as an astrological one, and consider an individual's susceptibility to plague as no different from that to gout.

Above all, to the physician it offered the apparent certitude of an effective system of practice. Its very antiquity, even to Galen, helped to confirm its authority, and its failures could be laid at the door of its practitioners, or its victims, rather than of the system itself. Its regularity provided a method for controlling health and disease, by both intervention and prophylaxis, while at the same time its emphasis on the individuality of each patient and ultimately of each condition gave ample opportunity for practitioners to display their skills and their learning in understanding that individuality and in prescribing accordingly. Yet, as a system, it was sufficiently simple for many patients to grasp, and even thereby to treat themselves, and hence to join with their physician in a combined attack on disease. The very accessibility of humoralism may have helped to establish the credentials of those who put its theories into practice at the bedside, and has given the patient added confidence in what was being done, simply through being able to follow what was being said or prescribed. (➤ Ch. 34 History of the doctor–patient relationship)

The downfall of humoralism has been a long time coming and, given the resurgence of interest in holistic medicine, humoral medicine without the humours, it may be postponed for some time yet. The flexibility of humoralism, which makes any discussion of its therapeutics extremely difficult, may in the end enable it to adapt successfully to the discoveries of modern medicine. (➤ Ch. 16 Contagion/germ theory/specificity)

FURTHER READING

The theory of humours is discussed in all works on Greek medicine. Most of the Hippocratic texts cited are available in English in the Loeb Classical Library series, translated by W. H. S. Jones and Paul Potter, or in the Penguin Classics *Hippocratic Writings*, which has a valuable introduction by G. E. R. Lloyd. The exceptions are *On Diseases, IV* and *On Generation*, for which recourse must be had to the translation and commentary by I. M. Lonie, *The Hippocratic Treatises 'On Generation', 'On the Nature of the Child', 'Diseases, IV'*, Berlin and New York, De Gruyter, 1981. Lonie's introduction, pp. 54–70, provides a masterly discussion of the development of the theory of humours and its relationship to contemporary philosophy. See also:

Flashar, Helmut, *Melancholie und Melancholiker in den medizinischen Theorien der Antike*, Berlin, Weidemann, 1966.

Kudlien, Fridolf, *Der Beginn des medizinischen Denkens bei den Griechen*, Zurich and Stuttgart, Artemis, 1967.

Thivel, Antoine, *Cnide et Cos?*, Paris, Les Belles Lettres, 1981.

For the later development of the theory, see:

Saxl, Fritz, Panowsky, Erwin and Klibansky, Raymond, *Saturn and Melancholy*, London, Nelson, 1964; the French translation (Paris, Gallimard, 1989) incorporates a few, generally minor, updatings.

Schöner, Erich, *Das Viererschema in der antiken Humoralpathologie*, Wiesbaden, Steiner, 1964.

Sears, Elizabeth, *The Ages of Man: Medieval Interpretations of the Life Cycle*, Princeton, NJ, Princeton University Press, 1986 (esp. chs 1 and 5).

A detailed (although far from convincing) discussion of Galen's theory of humours in modern clinical terms is given by Rudolph E. Siegel, *Galen's System of Physiology and Medicine*, Basle and New York, Karger, 1968.

Better is C. M. Brooks, J. L. Gilbert, H. A. Levey and D. R. Curtis, *Humors, Hormones, and Neurosecretions*, New York, State University of New York, 1962. The many publications of the Hamdard Institute, Karachi, (for example, its journal *Hamdard Medicus*), endeavour to relate the humoral medicine of the Galenic/Arabic tradition to the discoveries of modern medical science, with very variable results.

The survival of humoralism in popular thought is studied by Cecil Helman, ' "Feed a cold and starve a fever" – folk models of infection in an English suburban community, and their relation to medical treatment', *Medicine and Society*, 1978, 2: 107–37; and by Vicky Rippere, 'The survival of traditional medicine in lay medical views: an empirical approach to the history of medicine', *Medical History*, 1981, 25: 411–14.

15

ENVIRONMENT AND MIASMATA

Caroline Hannaway

In the late twentieth century, the effect of the environment on health and disease is once more to the fore of medical thinking. As degenerative and chronic diseases have become the primary causes of morbidity and mortality in Western society, attention to the extra-corporeal agents affecting human physiology and pathology has grown. (➤ Ch. 9 The pathological tradition) The rise to prominence of cancer, particularly, in the pantheon of mortality agents has been linked in numerous ways to environmental changes. (➤ Ch. 25 Cancer) Both chemical and radioactive substances, for example, are the subject of sustained scrutiny because of their perceived consequences over time for the environment and for human well-being. The century-long primacy of the micro-organism in thinking about disease causation is being eroded. Yet, looking to the environment as a determining factor in health and disease is, in certain senses, a reinstatement of long-held beliefs seeking to link people's functioning, or malfunctioning, to conditions in the surrounding world. From the time of the Greeks to the nineteenth century, medical writers and practitioners, and also their patients, did not hesitate to make correlations between changes in the environment and the occurrence of disease. The particular aspects of external conditions that are singled out and the significance attached to them may have shifted over the centuries, but not the making of the linkage.

The attention given to the environment in disease causation and occurrence over this long period was part of the endeavour to find natural explanations for disease – that is those expressed in terms of elements in the human world – rather than supernatural explanations (those having recourse to gods, demons, or punishments for sin) as causative agents. This approach has been identified as coming to the fore with the efflorescence of Greek science and medicine beginning in the fifth century BC. A hallmark of Greek thinking was its promotion of natural explanations for the phenomena of the world. For Greek medical authors, the imbalance in the four humours of the body caused the symptoms that characterized ailments, but the question remained of what put the humours out of kilter in the first place. (➤ Ch. 14 Humoralism) The non-naturals – air, food and drink, sleep, exercise, evacuations, and passions of the mind – were the first line of explanation, but beyond these external factors impinging most essentially on bodily functioning loomed those in the larger world. In a naturalistic account, the linkage of endemic disease with topography and weather served to round out the understanding of why certain ailments seemed to occur in certain locations on a continuing basis. The explanation of outbreaks of epidemic disease (that is, ones that affected large numbers of people with similar symptoms at the same time) was also amplified by reference to circumstances in the larger world. Climatic changes related to changing seasons, and special meteorological events, were looked to for determining the causes of unexpected outbreaks of generalized disease. (➤ Ch. 52 Epidemiology)

ENVIRONMENT IN THE HIPPOCRATIC CORPUS

The founding text for medical perceptions of the role of the environment in health and disease is part of the Hippocratic Corpus (fifth century BC). *Airs, Waters, Places* is believed to have been written to enable the Greek peripatetic physicians to anticipate what diseases they were likely to encounter when beginning practice in a new, unfamiliar town. Prognosis and the decision of whether to treat patients were important considerations, and a careful analysis of all factors assisting in this process was requisite for making sound judgements. The title of the work indicates the components of the environment to which it was judged most attention should be paid. *Airs* referred to winds and climatic effects according to season; *Waters* included both spring waters from the ground, and water from rain and snow; *Places* referred to the location of the town and the character of its site.

Airs, Waters, Places contrasts the healthiness and prevalence of particular disease conditions in towns subject to winds from the four directions. To give an indication of the character of this work, in the Greek settings described, south winds are hot and more unhealthy, and north winds cold and linked to certain ailments. Locale is significant in the equation of towns and airs. The unhealthiest waters are marshy stagnant waters; slightly less unhealthy are spring waters from rocky sites or waters from the earth that are either hot or whose source is in the vicinity of minerals; the best waters flow from high places and earthy hills. Not only the location of springs, but also the direction in which they face is important. While rain-water is praised as light, sweet, fine, and clear, its capacity to grow foul quickly is cited.

Water from snow and ice are both regarded as bad for health. Seasonal changes also figure in the description of factors to be assessed in disease incidence. If the weather in the different seasons follows a certain pattern, the year should be healthy. Deviations from such a pattern are likely to bring about disease. Violent changes of seasons at solstices, equinoxes, or other turning-points of the year, demarcated by the rising or setting of certain stars, are especially unpropitious.[1]

Airs, Waters, Places does not offer a systematic plan for studying disease causation. None the less, recurring themes of disease discussion in the Western tradition stem from these Greek medical ideas. One is the interconnectedness of seasonal and climatic change and shifts in the patterns of diseases affecting humans. A second is the necessity for an appreciation of topography. It must be noted at this juncture that *Airs, Waters, Places* is not a unified work. Indeed, it has been conjectured that it represents an amalgam of two essays, perhaps originally by different authors. The first eleven chapters, whose contents have been indicated above, provide the physician with the prognostic indicators for understanding disease in particular locales; the other thirteen, which have lacunae, discuss the differences between the peoples of Europe and Asia. The latter chapters are more geographical and anthropological than medical in character, and describe the physical and cultural characteristics of peoples as conditioned by the environment as a whole. The ideas in the first part of *Airs, Waters, Places* have been more medically influential over the centuries, but the belief that environment affects culture has been interwoven with the discussion of the interaction of humours and airs, waters, and places since antiquity, and forms part of the larger consideration of human beings in relation to nature that permeates Western thought.[2]

Other environmentally oriented Hippocratic texts are those on epidemics. *Epidemics I* and *III* both have series of individual clinical histories prefaced by accounts of weather and seasonal change throughout the year, with indications of common diseases. Here are seen exemplified ideas that have long-lasting ramifications in medical history. The pattern of seasons in each geographical location described has associated with it certain known changes in weather that have consequences for human health.[3] It is important for practitioners to be aware of the atmospheric constitution of the year (that is, the combination of weather and climate that give a distinguishing character to a period of time) in their expectations of disease occurrrence and their prognoses of disease outcome. Like the linkage of weather and disease, the concept of an atmospheric constitution remained in medical use into the nineteenth century.

THE CONCEPT OF MIASMA

A concept important in the continuing medical discussion of the relation of the environment and disease has been that of miasma. An idea of great antiquity and of shifting allusion over time, its original Greek meaning related to pollution or polluting agent. This encompassed both the notions of staining or tainting and also of physical or moral defilement. In the Hippocratic writings, miasma acquired further shades of reference. In the attempt to explain epidemics naturalistically, and not as punishments for sin or defilement, the air became significant as the cause of disease outbreaks and its tainting by miasmas the reason why a disease affected a number of people at the same time. The Hippocratic text *On the Nature of Man*, in which the humoral theory is elaborated, makes reference to bad air as a factor in disease causation and indicates corrupting elements.[4]

The exact nature or character of these miasmas remained undefined, but general sources of the putrefaction of the air included stagnant marshes and pools, vapours from a variety of sources including corpses of humans and animals, sick persons, excreta, spoiled foodstuffs, decaying vegetable matter, and exhalations that came from the ground through ruptures or clefts. This list contains sources of corruption that remained standard over the centuries and, as one or more of its elements could always be identified in a disease situation, they could form part of any attempt at explanation of disease causation. As is clear, sources of bad smells are primary candidates for undermining the healthiness of the air. The unhealthiness of fetid waters and their corruption of neighbouring air also continued to loom large in the specification of disease-ridden locations. (➤ Ch. 18 Ecology of disease)

In discussion of miasmas, it could not easily be spelled out exactly how bad air transmitted disease. This had to remain conjectural. Analogies with procedures of dyeing cloth, the tainting of substances, the effects of poisons, and the growth of a fire from an initial spark – that is, the spread of change in a medium and the affecting of a whole after an initial disruption – were called upon to answer the vexed question of what happened to the air to make it pathological. Expressions of ideas about seeds of disease carried in the air, found in authors such as Galen (AD 129-*c*.200/210) and Varro (127–16 BC), when examined in the larger context of Greek and Roman literature, cannot be identified as ancient forerunners of later animalcular theories of disease.[5] In causes of sickness external to the body, miasmas were predominant until well into the nineteenth century. And, like miasmas, the Latin term '*infectio*', which has also had a long history of use in medicine, has many parallel shades of meaning and similar functions in medical explanations to its Greek counterpart.[6]

AETIOLOGICAL THEORIES IN THE MIDDLE AGES AND RENAISSANCE

The notions outlined thus far were part of the textual tradition that was passed directly and indirectly through Arabic sources to Western medicine of the early Middle Ages. Humoral and environmental causes of disease continued as the dominant modes of explanation, and where new phenomena were encountered these were most frequently explained within the light of the existing texts. Strictly speaking, classical environmental medicine was structured around the interplay of the humours and surrounding elements. In so far as the seasons were thought to have an impact on disease conditions, notice was taken of those extraterrestrial signs that marked the passage of the seasons, such as solstices, equinoxes, and the rising and setting of certain stars or groups of stars in relation to sunrise and sunset. In medieval Europe, the influence of planets and stars in presaging the onset of disease was more fully elaborated. Thus explanations of the Black Death or other outbreaks of the plague sometimes invoked conjunctions of planets as precipitating causes, although corrupt air remained the underlying and most significant cause of disease outbreaks, and individual balance of humours the arbiter of contraction or avoidance of disease.[7] It could be debated whether such heavenly influences were part of a natural environmental explanation.

The revival of interest in anatomy and dissection in the Renaissance that peaked with Andreas Vesalius (1514–64) opened the way to new knowledge about the structure of the body and its functioning. (➤ Ch. 5 The anatomical tradition) It had little effect on received ideas about disease causation and the role of the environment. The virulent spread of syphilis from the late fifteenth century inspired discussion of issues relating to contagion and the transmission of disease, most notably with Girolamo Fracastoro (1478–1553), and of whether new diseases unknown to the ancients could appear, but did not seriously challenge received wisdom. Likewise, the revolutionary discoveries of William Harvey (1578–1657) in physiology, which marked an intellectual break with ancient thought, did not immediately influence disease theory. (➤ Ch. 7 The physiological tradition) In fact, it was in seventeenth-century England that the most notable new interest in Hippocratic ideas and methods in the study and treatment of disease occurred through the ideas of Thomas Sydenham (1624–89) that would significantly influence the study of disease for a century and a half.

MEDICAL METEOROLOGY

Two aspects of Hippocratic doctrines re-emphasized by Sydenham in his various writings were the need to have clinical histories of disease by close observation of patients and the need to examine the environmental factors of weather and seasonal conditions in disease appearance and incidence. His goal was better and more specific therapy. Sydenham, however, wanted to go beyond the individual case histories of the sort presented in the Hippocratic Corpus, and suggested their compilation into natural histories of diseases on the model of those relating to plants. This endeavour led him to study epidemics prevalent in London from 1661 to 1675. Out of this investigation came his distinctive view of the epidemic constitution of the atmosphere. In Sydenham's account, the epidemic constitution imprints the epidemic diseases of any given time with a special character. His idea then went beyond the atmospheric constitution of the Greeks. Thus in the years 1665–66, when the plague broke out in London, other epidemic fevers at the time had a pestilential character as well. (➤ Ch. 19 Fevers) A pestilential fever producing epidemic constitution of the atmosphere was responsible. Sydenham developed this notion in addition to the use of humoral theory and accepted environmental factors in explaining disease. He never clarified the mechanism of the generation of this influence, but it remains a property of the air. He did not rule out as a possibility the influence of conjunctions of heavenly bodies, but perhaps emphasized more the influence of effluvia or miasmas emanating from the bowels of the earth, the latter a source of modifications of the air being stressed by other contemporaries such as Robert Boyle (1627–91).[8]

Sydenham's importance in retrospect has less to do with the novelty of his ideas about causes of disease than the project he advanced for an observationally based history of disease correlated with a study of atmospheric conditions and seasons. He was not only called upon in his native land but had a significant and, some claim, a greater influence in continental Europe. The name of the 'English Hippocrates', as well as that of the ancient one, was summoned in many explorations of the role of the environment in health and disease throughout the eighteenth century.

At the same time as Sydenham was putting forward his ideas, the growth of the experimental sciences transformed the way in which the atmosphere and weather were studied. The development of instruments such as the thermometer, barometer, and devices for measuring rainfall and wind velocity brought attempts to quantify the condition of the atmosphere. With this came an expectation of a quantified meteorology instead of the qualitative descriptive one prevailing before. Rather than eclipsing the classical environmental medicine of the Hippocratic tradition, the new instrument-based meteorology gave renewed vigour to the quest for correlations between disease outbreaks and environmental conditions. Thus was launched an endeavour that gained momentum through the eighteenth century.

Members of the Royal Society of London such as Christopher Wren

(1632–1723), Robert Boyle, and John Locke (1632–1704) began urging in the 1660s the systematic collection of meteorological data to understand weather patterns, and the fashion for keeping meteorological journals began. Certain individuals suggested allying to this enterprise the recording of prevalent diseases, but such an initiative did not begin in earnest in Great Britain until the second decade of the eighteenth century. From then on, many physicians and lay people in a variety of provincial locations and in the capital maintained series of daily meteorological observations for long periods, some for thirty years or more. Some also recorded the names of concomitant diseases, especially those of the epidemic variety. Among these observers were John Huxham (1692–1768) at Plymouth, a keeper of records for over thirty-four years; Thomas Short (1690?–1772) at Sheffield for over thirty-three years; Clifton Wintringham (1710–94) at York, twelve years; and John Fothergill (1712–80) in London, four years.[9]

England was not the only country in which medical meteorology took root. In other European countries, most notably in France but also in Italy, in parts of Germany, and in Scandinavia, recorders shouldered a daily burden of instrument-reading and less frequent disease notation for considerable periods. In Italy, Bernardino Ramazzini (1633–1714) analysed the environmental elements involved in the epidemic constitutions of his town, Modena, for the years from 1690 to 1694 and also maintained a meteorological journal. Early German interest is demonstrated by the study by Friedrich Hoffmann (1660–1742) of Halle's epidemic constitution in 1700. French activity was stimulated at mid-century by the advocacy of members of the Academy of Sciences for studying the history of epidemics and collecting meteorological data, and gathered strength for the rest of the century.[10]

Europe was not the boundary for the endeavour. Meteorological data were also collected in the territories colonized by Europeans. Both the Caribbean and North America were a source of quantified weather observations accompanied in some instances by notations of current diseases. For example, the records of William Hillary (1697–1763) from Barbados for the years 1752 to 1758 provide weather and disease data, as does *An Account of the Weather and Diseases of South Carolina* (1776) by Lionel Chalmers (1715–77).[11] The public forum for these records of individuals everywhere, besides their own published works, were the learned journals and transactions of scientific and medical societies, which were also proliferating at that time.

By mid-century, suggestions were put forward that the observations of weather and disease made by isolated individuals might yield more fruitful insights into the understanding of disease patterns if systematically organized. With observers and their territories co-ordinated, the incidence of disease and its relation to the weather in a whole region, state, or country, it was argued, would be more readily ascertained. Despite the expressed desire of certain physicians of the potential merits of having a whole-nation survey in Britain, the lack of an institution or governmental structure to direct such an enterprise negated this ambition. The French were more successful. The Royal Society of Medicine of Paris organized an extensive network of observers in every province of France in the mid-1770s, whose task it was to make thrice-daily recordings of weather conditions and keep detailed lists of current diseases. To standardize the data, tabular forms were issued and recommendations for the type and use of instruments distributed. The aim was to understand weather patterns and develop a complete map of disease in France. This large-scale project yielded substantial amounts of data before the demise of the Society during the Revolution, but no easy means of interpretation.[12] The investigation of the climatic factors in the environment's role in medicine had gained new impetus from the developments in meteorology, but it did not lead to clarification or modification of explanations of disease causation.

Few showed recognition that the outcome of data collection was not obvious. Medical minds of the eighteenth century saw the problems of medical meteorology largely as ones of execution. One perceived difficulty was the requirement for diligence on the part of observers. Incomplete or short-term records were naturally regarded as of much less value than systematic long-term ones, but many busy observers found it difficult to make two or three meteorological observations at the same time of day every day for years on end, and reliable self-recording instruments did not appear before the nineteenth century. Other difficulties related to the instruments themselves. Standardization was unknown for most of the eighteenth century either in the design or the calibration of the instruments. In its large-scale project referred to above, for instance, the only solution the Royal Society of Medicine of Paris saw to this problem was to use one instrument-maker for all instruments used by its multiple provincial observers.[13] Where and when to make recordings were also matters of debate. For example, some observers read their thermometers indoors while others made outdoor readings, thus making agreement on temperature level difficult.[14] Medical meteorologists believed that most problems would be resolved by continued and more-regulated collection of data. The larger question of whether insights had been gained from this mass of material into prediction of the weather and therefore of potentially unhealthy situations, particularly those conducive to epidemics, was voiced only at the turn of the nineteenth century.

Other problematic issues related to the manner in which diseases were recorded. The need to develop common ground in the naming of diseases to assist the comparative examinations of their prevalence in different places was recognized by the mid-eighteenth century, but agreement on concepts and terminology proved hard to achieve. Disease definition and description remained governed by symptom complexes, and debate continued over how these should be grouped in categories. Establishing natural histories of disease was not a straightforward task. The ubiquitous 'fever' designation still held sway. The classificatory systems of men such as François Boissier de Sauvages (1706–67) in mid-century, and later of William Cullen (1710–90), had little effect on the medical meteorological venture.[15] (➤ Ch. 17 Nosology)

Then, too, while meteorological observations had acquired numerical values, disease observations had not. They remained at the level of generalized statements listing the diseases perceived to be common in a time period. Medical statistics to indicate incidence of disease were a product of the nineteenth century. No systematic registers of morbidity expressed in quantitative terms were maintained anywhere in Europe or elsewhere in the eighteenth century. Only particular institutions such as hospitals might be able to develop such information, and then only that pertaining to inmate populations. Some cities were certainly keeping records of births and deaths. The London Bills of Mortality, appearing sporadically in the sixteenth century and published regularly after 1603, are the best known, and there were calls for improving their accuracy and content in the middle of the eighteenth century, with an eye to making correlations with weather findings. But these suggestions were not pursued. Other European cities in Germany and France also began keeping data on population and causes of death, and Sweden set up a census in 1748.[16] (➤ Ch. 71 Demography and medicine) The concern of states for the health and welfare of their citizens according to mercantilist thinking was a spur to such initiatives. Contemporaries, however, could not utilize these records, even when available, to test larger hypotheses about patterns of disease, let alone the linkage of weather and disease. Inadequate mathematical tools proved to be the limiting factors in this instance.

MEDICAL TOPOGRAPHY AND GEOGRAPHY

In the interplay of the environment and health and disease, in addition to weather and seasonal changes, the Greek sources of environmental medicine had stressed locale. Certain town sites were unhealthier than others or more subject to particular disease problems because of their exposure to particular winds or because of their proximity to bodies of water regarded as likely sources of corruption of the air. The importance of an appreciation of location in matters of health was never entirely lost sight of, but these ideas took on new vigour in the enthusiastic revival of the exploration of disease and environment in the eighteenth century.

The concern with the medicine of places is seen in the growing popularity in the period of a genre known as the medical topography. These works usually focused on a specific town, sometimes a region, and described to a greater or lesser degree, depending on the author's abilities and resources, a wide range of elements in the surroundings and the environment that might impinge on health and disease. These could include the physical and geographical characteristics of the town or region's situation; the climate; the plants and animals common in the vicinity; the sources of water; the products of the area; the physical characteristics, way of life, and occupations of its inhabitants; the general size, layout, and institutions of the town; sanitary conditions; the number of residents, and the patterns of births and deaths, if such records were available; and, last but not least, the prevalent diseases. As this listing indicates, the range of factors considered worthy of notation has been much expanded beyond airs, waters, and places. In their exhaustive detail relating to locale, eighteenth-century medical topographies went much beyond the sketchier classical descriptions for the regions of Thessaly and Thrace. Social and hygienic aspects of the environment had now come into play.

While the Italians were amongst the pioneers of this genre of medical literature in the later seventeenth century – Ramazzini's work of 1695 on Modena is cited approvingly, for example – it was in the 1730s and 1740s that work began to proliferate delineating the medical topography of large numbers of towns and regions. Authors in all countries of both western and eastern Europe, and also in European colonies overseas, made contributions to what became an abundant literature.[17]

Many examples could be cited, but two initiatives should perhaps be singled out for expanding the topographical concept. The French deserve notice for going beyond the local or regional and seeking to understand disease distribution and prevalence, particularly for epidemic diseases, on a national scale. In the 1770s and 1780s, under the aegis of the Royal Society of Medicine of Paris, the attempt was made to develop a medical topographical appreciation of the entire country, and more than 225 memoirs covering most regions were collected.[18] The intervention of the French Revolution prevented the continuation of this project, and also of the organizers having to confront squarely the issue of what inferences they could draw from the copious information obtained. In Germany, the writing of topographies led to a more ambitious project and a change in scope of the genre. A series of topographies of individual German towns from the 1750s onwards culminated in a three-volume work by Leonhard Ludwig Finke (1747–1828) published in 1792–5. Finke's work was no longer entitled a medical topography, but a medical geography. In it, he sought to go beyond the boundaries of nations and understand disease and the environment on a worldwide scale.[19] Finke had certain difficulties in the execution of his work, and some information was extracted from travel literature, but it is not so much the book's content that is significant as the inspiration it gave to further investigations in the larger arena of medical geography. To name only one, in the German tradition, a link can be made between Finke and the massive compilation of August Hirsch (1817–94) entitled *Handbuch der historisch-geographischen Pathologie*, published in two volumes in 1859 and 1864. On the eve of the germ theory of disease, Hirsch sought to, first, describe the occurrence, distribution, and types of disease at different time periods and in various locations around the world; and second, to examine the relationship between these diseases and the environment in which those suffering from these diseases lived.[20] The appearance of this work in the mid-nineteenth century may in some respects seem surprising, but in fact medical topographical and geographical studies continued to be produced for a large part of the nineteenth century. Examination of the environment continued to loom large in disease aetiology until the theory of micro-organisms as causative agents became persuasive enough to hold sway. (➤ Ch. 16 Contagion/germ theory/specificity)

DISEASE AND ENVIRONMENT – THE NEW WORLD

The attempt to locate disease geographically, to which medical topographies and geographies are a testament, is in some senses the endpoint of an evolution in approach to disease that had begun with the Greeks. But at first sight this literature, especially the topographical, seems to make an analysis of environment and disease more confused. The interaction certainly becomes more complex. Medical topography includes all elements in the environment that might impinge on disease. However, the greater prominence of social and hygienic matters was to have an effect. The change that was eventually to make a difference in the discussion of disease causation was a movement from the traditional large-scale factors in the environment that were implicated in disease, and a focusing on more-specific ones.

The energy expended on investigating the relationship between disease and the environment documented in the quest for medical meteorology and the rise to prominence of medical topography was also fuelled by elements beyond those already described. From the sixteenth century on, European perceptions of the world were tempered by exposure to new climes. The opening of the New World and the imperial ambitions generated had changed the face of European politics and life. The struggle for power by European nation states led to the growth of navies and the conquest and colonization of territory in the Americas, the West and East Indies, Africa, India, and the Pacific. This expansion impinged on medicine in a number of ways. Of special note was the necessity for ensuring the health and well-being of soldiers and sailors in foreign lands and at sea for longer periods of time. In addition, the perception of detrimental mortality among colonists, and also slaves, inspired the detailed examination of weather, topography, and disease in new and very different environments to develop strategies for disease avoidance and therapy. (➤ Ch. 58 Medicine and colonialism)

By the eighteenth century, medical inquiries into these matters were regularly made at first hand. European-trained practitioners travelled with navies, accompanied troops garrisoned in new territories, and set up practice in colonies. During their overseas experience, they encountered different diseases, most notably yellow fever, but also others such as tetanus, yaws, and elephantiasis; they saw known ailments in new settings; and they tried to make sense of the patterns of incidence observed. Among the worrisome questions they had to confront were how to explain the causes of the heavy morbidity and mortality afflicting new arrivals, and the larger issue this raised of whether Europeans could adapt successfully to life in these very different environments.[21] (➤ Ch. 24 Tropical diseases)

In response to these colonial experiences, medical thinking on the environment and disease was modified. Clearly, the reports of these medical voyagers were a factor in the move to an expansionist view of the world and disease represented in the medical geographies. They also led to suggestions that changes in nosology were needed to accommodate new disease experiences, but the conviction that elements in the environment were significant in explaining the abundance of disease was in no way undermined; instead, in many senses, it was reinforced. Much of the colonial experience took place in the tropical zones, where the problems of coping with the effects of heat and humidity, noticeable in every aspect of life, powerfully impressed all observers. Moreover, the intense nature of these climatic factors was confirmed by measurements on the new eighteenth-century weather-recording instruments.

The medical response to the torrid conditions was, in fact, the development of a substantive literature on diseases of hot climates. *Essays on Diseases Incidental to Europeans in Hot Climates* by James Lind (1716–94) and published in 1768 is the best-known example of works on this topic. Other European powers had their contributors to the discussion as well – witness *Observations générales sur les maladies des climats chauds* by the Frenchman Jean Dazille (1732–1812) and published in 1785 – and a body of other authors from the seventeenth century wrote, sometimes at length, on particular locales.[22] In most of these works the palpably hostile climate figures as the primary cause of the multiple maladies besetting those transplanted to the tropics, throwing their bodily functioning into disarray. Other established causes such as stagnant waters and marshes also played a leading part as sources of the corruption of the air, especially under the strong rays of the sun, and the tropical environment was notable for the speed with which putrefaction set in in dead humans, animals, and plants – further sources of noxious miasmas. These elements, combined with the fact that European humoral sensibilities were naturally adapted to more temperate zones, were all called upon to explain the pathogenic nature of tropical climes.

The inability to control the climate or the geography meant that self-preservation or avoidance of disease had to focus on specific elements in the personal environment. The siting of housing on higher ground with ventilation designed to take advantage of winds, and changes in clothing and food, were among the primary recommendations for settlers. (➤ Ch. 53 History of personal hygiene) Other suggestions involved transfer to less deleterious locales. This advice, aimed at protecting the lives of troops stationed in the tropics, involved periods of respite in drier and preferably cooler locales. Works on military and naval medicine stemming from the colonial experience also emphasized the necessity for hygiene of location in maintenance of the health of personnel. The expansion of the world, then, did not undercut environmental medicine as a theory, but it did lead to an emphasis on attempted control of social and hygienic factors in the environment as the way to prevent disease.

THE AIR AS THE CAUSE OF DISEASE

As indicated thus far, elements in the environment remained closely linked with disease causation until well into the nineteenth century. The long heritage of Greek ideas of the significance of climate and place was accompanied by the belief that corruption of the air was an important factor in the explanation of disease, although the ways in which this occurred or its implications for disease transmission remained open to debate. The elusive concept of miasmas also maintained its place in the description of how the air was disrupted and caused disease by impinging on the humoral balance of individuals. Sources of such miasmas had been identified in classical times, many of them materials or situations creating a stench.

In the eighteenth-century revival of Hippocratic ideas, the atmosphere gained a predominant place. The air had moved to the forefront of scientific and medical attention in several ways. Beginning in the mid-seventeenth century, the physical properties of air were increasingly understood by experiments with the barometric tube and the air-pump. Air was shown to have its own physical law that related its pressure to its volume (Boyle's Law), and the pressure of atmospheric air came to be routinely measured by the barometer. Air became a quantifiable entity. That air was an essential component of life was dramatically demonstrated in animal experiments using the air-pump, but the essential ingredient for life was usually attributed to something in the air such as nitro-aerial spirits.[23]

In the mechanical view of air espoused by such figures as Boyle, the air was a matrix that could receive and contain minute corpuscles, spirits, and effluvia, some of which could be causative agents of disease. Boyle himself placed emphasis on subterranean emanations as implicated in disease.[24]

The influence of the experimental investigations of air are clearly seen in *An Essay concerning the Effects of Air on Human Bodies*, of 1733, by John Arbuthnot (1667–1735). He introduced such quantitative measures as atmospheric pressure and air density into the properties that define an environmental constitution. The air had a particularly important role in epidemic diseases for Arbuthnot because the human body continually absorbed air through its pores as well as breathing it. In addition to the properties and qualities of the air that are constantly changing, he pointed to the specific influence of emanations from the earth and waters that are constant at a given site. Arbuthnot believed that these latter might be subject to chemical analysis.[25]

The air itself became an object of chemical investigation in the second half of the eighteenth century. Building on the techniques and insights of Stephen Hales (1677–1761), who showed that air could be fixed in solid bodies, investigators such as Joseph Black (1728–99) and Joseph Priestley (1733–1804) demonstrated that atmospheric air was in fact a mixture of 'airs' or gases that had very different properties. Only one-fifth of the air, it turned out, was fit to support life, whilst the remaining four-fifths extinguished it. The former was known to Priestley as 'eminently respirable air', and Antoine Lavoisier (1743–94) would later call it oxygen. In addition to the distinction and isolation of the components of the atmosphere, many new artificially prepared 'airs' were collected and studied. Not only did the new pneumatic chemistry bring about a knowledge of new species of air, it also engendered a new confidence in the isolation and handling of gases.[26]

A direct application of these developments was the construction of the eudiometer, an instrument designed to measure the goodness of air. Such instruments, which varied in design and principle, were constructed so as to give a quantitative measure of the respirable part of the air. Priestley, Jan Ingenhousz (1730–99), and Felice Fontana (1730–1805) were leading designers of eudiometers, whose application in determining healthy or unhealthy environments was widely urged. They were deployed, above all, in enclosed spaces such as theatres, gaols, and hospitals, which could be particularly unhealthy environments.[27] The failure of the instrument, however, to register significant differences in the respirability of the air in different locations cut off the heralded promise that the new pneumatic chemistry held out for medicine. In fact, what this failure meant for the causation of disease was a turning away from the chemical composition of the atmosphere and a renewed emphasis on the evanescent miasmas.

The tracking down of the miasmas, which resisted detection by scientific instruments, invariably led back to their perceived source in a particular locale. What usually revealed their presence was a smell.[28] For this reason, such fetid sites as graveyards, tanneries, refuse dumps, cesspools, and so on, became the foci of attention of health reformers towards the end of the eighteenth and the beginning of the nineteenth centuries. There developed strong movements to clean these sites up. (➤ Ch. 51 Public health) It should not be thought that this increased emphasis on local and specific sites of contamination of the air was at the cost of the more global concepts of environmental medicine that had descended from the Greeks. The latter would remain a part of medical theory well into the second half of the nineteenth century, but practitioners with responsibility for public health increasingly came to concentrate on those more specific and localized sources of corruption that had always had a place in the larger theory. Down this path lay a new theory of disease causation in which the environment had a much lesser part.

NOTES

1   *Airs, Waters, Places*, in Hippocrates, *Works*, trans. by W. H. S. Jones, 2 vols, London, Heinemann, and New York, G. P. Putnam's Sons, 1923, Vol. I, pp. 65–137. For discussion about *Airs, Waters, Places*, see Genevieve Miller, ' "Airs, Waters, and Places" in history', *Journal of the History of Medicine and Allied Sciences*, 1962, 17: 129–40.

2   For the theme of human beings and their relationship to nature, see Clarence J. Glacken, *Traces on the Rhodian Shore: Nature and Culture in Western Thought from Ancient Times to the End of the Eighteenth Century*, Berkeley and Los Angeles, University of California Press, 1967. For Glacken's comments on *Airs, Waters and Places*, see pp. 82–8.

3   *Epidemics I* and *III*, in Hippocrates, *Works*, op. cit. (n. 1), pp. 139–287.

4   Owsei Temkin, 'An historical analysis of the concept of infection', in Temkin, *The Double Face of Janus and Other Essays in the History of Medicine*, Baltimore and London, Johns Hopkins University Press, 1977, pp. 457, 461; Vivian Nutton, 'The seeds of disease: an explanation of cantagion and infection from the Greeks to the Renaissance', *Medical History*, 1983, 27: 1–34, pp. 3, 13.

5   Nutton, ibid., pp. 1–11.

6   Temkin, op. cit. (n. 4), p. 457.

7   Nancy Siraisi, *Medieval and Early Renaissance Medicine: an Introduction of Knowledge and Practice*, Chicago, IL, and London, University of Chicago Press, 1990, pp. 128–9.

8   Kenneth Dewhurst, *Dr Thomas Sydenham (1624–1689): His Life and Original Writings*, Berkeley and Los Angeles, University of California Press, 1966, especially pp. 60–7; E. A. Winslow, *The Conquest of Epidemic Disease: a Chapter in the History of Ideas*, New York and London, Hafner, 1967, pp. 161–75.

9   Gordon Manley, 'The weather and diseases: some eighteenth-century contributions to observational meteorology', *Notes and Records of the Royal Society*, 1952, 9: 300–7; James C. Riley, *The Eighteenth-Century Campaign to Avoid Disease*, New York, St Martin's Press, 1987, pp. 19–20, 26–9; Frederick Sargent II, *Hippocratic*

Heritage: a History of Ideas about Weather and Human Health, New York and Oxford, Pergamon, 1982, pp. 292–5.

10 Riley, op. cit. (n. 9), pp. 32–4.

11 Sargent, op. cit. (n. 9), pp. 308, 311–19.

12 Caroline Hannaway. 'The Société Royale de Médecine and epidemics in the Ancien Régime', *Bulletin of the History of Medicine*, 1972, 46: 267–8.

13 Ibid., p. 268; Manley, op. cit. (n. 9), pp. 303–4.

14 Manley, op. cit. (n. 9), p. 302.

15 W. F. Bynum, 'Cullen and the study of fevers in Britian, 1760–1820', in W. F. Bynum and Vivian Nutton (eds), *Theories of Fever from Antiquity to the Englighten-ment, Medical History*, suppl. 1, London, Wellcome Institute for the History of Medicine, 1981, pp. 135–48.

16 Riley, op. cit. (n. 9), ch. 3.

17 Riley, op. cit. (n. 9), pp. 32–4, 42–4.

18 Hannaway, op. cit. (n. 12), pp. 267–8.

19 George Rosen, 'Leonhard Ludwig Finke and the first medical geography', in E. A. Underwood (ed.), *Science, Medicine, and History: Essays in Honour of Charles Singer*, 2 vols, London, Oxford University Press, 1953; Riley, op. cit. (n. 9), pp. 40–1.

20 Sargent, op. cit. (n. 9), pp. 269–79.

21 For discussion of acclimatization, see, for example, Karen O. Kupperman, 'Fear of hot climates in the Anglo-American colonial experience', *William and Mary Quarterly*, 1984, 41: 213–40.

22 Lind's work is described by Sargent, op. cit. (n. 9), pp. 196–200; and Bynum, op. cit. (n. 15), pp. 141–3.

23 Steven Shapin and Simon Schaffer, *Leviathan and the Air-Pump: Hobbes, Boyle, and the Experimental Life*, Princeton, NJ, Princeton University Press, 1985.

24 Riley, op. cit. (n. 9), pp. 9–13.

25 John Arbuthnot, *An Essay Concerning the Effects of Air on Human Bodies*, London, 1733; Riley, op. cit. (n. 9), pp. 10, 17–26.

26 Owen and Caroline Hannaway, 'La fermeture des innocents: le conflit entre la vie et la mort', *Dix-huitième siècle*, 1977, 9: 181–91.

27 A recent discussion of eudiometry is Simon Schaffer, 'Measuring virtue: eudi-ometry, enlightenment and pneumatic medicine', in Andrew Cunningham and Roger French (eds), *The Medical Enlightenment of the Eighteenth Century*, Cam-bridge, Cambridge University Press, 1990, pp. 281–318.

28 The concern with removal of smells is discussed fully in Alain Corbin, *The Foul and the Fragrant: Odor and the French Social Imagination*, trans. by Mirian Kochal Cambridge, MA, Harvard University Press, 1986. See also Riley, op. cit. (n. 9), ch. 5.

FURTHER READING

Airs, Waters and Places, Epidemics I and *III*, in Hippocrates, *Works*, trans. by W. H. S. Jones, Loeb Classical Library, London, Heinemann, and New York, G. P. Putnam's Sons, 1923, Vol. I.

Cassedy, James, 'Meteorology and medicine in colonial America: beginnings of the experimental approach', *Journal of the History of Medicine and Allied Sciences*, 1969, 24: 193–204.

Corbin, Alain, *The Foul and the Fragrant: Odor and the French Social Imagination*, trans. by Miriam Kocham *et al.*, Cambridge, MA, Harvard University Press, 1986.

Dewhurst, Kenneth, *Dr Thomas Sydenham (1624–1689): His Life and Original Writings*, London, Wellcome Institute, and Berkeley and Los Angeles, University of California Press, 1966.

Glacken, Clarence J., *Traces on the Rhodian Shore: Nature and Culture in Western Thought from Ancient Times to the End of the Eighteenth Century*, Berkeley and Los Angeles, University of California Press, 1967.

Jordanova, L. J. 'Earth science and environmental medicine: the synthesis of the late enlightenment', in Jordanova and Roy S. Porter (eds), *Images of the Earth: Essays in the History of the Environmental Sciences*, London, British Society for the History of Science, 1979, pp. 119–46.

Kupperman, Karen Ordahl, 'Fear of hot climates in the Anglo-American colonial experience', *William and Mary Quarterly*, 1984, 41: 213–40.

Miller, Genevieve, ' "Airs, Waters, and Places" in history', *Journal of the History of Medicine and Allied Sciences*, 1962, 17: 129–40.

Nutton, Vivian, 'The seeds of disease: an explanation of contagion and infection from the Greeks to the Renaissance', *Medical History*, 1983, 27: 1–34.

Riley, James C., *The Eighteenth-Century Campaign to Avoid Disease*, New York, St Martin's Press, 1987.

Sargent, Frederick II, *Hippocratic Heritage: a History of Ideas about Weather and Human Health*, New York and Oxford, Pergamon Press, 1982.

Temkin, Owsei, 'An historical analysis of the concept of infection', in Temkin, *The Double Face of Janus and Other Essays in the History of Medicine*, Baltimore, MD, and London, Johns Hopkins University Press, 1977, pp. 456–71.

Winslow, Charles-Edward Amory, *The Conquest of Epidemic Disease: a Chapter in the History of Ideas*, New York and London, Hafner, 1967.

16

CONTAGION/GERM THEORY/ SPECIFICITY

Margaret Pelling

The terms contagion and infection, although vague, convey a relatively straightforward meaning to the twentieth-century lay person. They refer to the fact that certain diseases, caused by living organisms, are passed from one person to another. It would generally be assumed that contagion is direct, by contact, and infection indirect, through the medium of water, air, or contaminated articles. Both are comprehended in the apparently simple question, is it catching? However, as recent attempts at health education in respect of AIDS have shown, this question is not simple at all. Moreover, 'infection' is applied in a more general sense; for example, for clean wounds that 'go bad'. Each concept has a long and complex history, which was temporarily simplified by the triumphs of bacteriology in the later nineteenth century. The twentieth century inherited a story involving a striking contrast, between the germ theorists (scientific, laboratory based, objective) and the sanitarians (bureaucratic, unscientific, politically motivated, bringing about improvement almost accidentally). The latter were miasmatists and believed that smells caused disease. (➤ Ch. 15 Environment and miasmata) This story, based primarily upon the two main phases of the British public-health movement, was reinforced by medical historians searching for early believers in germ theory who could be portrayed as lonely pioneers in a struggle between opposite points of view.[1] (➤ Ch. 51 Public health)

This retrospective account had many attractive features. It implied that the decline of infectious diseases was brought about by scientific progress in the field of medicine.[2] It laid stress on the importance of instrumentation, especially microscopy. (➤ Ch. 6 The microscopical tradition) Interest in germ theory appeared to have burgeoned with the renewed scientific spirit first of the Renaissance and then of the seventeenth and nineteenth centuries.[3] However, there were also many problems. One was that the classical world, in spite of laying the groundwork for modern science, did not appear to have evolved a concept of contagion. A second was that the status of the contributions of the early pioneers, notably Girolamo Fracastoro (1478–1553), has proved difficult to determine from the scientific point of view. Most importantly, detailed analysis has tended to show that even 'germ theorists' used the concepts of contagion, infection, and miasma as if they were difficult to distinguish, overlapping, or even interchangeable.

THE PROBLEM OF DEFINITION

If there is a single explanation for this difficulty it lies in the need for precise definition. As in the case of other long-lived and related concepts – for example, 'germ', 'species', 'virus', and 'spontaneous generation' – the concepts of contagion, infection, and miasma accumulated layers of connotation over time. Each period added its own attempts at definition, but was inevitably affected by the previous history of the concept. Attempts to replace such terminology for the sake of clarity usually failed.[4] It should be stressed that the historian's difficulty in arriving at workable definitions is often a reflection of contemporary lack of definition. For a number of reasons, this area of debate was particularly subject to confusion and ambiguity. In addition, many writers deliberately exploited this confusion, using over-simplification either to discredit ideas or to force their acceptance. One obvious way of doing this was not to distinguish between the new version of the concept, and the old.[5]

The first point of definition that needs to be made is that it is misleading to regard these concepts as purely medical. They have had a wide currency in a range of areas of thought and practice, which is reflected in an accretion of metaphor and analogy. Most of these analogies were not irrelevant to, but were part of, the argument. As we shall see, contagion and infection are intimately bound up with basic concepts of matter and purpose in the natural world, and at one level can be seen as part of élite culture. However, they are also closely related to (a) folk belief and practice; (b) practical experience in agriculture, horticulture, animal husbandry, and technologies such as dyeing and wine-making; (c) different crises of epidemic disease and shifts in the prevalence of endemic diseases at different periods; and (d) political, economic and epistemological conditions at a given time influencing the relationship between 'theory' and 'practice'. Ideas of contagion are inseparable from notions of individual morality, social responsibility, and collective action. This is shown most strikingly in respect of measures of isolation and quarantine, and the public health movements subsequent to industrialization.

CONCEPTS OF CONTAGION

The 'person-to-person' emphasis of the post-bacteriological period might lead us to see concepts of contagion as dependent upon high-density living or urbanization. (➤ Ch. 27 Diseases of civilization) However, it is more accurate to see contagion as reflecting the relationship between things in the world, as well as the influence upon human beings of factors in close and remote spheres of their environment. (➤ Ch. 18 Ecology of disease) In analysing humanity's situation, the classical period adopted a structure of causation which was elaborated in subsequent periods and continues to be relevant today. The history of the concept of contagion cannot be understood without reference to this traditional multifactorial structure of natural and supernatural causation, the validity of which was briefly obscured by the bacteriological period and by advocates of laboratory medicine. Laboratory science was successful in severely restricting, and hence manipulating, the number of factors involved in causing the phenomenon under investigation. Modern Western medical science has proceeded not by supplying full explanations, but by a process of specialization in which some categories of cause have been ignored or eliminated. In the later twentieth century, with the decline of most infectious diseases in the developed world, and the transition to chronic and degenerative diseases as dominant causes of death, there has been a gradual return to multifactorial explanations of disease more in accordance with traditional concepts. The 'exclusivity' of bacteriology was challenged by clinicians and epidemiologists from as early as the turn of this century.[6] It is arguable, however, that many medical scientists are still inclined to habits of thought which have also persuaded the lay person to expect both single-factor causes of disease and their corollary, 'magic bullets', as specific cures for such diseases. (➤ Ch. 39 Drug therapies)

This artificial simplicity in the explanation of disease is well represented by the aphorism of John Snow (1813–58), a major English epidemiologist: 'to be of the human species, and to receive the morbid poison in a suitable manner, is most likely all that is required'.[7] This formula seems inspired as well as straightforward in its attribution of cause and effect. However, even this statement is not as simple as it appears. What did it mean to receive the poison in a suitable manner? Why, if effect simply followed cause, was not everyone who was exposed to disease affected by it? To his contemporaries, there was a range of additional questions that Snow was simply choosing to ignore. Why did diseases prevail in some places and not others? Why did epidemics – or pandemics – rise and then decline, and affect the world at some times and not at others? Does disease consist of stimuli affecting the body, or the body's reaction to these stimuli? By the nineteenth century, these were long-established questions, which could be made to correspond to the traditional structure of causation. As in the case of Snow, conflicting views were often an effect of concentrating upon one among the possible range of causes at the expense of the others. (➤ Ch. 9 The pathological tradition)

Classical philosophy and epistemology made available to medicine an elaborate structure of explanation involving a hierarchy of causes.[8] First or primary causes were cosmological or divine (for example, the influence of stars and planets, the wrath of God or gods), and were more obviously subject to religious controversy. (➤ Ch. 61 Religion and medicine) The refusal to consider primary or remote causes is usually seen as an aspect of secularization and is identified with periods of particular conflict in Western thought between religion and science, but as a strategy it dates back to the classical period.[9] Remote causes related to the state of the atmosphere, or influences (such as volcanic action or the weather) broad enough in scope to bring about the rise and fall of epidemics. The 'epidemic constitution' of Thomas Sydenham (1624–89) is an example.[10] Exciting, efficient, or immediate causes related primarily to the more local environment or experiences of the diseased person, and were generally congruent with the 'non-naturals'. They could include factors such as diet, emotion (stress), or exposure to weather, but also injury, poisons, or other more specific agents of disease. Predisposing causes could overlap with this category, but were also invoked to cover characteristics of the individual's life or heredity that might render him or her unusually liable to a given disease. (➤ Ch. 20 Constitutional and hereditary disorders) Proximate causes came closest to defining the diseased state or process occurring in the diseased body.[11] Different periods are distinguished less by their answers to these questions, than by the questions that were selected as the most important. The first bacteriological explanations of disease in the nineteenth century tended to ignore proximate and predisposing causes, as well as primary causes, a strategy of which contemporaries were well aware, and which fuelled both resistance and reaction.

It follows that to compare a belief in epidemic constitutions with a belief in germ theory is not necessarily to compare like with like. Similarly, 'miasma' would tend to describe a more general level of cause, relating to locality, compared with contagion, which could best be seen as an exciting cause. Infection might be seen as bridging these two levels of cause. It should be stressed that an agent in one category of cause could be seen as also belonging to, or changing into, another category, as a result of a given set of circumstances. Causes could act singly or in concert in any given instance of disease. This traditional, inclusive form of analysis was often used tacitly or imperfectly, but was remarkably persistent. It helps to explain why in historical terms contagion and miasma have been more readily seen by theorists as alternative or complementary, rather than contradictory, factors in disease.

The notion of contagion also involved the question of how properties or qualities were transferred or propagated at the level of the ultimate constituents of matter. Contagion described an event in which an influence was 'increased' in some way. Historians of medicine looking for precursors of the germ theory tended to identify this increase as a crucial feature and one which should have suggested a form of multiplication peculiar to living organisms. It is, however, anachronistic to look at older ideas in this manner. The properties of living organisms were constantly being redefined and the boundaries between living and non-living entities constantly shifting. In the seventeenth century, for example, minerals were thought to grow in the earth, which could itself be seen as animate; and, as exploited by Donne ('Yea plants, yea stones detest/And love'), magnets apparently possessed some of the properties of life.[12] Multiplication was not definitively biological; the term 'biology' was itself not introduced until the late eighteenth century.[13] The enormous variety of complex phenomena involving such lower organisms as insects, parasites, and worms meant that different versions of the concept of spontaneous generation survived into the twentieth century.[14] Thus one form of life could dissolve by putrefaction, only to give rise to other forms. Moreover, multiplication did not need to be a material process. A range of concepts was available to describe phenomena involving the propagation of influence by 'action at a distance': the eye, for example, could transmit occult qualities affecting another individual.[15]

It is not too grandiose to relate views on contagion to classical philosophies regarded as basic to Western science. Natural philosophers of later periods theorized in the consciousness of alternatives stemming from Epicureanism and Aristotelianism, this was summarized by Cyril Dean Darlington (1903–81), a twentieth-century geneticist deploring the divorce between science and philosophy, as the choice between 'purpose and particles'. Aristotelianism is identified with biological models, Epicureanism or Greek atomism with physics. For Darlington, modern science represented a paradox: Aristotelianism and therefore teleology had been far more fruitful in the development of science, but modern scientific achievements, based on the atom, the molecule, the gene, and the organism, had endorsed instead the principles of Epicurus (341–270 BC) and Lucretius (c.99–c.55 BC).[16] In spite of its reference to the as-yet mysterious activities of living organisms, bacteriology came to be associated with this materialist, atomistic view of nature. As we shall see, some of those who theorized about contagion at different periods naturally gravitated towards views involving particles, of whom Fracastoro, for example, was avowedly Lucretian. For others, however, the myriad particles that might best explain the phenomena of infectious disease were most analogous to swarms of insects or other lower organisms, which had independent powers of movement.[17]

Certain homely analogies recur in the history of contagion. One example is that of rotting fruit: the observation that decay spread from one part of a fruit to another, and from one fruit to the next if they were in contact. Another persistent and even more important point of reference was the process of fermentation, especially of wine. Different interpretations of putrefaction and fermentation have been fundamental to theories of epidemic disease. Analogies to these processes were detected inside as well as outside the body. In each case, everyday events repeatedly demonstrated how a part could inform or affect the whole. Other analogies were found in the spread of odours, or the effects of the vapours of marshes, caves, and mines – what would now be ascribed to the laws of diffusion of gases. (Odours, it may be pointed out, are still little understood though some are of considerable potency.) Similar properties could be attributed to the animal breath. A final source of analogy, important in the classical period but relevant to homoeopathic ideas, was the effect of dyes in water, in which a small amount of material transmitted its main property to the whole mass. Parallels were constantly drawn between the spread of disease and the effects of poisons, where again an often tiny dose was able to affect the whole body, or to poison a well. The historical reference to poisons, including animal poisons such as the venom of snakes, is reflected in the co-option into the present day of the term 'virus'.[18] Predictably, historians have laid emphasis on terms used in the explanation of disease that seem to be biologically related – the two obvious examples being 'seed' and 'germ'. As already indicated, it is a matter of precise analysis of any given historical context (and of the appropriate language) to clarify whether these terms were being used so as to suggest the attributes of organisms in anything like the modern sense. The combination of bacteriology and popular belief has produced a simple equation between 'germ' and (fully developed) 'disease-causing organism'. Historically, however, 'germ' was borrowed from discussions to do with generation, growth, and differentiation. In the hands of nineteenth-century writers, it was applied to disease causation particularly in terms of the evolution of bodily products (including cells) into discrete entities capable of causing disease in a second person. In this context, 'germs' were by definition *not* fully developed organisms capable of causing disease; instead, some process of 'germination' was required, often outside the body, and with it a range of other factors or causes, usually environmental, before disease could result.

In the above discussion, it will be seen that attention readily shifts between agency and process in disease. This reflects another major difficulty in distinguishing concepts of contagion, infection, and miasma. Confusion arises from failure to distinguish between the *material* or *influence* (living or non-living) which is transmitted between persons or environments, and the *process* of transmission or affection, direct or indirect. Historically, there has been a tendency for contagion to imply the former, and infection the latter, but considerable freedom of usage has blurred this seemingly straightforward distinction.

THE CONCEPT OF SPECIFICITY

Specificity is another concept with a long history that has been subject to oversimplification.[19] Because animals and plants are said to belong to species, specificity in disease is readily seen simply as a function of causation by living organisms. The effect of the principles for the isolation of disease agents known as 'Koch's postulates' is for the presence of a given disease to be defined by the presence of a given bacterial or viral organism.[20] The twentieth-century lay person hardly sees it as appropriate to apply the concept of specificity to congenital, developmental, or degenerative diseases, or to disease states of even less integrity such as 'syndromes'. None the less, in historical terms the idea of specificity has had a broader meaning in which the infectious diseases appear as a special case. For older medical historians, the discovery of diseases that were the result of the invasion of the body by independent organisms represented a climax in the development of the modern, 'ontological' theory of disease. Ontology is concerned with essences of things and with individuality. The ontological view of disease stresses the realities of disease entities and therefore the constancy of any given disease from patient to patient. This contrasts with holistic interpretations, stressing instead the individuality of the patient and the uniqueness of his or her experience of disease. The ontological view chimes well with the idea of disease as invading the body from without, and implies that disease is characterized primarily by local, rather than whole-body, effects. By the nineteenth century, however, it was possible to transpose the ontological idea to the cellular level, so that disease could be seen as invasive within the interior environment of the body.[21]

The rise of the ontological theory of disease is associated with the challenge to Galenic humoralism mounted in the sixteenth and seventeenth centuries. (➤ Ch. 14 Humoralism) It is also associated with Baconian methods of observation and the compiling of case histories in order to arrive at a consistent picture of a particular disease.[22] Case histories stressed not only signs and symptoms, but also the course followed by a given disease over time. The infectious diseases seemed to show periodicity not only in the individual, but also in their epidemic rise and fall. However, the recognition of specific diseases, or at least specific disease states, was a feature of Arabic medicine and probably of ancient civilizations.[23] (➤ Ch. 31 Arab-Islamic medicine) The pitfalls of retrospective diagnosis from textual descriptions make this area a very difficult one for the historian. Nor should descriptions be isolated from the overall framework of interpretation of disease as it can be reconstructed for any given society. It is equally unsound to assume a priori that past societies lacked either the will or the ability to describe distinct diseases, or that each society had only one way of looking at disease.[24]

Specificity and the analogy with species of animals and plants came together in the work of Thomas Sydenham, the 'English Hippocrates'. That Sydenham was so described perhaps reflects the fact that he was more influential on the European continent, especially in Germany, than he was in England.[25] Sydenham's view that diseases had a character as constant as the immutable species of the organic world was deployed in the eighteenth century to create elaborate classifications of diseases analogous to the classifications of plants and animals.[26] (➤ Ch. 17 Nosology) However, the 'natural history' approach to disease, rather than leading directly to bacteriology, was taken to its logical conclusion in the early nineteenth century by exponents of *Naturphilosophie*, who saw diseases not only holistically, but *in toto* as organisms which grew and lived and died over long periods of time, parasitic upon a world that was itself living. For most practitioners of the time, specificity was a pragmatic concept, increasingly based on clinical observation, quantification, and pathological anatomy.[27] Paradoxically, the identification of the causes of major diseases as independent living organisms coincided with Darwinism and evolutionary theory, which stressed the mutability of species.[28] The relationship between disease theory and evolution is one requiring much further investigation.[29] It is not clear, for example, how ideas about the ascent if not the perfectibility of human beings, especially as social animals, were reconciled with the increasing conviction that the highest of organisms could be arbitrarily destroyed by the lowest. There is no doubt, however, that for some, bacteriology conveyed the gloomiest of messages, a kind of biological determinism, and that the lifting of this gloom was one reason for welcoming the findings of immunology, which stressed the human body's natural defences against disease.[30] (➤ Ch. 10 The immunological tradition)

CONTAGION THEORIES IN CHRONOLOGICAL SEQUENCE

It is not possible here to give a comprehensive account of ideas about contagion over time. In what follows, certain phases will be selected to give fuller illustration of points already made, and to provide a basic chronological framework.

THE CLASSICAL PERIOD

The classical period, as already indicated, has proved puzzling to lineally minded historians of germ theory because of its apparent failure to observe the contagiousness of disease. The favoured explanation of this lies in the supposed dominance of Hippocratic medicine, which saw an individual's diseases as unique to that individual, being compounded of factors in his or her constitution, personal history, and environment. The doctrine of humours included generalizations but was intended to express individuality. 'Lowest-common denominator' medicine, in which individuals were treated alike, was reserved for slaves and the military. Among the literate élite, therefore, differences rather than similarities would be stressed even in respect of a disease apparently spreading and affecting large numbers of people in a similar way. The two Hippocratic schools seemingly differed in the degree to which they were prepared to generalize about disease. Individuality was reinforced for the Western tradition by the synthesis of Galen (AD 129–c.200/210), who was vehemently opposed to the generalizing tendencies of the Methodists. Health, according to the Galenic tradition, was not merely the absence of disease. Rather, it was a balance actively maintained by a regimen designed to suit the individual.[31]

The classical contribution to concepts of contagion and infection related less to the individual than to the environment. The term 'infection' has a root meaning 'to put or dip into something', leading to *inficere* and *infectio*, staining or dyeing. This is a reminder that 'an infection is basically a pollution'. The same is true not only of 'contagion', but also of the noun 'miasma', which derives from the Greek verb *miaino*, a counterpart to the Latin *inficere*. Impurity is therefore a basic element in all three concepts.[32] These derivations hark back to empirical observation, but also evoke the broad spectrum of religious and moral ideas clustering around notions of pollution and taboo. Pollution is concerned not only with time and place, propriety and order, the material and the immaterial, but with the individual's sense of separateness from his or her environment and how this separateness is to be maintained or regulated.[33]

Finding or creating safe environments for human activity was an important preoccupation in classical literature. The Hippocratic emphasis on 'airs, waters, and places' is well known, but observations on health are made in other contexts, especially by agricultural writers, who mentioned dangers arising from swarms of insects, the poisonous emissions of marshes, and vapours from the earth. In such contexts, the term 'pestilential' is used to signify a concentrated degree of infectiousness. The air itself became infected. Of these writers, Varro (127–116 BC) is credited with a Lucretian explanation of natural phenomena and an idea of disease caused in particular localities by invisible animalcules taken in with the air, an idea both animalculist and miasmatist.[34]

THE MIDDLE AGES

The themes of shame, guilt, and pollution were continued under Christianity with the idea of disease as having followed the Fall. This did not, of course, mean that all disease was sinful; 'naturalistic' explanations were also common.[35] The Christian was expected to welcome trial by suffering, as well as earning grace by relieving the suffering of others. (➤ Ch. 67 Pain and suffering) Sin itself could be seen as contagious: one individual could mislead others, a false idea could spread, or the erring body could contaminate the soul.[36] Infectious diseases affecting the surface of the body became of considerable significance. The institutional isolation of lepers became the privilege and responsibility of the church. It is worth noting that lazar-houses were sometimes also used to confine the mentally ill. Leprosy, like syphilis later, differed from acute infectious diseases such as plague and smallpox by being gradual and lifelong.[37] Plague had a major effect in Europe from the fourteenth century and prompted administrative provisions affecting relations between towns, ports, and countries, as well as individuals.[38] A wide range of causes was invoked, but there was general agreement on isolation and quarantine. Such measures were probably from the beginning also used as a political and economic weapon. Having invented quarantine, Italy also originated public-health practices aimed at the control of disease inland and in towns.[39] Plague also initiated a special class of literature about infectious disease, the so-called plague tractates, which contained medical and spiritual advice and discussed rights and duties in times of pestilence. (➤ Ch. 52 Epidemiology)

THE RENAISSANCE

Notions of physical and moral contagion were recombined for Renaissance Europe by the sudden outbreak of syphilis, then also a disease drastically affecting the surface of the body.[40] Syphilis was associated with venery, but was thought also to spread by other means, as in the breath, by contaminated utensils, or in wet-nursing. The coincidence of this disease with the emergence of nation states was reflected in the names most commonly used for it, for example *morbus Gallicus* or the Neopolitan disease. Reference to venereal disease was widely deployed as a satirical weapon, notably in the rhetoric of anti-clericalism during the Reformation. Contemporaries also sardonically noted a tendency for euphemisms to emerge for use among the upper classes: traces of these can still be found in medical dictionaries as late as the nineteenth century. Syphilis thus provides an excellent example of cultural relativism in the diagnosis of infectious disease.[41] Contemporary fears about the increasing population of the poor, especially the vagrant poor, in part drew on the fear of disease. Syphilis was feared was well as plague.[42] (➤ Ch. 26 Sexually transmitted diseases)

Viewed retrospectively, the importance of this period for germ theory resides in the equivocal figure of Fracastoro, author of the poem of which the hero eventually gave his name to the disease, syphilis. Fracastoro is also credited with introducing the terms *fomes*, *fomites*, to refer to inert carriers (clothes etc.) of contagion. He has been alternatively ignored, eulogized, diminished, and merged into his context by successive generations of medical historians.[43] The problem is, in part, one of interpreting metaphor, but is also one of interpreting silence, since his works were little mentioned by later medical authors. Fracastoro appealed to historians seeking precursors of the germ theory because he drew upon Lucretian atomism and postulated 'seeds' of disease, which he probably did not regard as 'living' in the modern sense. Writing at a time when consciousness of both epidemic and endemic disease was high, Fracastoro also gave order to the phenomena to be explained and the possible explanations for them. He appeared to offer to bacteriology and epidemiology a pioneer of the scientific stature of Copernicus (1473–1543), Vesalius (1514–64), or William Harvey (1578–1657).[44] However, Fracastoro was not concerned to make the categorical distinctions between contagion, infection, and non-contagious disease which are so important from the modern point of view, and he included as contagious a range of occult influences characteristic of his period but alien to modern materialism.

The real importance of this period probably lies in the even more controversial figure of Paracelsus (*c.*1493–1541), a religious and medical reformer of great influence but blacklisted by traditionalist contemporaries as an alchemist and quack. Paracelsus's counter-philosophy undermined the intellectual credibility of Galenic humoralism and enfranchised generations of lower-order medical practitioners who wrote in the vernacular and promoted strong chemical remedies. As well as threatening the individuality and gradualness of the academic physician's approach to the patient, Paracelsus's natural philosophy favoured a view of diseases as having essences that influenced the body from without. The body was affected locally, not as a whole. However, Paracelsus was not particularly concerned with epidemic disease, and the influences he posited tended to be occult rather than material: religious or moral in origin and reflexively causing effects in the body paralleling the 'chemical' turbulences of stars.[45] Similar views were forwarded in the seventeenth century by Joan Baptista van Helmont (1579–1644), who continued the attack on Galenism and stressed local reaction in the body to pathogenic stimuli. This was, however, as much a spiritual as a material interaction. Galenic practice continued, but the two revolutionary medical philosophies of Paracelsianism and Helmontianism can be seen as the true foundations of the modern ontological view of disease.[46]

THE SEVENTEENTH AND EIGHTEENTH CENTURIES

Technical innovation, curiosity, and the stress on experience in the seventeenth century led to a range of microscopical observations. Interest in lower animals and plants ranged from the cosmological to the highly empirical, as with the 'little animals' of Antoni van Leeuwenhoek (1632–1723). As well as encouraging speculation about modes of generation, such observations prompted the formulation of 'animalcular' theories of disease.[47] Mostly, these were at the level of mind-games and not particularly central or influential. It is not clear to what extent ideas about disease were influenced by the rise of atomism and mechanistic explanations in natural philosophy.[48] It is notable that some observers brought into the literature of natural philosophy the accurate conclusions of popular belief about infectious disease or parasitism. Similarly, in the eighteenth century, Lady Mary Wortley Montagu (1689–1762) publicized in western Europe the Middle-Eastern technique of inoculation against smallpox; this transfer from popular practice was followed at the turn of the century by vaccination with cowpox, a technique also derived from popular observation.[49]

By the later eighteenth century, there was an awareness of a spectrum of infectious diseases stretching from smallpox at one end (highly infectious person to person, irrespective of locality), to malaria or ague at the other (not infectious person to person, but caught in particular localities).[50] These diseases appeared to have as their common denominator the generic disease process known as fever, in which the whole body was affected. (➤ Ch. 19 Fevers) Most of these diseases seemed also to be characterized by local effects, such as the pustules in smallpox. The disease process was still most commonly explained in terms of a febrile crisis within the body, involving a 'coction' of peccant matter, resolved by excretion of this matter through the body's pores or orifices. According to Sydenham's 'Hippocratic' view of disease, this process occurred naturally and it was the practitioner's task to enable and support it, not hinder it. This interpretation encouraged the already strengthening view that such diseases had a 'life of their own' in that they followed a specific course in the patient, which ought not to be cut short or diverted. However, for Sydenham, each case of disease, and each epidemic, remained a unique experience determined by a given set of circumstances.[51]

The infectious diseases came to illustrate major debates revolving around fever and inflammation: general and local phenomena, respectively, which seemed to constitute primary disease, or the body's first reaction to abnormal stimuli. The disease classifications produced in the eighteenth century by Sauvages (1706–67), Linnaeus (1707–78), and others were simplified and distilled for teaching purposes in the Scottish medical schools by the chemist and physician William Cullen (1710–90). Cullen placed most of the diseases now regarded as infectious in the category of pyrexiae or febrile diseases, differentiated by local inflammations. Within the pyrexiae, diseases spread by contact and well defined, such as smallpox, were attributed to specific contagions (and were also known as 'strictly contagious'). Between these and the diseases of locality at the other end of the spectrum (typified by ague or intermittent fever, associated with the vegetable putrefaction of marshes) lay the confusion surrounding the 'doubtful' diseases, which seemed to partake of the character of both. Some of these were attributed to 'common' contagions, a term reflecting two main ideas: first that, although definable, such diseases were modifiable by circumstances one into another; second, such diseases were intimately related to the environment, which could be responsible for the nature of their causes. According to a range of factors identified as affecting their behaviour and development, these diseases were, as repeatedly stressed, 'sometimes contagious and sometimes not'. This was a motley character alien to bacteriological specificity but compatible with long-established observations, especially those stressing pollution and putrefaction as factors in disease, as well as innumerable 'negative instances' or 'caprice' in the spread of diseases now known to be transmitted indirectly or through vectors. The most ill-defined members of this group were the continued fevers, which were later distinguished mainly into typhus, enteric (typhoid), and relapsing fevers. Possessing some of the same characteristics were the diseases apparently most closely related to common animal putrefaction – the 'septic' diseases, pyaemia, gangrene, septicaemia, scarlet fever, diphtheria, erysipelas, and puerperal fever. Experimental work in the eighteenth and early nineteenth centuries on putrid matters and the 'antiseptic' substances that seemed to control putridity was a reflection of broad-based attempts to identify, or substitute for, the power of living organisms to resist decay, but also contributed to ideas about disease. The eighteenth century also identified contaminated environments – crowded and confined gaols, ships, camps, mills, and hospitals – as capable of engendering contagious forms of disease, and practices of ventilation and disinfection as factors in preventing the concentration leading to contagiousness.

THE NINETEENTH CENTURY

For the nineteenth century, indigenous or endemic diseases (for example, continued fever, smallpox) were of major importance, as well as chronic diseases only gradually regarded as communicable, such as the many forms of tuberculosis. For the activists of the English sanitary movement, 'fever nests' and outbreaks of continued fever epitomized the preventable excesses of disease prejudicing the productivity of the labouring poor. The poor suffered a greater burden of disease than other classes, associated with the insanitary conditions in which they were forced to live. It was therefore the duty of government to intervene at this crucial point in the chain of causation of disease.[52] In theory, a multifactorial view was preserved; in practice and over time, stress came to be placed almost solely on the products of environmental putrefaction, especially of substances of animal origin. In many respects, this was a natural extension of approaches evolved in the eighteenth century. In other ways, however, it represented a departure which, at least in respect to some of its adherents, was described as 'anticontagionism'.

In the latter half of the seventeenth century, plague had withdrawn from western Europe and was replaced as a focus of concern by acute endemic infectious diseases such as smallpox and typhus. Until the early nineteenth century and the first pandemic of cholera, exotic epidemics threatened western Europe, but did not arrive (with the exception of cattle plague). There was less role for primary or remote causes, and more emphasis on factors influencing local outbreaks. However, the growth of intercontinental trade, as well as military and colonial activity, meant an enforced acquaintance with alien diseases such as yellow fever in their places of origin. (➤ Ch. 24 Tropical diseases; Ch. 58 Medicine and colonialism) Plague itself was increasingly seen as a disease of locality. A broad range of other trends influenced the development of environmental views, stressing in effect the intermediate range of causes.[53] Isolationist and coercive measures against plague were increasingly seen as primitive; quarantine measures were denounced by advocates of *laissez-faire* economics as politically suspect, inefficient, and obstructive to trade. Popular belief in contagion was seen as belonging to a primitive state of society, and as entailing a breakdown in social responsibility. English sanitarianism, which drew heavily upon the anticontagionism of the 1820s and 1830s, adopted less a causal than a correlative mode of reasoning. Its theorists, the most important of whom – the lawyer Edwin Chadwick (1800–90) and the physician Thomas Southwood Smith (1788–1861) – were also Benthamite utilitarians, sought to avoid speculation as to causes in a manner influenced indirectly by the sceptical philosophy of David Hume (1711–76).

The effect of such rationalist views on theories of disease was to push the 'doubtful' diseases such as plague, yellow fever, continued fever, influenza, and cholera along the spectrum of infectiousness towards the intermittent fevers, which were related to certain localities. Many anticontagionists could claim experience of the doubtful diseases in their alleged countries of origin, which influenced their views, but made it less likely that these views would be acceptable to orthodox metropolitan opinion in Europe. Stress on locality as forming the character of disease also meant comparative disregard for disease specificity as defined by the consistent clinical and pathological criteria being established in the European hospital-based medical schools. The energetic campaigning of the anticontagionists caused them to be identified by contemporaries as a particular body of opinion. Prominent among them were Benjamin Rush (1746–1813), Charles Maclean (c.1766–1825), Nicolas Chervin (1783–1843), and A. B. Clot (1793–1868).[54] It was in the interests of the anticontagionists to suggest that only two extremes existed with respect to the contagiousness of a given disease. Like some later germ theorists, the anticontagionists insisted that a disease was either contagious or it was not. Although both the sick body and the environment could contribute to the conditions bringing about non-contagious disease, diseases could not be of mixed character, or 'contingently contagious'. Popular beliefs (and administrative orthodoxy) tended to assume an epidemic disease was contagious; for anticontagionists, this character had to be proved. Most of their contemporaries, however, asserted that the notion of contagion opposed by the anticontagionists bore no resemblance to that currently held; rather, an antiquated view was deliberately being used so that controversial diseases like continued fever and cholera could be pushed into the non-contagious category. There was broad-based (if often inactive) agreement on the need for sanitary reform, and on the uselessness of quarantine; however, the anticontagionists, although influential, were, like the contagionists, very much in the minority, and their influence was never greater than at the time it was first asserted, in the 1820s and 1830s. The bulk of contemporary opinion preferred to consider each disease in the 'epidemic, endemic, and contagious' category individually, and to see the 'doubtful' diseases as contingently contagious.

The traditional multifactorial view was reinforced rather than otherwise by the characteristic nineteenth-century concern to make medicine more 'scientific'; a good example of this is the way in which statistical generalization was applied according to the French *méthode numérique*. The reaction against eighteenth-century systems in medicine encouraged an inclusive, fact-gathering methodology which was friendly to the broad generalizations of sanitarianism but inimical to its hardening into an exclusive system of explanation of infectious disease. This hardening was due not to the evolution of anticontagionist views nor to their increased influence, but to political and administrative constraints and the need to produce propaganda. The complexity – and confusion – of debates about epidemic disease in the nineteenth century arises not from any simple clash of opposite views, nor the conflict of the unscientific with the scientific, but from the general epistemological context (the nineteenth-century idea of a 'fact', for example), the special relationship between science and politics in the context of the public-health movement, and the frequent lack of real theoretical difference between the actual views being espoused.

The attempt to be sceptically scientific (in contemporary terms) meant that medicine was prepared to draw heavily upon other developing sciences, especially organic chemistry and gas chemistry, and such phenomena as electricity. Ironically, this caused frequent resort to argument by analogy, a procedure just as frequently deplored by contemporaries as unscientific. This dilemma, as well as the inclusive methodology adopted by the majority, is well illustrated by the framework of explanation of the infectious diseases evolved for England and Wales by the compiler of abstracts in the new Registrar General's Department, William Farr (1807–83).[55] Farr was required to produce a classification of diseases for national statistical purposes, and for a nomenclature which was later adopted internationally. He first grouped together as the 'epidemic, endemic and contagious' diseases all those which 'were of a specific nature, propagated in a peculiar manner and known by experience to become epidemic in unhealthy places and among the sickly classes, at greater or less intervals of time'. This group, the 'index to salubrity', was typified by smallpox but also included malaria.[56] A little later (in 1842), Farr redefined them as the 'zymotic' diseases, a term deliberately chosen to reflect an idea of the disease process as analogous to fermentation. As we have already seen, fermentation was a traditional point of reference for explaining the 'extension of influence' – or 'multiplication' – which seemed to characterize infectious disease as well as other bodily processes such as digestion. Although stressing (English) precursors, and a particular admirer of Sydenham, Farr was chiefly dependent upon the influential and comprehensive synthesis of the German chemist Justus von Liebig (1803–73). For his contemporaries in many countries, Liebig's theories redefined the relationship between the organic and inorganic worlds; they had great popular success and were extremely important in such areas as agriculture. Liebig did not reduce the living to the non-living, but suggested a molecular basis of continuity by which they could interact. He paid particular attention to fermentation, putrefaction, and decay. His formulations were thus ideally suited to explain diseases involving a continuity between the body and its physical environment. Liebig's chemical explanation of catalysis could also explain the process of increase of morbid matter, either in the body or outside it. (➤ Ch. 8 The biochemical tradition)

Farr recognized specificity in infectious diseases in terms less of their causes than of their predictable, law-like behaviour, both as epidemics and in the individual patient. On his own account, he recognized a 'species' 'whenever important pathological states and phenomena were isolated or could be individualised'.[57] In this, he was simply reflecting opinions typical of the 1830s and 1840s. On the one hand, he sought to distance himself from some 'natural historical' accounts of disease, and on the other, he was inclined to preserve for the infectious diseases the analogy Sydenham had drawn between them and plants and animals. However, his adaptation of Liebig also catered for specificity by proposing the existence in each case of a specific zyme, ferment or 'exciter', an organic poison affecting the blood but also showing a special affinity with certain organs or tissues. Unlike the mode of action of poisons, the process of zymosis could explain how (though not why) a disease suddenly became epidemic, or was more contagious in some circumstances than in others. By the 1840s, enough was known of the properties of gases to rule them out as the direct agents of infectious disease, in spite of the fact that such agents were usually seen as entering the body via the lungs. It seemed clear that the *materies morbi* was unlikely to be a simple, volatile substance, but rather 'highly organised particles of fixed matter', possibly resembling the pollen of flowers.[58] Such matter was in a state of pathological transformation at the molecular level. For Farr, however, non-specific decomposing organic matter was either a predisposing cause only, or a link in a chain of causation dominated by a zymotic exciter. Nonetheless, on epidemiological grounds, he felt obliged to retain the possibility of spontaneous generation.

Chemically influenced ideas about the pathological process, referring ultimately to the activity and selective affinities of organic molecules, dominated disease theory in the middle of the nineteenth century and were taken up even by those regarded as prototypical germ theorists, such as John Snow, who produced a whole essay on 'contagious molecular action'. Within this broad framework, the association of, for example, some processes of fermentation with the multiplication of micro-organisms appeared simply as a special case. Chemical theories also seemed better able to accommodate the possibility of spontaneous generation, detaching this concept from earlier versions of it seen by nineteenth-century writers as antique. However, enthusiasm for microscopical observation was also a feature of the second quarter of the century, and the emergence of cell theories coincided with a rash of claims for the role of organisms in skin diseases and diseases affecting lower animals and plants. Terms later used by bacteriologists, such as 'bacillus', and 'vibrio', were already current; 'bacterium' and 'spirochaete' were introduced at this time.[59]

'Fungi' were as characteristic a preoccupation of the nineteenth century as were animalcules of the seventeenth. Many observers, such as Louis Pasteur (1822–95), were investigating 'blights' and other diseases of considerable economic importance. Because fungi were proved to affect food plants, the idea that such agents might be connected with epidemic diseases of the gut such as cholera continued to be attractive until late in the century. Well-known 'germ theorists', such as William Budd (1811–80) and Joseph Lister (1827–1912), were inclined to be 'fungi theorists' in the 1840s and 1850s. A selection of the observations of this period (for example, that of Filippo Pacini (1812–83) of the cholera bacillus) are now regarded as having pre-dated the better-known work of the 1870s and 1880s. To the earlier decades also belongs work uncovering the complicated life-cycles of some parasites, and the puzzling phenomena of the 'alternation of generations', in which organic forms very dissimilar and appearing in unexpected locations were revealed to be related by unusual forms of reproduction. This not only increased scepticism about spontaneous generation, but also complicated the parasite analogy to which the germ theory (often to its disadvantage) was closely related.[60]

Between 1830 and the 1860s, repeated onslaughts of cholera encouraged speculation about epidemic disease. As with plague earlier, it is not surprising to find that some of these speculators opted for *contagium vivum*. It was usually felt that this option needed added justification because as an idea it seemed to be dredged up from the dim past, was heavily dependent upon analogy, and laid its author open to charges of being a vitalist. Moreover, the microscopical observations of the same decades, however suggestive, also encouraged critics to demand 'ocular demonstration' when agents like 'fungus germs' were posited. Thus it was held against the most prominent of these mid-century theorists, the pathologist and anatomist Jacob Henle (1809–85), that even he, an eminent microscopist, had been unable to demonstrate the existence of the 'epidemic infusoria'. Typically, Henle was given credit for 'ingenuity', a form of praise often implying marginalization. In the past, historians have given much credit to Henle as a prophet of germ theory, and particularly for his anticipation of 'Koch's postulates'; like Fracastoro, however, this aspect of his work has also been belittled. Henle did not so much state that contagions consisted of living organisms, as suggest how this might (in an ideal world) be established. Moreover, Henle reflected contemporary views in defining three categories of disease, the contagious, the miasmatic, and the miasmatic-contagious, of which the last, 'mixed' category was predictably the most problematic. Henle felt obliged to accept that some diseases could be both miasmatic and contagious, and that some development of the disease agent could take place outside the body.

For the mid-nineteenth century, the phrase 'germs of disease' would have conjured up, not the ingenious but self-sufficing hypotheses of theorists like Henle, but the beginnings of a disease outbreak, the onset of the pathological process, or a range of postulations suggesting the evolution of degenerate bodily products into agents of disease. Different versions of cell theory suggested how unorganized matter could take on form and differentiation. The ways in which organized matter broke down also attracted attention. Diseases in which decay seemed to begin in the living body were of special interest, as well as related bodily products such as pus. However, other diseases apparently involved not disintegration, but a special kind of growth in the body, such as with tuberculosis and cancer. The predominance of such concerns, which were related to major issues in biology, is evident when comparison is made with the peripheral position of a speculator like John

Grove (1816–95), a true 'germ theorist' who suggested that the ova of parasites and the spores of fungi normally circulated in the blood. Cellular and chemical pathology, on the other hand, had created a new microcosmic vision of the body in which its minute constituents themselves possessed many of the properties of independent life, exercised in an environment governed by the principles of chemical affinity and action at the molecular level.

That cholera and typhoid were described as 'filth diseases' until late into the century demonstrates the success of sanitary propaganda, which used oversimplified equations but was justified by accumulated evidence of correlation. In addition, the original utilitarian arguments for sanitary reform had been co-opted into a holistic religious and moral framework that resisted reformulation. Nevertheless, by about 1860, the position on 'filth' had become relatively refined. Although all forms of putrefaction involved hazards, epidemic disease was thought most likely to arise from changes in organic material that had once been part of the animal body. This view was able to accommodate the findings of epidemiologists suggesting, for example, the specific role of choleraic or typhoid discharges in the water supply.

The wide popularity of Liebig's chemical explanations of pathology and physiology was a measure of the strength of contemporary feeling that medicine and biology should achieve the same dignity as physics and mathematics and should be found subject to the same natural laws. The success of Pasteur's germ theory reveals the strength of feeling that this 'reductionism' could be taken too far, towards materialism and even atheism. In France, Pasteur's ideas were associated with anti-evolutionism, spiritualism, and conservative politics.[61] Pasteur had been committed since the 1840s to a programme of research in stereochemistry designed to separate 'the chemistry of non-living nature from the chemistry of living nature'.[62] From 1855, Pasteur's employment involved problem-solving in industrial contexts, in particular the production of wine, vinegar, and beer. His claim to originating 'pasteurization' – preservation by heating in closed vessels – began with a patent of 1865 for preserving wine. Pasteur's conclusion that fermentations could not take place in the absence of specific living organisms was based on notions of fact and experiment that contemporaries also found persuasive. In addition, Pasteur was a highly effective polemicist, able to simplify opposing views to good effect, and to represent his work as an issue affecting national self-respect. Although his and Liebig's views eventually emerged as being complementary, their debate remained competitive. Pasteur's explanation of varieties of fermentation offered a model for current preoccupations about disease, in suggesting the presence (varying with locality) of micro-organisms in the air; a specific, one-to-one relationship between the micro-organism and the type of fermentation; a similar specific dependency between the organism, its 'food', and other chemical features of the environment in which it multiplied; and methods by which the cause might be isolated and then made to reproduce the process for which it was responsible. In the early 1860s, Pasteur presented a similar explanation for putrefaction, suggesting a cycle, rivalling that of the chemists, in which 'life stems from death and death from life'. (➤ Ch. 13 Ideas of life and death) Pasteur underlined his biological explanation of the paradigmatic processes of fermentation and putrefaction by similar experimental findings with respect to economically important diseases of animals, especially anthrax. Effectively, Pasteur 'revealed the enormous medical and economic potential of experimental biology'.[63] The work relevant to germ theory was intimately connected to implications for the control of disease, although Pasteur himself developed only one treatment directly applicable to human disease (rabies).

The political, economic, and humanitarian potential of applying his ideas to specifically medical problems was obvious to Pasteur, but as a chemist he was relatively reticent to tackle the medical profession on its own territory. The germ theory was established as an issue of immediate clinical relevance to medical practitioners by the antiseptic methods of surgery advocated by Lister from the 1860s.[64] As Pasteur himself realized, Listerism involved acceptance that those who healed also caused disease, a dilemma in social and professional attitudes that had earlier destroyed Ignaz Semmelweis (1818–65), who had advocated hygienic procedures to reduce the incidence of puerperal fever.[65] (➤ Ch. 44 Childbirth) Lister, however, was not promoting cleanliness, but practices which could prevent infection by Pasteurian germs even in the absence of cleanliness; he therefore met the same kind of opposition as those who proposed the use of deodorizers and disinfectants as a substitute for the removal of filth and overcrowding. The debate over Listerism provides a focus of conflicting contemporary concepts of pollution. The moral absolute of purity was more compatible with the concept of asepsis, which rapidly followed Listerism and was ideologically more acceptable (although perhaps even more difficult to put into practice). Asepsis rather than antisepsis produced the stereotype of the masked surgeon in the bright white operating-theatre. Asepsis was also more compatible with traditional multifactorial interpretations of disease.[66] (➤ Ch. 42 Surgery (modern))

Pasteur's vision of specificity was based more on chemical process than on morphology. He was inattentive to problems of classification and to changing contemporary distinctions between microscopic animals and plants. Pasteur was perhaps the better able to reject – by 1872 – persistent claims by many observers that they had seen organisms at this level change one into another, claims which were cited in support of evolution. Overall, Pasteur tended to ignore rather than deny the implications of Darwinian evolution. He was strenuously opposing spontaneous generation from at least 1860, but even

Pasteur's 'victories' in this wide-ranging debate were more apparent than real, leading to reformulation rather than elimination of questions about the origin of life. His insistence on this issue undoubtedly helped to link disease specificity with the specificity of an invasive, disease-causing organism that reproduced itself consistently and showed 'normal' heredity. However, Pasteur was relatively casual about whether his *'germes'* were in any given instance latent precursors, or fully developed 'adult' organisms. His use of 'germ' prefigured the generalized popular usage of that term. That micro-organisms 'bred true' and did not normally transform themselves was established not by Pasteur, but by naturalists and botanists, in particular Ferdinand Cohn (1828–98) and Anton de Bary (1831–88), and in the context of disease causation primarily by the co-founder of modern bacteriology, Robert Koch (1843–1910).

Koch's first decisive contribution was published in 1876 and related to anthrax, an important disease of large animals and also of humans that had been a focus of observation and experiment for some decades.[67] Koch's work demonstrated the existence of a resistant spore phase, which explained puzzling aspects of the disease's behaviour; undermined chemical analogies and emphasized the role of biological reproduction by showing that virulence persisted even after extreme degrees of dilution; introduced the use of solid media that facilitated pure cultures; and established the experimental model by which a specific disease could be repeatedly induced in a sequence of susceptible subjects. Although the criteria of 'Koch's postulates' were not fulfilled in each case, even by Koch himself, the technical model he provided set off a chain reaction of findings in the 1870s and 1880s that constitutes the 'bacteriological revolution'. This revolution became international in scope but was mainly due to German investigators. As befitted his chemical background, Pasteur had always laid stress on the conditions necessary for the activity of micro-organisms, and under his direction the French school concentrated its attention on extending the principles of vaccination.[68]

Bacteriology created a new source of scientific authority for medicine, and made an enormous difference to its reputation for effectiveness in both prevention and cure. The historical reality behind these undoubted changes is inevitably more complex. Ironically, bacteriology did much to create a schism, evident today, between the laboratory scientist and the clinical practitioner.[69] More generally, bacteriological extremism seemed to deny the feasibility of modern urban society. Safety for the individual seemed to lie in extreme isolation, and a similar estrangement was implied between practitioner and patient. As long as bacteriology appeared to entail a kind of biological determinism, it gave radical new meaning to concepts of infection and contagion, pollution and taboo. These extremes were, however, rapidly modified, not only by immunology but by one of its corollaries, a reversion to the group as opposed to the individual. This reversion also marked a return to a more multifactorial, less exclusive approach.[70]

NOTES

1 See, for example, Charles Singer, quoted by M. Greenwood, 'Miasma and contagion', in E. A. Underwood (ed.), *Science, Medicine and History*, 2 vols, London, Oxford University Press, 1953, Vol. II, p. 501.

2 In what follows, the term 'infectious' will be used generically to embrace the whole group of epidemic, endemic, and contagious diseases caused by bacteria, viruses, and some other parasitic organisms.

3 See R. H. Shryock, *The Development of Modern Medicine*, 1936; repr. of 2nd edn, Madison, University of Wisconsin Press, 1979.

4 See, for example, (on 'species') J. Beatty, 'What's in a word? Coming to terms in the Darwinian revolution', *Journal of the History of Biology*, 1982, 15: 215–39.

5 See, for example, M. Pelling, *Cholera, Fever and English Medicine 1825–1865*, Oxford, Oxford University Press, 1978, pp. 262–3, 284–6.

6 O. Rosenbach, *Physician Versus Bacteriologist*, trans. by A. Rose, New York and London, Funk & Wagnalls, 1904; I. Galdston, 'The epidemic constitution in historic perspective', *Bulletin of the New York Academy of Medicine*, 1942 (2nd series), 18: 606–19.

7 Laid down (although with a qualifying footnote) in *On Continuous Molecular Changes* (1853); quoted in Pelling, op. cit. (n. 5), p. 206.

8 The ultimate reference is to the analysis by Aristotle (384–322 BC) of causes into formal, final, material, and efficient.

9 O. Temkin, *Hippocrates in a World of Pagans and Christians*, Baltimore, MD, and London, Johns Hopkins University Press, 1991, esp. chs 13–15.

10 D. Bates, 'Sydenham, Thomas', *Dictionary of Scientific Biography*, Vol. XIII, p. 215; E. W. Goodall, 'The epidemic constitution', *Proceedings of the Royal Society of Medicine (Section of Epidemiology)*, 1927–8, 21: 119–28.

11 The terminology used here reflects nineteenth-century usage. For a historically based exposition of aetiology aimed at twentieth-century medical students, see L. King, *Medical Thinking. A Historical Preface*, Princeton, NJ, Princeton University Press, 1982, ch. 10. See also M. Ullmann, *Islamic Medicine*, Islamic Surveys no. 11, Edinburgh, Edinburgh University Press, 1978, pp. 89–90.

12 C. Webster, review of W. Pagel, *William Harvey's Biological Ideas* (1967), *Ambix*, 1967, 14: 142; J. Donne, *Complete Poetry and Selected Prose*, ed. by J. Hayward, London, Nonesuch Press, 1990, p. 33.

13 P. J. Weindling, *Darwinism and Social Darwinism in Imperial Germany: the Contribution of the Cell Biologist Oscar Hertwig*, Stuttgart and New York, Gustav Fischer Verlag, 1991, p. 29.

14 J. Farley, *The Spontaneous Generation Controversy from Descartes to Oparin*, Baltimore, MD, and London, Johns Hopkins University Press, 1977.

15 K. Hutchison, 'What happened to occult qualities in the scientific revolution?', *Isis*, 1982, 73: 233–53; J. Henry, 'Occult qualities and the experimental philosophy: active principles in pre-Newtonian matter theory', *History of Science*, 1986, 24: 335–81.

16 C. D. Darlington, 'Purpose and particles in the study of heredity', in Underwood, op. cit. (n. 1), pp. 472–81. On the 1860s as 'the era of the particle', see J. K. Crellin, 'The dawn of the germ theory: particles, infection and biology', in F. N. L. Poynter (ed.), *Medicine and Science in the 1860s*, London, Wellcome Institute of the History of Medicine, 1968, pp. 57–76.

17 Pelling, op. cit. (n. 5), pp. 189–202; P. H. Futcher, 'Notes on insect contagion', *Bulletin of the Institute of the History of Medicine*, 1936, 4: 536–58.

18 Pelling, op. cit. (n. 5), ch. 4. On the modern history of viruses, see a series of articles by L. Wilkinson in *Medical History* from 1974, 18: 211–21; and works by S. S. Hughes, cited in Wilkinson, p. 211 n.

19 An exception is O. Temkin, 'The scientific approach to disease: specific entity and individual sickness', in Temkin, *The Double Face of Janus*, Baltimore, MD, and London, Johns Hopkins University Press, 1977, pp. 441–56.

20 On the postulates, named after the bacteriologist Robert Koch (1843–1910), see L. S. King, 'Dr Koch's postulates', *Journal of the History of Medicine*, 1952, 7: 350–61.

21 W. Pagel, 'The speculative basis of modern pathology. Jahn, Virchow, and the philosophy of pathology', *Bulletin of the History of Medicine*, 1945, 18: 1–43; cf. J. Bleker, 'Between romantic and scientific medicine: Johann Lukas Schoenlein and the natural history school 1825–1845', *Clio Medica*, 1983, 18: 191–201.

22 See K. Faber, *Nosography in Modern Internal Medicine*, London, Oxford University Press, 1923.

23 Ullmann, op. cit. (n. 11), chs 5 and 6.

24 See Temkin, 'Health and disease', in Temkin, op. cit. (n. 19), pp. 419–40.

25 F. N. L. Poynter, 'Sydenham's influence abroad', *Medical History*, 1973, 17: 223–34.

26 E. Goldschmid, 'Nosologia naturalis', in Underwood, op. cit. (n. 1), pp. 103–22.

27 G. A. Lindeboom, 'From the history of the concept of specificity', *Janus*, 1957, 46: 12–24; Pelling, op. cit. (n. 5), pp. 73 ff. and *passim*.

28 W. Collins (*Specificity and Evolution in Disease*, London, H. K. Lewis, 1884) argued for the obsolescence of specificity and for diseases being able to arise *de novo*.

29 Pelling, op. cit. (n. 5), pp. 254–6; W. F. Bynum, 'Darwin and the doctors: evolution, diathesis and germs in nineteenth-century Britain', *Gesnerus*, 1983, 40: 43–53.

30 See, for example, J. H. Baas, *Outlines of the History of Medicine*, trans. and enl. by H. E. Handerson, 1889; 2 vols, Huntington, NY, Robert E. Krieger, 1971, Vol. II, pp. 1008–10.

31 Temkin, 'An historical analysis of the concept of infection', in Temkin, op. cit. (n. 19), pp. 456–71; V. Nutton, 'The seeds of disease: an explanation of contagion and infection from the Greeks to the Renaissance', *Medical History*, 1983, 27: 1–34. See also A. C. Klebs, 'The history of infection', *Annals of Medical History*, 1917, 1: 159–73.

32 Temkin, op. cit. (n. 31), esp. p. 457.

33 Temkin, review of E. R. Dodds, *The Greeks and the Irrational* (1951), *Isis*, 1952, 43: 375–7.

34 S. Jarcho, 'Medical and non-medical comments on Cato and Varro, with histori-

cal observations on the concept of infection', *Transactions and Studies of the College of Physicians of Philadelphia*, 1976, 43: 372–8.

35 J. Kroll and B. Bachrach, 'Sin and the etiology of disease in pre-Crusade Europe', *Journal of the History of Medicine*, 1986, 41: 395–414.

36 An example of the persistence of these analogical concepts is A. Siegfried, *Germs and Ideas. Routes of Epidemics and Ideologies*, trans. by J. Henderson and M. Claraso, Edinburgh and London, Oliver & Boyd, 1965, esp. part 4.

37 A. Weymouth, *Through the Leper Squint: a Study of Leprosy from Pre-Christian Times to the Present Day*, London, Selwyn & Blount, 1938; S. N. Brody, *The Disease of the Soul: Leprosy in Medieval Literature*, Ithaca, NY, and London, Cornell University Press, 1974; K. Manchester, 'Tuberculosis and leprosy in antiquity: an interpretation', *Medical History*, 1984, 28: 162–73.

38 M. Dols, 'The comparative communal response to the Black Death in Muslim and Christian societies', *Viator*, 1974, 5: 269–97.

39 See, for example, B. Pullan, *Rich and Poor in Renaissance Venice: the Social Institutions of a Catholic State to 1620*, Oxford, Blackwell, and Cambridge, MA, Harvard University Press, 1971, part 2, esp. pp. 219–24, 248–52, 314–25; C. Cipolla, *Public Health and the Medical Profession in the Renaissance*, Cambridge, Cambridge University Press, 1976; R. Palmer, 'The control of plague in Venice and northern Italy 1348–1600', unpublished Ph.D. thesis, University of Kent, 1978; A. Carmichael, *Plague and the Poor in Early Renaissance Florence*, Cambridge and New York, Cambridge University Press, 1986. For a view of contagion and hence quarantine as purely political constructs, see C. Maclean, *Evils of Quarantine Laws*, London, T. & G. Underwood, 1824. See also G. B. Rothenberg, 'The Austrian sanitary cordon and the control of bubonic plague: 1710–1871', *Journal of the History of Medicine*, 1973, 28: 15–23.

40 C. Quétel, *History of Syphilis*, trans. by J. Braddock and B. Pike, Cambridge, Polity Press, 1990; Brody, op. cit. (n. 37); A. Foa, 'The new and the old: the spread of syphilis (1494–1530)', in E. Muir and G. Ruggiero (eds), *Sex and Gender in Historical Perspective: Selections from Quaderni Storici*, Baltimore, MD, and London, Johns Hopkins University Press, 1990, pp. 26–45.

41 M. Pelling, 'Appearance and reality: barber-surgeons, the body and disease', in L. Beier and R. Finlay (eds), *London 1500–1700: the Making of the Metropolis*, London, Longman, 1986, esp. pp. 89–103.

42 Pullan, op. cit. (n. 39), pp. 220–2, 245–52; M. Pelling, 'Healing the sick poor: social policy and disability in Norwich 1550–1640', *Medical History*, 1985, 29: 115–37; P. Slack, *Poverty and Policy in Tudor and Stuart England*, London and New York, Longman, 1988, esp. pp. 139 ff.

43 See for example C. Singer and D. Singer, 'The scientific position of Girolamo Fracastoro (1478?–1553)', *Annals of Medical History*, 1917, 1: 1–34; N. Howard-Jones, 'Fracastoro and Henle: a reappraisal of their contribution to the concept of communicable diseases', *Medical History*, 1977, 21: 61–8; V. Nutton, 'The reception of Fracastoro's theory of contagion. The seed that fell among thorns?', *Osiris*, 1990, 6: 196–234.

44 Singer and Singer, op. cit. (n. 43); C. Singer and D. Singer, *The Development of the Doctrine of Contagium Vivum, 1500–1750*, London (privately printed), 1913.

45 I am grateful to Charles Webster for his advice on Paracelsus's concept of

epidemic disease. See also Webster, *From Paracelsus to Newton*, Cambridge, Cambridge University Press, 1982.

46 W. Pagel, *Joan Baptista van Helmont. Reformer of Science and Medicine*, Cambridge, Cambridge University Press, 1982.

47 E. Gasking, *Investigations into Generation, 1651–1828*, London, Hutchinson, 1967; Singer and Singer, op. cit. (n. 44).

48 For a recent positive view see K. D. Keele, 'The Sydenham–Boyle theory of morbific particles', *Medical History*, 1974, 18: 240–8.

49 Baas, op. cit. (n. 30), Vol. II, p. 510; J. R. Smith, *The Speckled Monster: Smallpox in England, 1670–1970*, Chelmsford, Essex Record Office, 1987, pp. 30–33, 92–3.

50 For this and ensuing paragraphs, see Pelling, op. cit. (n. 5), with additional references as cited.

51 Temkin, op. cit. (n. 24), p. 427.

52 M. Pelling, 'Epidemics in nineteenth-century towns: how important was cholera?', *Transactions and Reports of the Liverpool Medical Institution*, 1983–4, 23–33.

53 L. J. Jordanova, 'Earth science and environmental medicine: the synthesis of the late Enlightenment', in Jordanova and R. Porter (eds), *Images of the Earth*, Chalfont St Giles, British Society for the History of Science, 1979, pp. 119–46; J. C. Riley, 'The medicine of the environment in eighteenth-century Germany', *Clio Medica*, 1983, 18: 167–78.

54 For European anticontagionism of the 1820s and 1830s, see E. Ackerknecht, 'Anticontagionism between 1821 and 1867', *Bulletin of the History of Medicine*, 1948, 22: 562–93.

55 On Farr, see Pelling, op. cit. (n. 5), esp. ch. 3; J. Eyler, *Victorian Social Medicine: the Ideas and Methods of William Farr*, Baltimore, MD, and London, Johns Hopkins University Press, 1979.

56 Pelling, op. cit. (n. 5), p. 93.

57 Pelling, op. cit. (n. 5), p. 94.

58 Pelling, op. cit. (n. 5), p. 107.

59 Baas, op. cit. (n. 30), Vol. II, p. 1003; W. Bulloch, *The History of Bacteriology*, London, Oxford University Press, 1960, ch. 8.

60 On the ambivalence of the parasite analogy see Pelling, op. cit. (n. 5), pp. 196 ff, 253–5, and *passim*; J. Farley, 'Parasites and the germ theory of disease', *Milbank Quarterly*, 1989, 67 (suppl. 1): 50–68.

61 See G. L. Geison, 'Pasteur, Louis', *Dictionary of Scientific Biography*, Vol. X, pp. 350–416, on which the following account of Pasteur is based: J. F. Hutchinson, 'Tsarist Russia and the bacteriological revolution', *Journal of the History of Medicine*, 1985, 40: 420–39.

62 N. Roll-Hansen, 'Louis Pasteur – a case against reductionist historiography', *British Journal of the Philosophy of Science*, 1972, 23: 351.

63 Geison, op. cit. (n. 61), pp. 364, 352.

64 See C. L. Dolman, 'Lister, Joseph', *Dictionary of Scientific Biography*, Vol. VIII, pp. 399–413; also D. Hamilton, 'The nineteenth-century surgical revolution – antisepsis or better nutrition?', *Bulletin of the History of Medicine*, 1982, 56: 30–40.

65 On Semmelweis's aetiological views see K. C. Carter, 'Ignaz Semmelweis, Carl Mayrhofer, and the rise of germ theory', *Medical History*, 1985, 29: 33–53.

66 N. J. Fox, 'Scientific theory, choice and social structure: the case of Joseph Lister's antisepsis, humoral theory and asepsis', *History of Science*, 1988, 26: 367–97.

67 For Koch see C. E. Dolman, 'Koch, Robert', *Dictionary of Scientific Biography*, Vol. VII, pp. 420–35.

68 Geison, op. cit. (n. 61), p. 388.

69 R. Maulitz, 'Physician versus bacteriologist: the ideology of science in clinical medicine', in M. Vogel and C. E. Rosenberg (eds), *The Therepeutic Revolution*, Philadelphia, University of Pennsylvania Press, 1979, pp. 91–108.

70 I. Galdston, 'Social medicine and the epidemic constitution', *Bulletin of the History of Medicine*, 1951, 25: 8–21; S. Kunitz, 'The historical roots and ideological functions of disease concepts in three primary care specialities', ibid., 1983, 57: 412–32.

FURTHER READING

Benton, E., 'Vitalism in nineteenth-century scientific thought: a typology and reassessment', *Studies in the History and Philosophy of Science*, 1974, 5: 17–48.

Douglas, M., *Purity and Danger: an Analysis of Concepts of Pollution and Taboo*, London, Routledge & Kegan Paul, repr. 1974.

Greenwood, M., *Epidemiology, Historical and Experimental*, Baltimore, MD, Johns Hopkins University Press, and London, Oxford University Press, 1932.

Long, E. R., 'The decline of chronic infectious disease and its social implications', *Bulletin of the History of Medicine*, 1954, 28: 368–84.

McDonald, J. C., 'The history of quarantine in Britain during the nineteenth century, *Bulletin of the History of Medicine*, 1951, 25: 23–44.

Morantz, R. M., 'Feminism, professionalism and germs: the thought of Mary Putnam Jacobi and Elizabeth Blackwell', *American Quarterly*, 1982, 34: 459–78.

Pagel, W. and Winder, M., 'Harvey and the "modern" concept of disease', *Bulletin of the History of Medicine*, 1968, 42: 496–509.

Parker, R., *Miasma: Pollution and Purification in Early Greek Religion*, Oxford, Clarendon Press, 1990.

Rosenberg, C., 'The cause of cholera: aspects of etiological thought in nineteenth-century America', *Bulletin of the History of Medicine*, 1960, 34: 331–54.

Sigerist, H., *The Great Doctors*, trans. by. E. Paul and C. Paul, New York, Doubleday Anchor Books, 1958.

Simon, J., 'Contagion', *British Medical Journal*, 1879, ii: 923–5, 973–5.

Stevenson, L. G., 'Science down the drain', *Bulletin of the History of Medicine*, 1955, 29: 1–26.

Warner, J. H., 'Science in medicine', *Osiris*, 1985 (2nd series), 1: 37–58.

17

NOSOLOGY

W. F. Bynum

I hope that Lord Grey and you are well – no easy thing seeing that there are above 1500 diseases to which Man is subjected.

(Sydney Smith to Lady Grey, 1 February 1836[1])

INTRODUCTION

'To name is to know', the old adage has it. 'A disease known is half cured', runs the proverb. Put these two together and nosology, the branch of medicine concerned with the classification of diseases, should have been the queen of the medical sciences. In practice, nosology was central to formal medical knowledge only during the eighteenth century, although under less grand titles such as the 'International Classification of Disease' it continues to be an object of attention, and throughout medicine's history, how doctors have named diseases offers a window on both their philosophical and practical preoccupations. Do diseases have existence apart from their idiosyncratic manifestations in individual sufferers? Are there essential characteristics to disease out there to be discovered, or is the naming of disease a nominalist exercise, done simply for convenience? How did Sydney Smith (1764–1840) know that there are 'above 1500' diseases in the world? What is the relationship between the 'disease' that the doctor diagnoses and the 'illness' that the patient experiences? Can disease be classified using similar criteria to those of a botanist classifying plants, or a zoologist, animals? What weight does the classifying (that is, naming) doctor give to the various manifestations of disease as seen in the individual patient? What is the difference between a 'disease' and a 'syndrome'; between a disease and a symptom; between a disease and its causes; between a disease and the person experiencing it;

335

between disease and sickness or illness? (➤ Ch. 12 Concepts of health, illness, and disease)

The very act of diagnosis carries with it nosological overtones, for calling a disease measles rather than smallpox, or phthisis rather than pleurisy, implies the existence of some classifying criteria, whether implicit or explicit. And this is so regardless of whether the diagnosing doctor holds to a 'physiological' or ontological concept of disease. Physiological (or 'biographical') concepts of disease imply that a disease cannot be understood apart from a particular individual suffering from it; within this framework, the line between health and disease is a continuous one, disease being a deviation from a state of health (or 'normality'). Within the ontological tradition, disease is posited to be some sort of entity which befalls a previously healthy person. As Henry Cohen summarized it:

> Many terms are used to cover these two concepts – e.g., *ontological* – indicating that independent self-sufficiency of diseases running a regular course and with a natural history of their own, as opposed to the *biographical* or *historical* which records the history of the patient. Other names arise from the founders of the schools of thought which appear to have given these concepts birth – e.g., *Platonic* and *Hippocratic;* from the philosophies from which they are primarily derived – the contrasting *realist* and *nominalist, rationalist* and *empirical, conventional* and *naturalistic* schools. The names are of little importance. The two notions varying a little in content and occasionally overlapping have persisted, the dominance of the one or the other at different epochs reflecting either the philosophy of the time or the influence and teaching of outstanding personalities.[2]

THE CLASSICAL TRADITION

On the above criteria, Hippocratic notions of diseases were physiological, and the Hippocratics had no interest in nosology *per se*. The theory that health results from a proper balance of the four humours, and disease from an imbalance or change in quality of them, located the disease to the particular person suffering from it. (➤ Ch. 14 Humoralism) Through their doctrine of the temperaments, the Hippocratics conceived that each person had a humoral balance which was correct for that individual; it was related to that person's 'naturally' dominant humour and his or her place within the life-cycle. The same cluster of factors – cold, sharp winds, bad air, injudicious eating – could, in particular circumstances, cause a variety of diseases, and the doctor would need to know the peculiarities of the patient's habits, recent history, life-style, temperament, etc., before being able to understand the disease and prescribe the proper course of treatment.

At the same time, the Hippocratic writings are full of clear discussions of a number of particular diseases, for which different nouns are used and, often, pathognomonic features described. That Hippocratic diagnostic categories do not always conform exactly with modern ones is not due to their lack of nosological sophistication, but to the differing features of their conceptual framework, diagnostic methods, and therapeutic aims. Many Hippocratic disease labels have remained – phrenitis, pleurisy, dropsy, gout – and through translation entered into later medical vocabularies, even if their actual meanings have changed.

The Hippocratic emphasis on bedside diagnosis and, above all, prognosis, meant that many of their writings were devoted to those activities; the Hippocratic work called *Aphorisms*, for instance, was filled with what today would be called 'clinical pearls' – useful diagnostic and prognostic tips which themselves were generalizations based on repeated observations. (➤ Ch. 35 The art of diagnosis: medicine and the five senses) These referred for the most part to specific diseases, and any further division of groups of diseases was limited to such things as the broad distinction between acute and chronic disorders, that between epidemic and endemic ones, or to categories such as diseases of women. Depending on circumstances, acute diseases could end in cure, relapse, or death, or turn into chronic ones.

Nor did Plato (427–347 BC) provide a systematic analysis of disease, despite the fact that his philosophy of ideas, and of the relationship between words and things, underpinned a good deal of the later history of essentialist thinking. Plato's notions of diseases, as elaborated in *Timaeus*, were basically Hippocratic, and his attempt to construct a more general classification of disease was not particularly coherent. He divided diseases into three classes: those resulting from excess or deficiency of one of the constituent elements of the body; those due to a reversed order in the formation of the structures; and those which result from 'breath'. The great philosophic ontologist actually produced a physiological nosology.[3]

Galen (AD 129–*c*.200/210) was a great admirer of Hippocrates (*c*.460–370 BC), and while he had much to say on the nature of disease, his comments on more general nosological matters were not particularly systematic. He distinguished between general and local diseases, and among the former provided an elaborate classification of fevers in a separate monograph, *On Different Kinds of Fever*. Another Galenic scheme divided deviations from health into congenital malformations, complexional imbalance, and trauma. In practice, the second of these categories was of most interest to physicians, and the third to surgeons. Complexional disorders (*mala complexio*) were directly related to Hippocratic humoralism.[4]

Galen did on occasion mention the 'seeds' of disease, which some historians have interpreted as a foreshadowing of the germ theory. However, as Nutton has recently shown, Galen never seriously deviated from the physiological mode of disease elaborated by the Hippocratics;[5] his 'seeds' are at best only one of a series of disease causes and must be interpreted as part of the internal processes of disease. The Roman poet Lucretius (c.95–55 BC), and various other medical writers, did speculate on the nature of these 'seeds' in the context of discussions why some diseases are contagious and others not, but ontological theories of disease never took root among classical authors. The micronosology of fever classification has a long and complicated history, but the referent was generally either observable phenomena associated with individual cases or, especially in later Galenists, the more abstract philosophical notions of form and quality.[6] (➤ Ch. 19 Fevers)

Consequently, the most common macronosological scheme to be used in the Middle Ages was the one that simply listed diseases serially, beginning with diseases of the head and working down to diseases of the feet. Since the humoral model could explain melancholy, hysteria, mania, and other conditions which we would describe as psychiatric, within the same framework as gout, fevers, and other 'physical' disorders, these could be included among diseases of the head (or reproductive organs) rather than as separate psychological complaints. This is not to say that doctors paid no attention to the role of the emotions (or passions) in the causation of disease. The passions were among the six 'non-naturals', the control of which played an important part in maintaining health. Nevertheless, the formal separation of mental from physical diseases was not a routine part of the classical tradition. (➤ Ch. 21 Mental diseases)

EARLY MODERN ONTOLOGICAL DISEASE CONCEPTS

A radical alternative to physiological models of diseases was enunciated by the complex, peripatetic mystic, theologian and doctor, Paracelsus (c. 1493–1541). Always an individualist, Paracelsus rejected the whole of the classical tradition and offered in its place his own natural philosophy, theology, and medical system. Drawing on a complex web of alchemy, astrology, analogy (for example, the doctrine of signatures, and the relationship between the microcosm and the macrocosm), observation, and experiment, he developed a cosmology in which three active principles – salt, sulphur, and mercury – condition the various states of matter. The causes of disease were to be found in minerals and in the atmosphere, which conveyed the poisons produced by astrological influences. These agents were distinct things (ens), with existence independent of the human sufferer. Disease was, then, a kind of parasitism, an invasion of the body by a specific foreign agent, which then set up court, disturbing normal function and threatening life itself.[7]

Paracelsus did not attempt a revised classification of disease based on this new model; indeed, he was rather vague about how such an enterprise would be carried out. Rather, its immediate consequences were therapeutic, for the object of therapy was to counteract directly the specific causative agents of disease. Specific rather than symptomatic therapy would be the order of the day. Through the doctrine of signatures (that substances with similar colours or shapes to the organs of the body were effective in diseases of those organs), and through the systematic search for specific active principles, he sought to turn traditional therapeutics on its head. He was appreciative of the value of plant remedies, but he also believed that chemical remedies found in the mineral kingdom were of equal importance. It was this latter emphasis on a chemical pharmacopoeia that differentiated later Paracelsians from the more traditional Galenists in the century after Parcelsus's death and provided an ongoing source of often acrimonious debates during the period: therapeutics rather than nosology was at stake.[8]

According to Walter Pagel, the Paracelsian idea of a disease ontology was fully realized by Johannes Baptista van Helmont (1579–1644). Although van Helmont was not simply a blind follower of Paracelsus, he was influenced by him and, like him, developed a highly idiosyncratic philosophy of nature. Van Helmont combined a personal mysticism with an actively enquiring mind. He conceived living bodies as functioning through the operation of a governing vital principle which, following Paracelsus, he called the *archeus;* in addition, individual organs possessed their own archei. Each disease was an external thing or *ens*, possessing a specific morbid seed or semen and capable of attacking and irritating the body, thereby causing disease, by the analogy of a thorn in the flesh. Through a complicated scheme, he grappled with the complexities of generalized and local disease, and with both the psychological and patho-physiological components of it. (➤ Ch. 7 The pathological tradition)

Both Paracelsus and van Helmont attracted many followers who clashed with upholders of traditional Galenic medicine. It was not simply through their ontological conceptions of disease, nor the new basis of therapeutics, that their challenge to medical orthodoxy was felt. Rather, they and their followers cast doubt on the whole basis of medical authority, education, and institutions. At a time of great political, social, and religious upheaval, they championed the right of the individual to explore new conceptions of nature and of human beings' relationship to God. (➤ Ch. 61 Religion and medicine) They are now seen as central to medicine's place in the Scientific Revolution, which in turn, is no longer viewed as simply the triumph of the 'mechanization of the world picture', but as a much more complex movement permeated by many religious, philosophical, social, and intellectual ferments.[9]

At the same time, while both Paracelsus and van Helmont offered new ways of conceptualizing the relationship between disease and patient, neither

339

left a systematic classification of disease. Within the Galenic tradition, Jean Fernel (1497–1558), who coined the words *physiologia* and *pathologia*, produced a classification that reiterated the increasing importance being attached to local diseases and their pathological changes. He divided diseases into general and special. Fevers provided the principal example of the former category, and these he divided into simple, putrid, and pestilential. Special diseases were divided into those affecting parts above the diaphragm, those below, and external diseases. He also distinguished between simple diseases, affecting part of an organ; compound ones, involving the whole organ; and complicated diseases, in which the relations between the parts were disturbed.[10]

Another progressive traditionalist, Girolamo Fracastoro (1478–1553), left a systematic account of the 'seeds of disease' in his treatise, *De Contagione et Contagiosis Morbis et Curatione* (1546). Two centuries of plague, and the more recent appearance of apparently new diseases, such as the English sweat and syphilis, had provided more urgency to the traditional question of why some diseases are contagious and some not, and posed the intriguing problem of whether diseases can appear *de novo*. The latter invited speculation on the relationship between the Creator and his creation (Would a benevolent God create yet more diseases to plague humans beyond those that came with the Fall?), as well as providing ammunition for those who held that not all necessary medical knowledge was contained in ancient writings. Contagious diseases required some model to explain what exactly was being spread and what its connection was to the cause of the disease in the original victim. The 'seed' model fitted, although neither Fracastoro nor his contemporaries had witnessed a disease-causing agent, and it is too easy to modernize him into a kind of proto-bacteriologist. Nevertheless, the Fracastorian 'seed' was an entity that bred true – plague was caught only from other plague victims – and provided a basis for a specific classification of contagious diseases, though not for a systematic ontological statement of disease in general.[11]

Despite the ease with which Fracastoro can be identified as the founder of much later parasitical theories of disease, he is probably more properly seen as a part of what could be called the 'virus' tradition, virus in this context having the older meaning of poison. The viral poison was the source of contagion, but it carried with it no necessary implications of being a living organism.

SYDENHAM

A central irony in the history of nosology rests in its being raised to medical prominence by the 'English Hipprocrates', Thomas Sydenham (1624–89). He was accorded that epithet mostly for the clarity of his clinical descriptions, but his affinities with the father of medicine went deeper, for Sydenham accepted the framework of Hippocratic patho-physiology, even if evidence that he was particularly concerned with the nuances of humoralism in the normal, healthy state, is lacking. In fact, his writings were virtually all concerned with diseases and their treatment. Nor is there any direct evidence that he saw himself continuing the Renaissance discussions originated by Paracelsus on the ontology of disease, or was influenced by van Helmont or more traditional writers such as Pieter van Foreest (1522–97), who had discussed the classification of fevers and the implications of 'new' diseases.[12] Sydenham quoted very few authorities in his writings, and from his attitude to formal medical education and book-learning, we can safely assume he was not particularly well versed in the literature of his profession.

Nevertheless, Sydenham advocated a programme for clinical medicine that was widely appreciated in the eighteenth century, and Knud Faber, in his classic study of the history of nosology, was correct to begin with Sydenham.[13] In essence, Sydenham's programme was simple: medicine is a craft activity and medical progress results from the accumulation of repeated careful observations of patients suffering from disease, and of the consequences of various treatments for their diseases. Medicine thus proceeded by a kind of trial and error, with the aim of matching better remedies to particular diseases, and the ultimate goal of discovering specific remedies, of which the best example was the use of Peruvian or Jesuit's Bark in cases of ague (or intermittent fever). Sydenham was one of the early enthusiastic advocates of the bark for ague, and his belief that the drug could stop the ague dead in its tracks – that is, was a *specific* – lay at the heart of his whole philosophy of medicine. Most remedies acted gradually, by helping the body get rid of the peccant humour that was the cause of the disease. The bark seemed actually to neutralize or root out the disease at its source. It was qualitatively different from ordinary remedies and encouraged Sydenham to hold that specific remedies could be found for other diseases. (➤ Ch. 39 Drug therapies)

The specific action of the bark would also have reinforced his notion that, despite their variable courses and symptoms in individual patients, diseases are specific entities which can be precisely described by astute clinicians. As Sydenham remarked, 'all diseases [must] be reduced to definite and certain *species*, and that, with the same care which we see exhibited by botanists in their phytologies'. The botanical analogy appeared again in his famous injunction to clinicians:

> Something in the way of variety we may refer to the particular temperament of individuals; something also to the difference of treatment. Notwithstanding this, Nature, in the production of disease, is uniform and consistent; so much so, that for the same disease in different persons the symptoms are for the most part the same; and the selfsame phenomena that you would observe in

the sickness of a Socrates you would observe in the sickness of a simpleton. Just so the universal characters of a plant are extended to every individual of the species; and whoever (I speak in the way of illustration) should accurately describe the colour, the taste, the smell, the figure, &c., of one single violet, would find that his description held good, there or there-abouts, for all the violets of that particular species upon the face of the earth.[14]

This was a much plainer statement than anything found in earlier writers, and while it made no claims for the ontological distinctness of the disease and the person suffering from it, it did insist that diseases are distinct and real categories which, despite individual variability, do possess qualities and natural histories that are unique to the specific disease in question.

In another, less frequently quoted passage, Sydenham was even more explicit about the patho-physiological processes that produced a specific disease:

Hence every specific disease is a disorder that originates from this or that specific exaltation, or (changing the phrase) from the specification of some juice in the living body. Under this head may be comprised the greatest part of those diseases that are reducible to some given form or type, in the production and maturation whereof Nature binds herself to a certain method as stringently as she does with plants and even animals. Each plant and animal has its proper and peculiar disorders. In like manner, each juice has its exaltations as soon as it has broken out into a species. Of this we have a clear, visible, and daily proof in the different species of excrescences, which trees and fruit exhibit in the shape of moss, and mistletoe, and fungi, and the like. Whether arising from a perversion and depravation of the nutritive juice, or from any other cause, these excrescences are, each and all, essences or species wholly distinct and different from the parent stock, whether tree or shrub.[15]

By evoking the analogy with mistletoe, Sydenham emphasized the distinctions of the disease from the person suffering from it, even while still operating within a traditional humoral framework.

Sydenham never attempted to base a whole system of medicine on this philosophy. Rather, his writings always related directly to his own clinical experience, including the careful observation of the prevalent epidemic diseases of London during his own practice in the 1660s and 1670s. These he related to a complex set of changing environmental conditions which he called the 'epidemic constitution'. (➤ Ch. 15 Evironment and miasmata) He left, in addition, vivid descriptions of a number of individual diseases, including smallpox, hysteria, St Vitus's dance, gout, and pleurisy; and some observations on the differences between acute and chronic diseases. Acute diseases, he reckoned, constituted two-thirds of the disorders that afflicted mankind; chronic diseases, such as gout and hysteria, made up the remainder. He was aware that on occasion an acute disorder could take root and become a more deep-seated chronic one, but he reckoned in general the causes of acute and chronic disease were radically different. Acute diseases were external, environmental in their origin, essentially acts of God with a tendency to manifest themselves in the form of epidemics. Chronic diseases originate within ourselves and can generally be related to the six non-naturals. This external–internal dichotomy was fundamental to Sydenham's perception of medical practice, although he was not sanguine that it was in the power of mortal humans to discover the ultimate, material cause of disease. This was one reason why he considered medicine to be essentially a craft activity, and doctors ever to be denied the knowledge of why the remedies they prescribed had their particular effects. Nevertheless, the careful doctor could know which specific diseases the patient was suffering from, and with time and observation, other specific remedies would be found, like the bark for ague.[16]

NOSOLOGY IN THE EIGHTEENTH CENTURY

Sydenham's writings established a European reputation. Hermann Boerhaave (1668–1738) admired the clarity of his clinical descriptions and the cogency of many of his therapeutic innovations. Giorgio Baglivi (1648–1701) echoed Sydenham's call for the practice of medicine to be reformed on the bedrock of careful and repeated bedside observations of disease and disease patterns. Both recognized that Sydenham had been merely putting into effect the earlier injunction of Francis Bacon (1561–1626) for doctors to collect 'histories of disease' as part of the latter's own vision of a Great Instauration, a new and more powerful understanding of the natural world based on the method of induction: the formation of general laws through the collection and analysis of numerous individual instances.

Both Bacon and Sydenham were assimilated into the vigorous Hippocratism which was so conspicuous a feature of Enlightenment medicine. At the same time, the towering figure of Isaac Newton (1642–1727) also cast a long shadow, offering encouragement to those who believed that massive, grand generalizations were possible in all areas of human enquiry, on the model that he had achieved for astronomy and natural philosophy in his *Principia* (1687). Baglivi and Boerhaave each stood in awe of Newton, and much of the physiological work was cast within the mechanical framework of medical Newtonianism, although Baglivi insisted that theoretical presuppositions should be put to one side when approaching the bedside.[17] (➤ Ch. 7 The physiological tradition)

The synthetic achievements of Newton encouraged doctors during the Enlightenment to produce their own grand versions of the medical knowledge within their ken. In particular, comprehensive nosologies of all human diseases became popular, especially after the work of the Swedish naturalist

Carl Linnaeus (1707–78) brought taxonomy to centre stage in the natural sciences. Although Linnaeus preferred to see himself as a second Adam (the first Adam having given names to plants and animals in the Garden of Eden) rather than a second Newton, he argued that proper classifications of the objects of scientific enquiry were a necessary precondition of reliable scientific knowledge. He introduced the system of binomial nomenclature whereby each species can be identified uniquely by its particular genus and species. Thus, human beings are members of the genus *Homo* and of the species *sapiens*, to distinguish them from all other species, including, in Linnaeus's scheme, the tailless apes that also occupy the same genus. Later naturalists have considerably revised Linnaeus's classification of the primates (a word he also coined), but his biological designation of human beings has been retained.[18]

Linnaeus devoted much of his creative energy to classifying plants and to expanding the theoretical principles underlying his taxonomic enterprise. As a young man, he went to Lapland, and he continued to send his students on specimen-gathering expeditions in many parts of the world, including Africa and the Far East. His success in fitting into his general taxonomic scheme the hundreds of new species of plants and animals then being examined in Europe for the first time gave great prestige to his endeavours, which raised again the question of artificial versus natural systems in taxonomy. Linnaeus argued that a natural system is possible, since there are 'natural' relationships between natural objects (such as species). By contrast, his great rival, the French naturalist Georges Buffon (1707–88), contended that nature 'knows only the individual', and that classifications are only heuristic devices, useful for many reasons but ultimately artificial (that is, synthetic.) In many respects, the Linnaeus–Buffon debate was the biological equivalent of the physiological–ontological dichotomy about diseases and their classification.

Linnaeus actually trained in medicine and left a disease taxonomy, as well as his botanical and zoological ones. His *Genera Morborum* (1763) divided all diseases into eleven major groupings, or classes, each with its essential defining characteristics, and further divisible into genera and species.[19] Throughout his work, Linnaeus used the Aristotelian principles of classification by downward division, whereby groups are successively differentiated by certain specified characteristics. Diseases proved less tractable than plants for this purpose. His broadest grouping was between febrile and non-febrile diseases, the fevers themselves being divided into three classes: exanthema, 'critical' fevers, and 'inflammatory' fevers. The first class was characterized by skin eruptions, the second by the presence of a red sediment in the urine, the third by a hard pulse and local pain. Overall, the fevers were to be diagnosed by the presence of a rapid pulse. Each class contained its own genera and species.

Among the eight classes of non-febrile diseases, four were disorders of nerves (disturbances of sensation, judgement, and movement), two of fluids, and two of solids. Those of the fluids were divided into suppressions and evacuations, suppressive diseases encompassing conditions such as coughs and constipation. Painful diseases appeared in various groups, as disturbances of sensation (gout thereby being a 'nervous' disease), but also contributed to the differentiae of inflammatory fevers, or in griping diarrhoea.

Linnaeus's disease classification was primarily symptom or sign oriented, and thus produced groupings which, by later criteria, were based on very superficial adventitious similarities. Athough he subsequently produced a second, expanded edition of his *Genera Morborum*, in this particular taxonomic endeavour he was a follower rather than a leader, for the French physician and botanist François Boissier de Sauvages (1706–67) had made nosology central to his medical practice and teaching. Although Linnaeus and Sauvages were correspondents, the first edition of the latter's *Nouvelles classes des maladies dans un ordre à celui des botanistes* was published in 1731, four years before Linnaeus's general taxonomic statement, the *Systema Naturae*. In its conception and basic structure, Sauvages' nosology thus drew upon local botanical traditions, and on the medical writings of Sydenham and Baglivi.[20] Sauvages identified some 2,400 different species of diseases, which he grouped according to various criteria. His classes were broadly similar to those that Linnaeus subsequently identified: fevers, inflammations, evacuations, paralysis, painful diseases, 'spiritual' and mental diseases, wasting diseases, and convulsive disorders. In the course of providing subsequent editions of his arrangement, he tinkered with the main groupings and fretted about some of the lower taxa, but the basic structure was still recognizable in 1763, when his five-volumed *Nosologia Methodica* announced his final, definitive classification. By then, the prestige of Linnaean taxonomy had made classification all the rage.

The nosologies of both Sauvages and Linnaeus are usually described as symptom based. Thus, for instance, they used varieties and locations of pain as a basis for classifying diseases. In other instances, they relied on what could be more accurately described as signs. Sauvages, for example, described jaundice as a kind of disease, which he broke into a number of species, depending on whether it was associated with obstruction, fever, plethora, or poison. Cough, too, he treated as a kind of disease, distinguishing seventeen different species. A different variety of features, including their course over time, informed his classification of fevers, all distinguished by the rapidity of the pulse, itself a sign. Sometimes he incorporated some element of cause, or aetiology, in the classificatory enterprise, and gross pathological changes – the *lesion* so important to clinicians from the early nineteenth century – also influenced some of his taxonomic decisions.

345

In carrying forward what he considered to be the Baconian programme of history-gathering, Sauvages developed considerable diagnostic skills. His approach encouraged him to be a splitter rather than a lumper, to differentiate an ever-expanding number of diseases based on slight differences in presentation, symptom, or outcome.

Sauvages was criticized in a number of ways by William Cullen (1710–90), but Cullen, too, saw the necessity of bringing order into a vast range of clinical observations through taxonomy. His own nosology reduced the number of disease classes to four, with the first three (pyrexiae, neuroses, cachexia) based on disturbances of the traditional classes of physiological functions (the vital, animal, and natural functions). His fourth class, 'local disease', occupied almost half of the number of genera he identified, and while it was a heterogeneous category, it did at least made some attempt to account for local pathological changes in disease classification. Cullen initially produced his nosology in a spare outline in 1769, but he subsequently used the framework it created in his *First Lines of the Practice of Physic* (1778–9), one of the most influential medical books of the century. Its multiple editions, adaptations, and translations, combined with Cullen's status as a teacher at the University of Edinburgh, ensured that thousands of medical students and practitioners throughout the world were familiar with his nosology and the therapeutic recommendations for the diseases he had described.[21]

Cullen was not an advocate of the ontological distinctness of disease, nor was he confident that the human mind could penetrate to the ultimate causes of things. Most diseases he believed to be caused by external influences – heat, cold, food, effluvia, dampness, etc. – and he was acutely aware that the same cluster of external factors could, under particular circumstances, cause different diseases in different individuals, or even in the same individual at different times. He thus became a keen student of the patho-physiological mechanisms of disease, though his physiology could best be described as the bedside variety, concerned with such traditional parameters as the pulse, the state of the blood vessels, and the nature of the various evacuations. Most of these patho-physiological processes were ultimately, he believed, under the control of the nervous system. In this, he was part of a widespread movement from the middle of the eighteenth century which emphasized the primacy of the nervous system. At a cultural level, this was related to a growing cult of sensibility and an enhanced consciousness of issues of refinement, class, gender, and nation in much of the historical, literary, and philosophical writing of the period.

Within medicine, these concerns found expression in a heightened awareness of the role of culture and refinement in producing 'nervous diseases', expertly analysed by Cullen's pupil Thomas Trotter (1760–1832) in his *A View of the Nervous Temperament* (1807). Another consequence was that no nosological category of Cullen had quite the same impact as his creation of a new class of nervous diseases, for which he coined the word 'neurosis'. At the same time he insisted that, in a manner of speaking, all diseases could be deemed 'nervous', so pervasive is the action of the nervous system. For Cullen, a neurosis was a disturbance of any of the functions of the nervous system, especially those of sensation and motion. He also grouped madness and other 'mental' disorders among the neuroses. During the nineteenth century, the meaning assigned to neurosis varied from author to author; never very precise, it assumed many of its modern implications through the work of Sigmund Freud (1856–1939) and his followers, acquiring in the process much more mentalist connotations than those envisaged by Cullen.[22] (➤ Ch. 43 Psychotherapy)

Another of Cullen's pupils, John Brown (1735–88), took the neurophysiology of his times in another direction, one with rather deliberate Newtonian overtones. Rather than creating new nosological schemes, Brown sought the underlying unities in all disease processes. He believed diseases could be recognized by their fruits, not their roots. Brown indentified the principle of life as a property that he called 'excitability', and considered that disease occurred when an excess or deficiency of this property was present. An excess produced a 'sthenic' disorder; a deficiency, an 'asthenic' one. There were thus just two basic kinds of disease, and, in practice, most diseases were asthenic ones, or diseases of debility. This could be the ultimate outcome even of sthenic disorders, for this property of excitability could soon become exhausted, with the production of asthenia, through what Brown called 'indirect debility'.

Just as Brown conceived of disease as the consequence of general pathophysiological disturbance, so therapy should be directed at restoring the proper balance of excitability. Therapeutic measures were thus of a general nature: depletives such as bloodletting and purgatives appropriate for sthenic complaints; stimulants such as opium and alcohol the treatment of choice in the instance of asthenic disorders (either direct or indirect). His own fondness (and later addiction) for opium and alcohol had been partially caused by what he held to be the successful treatment of his own case of gout, traditionally a quintessential disease of plethora or excess. Brown reckoned that it had produced an indirect debility, to which he attributed its successful management with opium and alcohol.[23]

The Brownian (Brunonian) system relegated nosology to a minor role and made the difference between health and disease a quantitative rather than a qualitative matter. It also made diagnosis and therapeutics relatively easy affairs. It achieved a good deal of popularity in Germany and Italy, although most doctors were suspicious of its simplicity and implicit populism. In the United States, Benjamin Rush (1746–1813) incorporated several Brunonian features in his own monolithic speculations on the nature of disease, although Rush was an enthusiastic bleeder. (➤ Ch. 40 Physical methods)

LESIONS AND DISEASES IN NINETEENTH-CENTURY MEDICINE

Although Cullen's *First Lines* continued to be published well into the nineteenth century, with translators and editors updating its contents, its function was more that of a general textbook then a theoretical guide to nosology. Within the context of the new 'hospital medicine', associated above all with the post-Revolutionary medicine school in Paris, the older symptom-based nosologies were seen as hopelessly unreliable and subjective. (➤ Ch. 49 The hospital) Instead, physical diagnosis, especially the development of percussion and auscultation, and the methods of clinico-pathological correlation, placed a new emphasis on the local lesion as the most important defining characteristic of disease. Temkin described the transformation as the incorporation of localist, surgical thinking into medicine; Ackerknecht as the development of hospital medicine; Foucault as the birth of the clinic.[24] Foucault summarized the shift by remarking that eighteenth-century physicians had asked their patients, 'what is the matter with you?'; nineteenth-century ones, 'where does it hurt?'; though with the insistence that the pain was not the disease, merely a guide to underlying pathology, which provided the only reliable, objective basis of diagnosing disease. Within the new mentality, pain and kindred signs and symptoms were not diseases to be classified, but pointers which directed the diagnosing doctor to the organs and, increasingly, to the tissues where disease was located. (➤ Ch. 67 Pain and suffering)

Consequently, nosology as a formal endeavour lost much of its lustre, although the development of the general textbook tradition (bearing such titles as 'A System of Medicine', or 'The Practice of Medicine') required classificatory schemes to organize diagnostic categories. In addition, continuities between eighteenth- and nineteenth-century concerns abound. *De Sedibus et Causis Morborum* (1761) by Giovanni Morgagni (1682–1771) was organ-based; and Philippe Pinel (1745–1826), one of the leading figures of Paris hospital medicine, published an influential *Nosographie Philosophique* (1798), which went into several editions. His five classes – fevers, inflammations, haemorrhages, neuroses, and organic lesions – bore important traces of his regard for Cullen (he had already translated the *First Lines* into French), but he also admired Morgagni. More than Cullen, Pinel struggled to reconcile pathology and clinical practice.

He also provided his pupil, Xavier Bichat (1771–1802), with a key stimulus in the elaboration of the tissue concept. Pinel had written, 'What matter that the arachnoid, the pleura, and the peritoneum reside in different regions of the body, since these membranes have general conformities of structure? Are they not affected by similar lesions in the state of inflammation [phlegmasis]?"[25] Bichat went on to identify (using only a hand-lens) twenty-one different kinds of tissue (fibrous, osseus, serous, mucus, synovial, glandular, etc.), each of which may be found in various organs or parts of the body. An early manifestation of Bichat's tissue concept can be seen in the treatise on heart disease (1806) by J. N. Corvisart (1755–1821), in which he identified diseases of the endocardium, myocardium, and pericardium, rather than simply discussing heart diseases *sui generis*. As Bichat insisted, pathological anatomy was the science of the future:

> This science is not only that of the organic changes which arrive slowly or as consequences in chronic diseases. It consists of the study of all possible alterrations of our bodies whenever we examine their diseases. With the exception of certain fevers and nervous diseases, almost everything in pathology is in its domain.[26]

Bichat was correct in identifying fevers and nervous diseases as two categories that were relatively intractable via the clinico-pathological method. Pinel had devoted almost one-third of his *Nosographie* to what he called the 'essential fevers', and his class 'Neurosis' included for the most part diseases he considered to be 'functional'. Although this class was much larger than diseases we would now call 'psychiatric', Pinel helped to formulate a notion of a 'mental' disease in his other major work, the *Traité médico-philosophique sur l'aliénation mentale ou la manie* (1801), produced as a result of his experiences as physician to the Salpêtrière. In it, he advocated a return to a simple Hippocratic nosology for insanity and related conditions, rejecting the complicated psychiatric classifications of late eighteenth-century authors such as Thomas Arnold (1742–1816). With the development of a specialism organized around the treatment of the insane, psychiatric nosology began to be hived off from more-general medical concerns. (➤ Ch. 56 Psychiatry)

'Essential' fevers continued to attract much comment, especially since they were a major source of mortality. The fever literature before the coming of bacteriology was often concerned directly or indirectly with the question of contagiousness, a debate which became much more urgent after cholera first struck Europe in the early 1830s. Since epidemic diseases by definition generally occurred in waves, they were relatively easy to diagnose, even if retrospective diagnosis in modern terms still often proves elusive. (➤ Ch. 52 Epidemiology) Clinico-pathological criteria allowed clinicians in France, Britain, and the United States more or less independently to distinguish between what are now called typhus and typhoid fever; and the increasing use of the thermometer ritualized by C. A. Wunderlich (1815–77) in Germany began to make the fever chart a routine part of a hospital stay and provided some basis for distinguishing the various febrile illnesses. Earlier, R. H. T. Laënnec

(1781–1826), inventor of the stethoscope, had developed what he believed to the pathognomonic criteria for diagnosing pulmonary phthisis during life. He also held that the formation of the small pathological processes called 'tubercles' anywhere in the body was symptomatic of a single disease. He thus created a disease category consonant with the modern diagnosis of 'tuberculosis' more than half-a-century before Robert Koch (1843–1910) indentified the tubercle bacillus. However, the nature and cause of the protean disorder long remained in dispute, and even Laënnec was dubious that its ultimate cause would ever be known. He recognized it only by its clinical and pathological consequences. His relutance to speculate on the ultimate causes of disease was shared by many of his French colleagues, for whom disease was to be diagnosed and thereby named from the lesions that it manifested. (➤ Ch. 36 The science of diagnosis: diagnostic technologies)

For the most part, then, the early nineteenth-century pathological tradition led doctors to eschew vast nosological schemes in favour of more focused studies of the diseases of a particular organ or system: for example, Corvisart on the heart; Laénnec on the lungs; and J. L. Alibert (1768–1837) on diseases of the skin. At the same time, F. J. V. Broussais (1772–1838) challenged the ontological orientation of the pathological anatomists with his own 'physiological' system. He accepted the importance of local lesions in the genesis of disease, but in his *Examen des doctrines médicales et des systèmes de nosologie* (1821) he argued that disease is never an ontological 'other', but simply the result of altered functions. In later works, he identified the ultimate source of disease as gastro-intestinal irritation, local manifestations being the result of sympathetic reaction to the primary lesion. His treatment of choice for virtually all diseases was leeching, which, he argued, produced counter-irritation and reduction of the inflammatory origin of the process.

Broussais produced one of the last monolithic systems of disease and treatment that can still be seen within the tradition of orthodox medicine. Although he had a number of followers in the 1820s and early 1830s, his direct influence was already on the wane by the time of his death. Indirectly, however, the issues he raised about disease as a process, and his critique of ontological formulations, continued to exercise medical thinking, even as anatomical pathology was extended through microscopy and chemistry. (➤ Ch. 6 The microscopical tradition; Ch. 8 The biochemical tradition)

Two developments lent substance to Broussais's contention that the transition from health to disease proceeded little by little, along altered physiological pathways. One was the mathematics of measurement and variability, from C. F. Gauss (1777–1855) to L. A. J. Quetelet (1796–1874) and beyond. Quetelet's social statistics examined various biological and social phenomena, elucidating a concept of the *mean* or *average*, which for many characteristics, such as height or weight, could be shown to fall out into the familiar (to us) bell-shaped (or Gaussian) curve. The equation of the average with the 'normal' was a relatively easy step, and the transition from the 'normal' to the 'abnormal' is, in the context of a Gaussian curve, a continuous one. The positivist philosopher Auguste Comte (1798–1857) generalized Broussais's medical philosophy, insisting that 'every modification – whether natural or artificial – of the real order concerns only the intensity of the corresponding phenomena'.[27] From this tradition emerged the concept that various physiological phenomena – the concentration of chemicals in the blood or urine, the ratio (and eventually, the number) of red and white blood cells, body temperature and metabolic rate, blood pressure – also varied around an average figure which could be related to age, sex, race, or even state of health. Early instances were the association by Richard Bright (1784–1858) of large amounts of albumen (protein) in the urine with diseases of the kidney; or the discovery by Rudolf Virchow (1821–1902) and John Hughes Bennett (1812–75) independently, that in a condition that Virchow first called leukaemia, the 'normal' ratio of red to white blood cells is reversed.

A second strand of argument followed from aspects of the first: the development of methods and procedures that promised to uncover the minute chain of events whereby normal structures became abnormal ones, turning into the lesions which were the footsteps of disease. Claude Bernard (1813–78) was suspicious of statistical truths (for him, one well-documented instance of a phenomenon was significant), but he argued vigorously on behalf of physiological explanations of disease processes. The static portraits of disease offered by pathological anatomy needed to be broken down into dynamic ones in the laboratory, with experimental physiology providing the bedrock on which the medicine of the future was to be built. Bernard's own work on sugar storage and use, and on the site of action of poisons such as curare and carbon monoxide, had clinical promise.[28]

Even within pathology, individuals like Virchow argued that disease was nothing but life under altered circumstances, and that cellular pathology offered the means to analyse the finer mechanisms of disease, henceforth to be located in the cells themselves. In a series of programmatic essays from the late 1840s, which culminated in his *Cellular Pathology* (1858), the young Virchow espoused the physiological standpoint in pathology, arguing that all diseases are reducible to active or passive disturbances of living cells, and that pathological formations are degenerations, transformations, or repetitions of normal structures.

Towards the end of his life, however, Virchow had modified his position, and insisted that cellular pathology was:

> expressly ontological. That is its merit, not its deficiency. There actually is an
> *ens morbi*, just as there is an *ens vitae*; in both instances a cell or cell-complex

has the claim to be thus designated. The *ens morbi* is at the same time a parasite in the sense of the natural-historical schools, not in the sense of the bacteriologists.[29]

Virchow's shift of opinion was essentially a pragmatic one, based on the vast changes in medicine he had witnessed, and the extent to which specific diseases did appear to exist, obeying explicable laws and capable of being defined (and diagnosed) with precision. Events in the clinic testified to the reality of the 'natural history' of diseases.

At the same time, Virchow was careful to distance himself from the simple parasitic model of disease of the bacteriologists. By the 1880s, the germ theory of Louis Pasteur (1822–95), Robert Koch, and others offered a new ontological paradigm of parasitism, equating the cause of disease after disease to invasion of external micro-organisms. Although the historical literature of the first half of the twentieth century sometimes exaggerated the extent to which bacteriology quickly triumphed over the resistance of old-fashioned doctors, the germ theory did offer a new way of thinking about disease specificity, particularly for the large group of 'essential' fevers which had always been nosologically awkward. It also promised to integrate a notion of cause into classification schemes: no tuberculosis without the tubercle bacillus. (➤ Ch. 16 Contagion/germ theory/specificity)

Nevertheless, it would be easy to overstate the actual impact of the germ theory on nosology *per se*. Most of the diseases in which bacteria, tropical parasites, and, later, viruses, were implicated already had reasonably specific clinical and pathological identities before the micro-organism was specified. (➤ Ch. 24 Tropical diseases) Indeed, for a number of diseases, a variety of micro-organisms was proposed before consensus was reached. In other instances, such as scurvy and beri-beri, micro-organisms were suggested as playing a causal role for diseases subsequently shown to have other aetiologies.[30] (➤ Ch. 22 Nutritional diseases) The article on 'Diseases, causes of', in the 1895 edition of Quain's *Dictionary of Medicine* listed living contagion last among a group of eighteen factors, including diet, cold, heredity, and temperament. The article on 'Disease, classification of' (there was none on 'Nosology') discussed a number of ways in which diseases had been grouped (general and local; organic and functional; hereditary and acquired; acute, subacute, and chronic), but concluded that none 'fulfils all that is required, or can be regarded as satisfactory'.[31]

By the end of the nineteenth century, most doctors would have been aware of the existence of agreed lists of acceptable diagnostic categories, since most developed countries were beginning to issue routine death certificates. In Britain, William Farr (1807–83) played the major role in drawing up these official nosologies, and he used his post at the Registrar General's Office as the base from which to comment, especially through his annual reports, on changing disease patterns in Victorian Britain. (➤ Ch. 51 Public health; Ch. 71 Demography and medicine) In the pre-bacteriological era, he coined the term 'zymotic', to describe those diseases whose causes he likened to fermentations, and he worked out elaborate mathematical formulae to relate the geographical distribution of cholera to the position of the water table in areas where it was prevalent. He encouraged his peers to base their final diagnoses on sound pathological criteria. Farr and the Swiss doctor Marc d'Espine (1806–60) also attempted to further an international standard nomenclature for diseases at the International Statistical Congress in 1853.[32] They discovered agreement even between themselves difficult, and obtaining a more general set of standard diagnoses still more awkward. Nevertheless, the very attempt at a transnational nosology suggests that medical science was beginning to provide a common vocabulary for medical communication. (➤ Ch. 59 Internationalism in medicine and public health)

THE CLINCAL SYNDROME

The germ theory did, in the end, provide for a certain number of diseases the desired goal of nosological schemes: one based on aetiology. Even for these parasitical diseases, however, no simple equation provided unambiguous guidelines. Even if there is no tuberculosis without the tubercle bacillus, individual response can and does vary from situation to situation, and from person to person. The total clinical picture may give the doctor confidence in diagnosis, but only statistical confidence in prognosis. And if this is true for the diseases caused by infections, it is even more the case for the chronic disorders which have come to predominate in developed countries in the twentieth century. Diagnostic techniques have made possible the naming of an ever-increasing number of diseases and syndromes, and medical science has come close to providing an international language among those who accept its precepts. Nevertheless, schizophrenia is more commonly diagnosed in the United States than in Britain, and French doctors and their patients relate more diseases to the liver than is common in other Western countries. Despite the efforts of international groups to set basic criteria for diagnosing a particular condition, the values of nation, specialism, or individual colour the relationship between the diagnosing doctor and the patient, and the label that the patient comes away with. (➤ Ch. 34 The history of the doctor–patient relationship)

Even without these filters, the basic language of modern clinical practice is widely recognized to be statistical, or probabilistic, in nature, especially when prognosis is being assessed.[33] Many older diagnostic categories – railway spine and flying gout, for example – have disappeared, but many more have been created during the past century, as new metabolic, biochemical, tomographic, and genetic techniques have developed. It is common for these to be called clinical syndromes rather than diseases, the word 'syndrome' referring to a set of signs and symptoms occurring together, but not carrying quite the biological connotations possessed by the word 'disease'. Even for disease categories, however, the simple causal model of the germ theory is not seen as appropriate. Most diseases, especially chronic ones such as cancers, arthritis, and cardiovascular disease, are multi-causal. Our forbears diagnosed 'essential' fevers; we diagnose 'essential' hypertension. (➤ Ch. 20 Constitutional and hereditary disorders; Ch. 25 Cancer)

At a more general level, the older debate about disease ontology has been replaced by concern about the social construction of diseases, the moral and political uses of diagnoses, the status of a whole series of issues such as, chronic fatigue syndrome, drug abuse, and the problem of scapegoating which the AIDS epidemic has highlighted. (➤ Ch. 37 History of medical ethics; Ch. 70 Medical sociology; Ch. 26 Sexually transmitted diseases)

NOTES

1 N. C. Smith (ed.), *The Letters of Sydney Smith*, 2 vols, Oxford, Clarendon Press, 1953, Vol. II, p. 637.
2 Henry Cohen, 'The evolution of the concept of disease', in Arthur L. Caplan, H. Tristram Engelhardt and James J. McCartney (eds), *Concepts of Health and Disease*, Reading, MA, Addison-Wesley, 1981, pp. 209–19, see pp. 210–11.
3 Walther Riese, *The Conception of Disease. Its History, its Versions and its Nature*, New York, Philosophical Library, 1953.
4 Ibid.
5 Vivian Nutton, 'The seeds of disease: an explanation of contagion and infection from the Greeks to the Renaissance', *Medical History*, 1983, 27: 1–34.
6 Aspects of this tradition are considered in W. F. Bynum and Vivian Nutton (eds), *Theories of Fever from Antiquity to the Enlightenment, Medical History*, suppl. 1, London, Wellcome Institute, 1981.
7 Walter Pagel, *Paracelsus – Introduction to Philosphical Medicine in the Era of the Renaissance*, Basle and New York, Karger, 1958.
8 See, for example, Allen G. Debus, *The English Paracelsians*, London, Oldbourne Press, 1965.
9 Walter Pagel, *Joan Baptista van Helmont. Reformer of Science and medicine*, Cambridge, Cambridge University Press, 1982; Pagel, 'Van Helmont's concept of disease – to be or not to be? The influence of Paracelsus', *Bulletin of the History of Medicine*, 1972, 46: 419–54.
10 Charles Sherrington, *The Endeavour of Jean Fernel*, Cambridge, Cambridge University Press, 1946.
11 Nutton, op. cit. (n. 5).
12 Vivian Nutton, 'Pieter van Foreest and the plagues of Europe: some observations

on the *Observations*', in H. L. Houtzager (ed.), *Pieter van Foreest*, Amsterdam, Rodopi, 1989, pp. 25–39.

13   Knud Faber, *Nosography. The Evolution of Clinical Medicine in Modern Times*, New York, Hoelser, 1930.

14   Thomas Sydenham, *Medical Observations Concerning the History and the Cure of Acute Diseases*, in *Works*, trans. by D. Greenhill, London, Sydenham Society, 1848, Vol. I, p. 15.

15   Ibid., p. 19.

16   Kenneth Dewhurst, *Dr Thomas Sydenham (1642–1689). His Life and Original Writings*, London, Wellcome Institute, 1966; G. G. Meynell, *Materials for a Biography of Dr Thomas Sydenham*, Folkestone, Kent, Winterdown Books, 1988.

17   M. D. Grmek, 'Georgius Baglio', in C. C. Gillespie (ed.), *Dictionary of Scientific Biography*, New York, Charles Scribner's Sons, 1970–80, Vol. I, pp. 391–2.

18   Ernst Mayr, *The Growth of Biological Thought*, Cambridge, MA, Harvard University Press, 1982, pp. 171–80.

19   Lester S. King, *The Medical World of the Eighteenth Century* Chicago, University of Chicago Press, 1958.

20   Julian Martin, 'Sauvages's nosology, medical enlightenment in Montpellier', in Andrew Cunningham and Roger French (eds), *The Medical Enlightenment of the Eighteenth Century*, Cambridge, Cambridge University Press, 1990, pp. 111–37.

21   John Thomson (completed by W. Thomson and D. Craigie), *An Account of the Life, Lectures and Writings of William Cullen MD*, 2 vols, Edinburgh, William Blackwood, 1859, remains a wonderful introduction to Cullen and his times.

22   José M. López Piñero, *Historical Origins of the Concept of Neurosis*, trans. by D. Berrios, Cambridge, Cambridge University Press, 1983.

23   W. F. Bynum and Roy Porter (eds), *Brunonianism in Britain and Europe, Medical History*, suppl. 8, London, Wellcome Institute, 1988.

24   Owsei Temkin, 'The role of surgery in the rise of modern medical thought', Temkin, *The Double Face of Janus*, Baltimore, MD, Johns Hopkins University Press, 1977; Erwin H. Ackerknecht, *Medicine at the Paris Hospital 1794–1848*, Baltimore, MD, Johns Hopkins University Press, 1967; Michel Foucault, *The Birth of the Clinic* trans. by A. M. Sheridan Smith, London, Tavistock, 1973.

25   Quoted in Foucault, op. cit. (n. 24), p. 132.

26   Quoted in Ackerknecht, op. cit. (n. 24), p. 55.

27   Georges Canguilhem, *The Normal and the Pathological*, trans. by C. R. Fawcett, New York, Zone Books, 1989, p. 48.

28   Claude Bernard, *An Introduction to the Study of Experimental Medicine*, trans. by H. C. Greene, New York, Dover Publications, 1957.

29   L. J. Rather (ed.), *Disease, Life, and Man. Selected Essays by Rudolf Virchow*, Stanford, CA, Stanford University Press, 1958, pp. 17 ff.

30   Kenneth J. Carpenter, *The History of Scurvy and Vitamine C*, Cambridge, Cambridge University Press, 1986.

31   Richard Quain (ed.), *A Dictionary of Medicine*, 2 vols, 2nd edn, London, Longmans, Green, 1895; for entries on 'Disease, causes of', and 'Disease, classification of', see Vol. I, pp. 507–16.

32   F. M. M. Lewes, 'Dr Marc D'Espine's statistical nosology', *Medical History*, 1988, 32: 301–13.

33   A. R. Feinstein, *Clinical Judgment*, Baltimore, MD, Williams & Wilkins, 1967.

FURTHER READING

Ackerknecht, Erwin H., *Medicine at the Paris Hospital, 1794–1848*, Baltimore, MD, Johns Hopkins University Press, 1967.

Canguilhem, Georges, *The Normal and the Pathological*, trans. by C. R. Fawcett, New York, Zone Books, 1989.

Caplan, Arthur L., Engelhardt, H. Tristram Jr and McCartney, James J. (eds), *Concepts of Health and Disease*, Reading, MA, Addison-Wesley, 1981.

Faber, Knud, *Nosography. The Evolution of Clinical Medicine in Modern Times*, New York, Hoeber, 1930.

Feinstein, Alvan R., *Clinical Judgment*, Baltimore, MD, Williams & Wilkins, 1967.

Foucault, Michel, *The Birth of the Clinic*, trans. by A. M. Sheridan Smith, London, Tavistock, 1973.

King, Lester S., *The Medical World of the Eighteenth Century*, Chicago, IL, University of Chicago Press, 1958.

——, *Medical Thinking. A Historical Preface*, Princeton, NJ, Princeton University Press, 1982.

Pagel, Walter, *Joan Baptista van Helmont. Reformer of Science and Medicine*, Cambridge, Cambridge University Press, 1982.

Riese, Walther, *The Conception of Disease. Its History, its Versions and its Nature*, New York, Philosophical Library, 1953.

Taylor, F. Kräupl, *The Concepts of Illness, Disease and Morbus*, Cambridge, Cambridge University Press, 1979.

18

THE ECOLOGY OF DISEASE

Kenneth F. Kiple

To write about the ecology of a single disease in its present state, to add something of its historical evolution and of the symbiotic relationships of parasite, vector, and host both endogenously and exogenously, and to include changing environmental as well as genetic and biochemical patterns, would require volumes and still be incomplete. Clearly to address the question of the ecology of disease (meaning all diseases) within a historical context in a single essay is an impossible task. None the less, with this caveat we can attempt to sketch in some broad, if often speculative, outlines.

THE ROLE OF DISEASE IN HUMAN EVOLUTION

To begin at the beginning, disease is a biological process that is considerably older than human beings; indeed, as old as life itself. The questions of where and how certain microbes became pathogenic to animals and later to humans may never be satisfactorily answered. It is generally conceded, however, that human pathogens are descended from free-living forms found in soil and water, and that the symbiosis between these forms and animals began many millions of years ago. Parasites and animals, in other words, evolved together. *Homo sapiens*, although a latecomer on the planet, is none the less the product of millions of years of evolution beginning with distant primate ancestors. Several million years ago, one species of these forest-living apes, called Australophines, left the forest to live on the plains and evolved into *Homo erectus*. At least the beginning of this evolutionary journey occurred in Africa, but *Homo erectus* later spread throughout much of the Old World. *Homo sapiens* has been identified from some 600,000 years ago. About 100,000 years ago these two merged with Neanderthal Man. Because *Homo sapiens sapiens* is thought to have evolved only about 40,000 years ago, it seems clear

357

that the human genetic constitution has changed relatively little in this short time-span, and thus we are mostly products of the distant as opposed to the recent past.[1]

Among other things, this means that despite a vast gulf of time separating us from the primates, our blood is extremely compatible with theirs (about 99 per cent). This suggests that a number of parasites that made (and make) a living off primate blood were (and are) more or less naturally adapted to parasitizing humans as well. In fact, it is doubtless the case that many human parasites are modifications of those that infected the remote ancestral primate from which all other primates including humans are descended.[2] We can divide parasitic infections very broadly into microparasites (bacteria, viruses, and protozoa) and macroparasites (parasitic helminths and arthropods). In general, microparasites are small, have very high rates of reproduction within a host, and tend to induce in survivors an immunity against reinfection. The macroparasites, by contrast, multiply at a much slower rate (if at all) within a host, and the immune response depends upon the number of parasites present and tends to be of short duration. Thus macroparasites can and do continually reinfect their hosts.[3]

Among the macroparasites that may well have kept evolutionary pace with humankind as we evolved from the primates are the *Enterobius* (pinworm or threadworm) and hookworm, while the microparasites include numerous protozoal infections, such as malarial parasites of the genus *Plasmodium*, and a considerable number of viruses including that of yellow fever. In addition, humans would have been affected by the parasites of other wild animals. An example here is African trypanosomiasis, or sleeping sickness, with the antelope being one of its reservoirs. Wherever the tsetse fly that spreads the disease abounded, sleeping sickness may well have placed definite limits on the areas into which hunter-gatherers would have expanded. In these early days, there were probably also wild-animal reservoirs for leptospirosis, relapsing fever, brucellosis, tularaemia, salmonellosis, and perhaps even plague. Still other ancient illnesses that found their way to humans include leishmaniasis, encephalitis, and hepatitis, as well as various parasites that entered the body via raw or under-cooked meat or water.[4] Still other diseases doubtless arose, a good example being the treponematoses. The original treponemes, which are believed to have caused yaws in early humans in the tropics and non-venereal syphilis in emerging villages during the early neolithic period, may have had an animal origin, but there seems to be fairly general agreement that they were probably micro-organisms that originally parasitized decaying organic matter, and later specialized in humans, entering their bodies through traumatized skin.[5]

All this having been said about human disease, it should be added quickly that so long as humans lived in small isolated bands their disease difficulties would have been largely limited to chronic infections with low infectivity. In small populations with few susceptible individuals, the illnesses that predominate are those in which the host can remain infective for long periods, such as amoebic dysentery, or diseases that have alternative hosts to serve as an additional reservoir, such as schistosomiasis. But these populations would not have been troubled with acute crowd infections such as measles or smallpox, which immunize survivors against future attacks and thus require large populations to support them.[6] Indeed it seems that hunger-gatherers, although not disease-free, were none the less not greatly troubled by many pathogens that would later on prosper in the bodies of their more sedentary descendants. In addition to living in small groups, they were constantly on the move. Thus they seldom remained in one spot long enough to foul their water supplies and let their garbage and excrement pile up to attract varmints that harbour diseases and the vectors that spread them. Nor until relatively recently did humans have the domesticated animals from which they have subsequently received so many of their illnesses.[7]

In addition, because hunter-gatherers ate such a wide range of foods, they would not have developed those nutritional-deficiency diseases that began to bedevil humans only as they became more 'civilized'. Interestingly, the remains of early humans suggest that, at least in terms of protein, their nutritional status was superior to that of practically all subsequent peoples, for it is only now that human stature is again approaching that of our ancient ancestors. Doubtless, there were food shortages from time to time as populations increased, and such shortages meant high mortality rates, especially among the old and the young, whose ability to compete for scarce resources was limited. Moreover, because infanticide was very likely the principal means by which small-scale societies remained small, one suspects that especially during a food crisis the very young were eliminated, and doubtless the elderly were often left behind to fend for themselves.[8]

Most of the evolutionary trek that led to humankind took place in the tropics, indicating that the original infections of those embarked on this journey were those of a warm and moist climate. But subsequent expansion across the globe that began with *Homo erectus* continued with human hunter-gatherers, as bands became too large and subdivided with new groups striking out into new lands, including those of the Americas, Australia, and Oceania: those stray chunks of Pangaea that had long before wandered away.[9] Indeed, it is a good bet that the pressure of growing populations *forced* individuals into these remote areas. These migrations occurred during the last ice age when the levels of the oceans were considerably lower – so low, in fact, that it was possible to walk from Siberia into North America. Similarly, because that ice age ended about 10,000 years ago, population pressure in the Old World, particularly on those individuals who had moved into the temperate zones, may well have forced the domestication of animals and the beginning of sedentary agriculture. One can presume the problem of population pressure, because if hunter-gatherer populations were not kept in check by disease in Africa, then those that drifted away from the tropics would have had even fewer checks on population growth. All pathogens requiring special vectors or intermediate hosts, such as the trypanosomes and arboviruses, would have been left behind, and the cooler temperatures would have proved discouraging to the vectors of many other ailments.[10]

With the domestication of plants and animals beginning in the Near East some 8,000 to 10,000 years ago, humans summoned forth a host of new diseases and in so doing set in motion changes in their disease ecologies that are ongoing today. As humans settled into sedentary agriculture and concentrated on a single crop, the immediate effect was food in such abundance as to foster still more of an increase in their numbers. It has been argued that the strenuous activities of hunter-gathers would have created an absence of female body fat that, in turn, would have limited female fertility. Conversely, as sedentary agriculturalists, females increased their body fat and consequently their fertility.[11] As village populations swelled, so did their capacity to host diseases, while the filthy conditions of those villages provided havens for rats, mice, ticks, fleas, and mosquitoes, all capable of harbouring and spreading a vast variety of ailments. New pathogens entered the environment in droves. The domesticated cows, pigs, sheep, cats, dogs, and goats all contributed their collections of pathogens to a swelling pool of diseases, as did domesticated fowl a bit later on. Thus the roundworm *Ascaris* began to evolve in humans, probably from the ascarids of pigs, and joined other, older helminthic parasites, such as the whipworm, pinworm, and hookworm, with the latter flourishing in the human faeces that were disposed of casually, if at all. Typhoid and other salmonella infections, along with amoebic dysentary, sprang from fouled water supplies; non-venereal syphilis passed from the mouths of dirty youngsters to other dirty youngsters and, perhaps along with leprosy, left an increasing number of disfigured and impaired individuals. Tuberculosis, a disease of animals prior to the advent of humans, was probably acquired from cattle and would have begun its insidious invasion of the human body at this time, if not before. Malaria and schistosomiasis took their tolls on workers where agriculture depended upon irrigation, as in Egypt, Mesopotamia, and India. In Africa south of the Sahara, attempts to farm within the forests with slash-and-burn agriculture created ideal conditions for the *Aedes aegypti* mosquito, the vector of yellow fever, and apparently encouraged the emergence for the first time of falciparum malaria, the most deadly of the malarial types.[12]

Sedentary agriculture with its concentration on a single crop that constituted the core diet of a people began to rob bodies of important nutrients and thus the ability to resist disease. At the same time, it introduced still other illnesses of a nutritional nature. The tall and robust hunter-gatherer was replaced with a progressively shorter and physically weaker farmer. In part, this decline in stature was the result of declining intakes of whole protein; and in part, it had to do with the synergistic relationship of diet and disease. As the intake of important nutrients declined, humans were taking on more and more helminthic boarders to share what nutrients were forthcoming. They were also acquiring other new infections that placed increasing demands on the body for protein in order to combat them.[13]

Thus, although populations continued to grow, the human body was now labouring for the first time under the twin stresses of a swiftly growing pool of diseases and a rapidly deteriorating diet. The body was not defenceless, however, because it is axiomatic that extended experience with a pathogen forces both host and pathogen to work out an immunological compromise. The illness will weed out the most susceptible individuals, while at the same time the most virulent strains of that illness will destroy themselves by destroying their hosts. Eventually, a state is reached where most hosts survive the pathogen and pass it along to another host. People, then, began the slow and painful process of building immunities to the collection of pathogens that reigned in their respective communities. (➤ Ch. 10 The immunological tradition)

At this point, however, these were still mostly chronic ailments that confronted humankind. Although populations were growing, they had yet to reach a density that could support the very acute and very transient infections, but doubtless such infections were even then in the process of evolving. Many pathogens of the newly domesticated animals must have tried and failed to invade humans. But occasionally one succeeded and adapted to them in such a way that, if it could be transmitted from one human to another, then it might well emerge as a new and specifically human pathogen at some time in the future. Humankind was at this stage incubating, as it were, diseases that would be specifically theirs and would burst upon them as soon as they were obliging enough to create communities sufficiently large to support these diseases, and other communities to which the pathogens could reach out. Measles was one of these – probably originally canine distemper, or rinderpest among cattle – that became so perfectly adapted to humans that an animal reservoir of the illness ceased to exist. Smallpox was another: its earlier animal host was probably the cow who had cowpox, although perhaps it was a disease of monkeys (monkeypox) as well. Diphtheria came from cattle. Influenza we can probably blame on swine, since we share the disease with them today. Indeed, it has been estimated that we share some 42 diseases with pigs, 50 with cattle, 65 with dogs (domesticated the longest), 46 with sheep and goats, 35 with horses, and 26 with poultry.[14]

We shall never know when these new plagues made their debut – probably not much before 3000 BC – but in some instances we can make a guess as to where. South Asia, for example, is a good suspect for being the cradle of smallpox. On the one hand, it was the first region to develop populations large enough to host the disease, and on the other, those ancient populations were the only ones with substantial cattle herds. When this evidence is viewed in the light of the existence in India of very ancient temples for the worship of a smallpox deity and the near certainty that smallpox inoculation was practised there during ancient times, there is clearly justification for the suspicion. (➤ Ch. 33 Indian medicine) Similarly, because smallpox and measles were not well distinguished until relatively recent times and, again, because of the significance of the early development of large populations, it seems a good guess that South Asia, and perhaps China, witnessed the rise of measles as well. In any event, smallpox and measles, together with influenza, chicken-pox, whooping cough, mumps, diphtheria, and a host of other diseases, arose with growing human populations. These were the illnesses that pass quickly and directly from human host to human host and need no intermediary carrier; in other words, they became the diseases of civilization. And in the areas where they arose they began to mount assaults on human immune systems.[15] (➤ Ch. 27 Diseases of civilization)

In most instances, such assaults would have produced a lifetime of immunity for survivors. Then, because of a lack of hosts, the diseases would either have died out or moved on to other host populations, only to return at a later date when enough non-immune individuals (created by either birth or migration) had once again accumulated. Presumably, such epidemics found their way to new host populations as the latter grew large and important enough to have contacts with the wider world. This, no doubt, often meant that such populations had grown to the outer limits of their food supply. The resulting competition for available food resources, in turn, would have effectively increased the pathogenicity of epidemic parasites. The consequence would have been to reduce the numbers of a host population again to a point considerably below the carrying capacity of its lands. In other words, from an ecological viewpoint, the epidemic diseases that we have called diseases of civilization arose with civilization to join limited food supplies in preventing human overpopulation.[16]

Pathogens also began to play a political role. As irrigation agriculture became more efficient in South and East Asia and the Middle East, cities developed and became magnets for myriad diseases. When this occurred, these pathogen-bearing multitudes became biologically dangerous to their neighbours, and indeed these pathogens must have frequently spearheaded efforts to conquer those neighbours. In this fashion, political consolidation led to more or less common disease pools in sections of South and East Asia and of the Middle East by about 500 BC, from which time ancient texts leave no doubt about the presence of epidemic pestilence.[17] (➤ Ch. 52 Epidemiology)

GRAECO-ROMAN PERIOD

At that time, another disease pool was still in a formative stage in the Aegean basin. The writings of Hippocrates (c.450–370 BC) and his followers leave no doubt about the citizens suffering from malaria, and the possibility of the presence of other major diseases such as tuberculosis, diphtheria, and influenza. But neither measles nor smallpox is clearly identified in the Hippocratic Corpus, despite their spectacularly visible symptoms. Indeed, the Athenian population seems to have been sufficiently disease-free to have managed significant growth despite its well-known propensity for war.[18]

During the Peloponnesian War (431–404 BC), however, which served to end Athenian imperial ambitions, an apparently new disease erupted to destroy a fair portion of the Athenian army, as well as a third or more of the population of Athens. Thucydides's famous description indicates that it arrived by sea. On the basis of symptoms described, plague, typhus, smallpox, measles, syphilis, and ergotism have been put forward as candidates. Whatever it was, it killed and immunized so many that it vanished, and stands in the history books as an odd occurrence among a people usually exempted from such epidemiological events.[19]

But the subsequent establishment of trade and travel across the Eurasian landmass meant that the succeeding world of the Romans enjoyed no such luxury, and from the second century AD onward, the populations of that world suffered from devastating epidemics. The first of these raged between AD 165 and 180 and a second held sway between 211 and 266. That these plagues were extraordinarily deadly is clear. The first may have killed between a quarter and a third of the people in affected areas, whereas the second reportedly killed as many as 5,000 a day in Rome during the height of the epidemic, while scourging the countryside as well. Obviously, the disease or diseases were extremely virulent among populations with little or no resistance, and although admittedly speculative, it seems likely that these epidemics signalled the addition of smallpox and measles to the Mediterranean disease pool. As well as these apparently new diseases, the Romans had to contend with malaria, a very old disease, which has been credited with playing a major role in the decline of Rome by decimating its population.[20]

THE MIDDLE AGES

Over the course of the next millennia, the Old World's four major disease pools, outside of Africa south of the Sahara, more or less merged while at the same time expanding outward – the latter accomplished partially by long-distance trade, the movement of missionaries, and fishermen. Perhaps most important, however, were the militant migrations from place to place of invaders such as the Magyars, raiders such as the Vikings, and crusaders like the soldiers of Islam. (➤ Ch. 31 Arab-Islamic medicine)

Such movement also facilitated the spread of still another deadly illness. Deadly, precisely, because it is not a disease of humans, but rather of rats, and because it infected humans only incidentally but with devastating consequences. Bubonic plague is suspected of first arising in north-western India, the original homeland of the species of black rat that is a principal carrier of the disease, although it also occurs in a variety of other rodents, as well as rabbits and related species. The first recorded epidemic, however, was that described by Procopius (d. AD c.563) in Constantiople in AD 542 (the Plague of Justinian), which at its height was reported to have killed some 10,000 people each day. By AD 547, it had reached western Europe, and for the next two centuries made frequent lethal excursions throughout the Mediterranean.

During these centuries, other epidemics of plague took place in Iraq and Iran, and it may have spread into China as well, although the history of disease there is unfortunately even more obscure than that in the West. Indeed, from the texts it might appear that this land of great antiquity was none the less disease-free until relatively recent times. For example, a sixth-century medical book claims that smallpox was introduced in AD 495, which seems very late given China's proximity to India. Or again, malarial fevers are said to have first made their appearance in Chinese medical texts in the seventh century, although at that time they had already doubtless been around for a millennium or two.[21] (➤ Ch. 32 Chinese medicine)

More readily believable is the late arrival of several diseases in the Japanese islands, which were sheltered by the sea from many of the epidemiological events of the mainland. Indeed, so virulent was the Great Smallpox Epidemic of AD 735–37 (killing between 25 and 35 per cent of the population) that it may represent the first assault of the disease on Japan – but not the last. Rather, epidemic followed epidemic in an age of plagues, which endured until around 1050. Measles was introduced during this era, as were influenza, mumps, and some sort of epidemic dysentery. Records from this period also indicate the presence of numerous endemic ailments such as malaria, hookworm, filariasis, leprosy, tuberculosis, and hepatitis.[22] Needless to say, such an onslaught thinned the population dramatically. But after 1050, population growth resumed (albeit in fits and starts) as Japanese immunological systems grew sturdier and as many of the ailments settled in to become endemic.

It is this taming of epidemic diseases by rendering them endemic that represents the next great change in the ecology of human disease. Such a phenomenon occurred gradually for, depending on the disease, between 5,000 and 40,000 new hosts are required annually for it to become endemic. But, sooner or later, cities that had previously suffered from epidemics, which killed or immunized so many that the diseases themselves disappeared for lack of hosts, became populous enough to produce through births enough non-immune individuals to retain the diseases permanently. In other words, diseases such as measles, smallpox, and numerous others that in the past had slaughtered people of all ages, now became childhood ailments. Most of these illnesses treat the young much more gently than adults, while providing them with immunity against future attacks. (➤ Ch. 45 Childhood) Moreover, as permanent reservoirs of these pathogens, the cities exported them continually to the countryside, so that epidemic diseases were tamed there as well.

It bears repeating that this was a gradual process and was dependent upon a number of variables besides the size of a population. In fact, such a process could still be seen at work in some places during much of the twentieth century. On the other hand, it happened relatively quickly in places such as Japan, with a dense and more or less closed population and thus little in-migration of disease-susceptible individuals. Indeed, from about the beginning of the thirteenth century onward, attacks of measles and smallpox in Japan were confined largely to children.[23]

There were other diseases, however, that humans could not tame or adapt to because they were not the primary target of the illness. Foremost in this category was bubonic plague, which in the fourteenth century launched itself on a new and extraordinary tour of the Old World. It is generally believed (although not without dispute) to have broken out somewhere east of the Caspian Sea, where it is enzootic, and then followed the trade routes to India and China, where it erupted in 1331. Certainly, some very deadly disease (or diseases) brought demographic disaster to China during the decades of the 1330s and 1340s. In the various parts of China where it raged, it was reported as killing up to two-thirds of populations. In any event, it very definitely was plague that broke out in the Crimea by 1346, and then spread throughout the Mediterranean and into the Middle East (where it took a heavy toll), and finally into northern and western Europe.[24] Doubtless, increased seaborne commerce had served to assist the black rat in establishing itself first in seaports, and then in spreading throughout much of the Old World. Another important factor was demographic. Europe, for example, was relatively crowded after a period of sustained population growth. Called the 'black death' (which was plague in its bubonic, pneumonic, and septicaemic forms), the disease is credited with reducing that population by about a third by 1353. Moreover, this was just the initial blow. Instead of vanishing from Europe as it had previously done, it continued to hammer away there until the eighteenth century, becoming a part of the disease ecology of the region for nearly half a millennium.[25] (➤ Ch. 72 Demography and medicine)

In addition to making a sizeable contribution to a European population decline for much of the period in question, the plague seems to have impacted on Europe's disease ecology in other, albeit mysterious, ways that remain to be explained. Leprosy for example, which had been present in Europe since at least the sixth centurty AD, receded after the middle of the fourteenth century while, by contrast, tuberculosis began an advance that would endure for centuries to come. Because tuberculosis provides some immunity against leprosy, perhaps its upsurge caused leprosy to fade. On the other hand, at about this time, Europe became cooler, causing people to wear more clothing, and obviously those people were far less crowded than before. Thus it has been considered by some that reduced bodily contact may have brought about leprosy's decline. Still another hypothesis is that the plague was directly responsible for killing off leprosy by killing off most of those who hosted it.[26]

THE FIFTEENTH CENTURY – EFFECTS OF EXPLORATION/COLONIZATION

The fifteenth-century Portuguese excursions along the coast of Africa and the inception of a slave trade to Europe, which helped to finance those voyages, brought many residents of the Old World face to face with pathogens that their distant ancestors had left behind. By the end of that century, blacks were so numerous in Spain and Portugal that in some places they outnumbered whites. Their treponemal infections arrived with them, especially yaws, which, in the more temperate climate of Iberia, according to E.H. Hudson, could have become the syphilis that would soon burst upon Europe.[27] (➤ Ch. 58 Medicine and colonialism)

A more immediate consequence, however, was the spread of falciparum malaria, by far the most deadly of the malarial types, which took firm root on the Peninsula, and is credited with depopulating the Tagus valley for a time. Yet malaria, even falciparum malaria, was no stranger to other parts of the Mediterranean region. Some peoples, such as the Italians and Greeks who lived on the sea, had long ago developed genetic defences against this virulent malarial type, thus documenting its antiquity among the Greeks and Romans. The Iberians had no such protection, however. Slightly later, the rest of Europe began to experience other types of malaria (presumably mostly vivax), which became widespread in England, France, Holland, and Germany. One wonders if it is mere coincidence that of these four countries, three had also become slave-trading nations.[28]

While Africans were adding pathogens to the European pool, the Europeans were making some contributions of their own to that of Africa south of the Sahara. Smallpox, long present in the north, doubtless had frequently reached those immediately to the south of the desert via the Muslims, who came to trade and raid and conquer and civilize. In some of West Africa and all of West Central Africa, however, the disease may well have been a European introduction. In any event, it was after the arrival of the Europeans that smallpox became a dreadful and much-feared scourge of many black Africans. Tuberculosis and bacillary pneumonia were two other illnesses unknown in black Africa prior to contact with the Europeans, and both combined eventually to make ailments of the lungs very prevalent destroyers of African lives.[29]

Yet despite the Africans' susceptibility to some illnesses of the Eurasian pathogenic pool, they were familiar with most of them because of long contact with the north. In fact, blacks relocated in the European disease environment of Iberia proved that familiarity by not only surviving, but by multiplying. In contrast, the few American Indians soon to be brought to Spain died at a terrible rate.[30]

Native Americans also died at awful rates in the Americas as the result of an onslaught of disease unleashed by the Europeans. Within a few short decades after their arrival in the New World, populations they had contact with are estimated by some to have been reduced by about 90 per cent in what was probably the worst holocaust of disease in the history of humankind.[31] It is not that the Americans were disease-free until 1492, but that they were free enough to emphasize the striking, evolutionary differences between the Americas and the Old World in the development of pathogens. Such differences arose after the breakup of the super-continent, Pangaea. South America preceded North America in becoming a separate continent by a considerable span of time, and broke free from Africa some 180 to 200 million years ago with dinosaurs and other large animals aboard. Also aboard were pathogens. A type of trypanosomiasis, for example, left the Old World to evolve in the New World; however, the vector of African trypanosomiasis, the tsetse fly, was not a successful immigrant to the latter. This forced the American trypanosome (*Trypanosoma cruzi*), which is harboured by a number of animals both domestic and wild as well as by human beings, to find another vector. That vector became reduviid bugs, and today the pathology of American trypanosomiasis is far removed from that of its African counterpart.[32]

Another disease that seems to be American is Carrion's disease or bartonellosis, which, like Chagas' disease, does not need a human reservoir. It is transmitted by the sand fly, as is leishmaniasis in an American form that differs considerably in its pathology from the Old World variety. A fourth disease whose pathogens apparently evolved in the Americas is pinta, a treponemal illness related to the yaws and non-venereal syphilis of the Old World, but which is of a much milder nature.[33] Significantly, these four diseases that evolved in the Americas did so in South America, that portion of the New World separated the longest period of time from the Old World. In view of the evidence of inflammatory response found in the bones of North American Indians, there may also be good reason to suspect the existence of yet one more treponemal infection in the Americas – one that produced syphilis or a syphilis-like infection.[34]

If the hypothesis of Hudson, that all treponemal infections are caused by the same pathogen, is accepted, and yaws, non-venereal syphilis, pinta, and syphilis are simply different manifestations of the same disease in different climatic circumstances, then perhaps the pinta of tropical South America could have become syphilis in the temperate climates of North America. Yet there is little evidence for the venereal transmission of treponematosis in pre-Columbian American skeletons. By contrast, C. J. Hackett (b. 1905), who viewed the clinical differences in the human treponemas as the result of mutations, believed that although pinta was the oldest type, arising before humans, venereal syphilis none the less developed in the Old World. (➤ Ch. 26 Sexually transmitted diseases) Originally it was a 'mild' disease, until the environmental and social circumstances of urban life in Europe transformed it into a much more virulent illness toward the end of the fifteenth century. Still another possibility is that two treponemal diseases, one that had either mutated or evolved in the Old World and the other in the New World, somehow fused after 1492 to become the new disease that burst upon Europe as the fifteenth century drew to a close.[35]

Bone evidence indicates that the pre-Columbian diseases of the Americas also included a tuberculosis-like infection among urban populations, and also arthritis, including rheumatoid arthritis, which some feel was a New World disease that subsequently spread to the Old World. Hepatitis, encephalitis, polio, and some varieties of intestinal parasites also tormented pre-Columbian populations, but, tragically, they had been exempted from experience with all of the epidemic diseases and with many of the chronic diseases that had forced the immunological systems of Old World peoples to erect defences against them.[36] The reasons for the exemption are not difficult to find. Although the antiquity of the human presence in the Americas remains controversial, there is no doubt that the early colonists were well established by 8000 BC, meaning that they arrived long before the epidemic diseases in question had even arisen in the Old World. Moreover, these first Amercians brought no domesticated animals with them to harbour disease, and presumably the rigours of the northerly latitudes would have weeded out most of the humans suffering from chronic ailments in traversing the Bering Straits. Although most of the new Americans maintained hunter-gatherer life-styles, complex civilizations based on sedentary agriculture did arise among the Mayas, Aztecs, Incas, and the Mississippian peoples, and animals such as dogs, turkeys, Muscovy ducks, guinea-pigs, and the llama were domesticated. (➤ Ch. 60 Medicine and anthropology) So although the New World was not nearly as rich in pathogens as was the Old World, there is no reason to believe that epidemic diseases similar to those of Eurasia would not have eventually evolved in the Americas had their inhabitants remained in isolation.[37]

That isolation, however, ended abruptly with European contact in 1492. If the Indians were immunologically naïve, it could be argued that the Europeans, and especially the Iberians, possessed the most alert and agile immunological systems in the world at that time. They had been in close touch with the outside world since Roman times, had experienced a succession of invaders after the fall of Rome, including the Muslims whose empire encompassed myriad peoples and their diseases, and had been in physical contact with Africa south of the Sahara for almost a century. The cities of Iberia, open sewers into which rodents burrowed and over which a host of insects swarmed at that time were clearing-houses of diseases that moved with trade from the north to the Mediterranean and back again. The human populations had routinely suffered from smallpox, measles, mumps, and countless other childhood ailments. They seldom bathed, and their skins, hair, bowels, and breath swarmed with pathogens. They were, to paraphrase Alfred Crosby, 'immunological supermen'.[38]

The slaughter began in 1493 among the Arawaks of the Caribbean. Swine influenza has recently been put forth as a candidate for the initial epidemic on the grounds that, among other things, it attacked the Spaniards as well as the Indians. Yet another possibility is typhus, which, although an Old World pathogen, had none the less just entered the western European disease environment. It apparently was brought from Cyprus to Spain, where it killed many soldiers on both sides during Spain's final effort in Granada to eject the Moors from the Peninsula. Smallpox made its American debut in 1518 if not sooner; measles followed, and within a few decades, most of Europe's diseases had been transplanted. Smallpox is credited with conquering the Aztecs for Cortez and his men, then racing ahead to soften up the Incas for Pizarro and his conquistadores.[39]

THE SIXTEENTH CENTURY – EFFECTS OF THE SLAVE TRADE

Yet if Old World diseases facilitated conquest, they also decimated a labour supply that the Spaniards had counted on to help in colonizing the vastness of their newly found empire. The problem became acute first in the Caribbean, where the Spaniards could not help noticing that the few blacks in their company, like themselves, were largely unaffected by the illnesses that were pulverizing the indigenous population. The result was a demand for

African imports, to which Charles I acceded in 1518 (the year smallpox slammed into the Caribbean), and the Atlantic slave trade was underway.[40]

African slaves, however, could not be divorced from African pathogens, and the result of this union was a profound change in the disease ecologies of the tropical and subtropical regions of the Americas. These regions, previously malaria-free, were soon teeming with falciparum malaria, which has been credited with depopulating a populous Amazon basin. The misnamed hookworm, *Necator americanus* must have arrived in the bodies of the first African immigrants, as did filariasis, schistosomiasis, and onchocerciasis. Yellow fever made a somewhat more tardy arrival because of the need to import its mosquito vector, *Aëdes aegypti*. This was accomplished at least by 1647, when that disease wrought havoc across the Caribbean basin.[41]

One consequence of the African diseases following closely on the heels of the pathogens imported by the Europeans was obliteration for the Indians of the Caribbean and for many natives of the low-lying areas surrounding it. In the higher, cooler, elevations of Mexico and Peru, by contrast, where the vectors of falciparum malaria and yellow fever rarely did their deadly work, core populations survived with immune systems that slowly began the process of catching up with those of European counterparts. The die-off, before population growth resumed, however, has been placed as high as 90 per cent, and not just for the Incas and Aztecs. Sooner or later, a demographic disaster of like magnitude was most likely the fate of almost all indigenous groups of the hemisphere.[42]

Another consequence of the migrating African pathogens was to accelerate the New World's demand for Africans. Europeans proved as susceptible as the Indians to malaria and yellow fever, which helped to destroy any notions that other Europeans following the Spaniards into the West Indies may have cherished of keeping their labour force white via systems of indentured servitude. Blacks, by contrast, seemed impervious to the 'fevers' that destroyed whites.[43] If malaria and yellow fever served to increase the value of blacks in the Americas, these fevers also delayed for centuries the time when Africa would be overrun by the Europeans. (➤ Ch. 19 Fevers) Africa very quickly developed a reputation among explorers and slave traders as 'the white man's grave', and with good reason in the light of later quantitative data which revealed the full extent of the risk of reaching that grave. During the early nineteenth century, the English sustained death rates upward of 700 men per 1,000 mean strength per annum when they stationed an army on the west coast of Africa. Clearly, Africa south of the Sahara possessed defences against outsiders that the Americas did not.[44] (➤ Ch. 15 Environment and miasmata)

The Americas may have had little to give the wider world in the way of pathogens, but this was not the case with foodstuffs. Manioc, maize, peanuts, and a number of varieties of yams and sweet potatoes found their way to

Africa where, ironically, they triggered population growth that was then drained off by the slave trade to the homelands of the plants in question. Moreover, the new plants represented a mixed blessing for other reasons. Diets that began concentrating too closely on manioc brought beriberi to the consumers; maize cursed others with pellagra and protein energy malnutrition, with kwashiorkor and marasmus its symptomatic poles to act in synergystic harmony with parasites in killing or enfeebling many of the African young.[45] (➤ Ch. 22 Nutritional diseases)

Maize, along with the potato, would also bring important nutritional changes to Europe that may have figured prominently in what has been called the European mortality decline. (➤ Ch. 73 Medicine, mortality, and morbidity) However, at the end of the fifteenth century, no such decline was in sight. Syphilis had just burst upon Europe, appearing in Italy during the Italian wars only to be spread to every nook and cranny of the land by disbanded soldiers at the end of the campaign. Smallpox, for reasons not yet understood, became substantially more virulent over the course of the sixteenth century, so that by the beginning of the seventeenth century it was accounting for 10 to 15 per cent of all deaths in some of the the western European nations. In fact, it is difficult to ignore the coincidence of the increased virulence of smallpox and the appearance of other 'new' diseases in Europe during the sixteenth century, and the rapidly increasing European contact with Africa and Africans as a result of the transatlantic slave trade. That trade, of course, brought about considerably more contact than ever before with what we might think of as the world's fifth important disease pool. In the case of smallpox, the disease is believed by some to have established an African focus at some time in the distant past, and one might speculate that this disease was, or became, variola major, which was imported to Europe to supplant variola minor, a much milder variety of the disease.[46]

THE SEVENTEENTH AND EIGHTEENTH CENTURIES

Typhus, another new illness for Europeans, followed up its debut in Granada by making regular appearances among armies, commencing with the Italian wars. It generally took more of a toll in lives than did the combatants. Plague continued as a serious threat, with notable outbreaks in Spain during the years 1596–1602 (perhaps as many as half a million died), followed by other appearances in 1648–52 and 1677–85, and the Great Plague of London of 1665.[47]

Meanwhile, the Portuguese, who led the European expansion, had added syphilis to the disease ecologies of Asia from India to Japan as the disease pools of the world continued to be pulled ever closer together by imperial ambitions. The Ottoman Turks swept west into the Mediterranean, the Portuguese were followed by other European powers into Africa and the Far East, and those same powers elbowed their way into the New World. In the latter, battles for control of the slave trade and for West Indian real estate immersed armies and navies in yellow fever and malaria. This brought immediate massive die-offs and also sent shock waves of yellow fever north to batter North American coastal cities and eastward to assault European cities.[48]

The voyages of James Cook (1728–79) to the Pacific during the second half of the eighteenth century opened the last of the isolated regions of Pangaea to its pathogenic mainstream with apparently the same lethal outcomes that had been sustained in the Americas. David Stannard has placed the die-off of the Hawaiian natives at about 90 per cent; in Australia, New Zealand, and the remainder of Oceania, the mortality precipitated by reunion with the rest of the world has probably been little different and is still ongoing. Indeed, throughout the twentieth century and even today in the Amazon basin, such immunological initiation has been observed by modern medicine as isolated groups have been discovered. Without the ability to resist the pathogens that also discover them, they seem to melt away almost overnight.[49]

In stark contrast, much of the rest of the world began to experience substantial population increases toward the end of the eighteenth century – a phenomenon that, with peaks and valleys, has continued to accelerate into the present. There has been much debate over the question of how it happened that so much of humankind was gradually released from the tyranny of disease ecologies that for so long had teased them by permitting populations to grow before suddenly and mercilessly butchering that growth. The only point of agreement seems to be that medicine, still mired in its own dark ages, had little to do with its inception, save for the contribution of the Jenner vaccine to the war against smallpox.[50] Certainly, a crucial factor was the ebb and flow of armies and navies, and traders and migrants who had directed most of the world's pools of pathogens into a common mainstream so that there were fewer epidemic surprises. In this same vein, the development of large urban areas across the globe to maintain diseases in epidemic form as childhood ailments was also vital.

Other factors played a role as well. Even if contact with the wider world was important for developing common immunities in the long run, from a short-term viewpoint it hardly seemed advisable to continue that contact when epidemic disease was on a nation's doorstep. Thus the rise of strong authoritarian governments to impose quarantines directly, or indirectly, in the form of port inspections for purposes of taxation was doubtless another factor of some importance, especially in keeping bubonic plague at bay. Moreover, those same governments could and did force the clean-up of cities. That they did it for aesthetic reasons none the less had an impact on health, as populations of disease-bearing insects and rodents were whittled down. Attention to the cleanliness of water supplies and sewage disposal, when it was forthcoming, was also of obvious salubrious advantage.[51] (➤ Ch. 51 Public health)

Even so, that some of the mechanisms bringing about the decline in mortality from disease remain mysterious can be seen in the example of tuberculosis. If people crowding into cities meant the taming of many illnesses, such a phenomenon also provided a fertile ground for tuberculosis, which spreads easily in such circumstances and quickly became a serious scourge of urban-dwellers across the globe. Yet beginning in the nineteenth century and continuing into the twentieth century, the disease receded dramatically, before medicine developed the 'magic bullet' to treat it. (➤ Ch. 39 Drug therapies) Tuberculosis is an infection that does most harm in the bodies of the badly nourished, and thus its decline lends credence to a growing conviction among scholars that improving nutrition played a crucial role in fundamentally altering the relationship of humankind with disease. Certainly, the importation of the New World potato made it possible for more of the common folk of northern Europe to eat more nutritiously; maize fed counterparts in sections of southern Europe, while New World crops – sweet potatoes, maize, and peanuts – caused Asian populations to increase. There was, in other words, a confluence of global foodstuffs as well as pathogens, although even this confluence brought disease, particularly in the nineteenth century. Milled rice and manioc triggered epidemics of beriberi from Brazil to Japan, and pellagra cursed many in the south of Europe and in the southern United States. In addition, both diseases ravaged black Africans, and their aetiologies were not fully unravelled until the discovery of vitamins during the pre-Second World War era.[52]

The vegetable foods, however, can also feed animals. Because they were gradually so employed, it was the greater availability of whole protein year-round in the form of milk, meat, cheese, and eggs that doubtless had much to do with providing older bodies with the ability to fight diseases successfully. More important from a population standpoint, that protein provided younger ones with the capability of surviving infancy and childhood. In circuitous fashion, then, the animals that gave humans so many diseases long ago, finally delivered up a means of combating them. Animals also helped to alter disease ecologies in other ways. Cattle herds grazing in northern Europe, in Asia, and later in the North American Midwest, for example, attracted the mosquito vectors of vivax malaria. Because that plasmodium does not live in cattle, the human-host–mosquito–human-host cycle was broken, especially in North America and Europe.

THE NINETEENTH CENTURY

The nineteenth century saw medicine breaking increasingly with hoary theories of the past while at the same time bringing scattered discoveries, including that of the microscope, to bear on the question of what causes disease. (➤ Ch. 6 The microscopical tradition) An immediate spur to this effort was the emergence of some new and exotic illnesses brought abruptly to the attention of medicine by colonialism. Foremost among these was Asiatic cholera. Although the disease had long been endemic in India and was witnessed there by the Portuguese in 1503, it had none the less been confined to India until British troop movements in 1818 first unleashed it on the wider world. This first pandemic raged in Asia and the Middle East. The second pandemic, beginning in 1827, embraced these regions and extended into Europe and the Americas as well. A third pandemic, starting in 1840, also spread worldwide, as did the fourth of the 1860s and 1870s. It was during the fifth pandemic (1881–96) that Robert Koch (1843–1910) isolated and identified the causative microbe. This pandemic, too, stretched around the globe but missed North America. A sixth pandemic (1899–1923) spared most of Europe and all of the Western Hemisphere.[53]

Although there are no precise calculations of deaths from cholera, which seems to have killed about half of those afflicted, it undoubtedly cost several million lives. But in return, cholera impelled science into the frantic research that led to the germ theory of disease, and people and governments learned to be considerably more careful about their water supplies and sewage disposal. (➤ Ch. 16 Contagion/germ theory/specificity)

In the late 1850s, with the establishment of cinchona plantations by the Dutch in Java, Europeans finally had a reliable supply of its first line of defence against malaria. Beginning in the 1870s, other drugs followed that would also help to preserve white health in the tropics. Thus armed, imperialist nations found Africa considerably more inviting than before, and it was soon shared up among them. Tropical medicine was an important arm of this effort, but more to preserve the health of the colonizers than of the peoples colonized. And to some immeasurable extent the colonizers improved the living conditions of a number of disease-bearing hosts and vectors by rearranging the African landscape for cash crops. The Americans also ventured into new subtropical and tropical territories taken from Spain, and joined in the business of tropical medicine. The methods by which malaria and yellow fever were spread were discovered at the turn of the century and, in the next few decades, the aetiology and epidemiology of numerous other tropical ailments were unravelled.[54] (➤ Ch. 24 Tropical diseases)

The greatest impact of these discoveries was the removal of yellow fever and malaria from the disease ecologies of North America and the introduction

of methods for controlling these illnesses in the rest of the Western Hemisphere. However, yellow fever remains very much alive in the jungles of
South America and of Africa, while malaria still kills millions worldwide each
year and debilitates tens of millions more.

THE TWENTIETH CENTURY

The twentieth-century war on contagious disease has seen the identification
of microbe after microbe, the subsequent control through vaccination of
disease after disease in the developed world, assaults on disease vectors like
the body louse, and new breakthroughs in therapy. The First World War
and its aftermath looms as a sort of epidemiological watershed. During that
war, typhus alone killed some two to three million individuals, and in its
aftermath, removed another three million people from Eastern Europe and
Russia. Meanwhile, as the war came to a close, the great influenza pandemic
that may have killed as many as thirty million in a worldwide rampage began.
Yet following these disasters, epidemics became something that, like famine,
only happened in the developing world. In the developed world, with the
temporary menace of polio successfully averted, medicine began to ignore
the threat of pathogens and self-confidently embarked on a crusade against
genetically based illnesses and chronic diseases such as cancer and heart-
related problems. (➤ Ch. 20 Constitutional and hereditary disorders; Ch. 25 Cancer)

Indeed, the dichotomy between the disease ecologies of the two worlds is
starkly illustrated. In only one does a significant portion of the population
live long enough to develop illnesses such as cancer, heart-related ailments,
and Alzheimer's disease, making these diseases the most significant problems
of health and outlets of life. In the developing world, pathogens remain by
far the most important cause of morbidity and mortality. In the developed
world, the major causative culprits have become factors in life-style and in
the environment that humans have so radically altered in the process of
becoming developed. Pathogens, by contrast, although they may play a role
in the production of some cancers, are viewed as of little consequence in
these newest human-made illnesses of civilization. (➤ Ch. 9 The pathological
tradition)

Yet smallpox (apparently now obliterated), along with measles, chicken-
pox, and all the rest of the old epidemic ailments that eventually became
childhood illnesses, were also human-made in the sense that they arose as
diseases of an advancing civilization that had learned to domesticate animals.
Thus it may well be axiomatic that radical changes in our cultural and
physical environment and social organization will bring concomitant changes
in our disease ecology. Moreover, after a brief respite from pathogenic peril
in the developed world, a new epidemic, that of AIDS, has surfaced to bridge

the gap between developed and developing world and to become a part of the disease ecologies of both.[55] That the AIDS viruses apparently evolved in Africa, the ancient homeland of humankind, and reached human beings via non-human primates brings us full circle by reminding us of where our distant ancestors acquired so many of their illnesses. In the developed world, however, the reaction to AIDS has been to view it like cancer and heart-related diseases as a disease of life-style – of drug use and homosexual behaviour – even though most of the millions of its victims in Africa, Brazil, and elsewhere do not use drugs and are not homosexual. To view AIDS in this light is comfortable because it implies that the individual has choices and thus control. But such a view tends to obscure most of what biology and history have taught us about diseases and disease ecologies. It tends to obscure our understanding that free-living forms can and do become diseases, especially in tropical regions. In the past, such spontaneously arising and evolving diseases probably did so mostly in the lower animals because they were by far the most numerous, but now humans are becoming increasingly numerous and there is no reason to believe that free-living forms may not do the same in human bodies. This does not seem to have been the case with AIDS, which arose in non-human bodies but only assumed a virulent form in humans. The monkeys that appear to have passed the viruses on to humans are seemingly not affected at all by its presence. These circumstances, of course, suggest that because the primates and the viruses in question are so well adapted to one another the viruses are not, in fact, new – just new for humankind.[56]

This, in turn, raises the question of how many other viral diseases are awaiting the opportunity to invade the human species, with AIDS appearing as merely the top of a viral iceberg. The answer is that we have already caught a glimpse of more than the tip. The Marburg, Lassa, and Ebola viruses all seem to have established themselves in non-human primates and all have already assaulted humans in Africa or in the laboratory with incredibly deadly consequences.[57] The fact that Africa, the home of humankind, is also the home of so many of humankind's most deadly diseases has to do with evolutionary forces as old as life itself. But the emergence of AIDS and these other viral illnesses to affect humans can be blamed largely on recent environmental changes and on the proposition that such changes, when radical, will bring forth new illnesses. In this case, as the Sahara expands and as humans have become ever more numerous in Africa, the forests are rapidly shrinking. Viral ailments are quite literally being squeezed from them. In addition, it has been estimated that there are many free-living viruses in the rainforests of Africa and South America that have the potential for becoming diseases. Receding forests and increasing human presence within those forests vastly improve their chances.[58]

376

The probability, then, of new diseases becoming a part of the human disease ecology is great. And great as well is the probability of the resurgence of many old diseases. We tend to forget that pathogens and their vectors are living things that have been forged in the evolutionary struggle to survive and that they have a considerable adaptive edge on humankind, some of them managing reproduction in less than half an hour. Thus typhus, during and after the Second World War, was brought more or less under control by the use of DDT to kill the body lice that carry it, but such an effort encouraged the evolution of body lice genetically resistant to DDT. It is not surprising then, that new strains of syphilis are appearing that have become resistant to antibiotics, and tuberculosis seems to be making a considerable comeback, to cite just a few alarming examples.

We have seen how diseases have arisen in humans in response to ecological changes and changing social organization. The first pathogens to adapt to humans probably evolved with them from the primates. Others adapted first in non-human primates and other wild hosts and were passed on to humans. With the domestication of animals, new diseases arose, first as epidemics, but later converted to endemic diseases as populations grew larger. Trade and imperial adventure drew the world closer together while unleashing terrible pestilence on those too long outside the Old World pathogenic mainstream, or as in the case of cholera, belatedly putting a disease in touch with that mainstream.

A more closely knit world also made it possible for illnesses such as plague and yellow fever, not normally diseases of humans, to seek out humans, with extraordinary lethality. Swelling populations provided a rapidly mutating swine influenza virus with hundreds of millions of hosts and tens of millions of victims in the early decades of the twentieth century. Yet despite these numerous lessons of the past, those in the developed world have been led to believe that if only the new chronic diseases could be subdued, their world, at least, would become essentially disease-free. That this is even a state we should wish for ignores the millennia of symbiotic evolutionary adaptation of humans and pathogens. It also ignores the experience of the American Indians.

NOTES

1 Thomas A. Cockburn, 'The evolution of infectious disease', *International Record of Medicine*, 1959, 179: 493–5; Thomas McKeown, *The Origins of Human Disease*, Oxford and New York, Basil Blackwell, 1988, pp. 1–2, 17–18.

2 Richard Fiennes, *Zoonoses of Primates: the Epidemiology and Ecology of Simian Diseases in Relation to Man*, Ithaca, NY, Cornell University Press, 1979, *passim*; Cockburn, op. cit. (n. 1), pp. 496–7.

3　Roy M. Anderson and Robert M. May, 'Population biology of infectious diseases: part 1', *Nature*, 1979, 280: 361–7.

4　Aidan Cockburn, 'Where did our infectious diseases come from? The evolution of infectious diseases', *CIBA Foundation Symposium*, 1977, 49: 103–12; William H. McNeill, *Plagues and Peoples*, Garden City, New York, Anchor Press/ Doubleday, 1976, p. 21; McKeown, op. cit. (n. 1), p. 39; Mark Nathan Cohen, *Health and the Rise of Civilization*, New Haven, CT, and London, Yale University Press, 1989, pp. 32–7.

5　Thomas A. Cockburn, 'The origin of the treponematoses', *Bulletin of the World Health Organization*, 1961, 24: 221–8; Corinne Shear Wood, 'Syphilis in anthropological perspective', *Journal of Physical Anthropology*, 1978, 12: 52.

6　Cohen, op. cit. (n. 4), pp. 32–42; Francis L. Black, 'Infectious diseases in primitive societies', *Science*, 1975, 476: 515–20.

7　McNeill, op. cit. (n. 4), p. 51.

8　McKeown, op. cit. (n. 1), pp. 20–1; Boyd S. Eaton and Melvin Konner, 'Paleolithic nutrition', *New England Journal of Medicine*, 1985, 312: 283–90; David R. Harris, 'The prehistory of human subsistence: a speculative outline', in Dwain N. Walcher and Norman Kretchmer (eds), *Food, Nutrition, and Evolution: Food as an Environmental Factor in the Genesis of Human Variability*, New York, Masson, 1981, p. 284; Geza Teleki, 'Primate subsistence patterns: collector-predators and gatherer-hunters', *Journal of Human Evolution*, 1975, 4: 125–84.

9　Thomas McKeown, 'Food, infection and population', *Journal of Interdisciplinary History*, 1983, 14: 241–2; Alfred W. Crosby, *Ecological Imperialism: the Biological Expansion of Europe, 900–1900*, London and New York, Cambridge University Press, 1986, pp. 14–16.

10　Cohen, op. cit. (n. 4), pp. 19–70; Cockburn, op. cit. (n. 4), p. 107.

11　L. L. Cavalli-Svorza, 'Human evolution and nutrition', in Walcher and Kretchmer, op. cit. (n. 8), p. 1; Rose E. Frisch, 'Population, food intake and fertility', *Science*, 1978, 199: 22–30; Mark Nathan Cohen, 'Speculations on the evolution of density measurement and population regulation in Homo Sapiens', in Mark Nathan Cohen, Roy S. Malpass and Harold G. Klein (eds), *Biosocial Mechanisms of Population Regulation*, New Haven, CT, and London, Yale University Press, 1980, pp. 291–7.

12　Folke Henschen, *The History and Geography of Diseases*, New York, Delacorte Press, 1962, p. 96; Stephen L. Wiesenfeld, 'Sickle-cell trait in human biological and cultural evolution', *Science*, 1967, 157: 1134–40; Frank B. Livingstone, *Abnormal Hemoglobins in Human Populations*, Chicago, IL, Aldine, 1967, p. 87.

13　Nevin S. Scrimshaw, Carl E. Taylor and John E. Gordon, *Interactions of Nutrition and Infection*, Geneva, World Health Organization, 1968, *passim*; Carl E. Taylor, 'Synergy among mass infections, famines and poverty', *Journal of Interdisciplinary History*, 1983, 14: 483–501; Nevin S. Scrimshaw, 'The value of contemporary food and nutrition studies for historians', *Journal of Interdisciplinary History*, 1983, 14: 529–34.

14　Cockburn, op. cit. (n. 4), p. 108; McNeill, op. cit. (n. 4), p. 51.

15　Sterling Hart, 'The historical impact of disease', *Strategy and Tactics*, 1977, 63: 24; Donald R. Hopkins, *Princes and Peasants: Smallpox in History*, Chicago, IL,

378

University of Chicago Press, 1983, p. 17; Roderick E. McGrew, *Encyclopedia of Medical History*, New York, McGraw-Hill, 1985, p. 313.

16 MacFarlane Burnet, *Natural History of Infectious Disease*, 3rd edn, Cambridge, Cambridge University Press, 1962, pp. 15–16.

17 McNeill, op. cit. (n. 4), p. 76 and *passim*.

18 McNeill, op. cit. (n. 4), 100–1; Frederick F. Cartwright, *Disease and History*, New York, Thomas Y. Crowell, 1972, pp. 6–7.

19 Cartwright, op. cit. (n. 18), pp. 7–8; Henschen, op. cit. (n. 12), p. 64.

20 McNeill, op. cit. (n. 4), pp. 115–23; Arturo Castiglioni, *Storia della Medicina*, Milan, Società Editrice, 1927, p. 251.

21 Angela Ki Chi Leung, 'Diseases of the premodern period in China', in Kenneth F. Kiple (ed.), *The Cambridge History and Geography of Human Disease*, 5 vols, Cambridge and New York, Cambridge University Press, 1992; Lu Gwei-Djen and Joseph Needham, 'Records of diseases in ancient China', *American Journal of Chinese Medicine*, 1976, 4: 3–16.

22 Wayne Farris, 'Diseases of the premodern period in Japan', in Kiple, op. cit. (n. 21).

23 Ibid.

24 Katherine Park, 'The black death', in Kiple, op. cit. (n. 21).

25 Ann G. Carmichael, 'Bubonic plague', in Kiple, op. cit. (n. 21).

26 Ann G. Carmichael, 'Leprosy', in Kiple, op. cit. (n. 21).

27 E. H. Hudson, 'Treponematosis and African slavery', *British Journal of Venereal Disease*, 1964, 40: 43–52.

28 Castiglioni, op. cit. (n. 20), p. 566; Ralph Linton, *The Tree of Culture*, New York, Knopf, 1955, p. 27; George Rosen, 'The biological element in human history', *Medical History*, 1959, 1: 158; Robert P. Hudson, *Disease and its Control: the Shaping of Modern Thought*, Westport, CT, Greenwood Press, 1983, pp. 44–7.

29 Kenneth F. Kiple, *The Caribbean Slave: a Biological History*, Cambridge and New York, Cambridge University Press, 1984, p. 13; Dauril Alden and Joseph C. Miller, 'The origins and dissemination of smallpox via the slave trade from Africa to Brazil', in Kenneth F. Kiple (ed.), *The African Exchange: Toward a Biological History of Black People*, Durham, NC, and London, Duke University Press, 1988, p. 39; Todd L. Savitt, *Medicine and Slavery*, Urbana, University of Illinois Press, 1978, pp. 36–7.

30 Crosby, op. cit. (n. 9), p. 198; A. J. R. Russell-Wood, 'Iberian expansion and the issue of black slavery: changing Portuguese attitudes, 1440–1770', *American Historical Review*, 1978, 83: 21–2; Levi Marreero, *Cuba: Economia y Sociedad*, Barcelona and Madrid, 1972, Vol. I, p. 158; Victor Alba, *The Latin Americans*, New York, Praeger, 1969, p. 24.

31 Crosby, op. cit. (n. 9), pp. 196–9 and *passim*; Henry F. Dobyns, *Their Numbers Become Thinned*, Knoxville, University of Tennessee Press, 1983, *passim*.

32 Burnet, op. cit. (n. 16), pp. 61–3; Philip D. Marsden, 'American trypanosomiasis', in G. Thomas Strickland (ed.), *Hunter's Tropical Medicine*, 6th edn, Philadelphia, PA, W. B. Saunders, 1984, pp. 565–73; Erwin H. Ackerknecht, *History and Geography of the Most Important Diseases*, New York, Hafner, 1965, pp. 128–30.

33 Thomas W. Simpson and Evan R. Farmer, 'Bartonellosis', in Strickland, op. cit. (n. 32), pp. 228–31; Wood, op. cit. (n. 5), p. 49.

34 Brenda J. Baker and George J. Armelagos, 'The origin and antiquity of syphilis:

paleopathological diagnosis and interpretation', *Current Anthropology*, 1988, 20: 703–37.

35 E. H. Hudson, 'Treponematosis', in Henry A. Christian (ed.), *The Oxford textbook of Medicine*, 8 vols, Oxford and New York, Oxford University Press, 1949, Vol. V, pp. 656 (10–122); C. J. Hackett, 'On the origin of the human treponematoses (pinta, yaws, endemic syphilis, and venereal syphilis)', *Bulletin of the World Health Organization*, 1963, 29: 7–41; Hudson, op. cit. (n. 27), pp. 43–52; Jane E. Buikstra, 'Diseases of prehistory in the Americas', in Kiple, op. cit. (n. 21); Baker and Armelagos, op. cit. (n. 34), pp. 703–37; Clarke Spencer Larsen, 'Bioarcheological interpretations of subsistence economy and behavior from human skeletal remains', *Advances in Archeological Method and Theory*, 1987, 10: 382–3.

36 B. M. Rothschild, R. J. Woods and K. R. Taylor, 'New World origins of rheumatoid arthritis', *Arthritis and Rheumatism*, 1987, 30: 61; Larsen, op. cit. (n. 35), p. 383; Lucille St Hoyme, 'On the origins of New World paleopathology', *American Journal of Physical Anthropology*, 1969, 31: 295–302.

37 Alfred W. Crosby, *The Columbian Exchange: Biological and Cultural Consequences of 1492*, Westport, CT, Greenwood Press, 1972, pp. 30–1; Buikstra, op. cit. (n. 35); Seonbok Yi and Geoffrey Clark, 'The Dyuktai culture and New World origins', *Current Anthropology*, 1985, 26: 1–20.

38 Crosby, op. cit. (n. 9), p. 34; Kiple, op. cit. (n. 29), pp. 7–9.

39 Francisco Guerra, 'The earliest American epidemic: the influenza of 1493', *Social Science History*, 1988, 12: 305–25; Hans Zinsser, *Rats, Lice and History*, 4th edn, London, Routledge, 1942, p. 241; P. M. Ashburn, *The Ranks of Death: a Medical History of the Conquest of America*, New York, Coward-McCann, 1947, *passim*; Crosby, op. cit. (n. 37), pp. 35–63.

40 Kiple, op. cit. (n. 29), pp. 12–13.

41 Kiple, op. cit. (n. 29), *passim*; Reinhard Hoeppli, *Parasitic Diseases in Africa and the Western Hemisphere: Early Documentation and Transmission by the Slave Trade*, Basle, Verlag für Recht und Gesellschaft, 1969, *passim*; Henry Rose Carter, *Yellow Fever: an Epidemiological and Historical Study of its Place of Origin*, Baltimore, MD, Williams & Wilkins, 1931, *passim*.

42 Kiple, op. cit. (n. 29), p. 11; Sherburne F. Cook and Woodrow Borah, *Essays in Population History: Mexico and the Caribbean*, 3 vols, Berkeley, University of California Press, 1971–79, Vol. I, *passim*; John Hemming, *Red Gold: the Conquest of the Brazilian Indians*, Cambridge, MA, Harvard University Press, 1978, p. 4; Dobyns, op. cit. (n. 31), *passim*.

43 Francisco Guerra, 'The influence of disease on race, logistics and colonization in the Antilles', *Journal of Tropical Medicine and Hygiene*, 1966, 69: 23–35; Kiple, op cit. (n. 29), pp. 14–22.

44 Philip C. Curtin, 'Epidemiology and the slave trade', *Political Science Quarterly*, 1968, 83: 191–216.

45 Kiple, op cit. (n. 29), pp. 25–6 and *passim*.

46 Lloyd Stevenson, 'New diseases in the seventeenth century', *Bulletin of the History of Medicine*, 1966, 39: 1–21; Crosby, op. cit. (n. 9), pp. 199–200; Cartwright, op. cit. (n. 18), p. 121.

47 Ackerknecht, op cit. (n. 32), pp. 33–5.

48 Crosby, op cit., (n. 37), p. 151; Guerra, op cit. (n. 43), pp. 23–35; Kiple, op cit. (n. 29), pp. 161–75.

49 David E. Stannard, *Before the Horror: the Population of Hawaii on the Eve of Western Contact*, Honolulu, University of Hawaii Press, 1989.

50 James C. Riley, 'Insects and the European mortality decline', *American Historical Review*, 1986, 91: 833–58; Hudson, op cit. (n. 28), p. 222.

51 Stephen J. Kunitz, 'Disease and the European mortality decline', in Kiple, op cit. (n. 21); E. A. Wrigley and Roger S. Schofield, *The Population History of England, 1541–1871*, Cambridge, MA, Harvard University Press, 1981.

52 Thomas McKeown, *The Modern Rise of Population*, London, Edward Arnold, 1976; Robert William Fogel, 'The conquest of high mortality and hunger in Europe and America: timing and mechanisms', Working Paper no. 16, Cambridge, MA, National Bureau of Economic Research, 1990; Daphne A. Roe, *A Plague of Corn: the Social History of Pellagra*, Ithaca, NY, Cornell University Press, 1973; W. R. Akroyd, *Conquest of Deficiency Diseases*, Geneva, World Health Organization, 1970.

53 Ackerknecht, op cit. (n. 32), pp. 22–31.

54 Gwyn Prins, 'But what was the disease? The present state of health and healing in African studies', *Past and Present*, 1989, 124: 160; Cartwright, op cit. (n. 18), pp. 137–66; Ashburn, op cit. (n. 39), pp. 230–8.

55 Frank Fenner, 'The effects of changing social organization on the infectious diseases of man', in S. V. Boyden (ed.), *The Impact of Civilization on the Biology of Man*, Canberra, Australian National University, 1970, p. 48.

56 J. Kanki, J. Alroy and M. Essex, 'Isolation of T-lymphotropic retrovirus related to HTLV-III-LAV from wild-caught African green monkeys', *Science*, 1985, 230: 951–4.

57 John C. N. Westwood, *The Hazard from Dangerous Exotic Diseases*, London, Macmillan, 1980; Wilbur G. Downs, 'Ebola virus disease', 'Lassa fever', and 'Marburg virus disease', in Kiple, op cit., (n. 21).

58 Wilbur G. Downs, 'The Rockefeller Foundation virus program: 1951–1971 with update to 1981', *Annual Reviews of Medicine*, 1982, 33: 1–29.

FURTHER READING

Ackerknecht, Erwin H., *History and Geography of the Most Important Diseases*, New York, Hafner, 1965.

Cohen, Mark Nathan, *Health and the Rise of Civilization*, New Haven, CT, and London, Yale University Press, 1989.

Crosby, Alfred W., *Ecological Imperialism: the Biological Expansion of Europe, 900–1900*, Cambridge and New York, Cambridge University Press, 1986.

Kiple, Kenneth F. (ed.), *The Caribbean Slave: a Biological History*, Cambridge and New York, Cambridge University Press, 1984.

——, *The Cambridge History World of Human Disease*, 5 vols, Cambridge and New York, Cambridge University Press, 1992.

McKeown, Thomas, *The Origins of Human Disease*, Oxford and New York, Basil Blackwell, 1988.

McNeill, William H., *Plagues and Peoples*, Garden City, New York, Anchor Press/ Doubleday, 1976.

19

FEVERS

Leonard G. Wilson

FEVER IN THE HIPPOCRATIC CORPUS

Fever has been since antiquity the paramount sign of disease in the body. In the Hippocratic writings (fifth–third centuries BC), disease was viewed as a process that followed a natural course and possessed, therefore, a natural history. The Hippocratic physician sought to learn the natural history of disease by careful observation so that when called to see a patient, the present stage of the disease might be recognized, its past history described, and its future course predicted. The practice of *prognosis* not only gave the patient confidence in the physician's judgement and skill, but it also determined treatment. Prognosis inevitably entailed a diagnosis of the disease afflicting the patient and its stage of development.[1]

The Hippocratic physician thought that diseases, and most especially fevers, were caused by a disturbance in the four fluids or humours of the body: yellow bile, black bile, blood, and phlegm. The choice of humours was based upon the body fluids or discharges, and the changes that seemed to occur in them during disease and recovery. (➤ Ch. 14 Humoralism) The humours might become disturbed by a badly regulated life, by excess in eating or drinking, exposure to heat or cold, violent exercise, or unusual fatigue (that is, by faulty regimen); or their fluctuations might be associated with the season of the year, with changes in the atmosphere and the weather, or with locality. Disturbance among the humours was primarily an imbalance resulting from an excess of one humour, which was present in what was called a raw or unconcocted state. Although the humoral theory has often been character-ized as purely speculative, it was, in fact, closely reasoned from much exact observation of the effects of disease on the bodies of patients, and the regular seasonal patterns in which disease occurred.

The establishment of disease, marked by excess of one humour, set in motion a struggle between the disease and the nature or physis of the body. The physis sought to restore the normal balance among the body fluids through the action of the innate heat, or natural warmth of the body. The increase of the innate heat during fever thus reflected an intense internal battle between physis and disease. The innate heat acted to concoct the humours, and by such coction or *pepsis* restore them to a healthy state. In the work *Ancient Medicine*, the Hippocratic writer described the changes that occurred in the nasal discharges during the course of a common cold as an example of how the physis of the body, acting through the innate heat, brought about coction (*pepsis*) of the humours to restore them to a healthy state. First, the profuse discharge from the nose was acrid, making the nose swell and inflame. The patient was then discharging raw, unmixed phlegm. Later, as the patient recovered, the nasal discharge became thicker and the inflammation subsided, a change resulting from coction and the restoration of a normal balance and mixture among the humours.[2] The process of coction was, therefore, the healing process within the body that brought about the change in the humours indicated by the change in the excretions. If the physis of the body won its battle with the disease, the excess harmful matter – raw unmixed humours – would be discharged. If, instead, the battle with the disease were lost, the patient would die. In treatment, the Hippocratic physician attempted to support the efforts of the body's physis to overcome the disease.

The theory of humours is stated most concisely in the treatise *On the Nature of Man*:

> The body of man has in itself blood, phlegm, yellow bile and black bile; these make up the nature of his body, and through these he feels pain or enjoys health. Now he enjoys the most perfect health when these elements are duly proportioned to one another in respect of compounding, power and bulk, and when they are perfectly mingled. Pain is felt when one of these elements is in defect or excess, or is isolated in the body without being compounded with all the others.[3]

The writer justified his selection of the four humours by showing that they might be found in the body at any time of the year. If the physician gave the patient a medicine that withdrew phlegm, the patient would discharge phlegm. If a medicine that withdrew bile was given, the patient would vomit yellow bile. By contrast, if given a medicine that withdrew black bile (apparently a purgative), black bile would be purged away. Black bile was the most obscure of the humours. It may have been associated with the dark colour of faecal matter, but its full significance for the Hippocratic physician can be appreciated only in relation to the pathological changes occurring in the diseases that were most frequently seen, in particular, the malarial fevers. As for the fourth humour, blood, it was always present, because blood always flowed from wounds. The four humours were to be found within the body at all times and were, therefore, its normal constituents.

The Hippocratic physicians developed their humoral theory from their observations of the diseases prevalent in ancient Greece and which fell into two principal groups: respiratory diseases and the malarial fevers. The respiratory diseases, including phthisis or pulmonary tuberculosis, were common, but the malarial fevers were nearly universal. In a malarious country, such as Greece was in ancient times and remained until very recently, almost every person at some time suffered from a series of attacks of chills and fever.

MALARIAL FEVERS

Malarial fevers are caused by one or other species of the microscopic proto-zoan parasite *Plasmodium*, which passes through the sexual stages of its life history within the body of an *Anopheles* mosquito, whose bite may transmit the parasites to humans. The parasites, known as sporozoites, are carried by the circulating blood to the parenchyma cells of the liver, where they multiply during a period of incubation lasting ten days to two weeks. After incubation, the parasites, now called trophozoites, return to the circulating blood, where each attacks and enters a red blood cell. Here, the trophozoite multiplies to produce twenty to thirty merozoites. After a period of incubation, which, depending on the species of *Plasmodium*, may be twenty-four, forty-eight, or seventy-two hours, the red blood cell breaks down, releasing its burden of parasites into the blood plasma. Each merozoite of the new generation thus released attacks another red blood cell, and the cycle is repeated. The release of each generation of merozoites into the blood plasma precipitates a severe chill followed by a high fever in the patient. When each merozoite is again safely ensconced within a red blood cell, the fever subsides, the patient breaks out into a profuse perspiration, and often falls into a deep sleep. On wakening, the patient is more or less well until the next chill occurs.

The various species of malarial parasites each have their own periodicity. *Plasmodium vivax*, the organism causing benign tertian malaria, has an incu-bation period of ten to seventeen days. The fever, which may rise to 104–106 °F, lasts from two to six hours and recurs every forty-eight hours (that is, on every third day). During the attack, nausea, vomiting, and diar-rhoea may commonly occur. If untreated, the attacks may recur every other day for two months or longer. As the disease progresses, the spleen enlarges, and, as a result of the excessive destruction of red blood cells, the patient becomes anaemic and occasionally may also become jaundiced.[4]

In malignant tertian malaria, caused by *Plasmodium falciparum*, the incubation period is shorter, the first attack of fever coming eight to twelve days after infection, the chill is less pronounced, and the fever is more prolonged and more variable. It may be continuous, remittent, or intermittent. *P. falciparum* proliferates very rapidly, producing a massive destruction of red blood cells and consequent severe anaemia. The spleen becomes enlarged, and frequently also the liver. The patient suffers from attacks of bilious vomiting and jaundice.

By contrast, quartan malaria, caused by *Plasmodium malariae*, is a milder disease.[5] The incubation period is longer than that of either benign or malignant tertian fever, extending as long as thirty to forty days. After premonitory symptoms of headache and vague aches and pains throughout the body, the patient may feel a chill lasting fifteen to forty-five minutes, accompanied by nausea and vomiting, and followed by a high fever lasting six hours or more. During the fever, the patient may experience further vomiting and diarrhoea. At the end of the attack, the patient sweats profusely as the temperature falls rapidly. On the fourth day, seventy-two hours after the first attack, a second attack of fever begins, and, if untreated, such attacks will recur every fourth day for as long as several months; quartan fever is the most persistent of the malarial fevers.[6]

Finally, malaria may appear as quotidian fever, in which there is a daily attack of fever lasting six to twelve hours. Quotidian fever may be the result of multiple infections of malarial parasites at different times.

Patients who have suffered from malarial infection for a prolonged period without treatment may develop malarial cachexia. Such patients are severely anaemic and their spleens greatly enlarged and hardened. The liver may also be enlarged. The skin has a saffron or dark lemon yellow tint.[7] After death, both spleen and liver are found darkened with a black pigment, the malarial pigment, which is haematin derived from the haemoglobin of the destroyed red blood cells.[8]

In addition to the fever and illness, the primary consequence of malarial infection is a massive destruction of red blood cells, producing anaemia and its accompanying weakness. In a healthy person, the red blood cells have an average life of 120 days, and when they break down, the haematin from their haemoglobin and other breakdown products are removed from the blood plasma by the reticuloendothelial cells of the spleen, the bone marrow, and, most importantly, the liver. In the liver, haematin is converted to pigments such as biliverdin and bilirubin, which are excreted in the bile. The bile pigments are carried with the bile into the intestine, where they are converted by bacteria into other pigments and are normally discharged in the faeces, to which they give the characteristic brown colour.

When, as in malarial fevers, the destruction of red blood cells is extraordinarily great, there will be a correspondingly large increase in the production of haemoglobin breakdown products. The liver, in attempting to remove the excessive haematin, may excrete increased amounts of bile pigments and the faeces may assume a darker colour than normal. At the same time, the levels of bile pigments in the blood plasma and the urine may be elevated, resulting in the yellowing of the skin, the fingernails, and the whites of the eyes; such a jaundiced appearance develops regularly in untreated falciparum malaria and occasionally in benign tertian malaria. The urine may also become more highly coloured. In prolonged or severe malarial infections, the destruction of red blood cells and the consequent release of haematin overwhelms the ability of the reticuloendothelial tissue to deal with it. In falciparum malaria, haematin accumulates in the spleen, the liver, and the bone marrow, turning the spleen and liver a dark-grey or even black colour. Black pigment may also be found in other tissues, including the brain. Occasionally, in falciparum malaria the patient's urine may turn completely black as a result of massive haemolysis, giving rise to the term blackwater fever. Mirko D. Grmek has pointed out that in ten of the case histories of patients with fever described in *Epidemics I*, by Hippocrates (c.450–370 BC), the patient's urine is described as black, and that the illness of Philiscus (*fl.* 410 BC), who lived near the recently built wall of Thasos in the northern Aegean, was clearly a case of blackwater fever.[9]

For malaria to be present in an area, not only the human population but also the population of *Anopheles* mosquitoes must become infected with malarial parasites, and the requirement gives certain distinctive characteristics to the epidemiology of the disease. In any one locality, the malarial infection will normally be transmitted to humans through the bites of infected *Anopheles* mosquitoes. Nevertheless, in temperate climates, adult *Anopheles* either die or go into hibernation each year with the onset of winter. The following spring, a new generation is hatched from eggs laid in water. *Anopheles* of the new generation will be free of malarial parasites until they bite people with malarial parasites in their peripheral blood. A curious feature of the parasite (*Plasmodium vivax*) implicated in benign tertian malaria is that patients who become infected in the late summer or autumn may not develop fever after the normal incubation period of ten to fourteen days, but instead after an interval of thirty to forty weeks; or, if they do develop fever at the end of the normal incubation period, they may have a relapse thirty to forty weeks after the initial infection. Thus, in a malarious district, an epidemic of benign tertiary malaria will occur each spring. The effect of either the delayed first attack or relapse after thirty to forty weeks is that the malarial parasite is carried over winter in its human host.[10] The reservoir of malarial infection, therefore, lies among malarial carriers in the human population rather than among *Anopheles*. In a malarious district with a subtropical climate, each spring will see the occurrence of an epidemic of benign tertian malarial fever as a result of infections that occurred the previous autumn. Following the spring epidemic, which appears usually during March and April in the northern hemisphere, there will be a lull for several weeks in the appearance of new cases of fever. In June, cases of a much more severe tertian fever (falciparum malaria) will again begin to occur and will increase in number through July, declining rapidly in August and September, until the onset of cool weather brings them to a halt.[11] As summer fades into autumn, patients who have suffered recurrent attacks of (untreated) malaria over many weeks will be anaemic, listless, and mentally depressed, with yellowed skins and enlarged and hardened spleens, and such effects will persist even after their fever subsides.

In 1909, the English classicist W. H. S. Jones (1876–1963) demonstrated from references in general Greek literature that in Homeric times malaria was rare or sporadic in ancient Greece, that it spread into Greece after 500 BC, and that by 400 BC malarial fevers had become endemic throughout the ancient Greek world.[12] Jones also argued that the numerous references to tertian and quartan fevers in the Hippocratic writings confirmed that malaria was endemic in Greece at the time they were written. More recently, Grmek has argued on a basis of palaeopathological evidence that, while benign tertian malaria and quartan malaria were probably already present, falciparum malaria reinvaded Greece early in the classical period, shortly before the writing of the Hippocratic *Epidemics I*, in which is described an epidemic of falciparum malaria on the island of Thasos.[13]

When malarial fevers are well established in an area, the frequency of their occurrence will depend largely upon whether mosquitoes are few or numerous. After a period of heavy rainfall, when much stagnant water is lying about in pools, puddles, and ditches, mosquitoes will breed very rapidly. The frequency of mosquito bites will rise and consequently so will the frequency of malarial infection. The Hippocratic physicians were familiar with the link between weather, season, and locality, as is reflected in the work Airs, Waters, Places, in which the author stated that if the rains occurred normally in autumn and winter, the year would likely be healthy. If, instead, the rains were delayed until spring, many cases of fever would occur during the summer. 'For whenever the great heat comes on suddenly while the earth is soaked by reason of the spring rains . . . the fevers that attack are of the acutest type.'[14] Cities that were well situated in relation to sun and winds and used good water were less affected in such a sickly year, but if they were located by marshes or stagnant water they would be more affected. 'If the summer proves dry,' the writer added, 'the diseases cease more quickly; if it be rainy, they are protracted.'[15] (➤ Ch. 15 Environment and miasmata) In the same work, the writer noted that in a poorly drained country, where the people drink marshy or stagnant water, 'the physique of the people must show protruding bellies and enlarged spleens'.[16]

SEASONAL INFLUENCES ON FEVERS

The Hippocratic physicians extended the relationship between warm, wet weather and fevers into a broad general relationship between the body's humours and the seasons. In each of the four seasons, one of the four humours was thought to predominate. Phlegm increased in winter because it was cold and wet and, therefore, akin to the cold and rainy weather of a Mediterranean winter. Consequently, the diseases produced by excess of phlegm, including colds, bronchitis, pneumonia, and consumption, tended to be more prevalent in winter, and people discharged more phlegm from their noses and in their sputum. When spring came, phlegm was still abundant, but the blood increased in quantity. The weather grew warmer, but rains still might occur; the countryside remained green and the streams continued to flow from the earlier winter rains. The spring season, therefore, was warm and wet, and since the qualities of blood were likewise warm and wet, the amount of blood in the body increased, and people were attacked by diseases resulting from excess of blood. These would include the spring outbreaks of fever (primarily relapses from the previous autumn of benign tertian malaria) and the dysenteries and nasal bleeding that might accompany them. As spring gave way to summer, the weather would become hotter and drier, and consequently yellow bile, which was hot and dry, increased and the diseases resulting from it prevailed, these being the severe fevers (falciparum malaria). Patients were hot, they vomited a yellowish fluid (which might be gastric juice or bile), and their skin tended to turn yellow. Their urine also might be yellower than normal.

As the summer waned in its turn and the weather, although remaining dry, grew cooler, the fevers lost their strength. Nevertheless, although the number of new cases might have declined, many patients would show the effects of repeated attacks through the weeks of summer. They would be weak, listless, their skins a dirty yellowish tinge, and their spleens enlarged and hardened. They might suffer from mental depression. The decline of fevers in autumn indicated to the Hippocratic physician that yellow bile had diminished in the body, while black bile, which, like the autumn, was thought to be cold and dry, increased. The Hippocratic writers saw a direct connection between black bile (*melaina chole*) and mental depression (*melancholia*). In *Epidemics III*, case II was a young woman who died on the eightieth day of a fever, her urine having been black throughout the course of her illness and her mind affected by melancholy.[17]

Black bile has seemed the most puzzling of the humours: its meaning must be seen in relation to the pathological effects of malarial fever, both the long-drawn-out effects of benign tertian or quartan malaria and the more rapidly inflicted consequences of falciparum malaria. Philiscus, whose illness is described in *Epidemics I*, suffered from black urine and his 'spleen stuck out, forming a rounded swelling'.[18] In the Hippocratic writings, the spleen was considered the seat of black bile. Although there is no mention of the performance of autopsies in the Hippocratic Corpus, there are references to the occurrence of tubercles in the lungs of hunchbacks (evidently victims of Pott's disease, tuberculosis of the vertebral column), knowledge of which could be obtained only by autopsy.[19] If a physician opened such a patient as Philiscus after death, he would have found the spleen dark grey or black in colour. Philiscus died during the epidemic of ardent fevers at Thasos during the third constitution described in *Epidemics I*.[20] Herepho, another victim of the same autumnal epidemic at Thasos, also had black urine, scanty black stools, and a swollen spleen.[21] These signs combined to argue that the fever was caused by an excess of black bile in its natural seat, the spleen.

From his observations of disease at Thasos over several years, Hippocrates, the presumed author of *Epidemics I* and *III* inferred a broad relationship between the occurrence of disease and the passage of the seasons. He wrote, 'For the coming on of winter resolves the diseases of summer, and the coming on of summer removes those of winter.'[22] In the treatise *On the Nature of Man*, written, according to Aristotle (384–322 BC), by Hippocrates's son-in-law Polybus (*fl*,. 370 BC), the occurrence of disease is correlated to the rise and fall of the humours with the passage of the seasons, and the nature of the universe. Each of the humours was always present in the human body, but as the year goes round, 'they become now greater and now less, each in turn and according to its nature'.[23] Each humour increased in the body when its qualities corresponded to the qualities of the season. Thus phlegm, which was cold and wet, increased in the body during winter, the cold wet season, and the associated diseases occurred more frequently. In spring when the weather continued wet, but grew steadily warmer, blood, which was hot and wet, increased, giving rise to dysenteries and haemorrhage from the nose. In the heat and drought of the summer, yellow bile, which was hot and dry, increased. Near the end of the treatise, Polybus revealed how the humoral theory was based upon the Hippocratic physicians' observations of the occurrence of malarial fevers. After asserting that the four kinds of fevers, the continued, the quotidian, the tertian, and the quartan, all came from bile, Polybus wrote:

> Now what is called the continued fever comes from the most abundant and the purest bile, and its crises occur after the shortest interval. For since the body has not time to cool it wastes away rapidly, being warmed by the great heat. The quotidian next to the continued comes from the most abundant bile,

and ceases quicker than any other, though it is longer than the continued, proportionately to the lesser quantity of bile from which it comes; moreover the body has a breathing space, whereas in the continued there is no breathing space at all. The tertian is longer than the quotidian and is the result of less bile. The longer the breathing space enjoyed by the body in the case of the tertian than in the case of the quotidian, the longer this fever is than the quotidian.[24]

The heat of the body in fever was thus the result of the excess amount of hot, dry, yellow bile in the body, and the vomiting and diarrhoea that accompanied fever represented the efforts of the body to discharge this.

By far the most protracted fever was the quartan fever, which might continue on through the autumn into winter. The heat of a quartan fever was less than that of a tertian, quotidian, or continued fever, and the interval during which the body might cool was longer. Polybus attributed the persistence of quartan fevers to black bile, which he said was the most viscous of the humours, and the slowest to be discharged. Quartan fevers resulted from black bile as well as yellow bile

> because it is mostly in autumn that men are attacked by quartans, and between the ages of twenty-five and forty-five. This age is that which of all ages is most under the mastery of black bile, just as autumn is the season of all seasons which is most under its mastery.[25]

The connection between black bile, quartan fever, and autumn again emphasizes that long-continued malarial infection tends to make its victims peculiarly liable to nervous irritability and mental depression (*melancholia*). By contrast, a person who was cheerful was considered to have the humours of his body in proper balance and was, therefore, said to be 'in good humour'.

TREATMENT

In the treatment of fevers, Hippocrates and his followers emphasized regimen, and particularly diet. They customarily gave acutely ill patients barley gruel or barley water, supplemented with hydromel (honey and water) or oxymel (honey and vinegar). The gruel was to be given according to the pattern of the patient's meals when in health and in quantities just enough to prevent 'severe pangs of hunger'.[26] The treatment for fever was thus to keep the patient on a semi-starvation diet while still providing adequate fluids, in order to reduce the amount of blood and bile in the body. Based as it was upon extensive medical experience, this treatment of malarial fevers may have been quite effective. In 1974 in eastern Niger, Dr M. John Murray and his colleagues observed that starving African natives who came into their mission hospital frequently developed malarial fevers about five days after they began to be fed.[27] The following year during a famine in the savannah country of eastern Ethiopia, the Murrays confirmed the same relationship among nomadic tribes-people of the Ogaden. So long as the people remained in a semi-starving state, they did not develop fever, even though they were infected with malarial parasites.[28] M. J. Murray and his team suggested that the depletion of iron in the body as a result of starvation inhibited the growth of malarial parasites in the circulating blood, and that when iron levels rose as a result of refeeding, the parasites multiplied rapidly.[29]

The effect of the severely restricted diet of barley gruel, supplemented by a little honey in water or vinegar – the regimen recommended for fevers by Hippocratic physicians – combined with the destruction of red blood cells by malarial parasites, would be to lower the iron levels in the blood. The iron deficiency would suppress further growth of the malarial parasites, thereby giving time for the patient's immune system to develop its defences. Thus the treatment of fevers described in 'Regimen in Acute Diseases' may have been helpful to patients suffering from a malarial fever.

A further means of lowering the iron levels of the patient's body might be by bloodletting. In *Epidemics I* and *III*, Hippocrates refers to bloodletting only occasionally, and not always in connection with acute fevers. A lack of connection between the treatment of fever and bloodletting was perhaps natural so long as blood was regarded as only one of the four humours, each of which waxed or waned in the body according to the season of the year. (➤ Ch. 40 Physical Methods) Nevertheless, as knowledge of the anatomy of the heart and blood vessels increased, blood gradually assumed primacy among the humours. (➤ Ch. 5 The anatomical tradition)

ANCIENT GREEK THEORIES OF ANATOMY AND PHYSIOLOGY

During the fifth and early fourth centuries BC, Greek physicians, including Hippocrates and his followers, possessed only fragmentary knowledge of the distribution of the veins throughout the body. They were acquainted with some of the superficial veins and were aware of the existence of the vena cava and the aorta in the interior of the trunk, but they did not understand how the various veins were interconnected.[30] At Athens during the later fourth century (perhaps two generations after Hippocrates), Aristotle carried out systematic anatomical dissections on animals that had been first starved and then strangled so as to retain the blood within the vessels. He revealed the veins as a connected system of vessels extending from the heart through-out the whole body. In his observations of the embryonic chick, developing within the egg, Aristotle saw that the beating heart was the first sign of life. From the moment it was visible, the heart contained blood and the embryonic chick appeared to develop within the skein of blood vessels extending out from the heart. To Aristotle, the heart became the centre of life and thought because it was the one organ at the centre of a system coextensive with the whole body. The blood contained within the heart and blood vessels became correspondingly important. Aristotle regarded blood as nourishment that the blood vessels absorbed from the intestine. Thus, blood provided the basis for the nutrition and growth of the body: 'This explains why the blood diminishes in quantity when no food is taken, and increases when much is consumed.'[31]

The physician Praxagoras of Cos (*fl.* fourth century BC) altered the anatomy of Aristotle by distinguishing arteries from veins. By definition, Praxagoras considered the arteries to be air tubes, like the trachea and bronchi, that served to conduct the breath or *pneuma* from the lungs to the left side of the heart and thence through the aorta and other arteries to the whole body. The arteries possessed their centre and origin in the heart; by contrast the veins arose from the liver, and their function was to carry the blood, formed from digested and assimilated nourishment, from the liver to the whole body. The interaction of blood and pneuma throughout the body generated the innate heat. If digestion was disordered, the nourishment might form excessive amounts of bile, thereby causing fever.[32]

Praxagoras's pupil, Herophilus of Chalcedon (*c.*355–*c.*280 BC), who spent much of his active career at Alexandria where he carried out extensive investigations of human anatomy, maintained the distinction of artery from vein and that the arteries carried pneuma. He showed that the walls of arteries were usually about six times as thick as the walls of veins.[33] Herophilus noted, too, that arteries pulsated whereas veins did not, and that in fever, the pulse became more frequent, larger, and stronger. He considered the pulse so important for the diagnosis of fever that he is said to have used a water-clock to count the number of pulsations in a measured period of time.[34]

Erasistratus of Chios (*fl.* 250 BC), who was active at Alexandria slightly later than Herophilus, demonstrated that the arterial pulse was dependent upon the heartbeat. He reasoned that each pulsation of the arteries resulted from their being filled with pneuma by the contraction of the left ventricle of the heart. Consequently, the stronger and more rapid pulse in fevers was the result of increased activity of the heart and an increased interaction between pneuma and blood throughout the body. Perhaps because he reasoned that in fevers there must be an increased consumption of blood as nutriment, Erasistratus opposed bloodletting as a treatment for fever. Nevertheless, he attributed fever to plethora, a condition resulting from an excess of blood in the veins. In plethora, some of the blood oozed through the synanastomoses into the arteries (normally filled only with pneuma). The blood in the arteries, being compressed by the pneuma pumped in from the heart, caused inflammation and fever. The proper treatment of plethora was the earlier Hippocratic treatment by starvation which, by emptying the veins gradually, would allow the blood to return from the arteries into the veins through the synanastomoses.[35]

GALEN'S INFLUENCE ON FEVER THEORIES

The concepts of fever developed by the early third century BC form the intellectual background to the thought of Galen (129-c. 200/210) in the second century AD, more than four hundred years later. Galen discussed his predecessors, and supported or contradicted their views, almost as if they were his immediate antecedents, if not his contemporaries. In a sense, the ideas of such men as Erasistratus were still contemporary in Galen's time, because they were upheld by a group of physicians active in the medical practice of Rome and elsewhere throughout the ancient world.

Galen retained the idea of blood as nourishment. Blood, he said, was formed in the liver from chyle; that is, the digested and assimilated food carried to the liver from the intestine through the portal vein. The liver was the head and origin of the veins, which distributed the blood throughout the body where it formed and nourished flesh and bone. Galen also retained the Hippocratic humoral theory, and attributed disease to an excess of yellow bile, black bile, or phlegm. In health, the humours were in proper balance and the treatment of disease, therefore, must be directed toward the restoration of balance.

Fever, according to Galen, might result from either an excess of yellow bile, black bile, or phlegm, a condition which he called a *cacochymia*, or from an excess of blood, a plethora. Excess humours might accumulate in one part of the body where they might cause putrefaction and excessive heat or fever. A body containing residues from over-indulgence was particularly liable to putrefactive fevers. To remove residues and to restore a healthy humoral balance, Galen advocated bloodletting. He thought that the physician should let blood not only when the patient was acutely ill, but whenever a fever was likely to occur.[36] He gave detailed indications as to when and how much blood to draw, according to the age and strength of the patient, the stage of the disease, the time of day, the season of the year, the weather, and the locality.[37] Galen used venesection in fevers in place of the earlier Hippocratic treatment by starvation, and accompanied it with cooling drinks. Venesection, he claimed, cooled the body and thus reduced the fever. The quantities of blood he took were often large.[38] Peter Brain has pointed out, on the basis of the observations of the Murrays in Africa and of others, that the reduction of the iron level in the body may have proved helpful in combating various infections, including both tuberculosis and malarial fevers.[39] Brain notes that women who had abundant menstrual bleeding and men who suffered from bleeding haemorrhoids both tended to escape many diseases.[40]

In late antiquity, Galen's extensive writings became the dominant authority in medical teaching. During the ninth century AD, the writings of both Hippocrates and Galen were translated from Greek into Syriac and Arabic in highly accurate versions by Hunain ibn Ishaq (808–73), and Arabic manuscripts of Hunain's translations became widely distributed throughout the Islamic world. (➤ Ch. 31 Arab-Islamic Medicine) Following the capture of Toledo by Norman crusaders in 1085, that city became a centre for the translation into Latin of both Arabic writings and Arabic versions of Greek writings. At Toledo during the twelfth century, Gerard of Cremona (c.1114–87) translated the works of Hippocrates and Galen into Latin, and his translations became the basis for medical teaching in universities during the thirteenth and fourteenth centuries. In the late fifteenth century, humanist scholars, seeking to recover the texts of ancient Greek authors in their original purity, began to make fresh translations of the works of Hippocrates, Galen, and other ancient medical authors directly from the Greek texts and to publish them in beautifully printed editions. By the mid-sixteenth century, the collected works of Galen were available in large printed folios, which were read by all serious students of medicine, and continued to form the basis of medical practice.

THOMAS SYDENHAM'S CONCEPTS OF FEVER

Thus, in the fever concepts of Thomas Sydenham (1624–89) in seventeenth-century England, despite the passage of 1,500 years, curiously little had changed. For Sydenham as for Galen, the writings of Hippocrates remained a source of valuable medical knowledge, although Sydenham also faithfully read Galen's works. Furthermore, just as in ancient Greece, through much of the English countryside in the seventeenth century the most prevalent diseases remained the malarial fevers: primarily benign tertian malaria, familiar to Sydenham as the annual spring epidemic of intermittent fever occurring from March to July.[41]

In 1655, newly married, Thomas Sydenham bought a house in King Street, Westminster, and began to practise medicine. Westminster was then a small community clustered about the great Abbey and the Palace and surrounded by open country, much of which was marshy and malarious. The epidemic of intermittent fevers each spring and early summer thus formed a large part of Sydenham's practice. The spring fevers were mild, and almost every patient recovered. Sydenham thought that they arose from the warmth of the sun acting on humours accumulated in the blood during the winter and treated them with 'a low diet without meat, a mild purge on the days of intermission, and a narcotic a little before the next fit'.[42] Hippocrates would have approved.

The annual spring epidemic of intermittent fever around Westminster in the 1650s conformed to what Gill has described as the epidemiological pattern of temperate-zone malaria and was entirely benign tertian malaria.[43] Beginning in September and through the autumn, Sydenham usually also saw a few cases of quartan fever. During the late 1650s, he also began to see an increasing number of cases of intermittent fever during the late summer and autumn, but in contrast to the spring intermittents, the autumnal intermittents were very severe, and a high proportion of those afflicted died. (➤ Ch. 52 Epidemiology) In 1661, the summer began early and was unusually warm. On 24 June, a woman in Sydenham's neighbourhood was seized with the first fit of a quartan ague. Ordinarily, quartan fevers did not begin to appear before September. About the beginning of July, a new epidemic of very severe intermittent fevers began and increased daily. 'By the month of August,' wrote Sydenham, 'they were doing fearful mischief. In many places the mortality was excessive, and whole families fell victims.'[44] Clearly, some time during the 1650s, or possibly earlier, England was invaded by falciparum malaria, and during the unusually warm summer of 1661 the epidemiological pattern of malarial fevers changed from that of temperate-zone malaria to that of the subtropical zone, in which the annual spring epidemic of benign tertian malaria is followed by an epidemic of malignant tertian (falciparum) malaria during the summer and autumn.[45] Falciparum malaria can only become epidemic when the average monthly temperature exceeds 68 °F.[46] In 1661, warm weather continued in England through the autumn into the winter, and the whole year was exceedingly sickly.[47] The set of circumstances created by a new invasion of falciparum malaria into England, witnessed by Sydenham at Westminster in 1661, were very similar to those encountered by Hippocrates at Thasos in Greece around 410 BC and described by him in *Epidemics I* and *III*. Sydenham thus shared with Hippocrates and other ancient Greek physicians the experience of living in a country where the most prevalent diseases were the malarial fevers and where most of the population became infected with malaria at some time. The presence of malaria imposed on the occurrence of fevers a regular pattern that followed the succession of the seasons.

The epidemic of malignant tertian fever that ravaged England during the summer and autumn of 1661 was not repeated the following year, when the autumnal epidemic included only cases of quartan fever. During the winter of 1661–2, the prevalent disease was a continued fever. Sydenham is vague as to the prevalence of autumnal intermittents in 1663 and 1664, but he may have seen at least some cases in those years. In his *Medical Observations* of 1674, he devoted considerable discussion to the treatment of autumnal intermittents, but confessed that he had 'not yet been fortunate enough to cure autumnal intermittents by any sure practice'.[48]

The prolonged and consistent character of the intermittent fevers and their association with season, weather, and locality, which Sydenham observed around Westminster from 1661 to 1664, may have been influential in leading him to observe disease systematically and to consider it rationally, as the intermittent fevers had served for Hippocratic physicians two thousand years earlier. Furthermore, Sydenham drew from his prolonged observation of intermittent fevers the conclusion that the various forms of fever were each distinct and specific: 'Nature in the production of disease is uniform and consistent.'[49] As an example, he cited the case of quartan fever:

> It begins almost always in autumn; it keeps to a regular course of succession; it preserves a definite type; its periodical revolutions, occurring on the fourth day, . . . are as regular as a watch or any other piece of machinery; it sets in with shivers and a notable feeling of cold, which are succeeded by an equally decided sensation of heat, and it is terminated by a most profuse perspiration. Whoever is attacked must bear his complaint till the vernal equinox, there or thereabouts.
>
> Now putting all this together, we find reasons for believing that the disease is a species equally cogent with those that we have for believing a plant to be a species.[50]

Nevertheless, in contrast to species of plants and animals, each of which lived independently, each species of disease was dependent upon the humours of the body that engendered it.

Sydenham adopted the ancient humoral theory of disease (it fitted the observed phenomena of fevers too well for him to do otherwise), but he adopted it with a significant difference. Among the four humours (phlegm, blood, yellow bile, and black bile), Sydenham emphasized one: namely, blood. The others must be contained in, or derived from, the blood. He saw clearly that the meaning of the discovery of William Harvey (1578–1657) of the circulation of the blood was that the fluids in the body must either be blood, or must originate from the circulating blood. Every disease, therefore, must be a disorder of the blood.

Sydenham retained the Hippocratic concept of the elimination of harmful matter in disease. Disease, he said, 'is nothing more than an effort of Nature . . . to restore the health of the patient by the elimination of the morbific matter'.[51] Diseases arose, he thought, partly from particles of the atmosphere which might enter and become mixed with the juice (humours) of the body and with the blood, which would spread the disease throughout the body. Disease might also arise from 'fermentations and putrefactions' of the humours, when the powers of the body proved inadequate to digest or to excrete them. In bubonic plague, the disease discharged the harmful matter through abscesses. In fevers, the processes of sweating, diarrhoea, or other evacuations served to remove the harmful particles from the blood; in smallpox, the eruption on the skin performed the same function. Sydenham referred repeatedly to what he called the 'despumation of the blood'. Despumation is the clarification of a heated liquid by skimming off the foam or scum from the surface. To assist the despumation of the blood, Sydenham said that the physician possessed two resources, bleeding and purging. He was cautious in advocating their use, but following an autumnal intermittent fever, the patient should be purged to prevent its recurrence. Bleeding might also be used to assist the purification of the blood in pleurisy or pneumonia. Sydenham's confidence in the specific nature of diseases was strengthened by his successful use in 1663 of Peruvian bark to cure a quartan fever. If diseases were specific, then each might have a specific remedy, and Peruvian bark was a specific remedy for quartan fever. (➤ Ch. 9 The pathological tradition; Ch. 39 Drug therapies)

The severe cold of the winter of 1664–5 in England brought an end to the great epidemics of fevers of the preceding four years. In May 1665, the plague, which had reappeared briefly in London the previous autumn after an absence of sixteen years, broke out again. Few at first, the cases of plague increased explosively in July, and by September plague was causing 7,000 deaths a week. Before the epidemic ended in November, about a fifth of the population of London is estimated to have perished.

In June, shortly after the plague appeared in London, the court and all the officers of government left Westminster for the countryside. Sydenham also went with his wife and children. When he returned to Westminster in the autumn of 1665, he was struck by the fact that whereas he saw many cases of plague, he saw almost none of fever. The plague seemed to have driven away the fever. Sydenham attributed this change to some obscure alteration in what he called the *epidemic constitution* of the atmosphere. 'This is how it is', he wrote later. 'There are different constitutions in different years. They originate neither in their heat nor their cold, their wet nor their drought; but they depend upon certain hidden and inexplicable changes within the bowels of the earth. By the effluvia from these the atmosphere becomes contaminate, and the bodies of men are predisposed and determined ... to this or that complaint.'[52] (➤ Ch. 18 The ecology of disease)

BOERHAAVE AND HIS FOLLOWERS

At Leiden in June 1701, Hermann Boerhaave (1668–1738) began to lecture on the institutes of medicine. He sought to incorporate into medical thought the multitude of new discoveries in anatomy and physiology made during the seventeenth century. These created a new anatomy and physiology, and it was clear to Boerhaave that scientific physiology must have a bearing on the understanding of disease and its treatment. He therefore sought to unite the new science with the older tradition of clinical medicine. (➤ Ch. 7 The physiological tradition)

In 1714, Boerhaave was appointed Professor of the Practice of Medicine in Leiden University and began clinical teaching at the St Cecilia Hospital. In his teaching Boerhaave praised Sydenham for his accurate observation of the natural history of diseases.[53] In his discussion of fever, Boerhaave described continued fever, ardent fevers, and intermittent fevers.[54] Like Sydenham, he distinguished the autumnal intermittents from the vernal ones, a distinction necessary because of their different symptoms, duration, and treatment. The autumnal intermittents resembled continued fevers in their onset, and Boerhaave recommended the prompt use of Peruvian bark for them.[55] The prime symptom of fever was an accelerated pulse and heartbeat, arising, he thought, from a stagnation of the blood at the ends of the capillaries and accompanied by an irritation of the heart – an explanation of fever in terms of the new physiology.[56] There was an increased body heat, which Boerhaave measured by means of an alcohol thermometer held in the patient's hand.[57] (➤ Ch. 35 The art of diagnosis: medicine and the five senses)

From 1701 until his death in 1738, Boerhaave was the most influential medical teacher in Europe, his students coming from almost every European country. Boerhaave's high respect for Sydenham was particularly significant for his English-speaking students, who were thereby encouraged to read Sydenham.[58] The multitude of eighteenth-century works on fever tend either to reflect Boerhaave's teaching in varying degrees or to build upon it.[59]

One of Boerhaave's English students was John Huxham (1692–1768), who matriculated at Leiden in May 1715. In 1717, he began medical practice at Plymouth, and in 1739 he published a work on the relation of epidemic diseases to weather. In 1755, he published a work on fevers.[60] Huxham began by citing Boerhaave's *Aphorisms*, and, like Boerhaave, he thought that the accelerated pulse and heartbeat, increased body heat, and flushed skin in fevers reflected both a stimulated state of the heart and an increased resistance to the flow of blood through the capillaries. Among the continued fevers, he distinguished a slow nervous fever from the putrid, malignant or pestilential fever, noting that the latter was caused by contagion. At Plymouth, he saw cases of the 'putrid, malignant, or pestilential fever' among men brought ashore from naval ships, its contagious character permitting it to spread rapidly among a ship's crew, as it did also in military camps, hospitals, and prisons, so that it became known as ship fever, camp fever, or prison fever.

Another Boerhaave student, Sir John Pringle (1707–82), who observed epidemics of such fever extensively during military campaigns in the 1740s, thought it could occur wherever men were crowded together in a dirty, badly ventilated place. Pringle noted that the fever was highly contagious.[61] During the Seven Years' War (1756–63), epidemics of fever occurred among many ships of the British Navy, especially in the large fleets sent to North America.[62] In 1763, James Lind (1716–94), Physician to the Haslar naval hospital at Portsmouth, observed that many of the fever patients from naval ships had not changed their clothes for over four months, and their 'unshifted linen and rags were sufficient to have bred an infection'.[63] (➤ Ch. 53 History of personal hygiene) Nevertheless, he observed that fever epidemics occurred on some ships but not on others, and when men from a healthy ship were ordered on board a fever-laden ship to relieve the shortage of crew, they too came down with fever.[64] The contagiousness of the fever was more observable in a fleet because a ship's crew lived closely together under the same conditions, eating the same food, and yet was isolated both from the land and from the crews of other ships.[65] The fever was marked by a characteristic rash of large reddish or bluish spots on the skin that often caused it to be called spotted or petechial fever.

In the late eighteenth century, epidemics of the same putrid, petechial, or malignant fever occurred also among the poor of English cities such as London and Liverpool.[66] Such epidemics, like those on ships, in hospitals, military camps, or prisons, reflected a fundamental change in the pattern of prevailing diseases that accompanied the rise in population, the growth of towns, the founding of hospitals, and the great wars of the eighteenth century. It was a shift from the diseases of the countryside, dominated by the seasonal epidemics of intermittent fevers, to the diseases of cities, among which the most common were continued fevers. Whereas the pattern of diseases that Sydenham observed around Westminster in 1661 was essentially identical to that described by Hippocrates at Thasos in the fifth century BC, by 1800 the diseases of London were very different from the Hippocratic pattern. Although intermittent fevers might persist in parts of the countryside, they were gone from the cities; in their place were the continued fevers, consumption, and smallpox. (➤ Ch. 27 Diseases of civilization)

CULLEN'S INFLUENCE ON FEVER THEORIES

The concepts of fever most widely accepted by British physicians in 1800 were those of William Cullen (1710–90), Professor of Medicine in the University of Edinburgh from 1773 to 1790. Cullen distinguished a simple inflammatory fever (such as might accompany a cold or pneumonia), with a strong hard pulse, but no delirium, as 'synocha'. If a fever was accompanied by delirium or stupor, he called it 'typhus'. In Scotland, the most common form of continued fever seemed to be a combination of synocha and typhus that Cullen called 'synochus'. Although he thought of fever as a general disease that might assume various forms, the common underlying phenomenon was a spasm of the arteries. A fever developed in three stages: first, a stage of weakness or debility, with relaxation or atony of the arteries; second, a stage of irritation, corresponding to the shivering or chill that resulted from irritation; and third, the hot stage resulting from the spasm of the arteries following their irritation.[67] Cullen thought that fevers might be caused by matter floating in the atmosphere: if the source of the matter arose from the bodies of the sick, it would be called contagion; if it arose from marshes and moist ground, it would be called miasma. A contagion or miasma exerted a sedative influence on the body, inducing debility, and Cullen emphasized supportive treatment to overcome this. He also used bloodletting in moderation to relieve spasm of the arteries, but continued to rely on the healing power of nature. (➤ Ch. 17 Nosology)

Cullen's student, John Brown (1735–88) repudiated Cullen's faith in the healing power of nature and urged that the physician intervene actively in the disease. Brown postulated a principle of excitability in living matter that was consumed to generate excitement, or vital activity. Excessive stimulation, a sthenic diathesis, would exhaust excitability and produce excessive excitement; by contrast insufficient stimulation, an asthenic diathesis, would allow the accumulation of excitability, but would generate insufficient vital activity. Excessive excitement of the body was followed by debility and hence fever.

Benjamin Rush (1746–1813), Cullen's American student, adopted Cullen's and Brown's theories with some modification. Rush thought that fever was preceded by debility that caused excitability to accumulate, making the body susceptible to such pathogens as contagia, miasmata, or injury, any of which could bring about an irregular action of the arterial system. Rush conceived that treatment should combat both the debility that predisposed the body to disease and the irregular arterial action that resulted from debility. To combat debility, he used stimulating medicine, such as alcohol and calomel (mercurous chloride), and bloodletting. Rush believed in the unity of fever, opposing any attempt to discriminate among fevers, and his treatments were general. He thought that Peruvian bark was effective because it was bitter and astringent and, therefore, exerted a tonic effect on the fibres of the body. As Professor of Medicine at the University of Pennsylvania from 1789 until his death in 1813, and as a prolific author, Rush was the most influential medical teacher in America, and his advocacy of the vigorous use of calomel and bloodletting was widely accepted by American physicians in the early nineteenth century.

THE NINETEENTH CENTURY

During the early nineteenth century, British physicians also tended to believe that continued fever was a general disease that might assume various forms and might become complicated by local inflammation, its variable manifestations influenced by the prevailing epidemic constitution of the atmosphere. The fever that British physicians called typhus became increasingly common with the growth of towns and cities following the Industrial Revolution. Typhus was almost constantly present in the crowded slums of cities, and it occurred frequently also in the new villages built around mills and factories in the countryside, both as sporadic cases and in epidemics. Fever epidemics were sensitive to economic conditions, and the severe economic depression following the peace of 1815 was accompanied by widespread outbreaks throughout the British Isles from 1816 to 1819. (➤ Ch. 52 Public health) The fever was clearly contagious, and on post-mortem examination showed no particular lesion, although physicians occasionally found that fever patients who had suffered from diarrhoea might show lesions in the small intestine. They thought intestinal inflammation was merely an incidental feature of the fever.[68]

RESEARCH ON TYPHOID AND TYPHUS FEVERS

By contrast, during a fever epidemic in Tours, France, in 1816, Pierre Bretonneau (1778–1862) found that victims of continued fever showed lesions of the small intestine so consistently that he named the disease for its lesion: *dothienenteritis* (that is, intestinal boils).[69] At La Charité hospital in Paris during the 1820s, Pierre Louis (1787–1872) conducted a systematic study of patients with continued fever, and in 1829 published his classic study of 138 cases of what he called typhoid fever, by which he understood a continued fever identical with the typhus fever described by British authors.[70] He found that every patient who died from typhoid fever had the characteristic lesions of the Peyer's patches in the wall of the small intestine described earlier by Bretonneau. Furthermore, by systematically recording his observations of the signs, symptoms, and course of patients with typhoid fever, compared with those of patients suffering from other acute diseases, he was able to form a complete picture of the clinical history of the disease. He showed that typhoid fever followed a remarkably consistent course of about twenty-eight days that could not be interrupted or shortened by treatment. It attacked young adults, usually in their early twenties, who had recently come to Paris. As a rule, the younger the patient was when attacked, the milder was the disease.

Louis described the clinical and pathological features of typhoid fever so clearly and completely that it could be recognized wherever it might occur.

Thus when in August 1832 James Jackson Jr (1810–34) returned to Boston, Massachusetts, from Paris, after several months spent in clinical study with Louis, he found that the epidemic of 'autumnal fever' then occurring in Boston was identical to the typhoid fever described by Louis. Similarly, in Philadelphia in 1834, William Wood Gerhard (1809–72), another student of Louis, identified cases of continued fever among Irish immigrants brought into the Pennsylvania Hospital as identical to Louis's typhoid fever. Gerhard's patients were also very young – their average age was twenty – and had been in Philadelphia only one or two months before they fell ill. Gerhard demonstrated, too, that typhoid fever was entirely distinct in its symptoms, course, and pathology from remittent fever, which throughout much of the southern and western United States was often called autumnal fever. At the Blockley Hospital in Philadelphia during the winter of 1836, Gerhard studied an epidemic of a continued fever very different from typhoid fever. In autopsies of about fifty patients, he found no lesions in the intestines. The course of the fever was shorter than that of typhoid fever, although more fatal, and patients consistently developed a peculiar eruption of reddish or purple spots. The fever was highly contagious, while typhoid fever was not. Gerhard concluded that the Philadelphia epidemic of 1836 was the true typhus of the British Isles, identical to the ship fever, jail fever, camp fever, or petechial or spotted fever described by eighteenth-century writers.[71]

Although Gerhard provided clear and compelling evidence for the existence of two specific kinds of continued fever, his evidence did not immediately persuade the British medical world. Hospitals in British cities received many fever patients. Some at autopsy showed lesions of Peyer's patches; others did not. The intestinal lesions, therefore, seemed to British medical practitioners a variable rather than a constant feature of continued fever, and most British physicians continued to believe that typhoid and typhus fevers were identical.

At the London Fever Hospital, William Jenner (1815–98) began in 1847 to study continued fever. In 1849, he published the results of his study of sixty-six fever patients upon whom he had performed autopsies.[72] Jenner found that they suffered from two distinct diseases, typhus fever and typhoid fever, which he could distinguish readily during life. Like Louis, Jenner found that the typhoid fever patients were young, with an average age of twenty-two years, whereas typhus fever affected all age groups. The onset of typhoid fever was gradual, that of typhus fever sudden; the eruption on the skin was quite different in the two diseases. The duration, symptoms, and courses of the two fevers were also distinct, as was their pathological anatomy, with typhoid fever victims alone having the characteristic lesions in the Peyer's patches of the small intestine. Jenner's work confirmed the earlier work of Gerhard and others. His extensive observations were carried out in England where the two diseases had been confused, and he presented his results with extraordinary clarity.

Jenner took particular pains to answer the arguments of British physicians who insisted that typhoid fever was merely typhus fever complicated by a particular lesion, or that they were merely variant forms of a single disease, their variations influenced by changes in the epidemic constitution of the atmosphere. He noted that most of his cases had occurred during the same epidemic constitution and that from 1847 to 1849 there had been no change whatever in the characteristics of typhus and typhoid fevers as they were seen at the London Fever Hospital. Jenner said that typhus and typhoid fever were distinct diseases, just as were smallpox and scarlet fever.

Adhering to standards established by Louis, Jenner recorded the symptoms of each patient, so that he could state the proportion of patients who showed any particular symptom on any particular day after the onset of illness. Similarly, at autopsy, Jenner recorded the state of all the organs, whether healthy or diseased. His 1849 paper thus reflects the influence of Louis's methods of clinical investigation on British medicine.

The recognition that typhus and typhoid fevers were each distinct and specific diseases had profound practical consequences for medicine. Louis had shown that the course of typhoid fever could neither be interrupted nor shortened by treatment, and his conclusion was supported by the earlier experience of Nathan Smith (1762–1829) with typhoid fever (which Smith called typhous fever) in New England villages.[73] In a statistical study of the effect of bloodletting on typhoid fever, Louis showed that while mild bloodletting in the very early stages of the disease might be slightly beneficial, at later stages it was harmful. Since the course of typhoid fever was unalterable, Nathan Smith and others learned that the best treatment was mild and supportive. In contrast to the malarial fevers, typhoid fever patients benefited from a generous diet. In Boston, Massachusetts, in 1835, Jacob Bigelow (1786–1879) argued that since many diseases, including pneumonia and typhoid fever, followed a natural course tending toward recovery, they should be considered self-limited diseases.[74] The physician could do little to influence the course of a self-limited disease, and ought, therefore, to depend mainly on the healing power of nature.

In London, William Jenner saw a still more far-reaching significance to the distinct and specific character of typhus and typhoid fevers. If each disease were distinct and specific, then each must have its own specific cause. Cases of typhus and typhoid fever came into the London Fever Hospital at every season of the year and always manifested the same distinct sets of characters. Especially for typhus fever, the houses from which patients came showed that patients tended to have a history of previous contact with another case. Jenner considered typhus fever very contagious; typhoid fever was much less so, but was still capable of being communicated by contagion. Since the two fevers were distinct, each must result from its own specific contagion. The establishment of typhus and typhoid fevers as distinct individual diseases thus became evidence for the theory of contagion. (➤ Ch. 16 Contagion/germ theory/specificity)

The question of the cause of continued fevers was of grave urgency to nineteenth-century physicians because of the vast extent and high mortality of such diseases. In 1856, William Budd (1811–80) estimated, conservatively, that each year 20,000 people died of typhoid fever in Great Britain and at least 100,000 people passed through the disease:

> No one can know what these figures really imply who has not had experience of this disorder in his own home. The dreary and painful night-watches, the unusual length of the period over which the anxiety is protracted, the long suspense between hope and fear, and the large proportion of cases in which hope is disappointed ... make up a sum of distress ... scarcely to be found again in the history of any other acute disorder.[75]

Typhoid fever tended to occur sporadically, or in small, circumscribed epidemics as much in small towns and country villages as in large cities, and in all classes of society. It most frequently attacked young people, often those who had recently moved to a city. Medical students were frequently its victims. Although typhoid fever might occur at any season of the year, it tended to occur so frequently and regularly during the late summer and autumn that it was known as autumnal fever.

In contrast to the regular occurrence of typhoid fever, typhus fever and relapsing fever occurred irregularly in great epidemics, often during times of economic distress. In Great Britain, widespread epidemics of these fevers had occurred in 1817–19, 1826, 1836, 1843, and 1856. They were pre-eminently diseases of the poor and unemployed in crowded manufacturing towns and large cities, occurring only rarely in the countryside or among members of the upper classes. Typhus fever was associated especially with overcrowding, while relapsing fever accompanied destitution and hunger so frequently as to be called famine fever. In Ireland during the famine years of the 1840s, relapsing fever was especially common, and it was often carried by Irish emigrants to Scotland, England, and North America. Typhus fever and relapsing fever were both recognized to be highly contagious from the experience in hospitals of their frequent transmission to nurses and physicians.

In 1855, Charles Murchison (1830–79), a young Scottish physician, returned from India to settle in medical practice in London and in 1856 became an assistant physician at the London Fever Hospital. In 1858, he argued that typhoid fever ought more properly to be called pythogenic fever (from πυθων = putrefaction, and γενης = generation) because it was caused, he believed, either by emanations from putrefying organic matter or by organic impurities in drinking-water.[76] This theory influenced the belief, then widely held in Great Britain, that bad smells arising from privies, drains, or cesspools might by themselves cause fever. In 1862, Murchison expanded and supported his concept of the pythogenic origin of typhoid fever in a large monograph on the continued fevers of Great Britain.[77] In contrast to Murchison's pythogenic theory, William Budd of Bristol argued in successive publications from 1856 onward that while the contamination of drinking-water by sewage might communicate typhoid fever, it could do so only when the sewage contained the specific poison of typhoid fever. Budd gained his conviction of a specific cause for typhoid fever from an epidemic at the village of North Tawton in Devonshire in 1839. He showed that the intestinal discharges of patients were the specific vehicle by which the disease was transmitted, and he compared the intestinal lesions in typhoid fever with the lesions on the skin in measles, smallpox, or other specific contagious diseases.

During the 1860s and 1870s, Budd's view was supported repeatedly by the study of typhoid fever epidemics caused by contaminated drinking-water. In 1886, C. Hilton Fagge (1838–83) described eleven epidemics of typhoid fever spread through drinking-water and three epidemics spread through contaminated milk, the latter usually having arisen from a particular source of water used to wash pails or cans.[78] In 1873, Murchison investigated one such milk-borne epidemic of typhoid in his own household and the vicinity of Cavendish Square.[79] At Zurich in 1880, Carl Joseph Eberth (1835–1926) described a bacillus that he had found consistently in the lesions of twelve cases of typhoid fever; and at Berlin in 1884, Georg Gaffky (1850–1918) succeeded in growing Eberth's bacillus in pure culture. Gaffky was unable to prove conclusively that this was the cause of typhoid fever because he could find no experimental animal in which he could produce the disease by inoculation. Nevertheless, the constant association of the bacillus with cases of typhoid fever gradually persuaded physicians that it was the actual cause, and in 1896 that belief was confirmed when, independently, Richard Pfeiffer (1858–1945) in Berlin and Max Gruber (1853–1927) in Munich observed that the blood serum of typhoid fever patients caused broth cultures of Eberth's bacillus to clump together and precipitate; and within a few months, Fernand Widal (1862–1929) in Paris made the reaction a diagnostic test for typhoid fever.

The large annual prevalence of typhoid fever in nineteenth-century cities combined with the month-long duration of the disease in each patient combined to make it the overwhelming preoccupation of the medical profession. The fixed and invariable course of the disease, recognized early by such physicians as Nathan Smith and Pierre Louis, emerged even more strikingly in 1868 when Carl Wunderlich (1815–77) published temperature charts for various fevers based upon the records of more than 25,000 patients observed in his clinic at Leipzig. (➤ Ch. 36 The science of diagnosis: diagnostic technology) The chart for typhoid fever consistently rose and declined from the first to the twenty-second day along an almost parabolic curve.[80] Such regularity gradually convinced physicians that typhoid was not to be treated by medicines. Both Fagge in 1886 and William Osler (1849–1919) in 1892 advocated treatment by diet, with a strong emphasis on milk, chicken or beef broths, and fruit juices or other liquids. Osler also described the value of the cold-water bath introduced by James Currie (1756–1805) in Liverpool in the 1790s to bring down the temperature of patients. Although the cold-water treatment appeared to lower mortality, said Osler, it was, harsh and patients complained of it bitterly.[81] In private practice he never used it. 'It would almost appear to be the mission of typhoid fever,' Lloyd Stevenson has written, 'to teach to nineteenth-century medicine once again the healing power of nature, shaking its faith in drugs and adding immeasurably to its skepticism.'[82]

CONCLUSION

The development of sewerage and supplies of pure, piped water in cities greatly reduced the incidence of typhoid fever in the early twentieth century, and it is now rare in advanced countries. Similarly, the discovery of the rickettsial cause of typhus fever and the spirochaete causing relapsing fever, together with the discovery that both organisms are transmitted by the body louse, have permitted the virtual elimination of epidemics of typhus fever and relapsing fever, except during wartime or in other circumstances of social chaos. (➤ Ch. 66 War and modern medicine) Meanwhile, throughout the nineteenth century, the malarial fevers remained widely prevalent, especially in warm temperate, subtropical, and tropical countries. In Constantine, Algeria, in 1880, Alphonse Laveran (1845–1922) first observed malarial parasites in human blood; and in subsequent years the life history of the malarial parasite was worked out, culminating in 1897 in the discovery by Ronald Ross (1857–1932) of the sexual stages in the *Anopheles* mosquito. Ross realized promptly that the key to the prevention of malarial fevers lay in the control of *Anopheles*, and in Sierra Leone in 1899 he gave a practical demonstration of how the elimination of mosquito breeding-places near dwellings was followed by the disappearance of malaria. The following year in Havana, influenced by Ross's work, Walter Reed (1851–1902) and his co-workers discovered the transmission of yellow fever by *Stegomyia* mosquitoes; and in 1901, William C. Gorgas (1854–1920) directed a vigorous campaign to eliminate the breeding-places of mosquitoes that resulted in the eradication of yellow fever and a great reduction in malaria. Later, Gorgas used similar methods to prevent both yellow fever and malaria during the building of the Panama Canal. (➤ Ch. 24 Tropical diseases)

In the United States, the lower Mississippi and Ohio valleys and large areas of the rural South remained as malarious in 1900 as they had been in the early nineteenth century. In 1913, the Rockefeller Foundation began experimental projects on mosquito control in Arkansas. The marked success of the early projects led to their wide extension, and subsequently the Foundation's work was supported and extended by the United States Public Health Service, so that by 1940 the systematic control of mosquitoes had spread throughout much of the southern United States and the incidence of malarial fevers had fallen to a very low level. In Europe, the Rockefeller Foundation carried out similar campaigns, although these were interrupted by the Second World War. After 1945, anti-malaria campaigns relied heavily on spraying with DDT, but this proved to have two fatal flaws: it led to the emergence of DDT-resistant strains of mosquitoes, and at the same time did such serious damage to other animal life that the practice had to be abandoned. At the end of the twentieth century, rural areas in many less-developed countries remain malarious, and malarial fevers continue to be a serious health problem.

NOTES

1 In contrast to the widespread opinion among students of Greek medicine that Hippocratic physicians were not interested in diagnosis of diseases, Grmek has argued convincingly that they did practise diagnosis in order to achieve the ability to make a prognosis: see Mirko D. Grmek, *Diseases in the Ancient Greek World*, trans. by Mireille Muellner and Leonard Muellner, Baltimore, MD, and London, Johns Hopkins University Press, 1983, pp. 292–5.

2 'Ancient Medicine', in *Hippocrates, Works*, trans. by W. H. S. Jones, 4 vols, London and Cambridge, MA, Loeb Classical Library, 1923–31, Vol. I, pp. 3–64, see pp. 47–9.

3 'On the Nature of Man', in *Hippocrates, Works*, Vol. IV, pp. 2–41, see pp. 11–13.

4 Brian Maegraith, *Pathological Processes in Malaria and Blackwater Fever*, Oxford, Blackwell Scientific, 1948, pp. 4–8.

5 Ibid., pp. 12–16.

6 Maegraith, op. cit. (n. 4), pp. 8–12.

7 William Osler, *The Principles and Practice of Medicine*, New York, Appleton, 1892, pp. 145, 153.

8 Maegraith, op. cit. (n. 4), pp. 65–7.

9 Grmek, op. cit. (n. 1), pp. 284–300.

10 L. W. Hackett, *Malaria in Europe: an Ecological Study*, London, Oxford University Press, 1937, pp. 156–8.

11 W. H. S. Jones, *Malaria and Greek History*, Manchester, Manchester University Press, 1909, pp. 23–59.

12 Clifford Allchin Gill, *The Seasonal Periodicity of Malaria and the Mechanism of the Epidemic Wave*, London, J. & A. Churchill, 1938, pp. 35–47.

13 Grmek, op. cit. (n. 1), pp. 275–83.

14 'Airs, Waters, Places', in *Hippocrates*, op. cit. (n. 2), Vol. I, pp. 66–137, see p. 99.

15 Ibid., p. 103.

16 op cit. (n. 14), p. 135.

17 Grmek, op. cit. (n. 1), pp. 284–5.

18 'Ancient Medicine', in *Hippocrates*, op. cit. (n. 2), pp. 261–3.

19 'On Joints, 41', in *Hippocrates*, op. cit. (n. 2), Vol. III, pp. 279–83, see p. 281; Hippocrates, *'De Morbis*, I, 19', quoted in C. R. S. Harris, *The Heart and Vascular System in Ancient Greek Medicine from Alcmaeon to Galen*, Oxford, Clarendon Press, 1973, p. 100.

20 'Epidemics I', in *Hippocrates*, op. cit. (n. 2), Vol. I, pp. 141–211, see p. 167.

21 'Epidemics III', in *Hippocrates*, op. cit. (n. 2), p. 191.

22 op. cit. (n. 20), p. 255.

23 'On the Nature of Man', op. cit. (n. 3), pp. 21–3.

24 'On the Nature of Man', op. cit. (n. 3), pp. 39–41.

25 'On the Nature of Man', op. cit. (n. 3), p. 41.

26 'Regimen in Acute Diseases', in *Hippocrates*, op. cit. (n. 2), Vol. II, pp. 63–125, see p. 71.

27 M. J. Murray, A. B. Murray, N. J. Murray and M. B. Murray, 'Refeeding-malaria and hyperferraemia', *Lancet*, 1975, 1: 653–4.

28 M. J. Murray, A. B. Murray, M. B. Murray and C. J. Murray, 'Somali food shelters in the Ogaden famine and their effect on health', *Lancet*, 1976, 2: 1283–5; M. J. Murray and A. B. Murray, 'Starvation suppression and refeeding activation of infection: an ecological necessity', *Lancet*, 1977, 1: 123–5.

29 M. J. Murray, A. B. Murray, M. B. Murray and C. J. Murray, 'The adverse effect of iron repletion in the course of certain infections', *British Medical Journal*, 1978, 2: 1113–15.

30 See Harris, op. cit. (n. 19), pp. 1–96.

31 Aristotle, *De Partibus Animalium II*, 3 650 a 36–40, trans. by William Ogle, in *Aristotle, Works*, eds J. A. Smith and W. D. Ross, 12 vols, reprint edn, London, Oxford University Press, 1958, Vol. V.

32 Fritz Steckerl, *The Fragments of Praxagoras of Cos and his School*, Leiden, E. J. Brill, 1958, pp. 7–32.

33 *Herophilus: the Art of Medicine in Early Alexandria*, ed. and trans. by Heinrich von Staden, Cambridge, Cambridge University Press, 1989, p. 221.

34 Ibid., p. 354.

35 *Dictionary of Scientific Biography*, s.v. 'Erasistratus' by James Longrigg. Cf. Longrigg, 'Anatomy in Alexandria in the third century BC', *British Journal of the History of Science*, 1988, 21: 455–88.

36 Peter Brain, *Galen on Bloodletting: a Study of the Origins, Development and Validity of his Opinions, with a Translation of the Three Works*, Cambridge, Cambridge University Press, 1986, pp. 80–1.

37 Ibid., pp. 86–99.

38 Brain, op. cit. (n. 36), pp. 122–34.

39 Brain, op. cit. (n. 36), pp. 158–72.

40 Brain, op. cit. (n. 36), p. 170.

41 Benign tertian malaria in England followed the epidemiological pattern of temperate zone malaria described by Gill, op. cit. (n. 12), pp. 18–34.

42 Thomas Sydenham, *Methodus Curandi Febres Propriis Observationibus Superstructura*, trans. by R. G. Latham, Folkestone, Winterdown Books, 1987, p. 107.

43 Gill, op. cit. (n. 12), pp. 18–34.

44 Thomas Sydenham, 'Medical observations concerning the history and the cure of acute diseases' [1676], in Thomas Sydenham, *Works*, trans. by R. G. Latham, 2 vols, London, Sydenham Society, 1848, Vol. I, pp. 3–268, see p. 41.

45 Gill, op. cit. (n. 12), pp. 35–47.

46 Ibid., p. 10.

47 Samuel Pepys, *Diary*, ed. Robert Latham and William Matthews, 11 vols, Berkeley and Los Angeles, University of California Press, 1970–83, Vol. III, p. 10.

48 Sydenham, op. cit. (n. 44), p. 81.

49 Sydenham, op. cit. (n. 44), p. 15 (preface).

50 Sydenham, op. cit. (n. 44), pp. 19–20 (preface).

51 Sydenham, op. cit. (n. 44), p. 29.

52 Sydenham, op. cit. (n. 44), pp. 33–4.

53 Hermann Boerhaave, *A Method of Studying Physick*, trans. by Samber, London, 1719, pp. 316–18. Cf. Boerhaave, *Boerhaave's Orations*, trans. by E. Kegel-Brinkgreve and A. M. Luyendijk-Elshout, Leiden, E. J. Brill, 1983, pp. 139–40, 262.

54 Hermann Boerhaave, *Aphorisms: Concerning the Knowledge and Cure of Diseases*, trans. from the Latin edn, Leiden, 1728, London, 1735, pp. 137–201, Aphorisms 558–782.

55 Ibid., pp. 194–5, Aphorism 767.

56 Ibid., pp. 139–40, Aphorisms 571–77.

57 Ibid., pp. 167–8, Aphorism 673.

58 E. Ashworth Underwood, *Boerhaave's Men at Leyden and After*, Edinburgh, Edinburgh University Press, 1977.

59 John Huxham, *An Essay on Fevers*, London, 1755.

60 Ibid.

61 John Pringle, *Observations on the Nature and Cure of Hospital and Jayl Fevers*, London, 1750; Pringle, *Observations on the Diseases of the Army in Camp and Garrison*, London, 1752.

62 James Lind, *An Essay on the Most Effectual Means of Preserving the Health of Seamen in the Royal Navy*, London, 1757.

63 James Lind, *Two Papers on Fevers and Infection*, London, 1763, pp. 10–11.

64 Ibid., pp. 21–2.

65 Lind, op. cit. (n. 63), p. 36.

66 Charles Creighton, *A History of Epidemics in Great Britain*, 2 vols, London, 1894, Vol. II, pp. 133–4.

67 William Cullen, *First Lines of the Practice of Physic*, 2nd edn, 2 vols, Edinburgh, 1778, Vol. I, pp. 59–61. Cf. Dale C. Smith, 'Medical science, medical practice, and the emerging concept of typhus in mid-eighteenth-century Britain', in W. F.

Bynum and V. Nutton (eds), Theories of Fever from Antiquity to the Enlightenment, Medical History, suppl. 1, London, Wellcome Institute for the History of Medicine, 1981, pp. 121–34.

68 Leonard G. Wilson, 'Fevers and science in early nineteenth century medicine', *Journal of the History of Medicine*, 1978, 33: 386–407.

69 Armand Trousseau, 'De la maladie à laquelle M. Bretonneau a donné le nom de dothinentérie ou dothinentrite', *Archives générales de la médecine*, 1826, 10: 67–78, 169–216.

70 Pierre Louis, *Recherches anatomiques, pathologiques et thérapeutiques sur la maladie connue sous les noms de gastro-entérite, fièvre putride, adynamique ataxique, typhoïde, etc. etc., comparée avec les maladies aiguës les plus ordinaires*, 2 vols, Paris, 1829.

71 W. W. Gerhard, 'On the typhus fever which occurred at Philadelphia in the spring and summer of 1836', *American Journal of Medical Science*, 1837, 20: 289–322.

72 William Jenner, 'On typhoid and typhus fevers', *Edinburgh Monthly Journal of Medical Science*, 1849, 9: 663–80.

73 Nathan Smith, *A Practical Essay on Typhous Fever*, New York, 1824.

74 Jacob Bigelow, *A Discourse on Self-limited Diseases*, Boston, MA, 1835.

75 William Budd, 'On intestinal fever: its mode of propagation', *Lancet*, 1856, 2: 694–5, see p. 694.

76 Charles Murchison, 'Contributions to the etiology of continued fever: or an investigation of various causes which influence the prevalence and mortality of its different forms', *Medico-Chirurgical Transactions*, 1858 (2nd series), 23: 219–306.

77 Murchison, *A Treatise on the Continued Fevers of Great Britain*, London, Parker, Son & Bourn, 1862.

78 Charles Hilton Fagge, *The Principles and Practice of Medicine*, 2 vols, Philadelphia, PA, P. Blakeston, 1886, Vol. I, pp. 190–5.

79 Ernest Hart, 'The outbreak of typhoid fever from the distribution of infected milk', *British Medical Journal*, 1873, 2: 206–7.

80 C. A. Wunderlich, *On the Temperature in Diseases: a Manual of Medical Thermometry*, 2nd edn, trans. by W. Bathurst Woodman, London, New Sydenham Society, 1871, pl. II, fig. 1.

81 Osler, op. cit. (n. 7), pp. 34–6.

82 Lloyd G. Stevenson, 'Exemplary disease: the typhoid pattern', *Journal of the History of Medicine*, 1982, 37: 159–82, see p. 180.

FURTHER READING

Ackerknecht, Erwin H., *Malaria in the Upper Mississippi Valley*, Baltimore, MD, Johns Hopkins Press, 1945.

——, 'Broussais, or a forgotten medical revolution', *Bulletin of the History of Medicine*, 1953, 37: 320–34.

Brain, Peter, *Galen on Bloodletting: a Study of the Origins, Development and Validity of his Opinions, with a Translation of the Three Works*, Cambridge, Cambridge University Press, 1986.

Bruce-Chwatt, Leonard Jan and Zulueta, Julian de, *The Rise and Fall of Malaria in Europe: a Historico-Epidemiological Study*, Oxford, Oxford University Press, 1980.

Budd, William, *On the Causes of Fevers*, ed. by Dale C. Smith, Baltimore, MD, Johns Hopkins University Press, 1984.

——, *Typhoid Fever: its Nature, Mode of Spreading and Prevention*, London, Longmans Green, 1873; reprinted New York, 1931.

Childs, St Julien Ravenel, *Malaria and Colonization in the Carolina Low Country*, Johns Hopkins University Studies in Historical and Political Science, no. 58, Baltimore, MD, Johns Hopkins Press, 1940.

Gill, Clifford Allchin, *The Seasonal Periodicity of Malaria and the Mechanism of the Epidemic Wave*, London, J. & A. Churchill, 1938.

Grmek, Mirko D., *Diseases in the Ancient Greek World*, trans. by Mireille Muellner and Leonard Muellner, Baltimore, MD, and London, Johns Hopkins University Press, 1983.

Hackett, L. W., *Malaria in Europe: an Ecological Study*, London, Oxford University Press, 1937.

Hippocrates, *Works*, trans. by W. H. S. Jones, 4 vols, London and Cambridge, MA, Loeb Classical Library, 1923–31.

Jones, W. H. S., *Malaria and Greek History*, Manchester, Manchester University Press, 1909.

King, Lester, S., *Transformations in American Medicine: from Benjamin Rush to William Osler*, Baltimore, MD, Johns Hopkins University Press, 1973.

Maegraith, Brian, *Pathological Processes in Malaria and Blackwater Fever*, Oxford, Blackwell Scientific, 1948.

Risse, Guenter, B., 'The Brownian system of medicine: its theoretical and practical implications', *Clio Medica*, 1970, 5: 45–51.

——, 'Epidemics and medicine: the influence of disease on medical thought and practice', *Bulletin of the History of Medicine*, 1979, 53: 505–19.

——, *Hospital Life in Enlightenment Scotland: Care and Teaching at the Royal Infirmary of Edinburgh*, Cambridge, Cambridge University Press, 1986.

Smith, Dale C., 'Quinine and fever: the development of the effective dosage', *Journal of the History of Medicine*, 1976, 31: 343–67.

——, 'Gerhard's distinction between typhoid and typhus and its reception in America, 1833–60', *Bulletin of the History of Medicine*, 1980, 54: 368–85.

Stevenson, Lloyd G., 'A pox on the ileum: typhoid fever among the exanthemata', *Bulletin of the History of Medicine*, 1977, 51: 496–504.

——, 'Exemplary disease: the typhoid pattern', *Journal of the History of Medicine*, 1982, 37: 159–82.

Sydenham, Thomas, *Methodus Curandi Febres Propriis Observationibus Superstructura*, trans. by R. G. Latham, Folkestone, Winterdown Books, 1987.

Warner, John Harley, *The Therapeutic Perspective: Medical Practice, Knowledge, and Identity in America*, Cambridge, MA, Harvard University Press, 1986.

20

CONSTITUTIONAL AND HEREDITARY DISORDERS

Robert C. Olby

> If such men happen, by their native *constitutions*, to fall into the gout, either
> they mind it not at all, having no leisure to be sick, or they use it like a dog.
> (Sir William Temple (1628–99), quoted in Samuel Johnson's *Dictionary*)

Charles Darwin (1809–82) reckoned that 'a long catalogue could be given
of all sorts of inherited malformations and of predisposition to various diseases', and he continued: 'Striking instances have been recorded of epilepsy,
consumption, asthma, stone in the bladder, cancer, profuse bleeding from
the slightest injuries, of the mother not giving milk, and of bad parturition
being inherited.'[1] Clearly, he was writing at a time when ideas about heredity
were, by contrast with modern knowledge, very confused. His discussion of
the subject displays an amalgam of scattered empirical data, adherence to
the inheritance of acquired characters, the hereditary effect of use and disuse
of organs, and an understandable 'failure' to distinguish between diseases
due to infection and those which we know to be genetically determined. Nor
should he be considered exceptional in holding such views. Consider his
expert informant, Sir Jonathan Hutchinson (1828–1913) FRS, who in 1881
lectured to the Royal College of Surgeons on 'The Pedigree of Disease' and
described the inheritance of scrofula, gout, tuberculosis, leprosy, scurvy, and
rickets. Although Hutchinson admitted the power of diet to cure the latter,
he assured his listeners that it is definitely a 'diathesis', that is, 'any bodily
condition, however induced, in virtue of which the individual is, through a
long period, or usually through the whole life, prone to suffer from some
peculiar type of disease'.[2] Diatheses can be acquired and they can be
inherited. Some, like gout, are first acquired, then inherited. Others are
passed on to the progeny by infection, but not through the germ, such as
with syphilis for example. The underlying theory is clear: environmental insult

leading to the establishment of the diathesis, which then persists, often becoming strongly inherited. The aim of this essay is to locate the amalgam of concepts which is found in the literature of the nineteenth century concerning constitutional and hereditary disorders, to indicate their probable origins, and to trace their evolution and clarification as the modern science of human genetics became established.

THE CONCEPT OF CONSTITUTION

The view of the body as an organized structure, acting as a whole, its constituent traits being inherited *en bloc*, is what is meant by the term constitution. This organization, it was alleged, gave rise to a vigorous or weak constitution, resistant or susceptible to disease as the case may be. The physician, alienist, and anthropologist James Cowles Prichard (1786–1848) held such a view. His distinction between congenital and acquired varieties of structure issued from his conception of hereditary constitution. He wrote:

> All varieties of structure, which are congenital or a part of the original constitution impressed upon an individual from his birth, or arising from the development of a natural tendency, are hereditary, or liable with a greater or less degree of certainty, to be transmitted to the offspring.[3]

Later in the same work, he returned to these 'laws of organization impressed upon its [the individual's] original germ', and he added:

> These inbred or spontaneous tendencies, governing the future evolution of the bodily fabric, cause it to assume certain qualities of form and texture at different periods of growth. From these predispositions are derived the characteristic differences, and the peculiarities of individual beings.

Among the examples of congenital varieties he mentioned the Negro and albino. Dismissing the view that these were simply cases of disease, he pointed to the constitutional features associated with the absence of pigment:

> The want of secretion which gives colour to the hair, eye, and skin is connected with a peculiar delicacy of constitution. . . . Persons of very fair complexion are often less robust than those of more swarthy hue; and they are more subject to a variety of diseases. Men of the choleric and melancholic temperaments, which are both characterized by black hair, are well known to have generally sounder and more vigorous constitutions, and to be less susceptible to morbific impressions from external causes than the sanguine. The Negro constitution has some peculiar morbid predispositions, but in many respects is endowed with greater vigour than that of lighter complexion.

Prichard's use of the terms 'choleric' and 'melancholic' remind us that these classifications of temperament derive from the Hippocratic Corpus (fifth to third centuries BC). There the humoral theory was expounded, in which four

413

humours establish an equilibrium in the body, the relative dominance of any one humour defining the corresponding temperament of the individual – excess of blood giving a sanguine temperament, yellow bile a choleric one, black bile a melancholic one, and phlegm a phlegmatic one. (➤ Ch. 14 Humoralism) The tendency to disease of these differing humoral constitutions paralleled the differing temperaments, thus an excess of yellow bile made the individual prone to choleric diseases. In 'Airs, Waters, Places', the Hippocratic writer attributed many medical disorders to the constitution of the body, and this in turn to the quality of the soil, water, air, climate, and mode of life. This predisposing of the individual to specific disorders and diseases by virtue of his or her constitution gave rise to the nineteenth-century concept of 'diathesis', and this was used to refer chiefly not to acute but to chronic conditions which progressively or intermittently affected the individual, such as gout, epilepsy, asthma, tuberculosis, and cancer. The diathesis, once established, tended to be inherited.

Diathesis is not a recent term, but can be traced back to the Hippocratic Corpus. There, and in the writings of Aristotle (384–322 BC) and Galen (AD 129–c.200/210), it is used inconsistently, having a variety of meanings. In the seventeenth and eighteenth centuries, Galen's term 'temperament' (produced by the particular mixing of the four humours) was popular, but early in the nineteenth century the old Greek term diathesis, according to Erwin Ackerknecht, 'acquired a very definite meaning in Paris', 'the new capital of pathological anatomy, localism and solidism!' The *Dictionnaire des sciences médicales* (1812) defined it as: 'that state of the body which makes it acquire certain diseases'. Born of the humoral theory, the concept was expropriated by pathologists in an age of increasing solidism; it offered 'a way out of the etiological dead end into which the abandonment of the humours has led in the field of general diseases'. (➤ Ch. 9 The pathological tradition)

Prichard considered that the differing susceptibilities to diseases could be correlated with external differences: colour of skin and hair. Thomas Laycock (1812–76) was of a similar opinion, but Hutchinson disagreed. He drew a distinction between the 'peculiarities incident to race and family, which, for the most part, entail no morbid proclivity whatever', and 'the various common causes of disease acting, perhaps, through many generations'. Thus, what has been called temperament 'divides itself naturally into these two parts, race and diathesis'. He concluded:

> We shall see that the connection between special diseases and the external configuration of the body is less close than has been assumed, and that the best plan is to study carefully the scope of power of each kind of morbid influence under the varied circumstances which may attend its action.

Hutchinson went on to distinguish between temperament, idiosyncrasy, and diathesis. He did not deny the reality of temperament, 'the original vital endowment of the individual', but he doubted man's ability to discriminate it. He held that temperament and idiosyncrasy were purely hereditary, but that diatheses could be hereditary or acquired. An acquired diathesis, given enough time, would become hereditary. It could also develop into an idiosyncrasy, for this was 'diathesis brought to a point', as when an individual apparently just like those around him 'is poisoned by the smallest quantity of some ordinary drug', or fails to digest an item of diet 'which is daily food to his companions'. Or it could be the virus of some specific fever that 'either produced on him no apparent effect, or may be attended by symptoms of tenfold their usual violence. Sometimes it is an extraordinary immunity which is revealed, and sometimes an almost incredible degree of susceptibility.'[4] This category embraced what we would call food and drug allergies – he mentioned iodide rash and iodide coryza, conjunctival pains following the administration of arsenic, and sensitivity to eggs, fish, coffee, and tea, and 'various forms of alcoholic beverages'.

Diatheses that Hutchinson considered to be of well-nigh universal occurrence he classified according to their causes. As an example of a diathesis caused by climate, he cited malaria due to the emanation from marshy ground, swamps, and jungles; and cretinism due to 'certain telluric conditions, and especially to mountains and valleys'. The most extreme examples of cretinism were produced only when the condition had been transmitted through several generations. The most important of the diatheses produced by diet, said Hutchinson, is gout. Once this disorder is established, he added, it is very difficult to eradicate, 'even after several generations of strict temperance'.

Although gout was the most common affliction, cretinism supplied the most striking example of an allegedly hereditary taint. (➤ Ch. 23 Endocrine diseases) In *The Country Doctor*, Honoré de Balzac (1799–1850) described the surprise and horror with which the cavalry officer chances upon an old cretin:

> At the sight of the deep, circular folds of skin, on the forehead, the sodden, fish-like eyes, and the head, with its short, coarse, scantily-growing hair . . . who would not have experienced . . . an instinctive feeling of repulsion for a being that had neither the physical beauty of an animal nor the mental endowments of a man, who was possessed of neither instinct nor reason, and who had never heard nor spoken any kind of articulate speech.

Here we have the model for both diathesis and degeneration. Some environmental poison produces the disorder, and in the course of several generations it becomes fixed as a hereditary tendency which resists our efforts to remove it. The fear that such tendencies, as they accumulated, would in the long run bring about the extinction of whole nations, was genuinely entertained by those who subscribed to the theory of degeneration.

Clearly, this nineteenth-century theory of diathesis was used to account for a mixed bag of disorders, including many that in the latter part of the century were shown to be due to microbial pathogens. However, we should be wary of simply treating diathesis as 'a cemetery of dead medical concepts' as Ackerknecht suggested. The establishment of the germ theory of disease did not banish talk of diathesis and degeneration. (➤ Ch. 16 Contagion/germ theory/specificity) The evidence of familial tendency to disease and of differing susceptibility of individuals continued to invoke constitutional and hereditary factors. Although authorities like Hutchinson distinguished between transmission from parent to offspring by infection, as in the case of syphilis, and by heredity, as in gout, and despite recognizing Prichard's distinction between congenital and acquired disorders, the conceptions of inherited human diseases of the late nineteenth century differed markedly from those of the twentieth century. The dominant view represents a combination of environmental and hereditarian concepts, environmental because environmental and dietary poisons cause a hereditary 'taint', hereditarian in that the taint is persistent. The advent of the germ theory served to introduce a specific agent which could take over the role of environmental factors such as miasmas, but the hereditary diathesis remained to account for the familial incidence and differing susceptibilities of individuals. (➤ Ch. 15 Environment and miasmata)

THE CONCEPT OF DEGENERATION

We should remember, too, that there was a concept that drew on the theory of hereditary constitution and was pervasive in nineteenth-century culture. This was degeneration. Daniel Pick has demonstrated this in the writings of Conan Doyle, Joseph Conrad, H. G. Wells, Hippolyte Taine, and Emile Zola, and also in the medical, psychiatric, and psychoanalytic literature of the Victorian and Edwardian periods. (➤ Ch. 65 Medicine and literature)

The medical authority who wrote most extensively on degeneration was the French alienist Benedict Augustin Morel (1809–75), whose *Traité des dégénérescences physiques et morales* (1857) sought to demonstrate the process of formation of the morbid varieties in the human species. Morel claimed that the symptoms of insanity were the same the world over. (➤ Ch. 21 Mental diseases) The prognosis of the disease, the expression of the features, even the shapes of the head, were all due to the same 'severe degenerative cause'. But he was not speaking of degeneration in the old sense of the word, where climate causes changes in the species which could return to the original type by interbreeding with the original stock. Morel's degeneration showed a progressive decline in both adaptation and fertility. It was not adaptive, but 'maladive'. Abandoned to itself its reproductive capacity declined, so that its ultimate duration was limited 'like that of all monstrosities'. To the extent that such degenerations had reproductive contact with the same part of the population, however, they constituted the greatest obstacle to the progress of humanity. Formerly, such degenerations were the exclusive lot of the rich and indifferent class, but now, claimed Morel, they were attacking the constitution of the workers and country people to a disturbing extent.

He was confident that the process of degeneration was of the same nature as the development of chronic alcoholism. Using the account by the Swedish physician Magnus Huss (1807–90) in his book *Alcoholismus Chronicus* (1852), Morel described the progressive degeneration: the diminishing strength, the muscular tremble, the painful spasms, the lasciviousness and eroticism yet enfeebled generative powers, and finally the delirium tremens. The children of chronic alcoholics, he claimed, tended to suffer either from congenital idiocy, or to develop it after a number of years. Thus the hereditary constitution of the stock had been damaged by the 'intoxicating principle' – that is, alcohol.

Morel's study of cretinism led him to conclude that, here again, an 'intoxicating principle' was at work, possibly magnesium in the calcareous soils in the high narrow valleys of the Vosges, Alps, and the Savoie, where villages contained families with many affected persons. In this, he agreed with the Archbishop of Chambéry; but these two disagreed over the prognosis of cretinism. Whilst the archbishop recognized that treatment could alleviate the condition, Morel denied the possibility of recovery of the genuine cretin, and seeing this application as an indicator of degeneration, he urged segregation of the affected so as to prevent its spread through parentage to the next generation. Segregation was equally desirous, he felt, for those whose degeneration showed itself in madness. In so far as it resulted from the actions of toxins like alcohol, opium, and tobacco, its increasing incidence was to be expected, for 'pernicious liquor' was being manufactured on a large scale and sold cheaply. Since he believed that degeneration leads ultimately to sterility, it could threaten the future of European nations.

Ian Dowbiggin has argued that Morel and other alienists attributed these examples of degeneration to hereditary taint because they were unable to find any specific organic lesions to which these mental and physical defects could be attributed. They were concerned that psychiatry should not become separated from medicine, and by invoking 'morbid heredity' they were able to offer an organic cause in the absence of evidence from traditional pathology. (➤ Ch. 56 Psychiatry) J. M. Charcot (1825–93) was later to do as much when he distinguished functional from organic neuroses. Nor did Sigmund Freud (1856–1939) fail to stress the importance of heredity as a causal factor in the incidence of hysteria in 1896. Morbid heredity as a cause of degeneration had the advantage, Dowbiggin suggests, that it was 'elastic' enough to accommodate psycho- and neuropathological considerations and thus to make mind–body dualism acceptable. Heredity, as many pictured it, was not due to a set of material particles, but was akin to memory – both organic and psychic.

THE CONCEPT OF HEREDITY

In Morel's concept of degeneration we have a pathological process acting in a unitary manner and producing a wide range of symptoms. Turning to the extensive book by Prosper Lucas (1805–85), *Traité philosophique et physiologique de l'hérédité naturelle* (1847–50), we again find a dynamic conception of heredity. Lucas followed the traditional analogy between heredity and a balance of forces and he set it in a creationist framework that served to relate the 'facts' of creation and of procreation. How could the empirical date of variability be accommodated to the accepted fixity of species? He introduced two primordial laws or principles: the law of *innéité* which governed the individual and represented the activity of invention or imagination, nature creating or improvising; and the law of *hérédité*, which governed the species and represented the activity of imitation or memory.

In the beginning, the force of 'direct creation' formed species of living things by invention or imagination. Since that time, life had continued under a second form of generation – procreation. In this transition from creation to procreation, the law of invention became *innéité*, representing what there was of originality, of imagination, and the liberty of life in the mediate generation of being. The law of imitation became *hérédité*, representing what there was of repetition and of memory of life in procreative generation. But the law of invention had been restricted in procreation so that it affected characteristics non-essential to the species, leaving the specific type unchanged and totally under the influence of the law of imitation. Individual variability within the species was thus due to *innéité*, constance of specific type to *hérédité*.

This summary of Lucas's conceptual scheme illustrates the model of opposing forces and also the influence of mind upon matter, in terms of the two fundamental mental faculties of imagination/invention and imitation/memory. The association of heredity with memory leading to the concept of organic memory was undoubtedly influential in nineteenth-century biology as well as in twentieth-century psychoanalytic theory. For Lucas, it was central to his conception of heredity. Like Morel, Lucas was concerned about the future constitution of European nations; however, rather than attributing all defects to one process of that degeneration, he treated them separately, recording their appearances in successive generations to demonstrate the strength of their hereditary transmission. He believed that variability is necessarily contingent on reproduction, that acquired characters are inherited, including mutilations. He concluded with some eugenic proposals to mitigate the accumulation of hereditary defects that he believed was taking place.

PERFECTIBILITY AND HEREDITARIANISM

The gloom that pervades these nineteenth-century writings on constitution and heredity alerts one to the possibility that it represents a swing of the pendulum, that this pessimism was a reaction to previous over-optimistic claims for the future of people in western Europe. Did not the *encyclopédistes* preach the perfectibility of humans? In a Lockean world where British empiricism ruled, anything could be achieved by social engineering – the enhancement of intelligence by education, of physical constitution by diet and exercise, and the ever-increasing longevity that medical science and public health policies could provide? Had not William Godwin (1751–1836) looked forward to the day when people could expect to live naturally for ever? (➤ Ch. 46 Geriatrics)

It was in opposition to such claims that hereditarian doctrines were fashioned. Although nineteenth-century hereditarianism is usually associated with the views of Francis Galton (1822–1911), he represented the extreme of a spectrum of positions on the relation between nature and nurture for so-called 'hard' to 'soft' heredity. Many authorities who believed in the strength of heredity also believed that acquired characters can, in the course of generations, become strongly inherited. (This is illustrated in Hutchinson's view that an acquired diathesis can become hereditary.) What particularly concerned these hereditarians was the evidence which they believed showed that the many defects produced in humans, allegedly as a result of their urban-industrial mode of existence, become heritable. Thus the surgeon Sir William Lawrence (1783–1867) complained that:

> A superior breed of human beings could only be produced by selections and exclusions similar to those so successfully employed in rearing our more valuable animals. Yet in the human species, where the object is of such consequence, the principle is almost entirely overlooked. Hence all the native deformities of mind and body which spring up so plentifully in our artificial mode of life, are handed down to posterity, and tend, by their multiplication and extension, to degrade the race.[5]

The phrenologists, too, opposed to the claims of the perfectibilists the 'facts' of organic inheritance.[6] They did not deny that acquired characters may be inherited, but they stressed the difficulty of eradicating such characters. This is why there have been many hereditarians and eugenists with Lamarckian leanings. These accepted that injuries are not inherited, yet that constitutions damaged by the effects of pernicious liquors would be inherited, especially if such a life-style were continued over several generations.

The increasing support for hereditarian explanations that we note as the nineteenth century progressed is attributed by Daniel Pick to more than merely professional interests. Political events created political currents favourable to the spread of hereditarianism, and belief in degeneration in particular. Thus in France there was considerable pessimism about the future of democracy following the 1848 revolution. In place of the fond aspirations of the Liberals, Charles de Remusat (1797–1875) remarked that many of the French concluded that modern democracy was simply 'turbulent decadence'. In the 1890s and Edwardian Britain, the terms 'decadence' and 'degeneration' were much used. Royal commissions were set up to report on inebriation, lunacy, physical deterioration, and feeble-mindedness. The turn of the century marked the advent of the 'new Liberalism', which replaced self-help and minimal interference by the state with welfare provision and state planning. Science was increasingly recognized as a resource needed in formulating government policy. This was the reason for the support that the Conservative politician A. J. Balfour (1848–1930) gave to the establishment of the Arthur Balfour Chair of Genetics at Cambridge University in 1912. And was it not Galton's perception of this change in the political climate that encouraged him to deliver his address on eugenics in 1902? If the French felt a mood of pessimism following the 1848 revolution and one of humiliation after the Franco-Prussian war of 1870, the British knew what it was like to have their pride wounded when they fought the Boers in South Africa. The discovery that only one in two of the volunteers from the working class was fit enough to be accepted into the Army served to assure the hereditarians that their worst fears about the extent of the hereditary degeneration of the British nation were justified.

A like transition from liberal to interventionist policies or 'corporatism' took place in Germany. In his account of this phenomenon, Paul Weindling has shown the presence of important parallels between this change in the political sphere and changes in the character of the medical and biological sciences in Germany. The same era that witnessed the erosion of individualistic liberalism saw also the rise of scepticism towards the effectiveness of bacteriological science, and enthusiasm for the hereditarian doctrine of constitutional susceptibility to infectious diseases. (➤ Ch. 10 The immunological tradition) The assumption that such susceptibility was due to tainted heredity – resulting from exposure to 'racial poisons' – had the effect of stimulating initiatives in public hygiene. From the 1890s, many sanatorium and clinics were established in the effort to reduce the incidence of venereal disease and tuberculosis. At the same time, the eugenic movement gained strength. Unlike the British eugenists, however, their German colleagues were especially concerned with the biology of race, and their society – the first eugenic society to be formed – was called the Deutsche Gesellschaft für Rassenhygiene. (➤ Ch. 37 History of medical ethics)

THE NATURE–NURTURE CONTROVERSY

The very term 'inheritance' has Lamarckian undertones. Borrowed from the land-owning aristocracy, it was a metaphor that proved misleading. For did not a testator pass to his descendents what he had acquired as well as what had been bequeathed to him? Perhaps this explains why the French term *hérédité* became popular instead. Although Galton still used the old term in 1889 in his book *Natural Inheritance*, it contained a precise and novel conception of the subject; namely, the study of the statistical relations between the distribution of characters in successive generations. This was a much narrower view of the subject than had been entertained hitherto, for traditionally, inheritance was seen as just one aspect of the grand subject of generation. What had focused Galton's mind in this way was the disagreements over the nature and extent of heredity. This he discussed under the two terms, nature and nurture, possibly following Shakespeare's example. In *The Tempest*, Prospero described Caliban as: 'A devil, a born devil, on whose nature nurture can never stick.' The perfectibilists claimed that human beings had reached a high state of civilization because they were subjected to education and training for that end. Nurture was all-important. Furthermore, some of the effects of such upbringing became subject to heredity and therefore were incorporated into the stock. The perfectibilists thus saw in ameliorative policies and social engineering the route to the enhancement of the human constitution.

The historian H. T. Buckle (1821–62) was sceptical towards claims of heritability. Testily he remarked:

> We often hear of hereditary talents, hereditary vices and hereditary virtues; but whoever will critically examine the evidence will find that we have no proof of their existence. The way in which they are commonly proved is in the highest degree illogical; the usual course being for writers to collect instances of some mental peculiarity found in a parent and in his child, and then to infer that the peculiarity was bequeathed. By this mode of reasoning we might demonstrate any proposition; since in all large fields of inquiry there are a sufficient number of empirical coincidences to make a plausible case in favour of whatever view a man chooses to advocate.[7]

G. H. Lewes (1817–78) objected to Buckle's scepticism. Surely there was no doubt that organization is inherited, and don't 'the tendencies and peculiarities of men depend on their organizations?' he asked.[8] Buckle, suggested

Lewes, had been misled by the evident frequency with which offspring appear not to resemble either parent. But talent does run in families and we do inherit our parents' organizations. Our resemblances to them, however, may be a compounding of the two or a distribution of the organs of the one and of the other.

In his travels in Africa, Galton came to the conclusion that human beings' mental and physical characters are inherited. It was the expectation that the likeness should be between parent and offspring. He revised this view in two ways. First, the relation of inheritance was between *ancestors* and offspring, therefore one should not expect to find a constant direct likeness between parents and offspring. Second, he realized that the student of heredity was dealing with the products of a stochastic process – that is, one governed by chance. In order to demonstrate the presence of a law governing these data, therefore, he would have to use the statistical methods recently introduced by the Belgian Adolph Quetelet (1796–1874). Galton's application of Quetelet's methods to the study of heredity was a significant innovation. He claimed that the result of these efforts was a demonstration that constancy of type was achieved by a process which he first called 'reversion' and later 'regression'. This process pulled back the extremes of a character – for instance, very short and very tall stature – towards the mean of the population. But it was not really a force, it was the 'weight' of all the ancestral contributions. To illustrate the relationship between generations, he pointed to the necklace consisting of a continuous chain and the pendants attached to it. The chain corresponded with the germinal material or the 'stirp' as he called it, and the pendants represented the individuals who were thus only indirectly connected one to the other through the germinal material. This was an anticipation of the concept of August Weismann (1834–1914) of the isolation of the germplasm. It was important in two other respects: it was a particulate theory, in that hereditary transmission was due to the numerous independent material particles in the germinal material; and it was unitary, in that variation (other than 'mere fluctuating variability' attributable to the environment) and also reversion were manifestations of heredity, not of the alleged opposing forces of variation.

In his search for crucial evidence with which to decide the relative importance of nature and nurture, Galton found identical and non-identical twins. He assumed that the cause of the difference between the two groups was that of issuing from the same fertilization (identical, now termed monozygotic twins), and from two different fertilizations (non-identical or dizygotic twins). Camille Dareste (1822–99) had given this explanation only two years before when he reported it to the Société d'Anthropologie in 1874.[9] Although the methodology for making the distinction between these two classes was established by H. W. Seimens (b. 1891) in 1924, the status of twin studies has since been tarnished due to the abuse they have suffered at the hands of the hereditarians anxious to demonstrate the high heritability of intelligence.

CONSANGUINITY

The topic of major concern to students of human heredity in the nineteenth century was the effects of inbreeding or consanguinity. It was canvassed as one of the causes of hereditary degeneration. Marriages between close relatives have long been discouraged and in many countries forbidden. Since the sixth century, the Catholic church has ruled against consanguinity with varing degrees of severity. In the twentieth century, first-cousin marriages require a special dispensation. In the USA, one-third of the states prohibit such marriages. It is common knowledge that marriages between parent and child, brother and sister, niece and uncle, nephew and aunt are also forbidden. Not all such prohibitions have had a rational biological justification, and where such is lacking the result has been a flouting of the law. Thus the statute, dating back to Henry VIII (r. 1509–47), against the marriage of a widower with his deceased wife's sister did not prevent one in thirty-three widowers from marrying their sisters-in-law, a fact that impressed the Royal Commission on Marriage Law in 1848.

Charles Darwin's extensive researches into the mechanisms in the animal and plant kingdoms that hinder or prevent self-fertilization were strongly supportive of the view that 'nature abhors inbreeding'. It was natural to conclude that the act of inbreeding, if continued long enough, led to deterioration and sterility. Animal breeders had long known of the enfeebling effects of continued inbreeding. Thus Sir John Sebright (1767–1846) rejected the claim by Robert Bakewell (1725–95) that inbreeding did not necessarily cause degeneration, and pointed to the poor state of the descendents of Bakewell's Leicester sheep and of his own inbred stocks of spaniels and fancy pigeons. Darwin, always an admirer of the breeders' practical experience, elevated their opinion into a great law of nature, but he noted that:

> Many physiologists attribute the evil exclusively to the combination and consequent increase of morbid tendencies common to both parents: that this is an active source of mischief there can be no doubt. It is unfortunately too notorious that men and various domestic animals endowed with a wretched constitution, and with a strong hereditary disposition to disease, if not actually ill, are fully capable of procreating their kind. Close interbreeding, on the other hand, induces sterility; and this indicates something quite distinct from the augmentation of morbid tendencies common to both parents.[10]

On the other hand, he doubted that the prohibition in so many societies of closely related marriages was due either to the observation of their biological ill-effects or to the recognition of the effects of consanguinity on the descent of property. Therefore it was not possible to cite the widespread prohibitions of consanguineous marriages as decisive evidence that they were injurious. Darwin doubted that the question would ever be answered by direct evidence, for humans 'propagates [their] kind so slowly and cannot be subjected to experiment'.

Added to his long-held interest in the subject of inbreeding and outbreeding, Darwin had a personal interest in the subject of consanguinity, for he had married his own first cousin. When he learnt that the census of 1871 was to be debated in Parliament, he wrote to his friend Sir John Lubbock (1834–1913), asking him to make a case for the inclusion of questions about consanguineous marriages in it. Lubbock obliged, but his request was voted down. Two years later, Darwin's son, George (1845–1912), hit upon an ingenious method for supplying statistics on the subject. By determining the frequency of first-cousin marriages between persons with the same surname in sample populations, he derived from the known frequency of same-name marriages the probable frequency of first-cousin marriages in given classes and in given localities. Not surprisingly, the highest frequency was among the aristocracy, and the lowest in the population of London. The parents of inmates of asylums did not show a significantly higher average of consanguineous marriages than the rest of the population. In the case of the parents of deaf-mutes, he found no difference.[11] During the 1880s and 1890s, Darwin's paper became widely known and may well have been, as Alfred Huth (1850–1919) claimed, a major influence in changing public opinion on the effects of consanguinity. Instead of being regarded as harmful in its own right, the view gained credence that any harm was due solely to the intensification of 'hereditary taint' already present, though not manifest, in the parents. The likelihood that such a taint was present in both parents was clearly greater for first-cousin spouses than for unrelated spouses. The progeny of the former were therefore more likely to show hereditary taint than those of the latter, but it was not inevitable that consanguineous marriages should yield defective offspring. It was also the view of Vilhelm Uckermann (1852–1925), whose magnificent study of deaf-mutism in Norway constitutes possibly the most comprehensive analysis we possess of inbreeding in a large human population. He expressed the theory of intensification in the words: 'L'intensité de l'hérédité croit avec la proximité du sang'; and believed that consanguinity was four times more frequent among the parents of deaf-mutes in Norway than among the parents of hearing children.[12] So striking was this contrast that he reckoned the incidence of deaf-mutism could be used as an index of consanguinity. By studying the local distribution of deaf mutism and consanguinity, he came to the conclusion that these local differences were due to differing degrees of communication in different territories which affected the degree of inbreeding, and he concluded by urging as the most efficacious remedy the improvement of communications.

THE IMPACT OF MENDELISM

In 1900, the paper that Gregor Mendel (1822–84) had published in 1866, describing his study of hybrids of the edible pea, was discovered, and his results replicated by three botanists, Hugo de Vries (1848–1935), Carl Correns (1864–1933), and Erich Tschermak (1871–1962). In the same year, the Cambridge zoologist William Bateson (1861–1926) introduced Mendelism to England. Six years later, Bateson felt confident enough to introduce a term to describe the new discipline that he saw emerging. He chose the word 'genetics', which he defined as: 'The elucidation of the phenomena of heredity and variation: in other words, the physiology of descent, with implied bearing on the theoretical problems of the evolutionist and systematist, and applications to the practical problems of the breeders, whether of animals or plants'.

Although Bateson did not mention humans in this definition, he was soon eager to discover examples of Mendelian inheritance in them. Nor did he have to wait long. In 1902 he learnt of the work by Archibald Garrod (1857–1935) on alkaptonuria. Advised by Bateson, Garrod had looked for and found that three out of the four families he had described in 1901 were first cousin marriages. While the effects of consanguinity, as we have seen, were much discussed in the nineteenth century, it was Mendelism that offered a theoretical explanation. What had been called 'intensification' of heredity in such marriages was attributed by the Mendelians to the association of recessive characters. Garrod agreed with Bateson that the Mendelian theory of the double recessive offered a plausible explanation for the paradox of the rarity of the constitutional diseases he described in the general population and their much higher frequency among the issue of first-cousin marriages.[13]

In 1906, Bateson was invited by the Neurological Society of London to speak on the application of Mendelian heredity to humans. Aided by medical authorities he began the study of pedigrees of disease. The resulting address was modest in its claims: 'Application is rather for the future than for the present. The application of Mendelian rules to mankind has not made the progress that was to have been expected.'[14] His strategy was to cite the recent paper of William Curtis Farabee (1865–1925) on the inheritance of brachydactyly and the report by Edward Nettleship (1845–1913) on presenile cataract, the pedigrees of both of which conformed with the expectation for a dominant Mendelian factor, the normal condition being recessive. He went on to describe the range of examples found in animals and plants that were relevant to human heredity – the inheritance of sterility and resistance to disease in plants, of coat colour and behaviour in mammals (the waltzing mice) – and the complexities introduced by multiple-factor inheritance, sex limitation, and interaction of factors, and changes in the dominant/recessive relationship depending on the sex.

Bateson expanded this account in chapter xii of his well-known *Mendel's Principles of Heredity* (1909). Always thoughtful and critical, he remarked on the discrepancy between the wealth of knowledge of the genetics of 'striking peculiarities which are of the nature of deformity or disease' as compared with the dearth of that of normal characters. Skin colour and stature clearly involved several factors, and hair colour showed some evidence of segregation, while only eye colour was comparatively simple. But there were fresh pedigrees of hereditary disorders, notably Nettleship's study of congenital stationary night-blindness, which included 2,116 individuals covering nine generations stretching back to an ancestor born in 1637.[15] Striking though such cases were of the power of inheritance, not all of them offered the numerical support for the operation of Mendel's laws in humans that Bateson had hoped for. While in the case of brachydactyly the many pairings of an affected parent (heterozygote) with an unaffected one (double recessive) gave 39 affected to 32 normal, thus roughly supporting the Mendelian prediction of a 1:1 ratio, the corresponding numbers for such pairings in the case of night-blindness were 130 and 242. Here, as in the case of some recessive disorders, under-reporting of affected individuals was suspected. In other cases, pedigrees contained an excess of affected individuals. Thus when Bateson added up the cases of albinism in Dr Magnus's ten pedigrees, he found 174 normal to 115 albino, but for this recessive condition he reckoned that the figure should have approached 216:72 or 3:1. The Mendelians could offer explanations for these departures, but their opponents were not impressed. Quite apart from the special limitations which the study of human heredity imposed, there was also the confusion caused by the assumption of these early Mendelians that they could treat the numerical date from random-breeding populations in the same way as they treated the data from a Mendelian experiment. When Bateson's colleague, R. C. Punnett (1875–1967), addressed the Royal Society of Medicine on 'Mendelism in relation to disease', the statistician Udny Yule (1871–1951) tackled him on this point. He explained:

> Assuming that brown or duplex eye colour was dominant over blue, if matings of persons of different eye-colours were random ... it was to be expected that in the population there would be three persons with brown eyes to one with blue; but that was not so. There were more blues than brown. The same applied to the examples of brachydactyly.[16]

All Punnett could reply was that maybe the nation was slowly becoming brown-eyed and brachydactylous. Afterwards, he took the problem to the

Cambridge mathematician G. H. Hardy (1877–1947), who then set out the famous equilibrium principle that bears the names of both him and Wilhelm Weinberg (1862–1937). This states simply that in a random-breeding population, the distribution of normal and affected individuals represents an equilibrium between the two genetic factors concerned, which is dependent on their initial frequencies and remains constant in successive generations, assuming, of course, there is no selective advantage to the one or to the other. This means that such constancy in the distribution is consistent with Mendelian transmission, although the distributions of 3:1 or 1:2:1 are not found in the population as a whole. Even with this important theoretical development, however, the study of human genetics did not make significant advances until the close of the First World War, with the investigation of the distribution of blood groups in the soldiers of the many nations gathered in Europe in 1918.[17] Such massive and striking data offered the empirical basis for reliable interpretation of the growing body of factual information on hereditary transmission in humans.

METHODOLOGY AND THE DEBATE OVER TUBERCULOSIS

Although H. T. Buckle long ago stressed the weakness of pedigrees as evidence for heredity, it was not until the last decade of the nineteenth century that such criticism became a salient feature of the debates on the heritability of characters in humans. Controversy over the aetiology of tuberculosis was central to these debates, for the issue was not simply whether the disease is caused by a germ or by a miasma (environmental poison) but whether it resulted from an inherited constitutional diathesis. Thus William Dale (*fl.* 1891), physician to the West Norfolk and Lynn Hospital, reckoned it would not be long before 'the bacteria phantasm will have ceased to trouble or perplex us, and that the medical man of the future will stand amazed at our exceptional credulity'.[18] He did not deny that the Koch bacillus was present in tuberculous individuals, but he doubted it was the *vera causa* of the disease. Instead, he classified consumption among the constitutional and non-infectious diseases. 'Damp, dark, and crowded rooms, with insanitary surroundings', he decided, were a potent factor in developing the predisposition. Such peculiarities of constitution, he continued, were 'certain latent conditions in the human frame which are inherited, and which render it liable to special and peculiar diseases'. It was not that the diseases themselves were transmitted. Whereas tuberculin had proved unsatisfactory, and sometimes fatal, treatment that strengthened and altered the system had, according to this constitutive theory, the hope of 'extinguishing, or at least modifying its morbid tendencies'.

In Germany, Alexander Riffel (1832–1922) also argued against the Koch theory and in favour of a hereditary diathesis. The familial incidence and varied susceptibility strongly supported such a view. Instead of studying isolated pedigrees, or experimenting with animals – those investigations he conducted did not confirm the claims for the infectious nature of consumption – he studied whole populations. He took the stable populations of small communities and recorded the disease incidence of all the families. The result, he claimed, did not support Koch's theory, but did support his theory of hereditary predisposition.[19] (➤ Ch. 71 Demography and medicine)

Riffel's work was soon strongly criticized, but together with the similar studies of Otto Ammon (fl. 1890) it stimulated Wilhelm Weinberg to look closely at the incidence of diseases in families. He approved of the acceptance by Ottokar Lorenz (1832–1904) of August Weismann's views of heredity, and Lorenz's criticism of the use of pedigrees, but he did not accept this famous genealogist's advocacy of genealogies.[20] After cataloguing the many pitfalls in collecting the data of heredity in humans, Weinberg discussed Riffel's study of whole populations. This involved the pursuit of data from previous generations by the use of local registers. Riffel took such searches from one family into many others, and finished up over-recording the data, an error which his bacteriological critics treated with severity. Weinberg realized that the subject of human genetics had stood still because of these numerous errors, which, he explained, were all 'situated in the domain of method'.

Weinberg therefore searched for a characteristic, claimed to be inherited, for which there would be good records, and which was not subject to selection in the choice of mates. He found it in twinning. Further, he realized that non-identical twin-bearing, if a heritable characteristic, would be due only to the mother. At this juncture (1905), he heard a lecture by Heinrich Ernst Ziegler (1858–1925) in which Mendel's theory was described and an attempt made to relate it to the facts of gamete formation and fertilization.[21] Impressed by this, Weinberg responded positively when it was suggested that he should look for evidence that this twinning showed a Mendelian form of inheritance. As Weinberg recalled:

> it would have been very difficult to collect a sufficient number of cases in which children of mothers of twins had married each other and then determine the frequency of twin births among their children [which conforms to a Mendelian experiment]. I have therefore tried to construct a formula for the frequency of dominant and recessive traits among the mothers, daughters, and sibs of persons affected with such traits of the same character under the assumption that absolute panmixis is present.[22]

The result was the famous Weinberg equilibrium formula:

$$m^2AA + 2mnAB + n^2BB$$

where A is the frequency of the dominant factor and B that of the recessive. [The modern notation is: $p^2 + 2pq + q^2$.] Weinberg's paper of 1908 was the most trenchant critique of the study of inheritance in humans and at the same time the most creative and positive contribution to the subject in the opening decade of Mendelian genetics.

To overcome the problems in data collection that Weinberg had exposed in the case of the study of the inheritance of diseases was very difficult. Whilst bacteriological and veterinary research established Koch's theory, debate over the inheritance of differing susceptibilities to tuberculosis persisted. In his authoritative *Handbook of Geographical and Historical Pathology* (1886), August Hirsch (1817–94) had declared 'that the severest sceptic can hardly venture to deny an hereditary element in the case'.[23] But attempts to establish this claim have continued to the present day. In 1990 the *New England Journal of Medicine* carried a paper on the greater incidence of tuberculosis among blacks than among whites in racially integrated nursing-homes in Arkansas, and attributed it to racial differences in infectibility.[24] This prompted a lively correspondence, which shows that there is not yet a consensus among experts on the subject.

The history of the relation has been marked by two opposing tendencies. On the one hand, many allegedly hereditary diatheses have been exposed as externally induced diseases, and on the other, many disorders assumed not to have any genetic basis are now claimed to have one. Admittedly, the concept of diathesis implicates external factors as well as internal ones, but the emphasis that was placed by many authorities on the latter suggests that the culture of late nineteenth-century Europe favoured hereditary explanations. Both hereditarian and evolutionary theory had an impact in many areas outside academic zoology and botany. Thus the literature of the period contains many examples of characters who suffer from 'hereditary taint'. Or consider the use made of the notion of atavism by Cesare Lombroso (1835–1909) in his study of criminals, and in the account by John L. H. Down (1828–1909) of a group of feeble-minded children whom he called 'mongol' because he believed they resembled the Mongolian race in their external features. Atavism, or the reversion to ancestral/primitive types, was considered the cause of many congenital abnormalities which have since been attributed either to gene mutations or to chromosomal abnormalities. Down suggested that the initiating event in the production of a mongol child might be tuberculosis in the parents. This 'is able to break down the barrier ... of racial differences' and thus to reveal the common origin of the different human races.[25] A review of 1958 cited some forty theories that had been advanced to account for Down's syndrome, but in 1959 the presence of an extra chromosome discovered in the cells from affected children,[26] which was soon confirmed by other research, suggested that the syndrome was caused by developmental errors arising from defects in the nucleus, due possibly to the advanced age of the mothers at the births of these children.

THE IMPACT OF MOLECULAR GENETICS

Many of the early geneticists, including Wilhelm Johannsen (1857–1927) author of the term 'gene' for the Mendelian 'factors', did not want to discuss its material basis. Even T. H. Morgan (1866–1945), who with his colleagues at Columbia University, New York, provided the evidence for associating genes with the thread-like chromosomes found in the nuclei of cells, urged that 'it does not make the slightest difference whether the gene is a hypothetical unit, or . . . a material particle. In either case the unit is associated with a specific chromosome, and can be localized there by purely genetic analysis.'[27] Working with the fruit fly, *Drosophila*, the Columbia group succeeded in 'mapping' genes on the four pairs of chromosomes, using as their yardstick the extent to which characters were 'linked' to one another in hereditary transmission. Further progress was made in the detailing of these maps following T. S. Painter's (1889–1969) realization in 1933 that the serial order of the genes established by linkage studies could be correlated with the succession of bands on the 'giant chromosomes' observable in insect salivary glands. Moreover, their 'annulated structure', as he described these bands, could be used to identify any rearrangements of chromosome segments that occurred.

The task of mapping the genes in humans proved much more difficult. Indeed, there was a lengthy controversy over the number of chromosomes present in human beings and over the nature of sex determination. In insects, sex was found to be determined by the chromosomes in more than one way: two different sex chromosomes (X and Y) for males and two the same for females (X and X), or the reverse. Or the difference was produced by the presence or absence of one sex chromosome (X). For four decades, the number of chromosomes in human beings was widely believed to be 48, but Joe Tjio and Albert Levan (b. 1905) could only find 46 when they used a new technique in 1956. Although they described this result as 'very unexpected', they found it 'hard to avoid the conclusion that' the diploid number (2n) was 46.[28] This discovery, once accepted, clarified the subject. Both sexes have 46 chromosomes (not 48 in the female and 47 in the male) and males have the X and Y chromosomes and females the two X chromosomes. Armed with the new techniques of preparing chromosomes and growing human cells in tissue culture to provide them, the chromosomal basis of several conditions was revealed in 1959. (➤ Ch. 11 Clinical research) We have already mentioned

Down's syndrome (see p. 429). In the same year two intersexes, Klinefelter and Turner syndromes, were shown to possess abnormal complements of sex chromosomes, the former being XXY and the latter XO.[29] Here was suggestive evidence that failures in the equal distribution of chromosomes to daughter cells (non-disjunction) could cause abnormal development.

Admittedly, progress in the mapping of human genes was slow. The association of heritable characters with one sex provided a starting-point. The discovery in 1919 of racial differences in the frequency of the blood groups A, B, and O provided a second very useful set of markers that was pursued especially by British geneticists in the inter-war years. A third marker was provided by the histocompatability genes, which control the power of the individual to 'recognize' and reject foreign cells. Nor should we forget the clues provided by major chromosome rearrangements: deletions, insertions, and inversions. Yet in spite of all these clues, success was virtually limited to the location of dominant genes and those recessive genes that reside on the X chromosome. This situation was changed when the new recombinant DNA technology was introduced. This was the fruit of the molecular approach in genetics. Until the late 1940s, there was a broad consensus that genes are made of protein, or at least that the 'codescript' of the gene is protein. By 1950, however, the other constituent of chromosomes – nucleic acid – became a candidate for this role, rather than being merely a supportive structure for the genes. The publication of a highly suggestive model of the nucleic acid of the chromosomes – deoxyribonucleic acid (DNA) – by James D. Watson (b. 1928) and Francis Crick (b. 1917) in 1953 served greatly to strengthen its candidacy.[30] The model consisted of two long chains of units called the 'bases': adenine (A), thymine (T), guanine (G), and cytosine (C). The bases on one chain were paired with the bases on the other, A with T and G with C. These pairing rules have proved to be the secret behind the fidelity with which the genes duplicate and express their 'information', and they underlie the success of recombinant DNA technology.

Within a decade, the molecular biology of DNA and its relation to the proteins had become a very fashionable field of research, the crowning achievement of which was the unravelling of the genetic code and of the sequences of amino acids that make up the large and complex protein molecules that are the products of the genes. It became possible to describe the structure and action of the gene in molecular terms: the arrangement of the bases on the chains of DNA contains the information in the gene; three neighbouring bases constitute a 'codon' that 'spells' a particular amino acid in the protein specified by the gene.

On the basis of the conception of the gene as a genetic code and the gene product as a protein with a specific sequence of amino acids, one could predict that changes in the bases of DNA could cause mutations because they could lead to the specification of amino acids differing from those normally present in the protein gene product. In 1956, this was dramatically shown in the case of sickle-cell anaemia, when Vernon Ingram (b. 1924) identified one amino acid substitution in the haemoglobin of those suffering from this debilitating disease.[31] Some years later, when the gene involved had been sequenced, the base change producing this disease was identified. Because of the intense interest in haemoglobin pathologies, the molecular genetics of the haemoglobins has often led the way, as in this case. If these sequences could be discovered, it might become possible to make genes. Whilst the sequencing of proteins became a routine task, methods for sequencing the DNA in chromosomes did not become available until 1975, and even then the task remained difficult. During the 1970s, however, recombinant DNA technology came dramatically into existence to revolutionize genetics and to open up the possibility of sequencing the DNA of all the chromosomes of human beings. Thus has arisen the human genome project, a massive, long-term programme to sequence the three billion base pairs of human beings' DNA.

The task of identifying the genes responsible for congenital defects and for susceptibility to cancers and infectious diseases could not wait until this programme would be completed. (➤ Ch. 25 Cancer) The new technology could help here by finding markers other than the blood group and histocompatibility genes. Candidates for such markers should be present in all individuals and show variations from one individual to another. Here, the idea arose to use some of those stretches of DNA that did not appear to code for any structural or regulatory genes. In these regions, scattered along all the chromosomes there were slight variations – a different base here or there – in different individuals. Such differences would allow the tracing of paternal and maternal DNA through their descendants. The suggestion to use these regions of DNA as markers was published in 1980 and the term restriction fragment length polymorphism (RFLP), was coined to describe them.[32] The techniques of recombinant DNA science needed to identify these markers had been developed over the previous decade, so there was no delay in the response to the RFLP paper. The progress made since that time has been remarkable. The genes for Duchenne muscular dystrophy, Huntington's chorea, retinoblastoma, cystic fibrosis, polycystic kidney disease, myotonic dystrophy, and Wilson's disease have been identified and sequenced. Now it is possible to use 'reverse genetics': that is, starting with the DNA sequence to predict the constitution and properties of the protein gene product. In this way, information has been obtained concerning the mechanism of diseases like cystic fibrosis, hitherto shrouded in mystery. In the case of Duchenne muscular dystrophy, dystrophin, the protein encoded by the normal gene, was found to be absent from affected persons. Its function in the contractile process of muscle tissue is being investigated.

One result of the identification of these genes has been the production of 'probes', which can detect the presence of the genes in the offspring of affected persons and carriers. Not surprisingly, the new power that these tools affords the medical and legal professions has excited concern. (➤ Ch. 69 Medicine and the law) A.G. Motulsky (b. 1923) responded to critics who claimed that molecular geneticists were playing God:

> But what is meant by playing God? Is not out increasing control of the environment and human destiny playing God? Is not curative and preventative medicine playing God? Is not the cleaning up of the unhealthy environment that caused a large proportion of infants to die of diarrhoea playing God?[33]

CONCLUSION

The notion of the hereditary diathesis has been transformed rather than buried. True, the unitary notion of constitution has been replaced by that of discrete elements – extra chromosomes, chromosome translocations, and mutated genes – which have specific effects on development as in Down's syndrome, cause biochemical abnormalities as in the 'inborn errors of metabolism' studied by Garrod, and affect susceptibility to disease as in sickle-cell anaemia. But the fundamental idea of different susceptibilities to external pathogenic agents, be they physical or chemical, bacterial or viral, has survived. (➤ Ch. 8 The biochemical tradition)

We have also seen that controversy over the heritability or non-heritability of a whole range of disorders was already in play in the nineteenth century, as was the vexed question of the effects of inbreeding. Here, it was concluded that the process of inbreeding did not *itself* cause degeneration and weaken the hereditary constitution. The introduction of Mendelian heredity sharpened the debate by introducing fresh criteria for the acceptance of a condition as heritable, but the unacceptability of experimentation on humans made progress more dependent on the theoretical development of population genetics than on experimental genetics. Here, the Hardy-Weinberg equilibrium law, which arose out of the debate over the heritability of chronic diseases was of central importance. Histories of human genetics have tended to neglect this point and instead to concentrate upon the role of evolutionary concerns. Consideration of the history of constitutional diseases is thus timely.

The problem of finding markers with which to map human genes has been an important factor in determining the progress of human genetics. The very recent history demonstrates this point by showing what could be achieved in a short time once the RFLP technique was introduced. Clearly, historians would do well to promote the preservation of documents from this dramatic period in the history of human genetics. Not only have the achievements of the 1980s revealed the power of recombinant DNA technology, they have also provided empirical support for some of the old ideas, albeit now rendered precise and free from Lamarckian assumptions. Thus a predisposition to suffer from cancer, and the existence of conditions that can be both acquired and hereditary, as in retinoblastoma, can be understood in terms of molecular genetics. Finally, the recent developments hold out the possibility of tackling the hereditary factors allegedly involved in the incidence of common diseases. At the beginning of this century, it was the inability of Mendelism to deal with such diseases that disposed many in the medical professions to view this new doctrine with considerable scepticism. How the subject has been transformed! The control and manipulation of the hereditary constitution of humans often seems close at hand. Gene therapy has made its entry into medical practice; the subject that once found no place in medical education can today make claims for its potential to transform treatment. The power this could give to those in charge of our health has caused public concern, however, as expressed in 1986 in the form of an anti-genetic 'Counter Congress', which was held in Berlin during and alongside the Seventh International Congress of Human Genetics.[34] (➤ Ch. 68 Medical technologies: social contexts and consequences)

NOTES

1   Charles Darwin, *The Variation of Animals and Plants under Domestication*, 2 vols, London, John Murray, 1868, Vol. II, pp. 7–8.

2   Jonathan Hutchinson, *The Pedigree of Disease*, London, 1884, p. 3.

3   J. C. Prichard, *Researches into the Physical History of Mankind*, 3rd edn, 5 vols, London, 1836–47, Vol. I, p. 366.

4   Hutchinson, op. cit. (n. 2), p. 26.

5   William Lawrence, *Lectures on Physiology, Zoology, and the Natural History of Man*, London, 1819, p. 459.

6   V. L. Hilts, 'Obeying the laws of hereditary descent: phrenological views on inheritance and eugenics', *Journal of the History of the Behavioural Sciences*, 1982, 18: 62–77.

7   H. T. Buckle, *History of Civilization in England*, London, Routledge, 1857, Vol. I, p. 162 n. 12; this passage is reprinted in R. C. Olby, *Origins of Mendelism*, 2nd edn, Chicago, IL, Chicago University Press, 1985, pp. 168–70.

8   G. H. Lewes, *The Physiology of Common Life*, Edinburgh, 1859–60, Vol. I, p. 382. reprinted in Olby, op. cit. (n. 7), pp. 170–4.

9   Camille Dareste, 'Mémoire sur l'origine et le mode de formation des monstres doubles', *Archives zoologiques expérimentales*, 1874, 3: 73–118.

10   Darwin, op. cit. (n. 1), p. 116.

11   G. H. Darwin, 'Marriages between first cousins and their effects', *Journal of the Statistical Society*, 1875, 38: 172.

12 V. K. Uchermann, *Les Sourds-muets en Norvège. La Sourd-muetité, sa distribution, ses causes, ses symptôms, son rapport avec les unions consanguines, conditions sociales des sourds-muets avec remarques sur la diagnose, la prophylaxie et le traitement de la sourd-muetité*, Christiania, 1901, p. 111.

13 A. E. Garrod, 'The incidence of alkaptonuria: a study in chemical individuality', *Lancet*, 1902, 2: 1618; reprinted in S. H. Boyer IV (ed.), *Papers on Human Genetics*, Englewood Cliffs, NJ, Prentice-Hall, 1966, pp. 88–9. See also Garrod, *Inborn Errors of Metabolism*, London, 1909; reprinted in H. Harris (ed.), *Garrod's Inborn Errors of Metabolism*, London, 1963. For Garrod's discussion of diathesis see Garrod, *The Inborn Factors of Disease. An Essay*. Oxford, Clarendon Press, 1931.

14 William Bateson, 'An address on Mendelian heredity and its application to man', *Brain*, 1906, 2: 157; reprinted in Beatrice Bateson, *William Bateson, F.R.S. Naturalist. His Essays and Addresses together with a Short Account of His Life*, Cambridge, Cambridge University Press, 1928, pp. 181–200.

15 E. Nettleship, 'A history of congenital stationary night-blindness in nine consecutive generations', *Transactions of the Ophthalmic Society of the United Kingdom*, 1907, 27: 269–93.

16 G. U. Yule, 'Contribution', *Proceedings of the Royal Society of Medicine*, Epidemiological Section, 1908, 1: 165. This follows the paper by R. C. Punnett, 'Mendelism in relation to disease', ibid, pp. 135–61.

17 L. and H. Hirschfeld, 'Serological differences between the blood of different races', *Lancet*, 1919, 2: 675–9; reprinted in Boyer, op. cit. (n. 13), pp. 32–43.

18 W. Dale, *Inherited Consumption and its Remedial Management*, London, 1891, p. 28.

19 A. Riffel, *Die Erblichkeit der Schwindsucht und tuberkulösen Prozesse, nachgewiesen durch zahlreiches statistisches Material und die praktische Erfahrung*, Karlsruhe, 1891, p. v.

20 Ottokar Lorenz, *Lehrbuch der gesammten wissenschaftlichen Genealogie. Stammbaum und Ahnentafel in ihrer geschichtlichen, sociologischen und naturwissenschaftlichen Bedeutung*, Berlin, Verlag von Wilhelm Herz, 1898.

21 H. E. Ziegler, 'Ueber den derzeitigen Stand der Vererbungslehre in der Biologie', *Verhandlungen des Kongresses für innere Medizin*, 22nd Kongress, Wiesbaden, 12–15 April 1905, pp. 29–53. This address was expanded in Ziegler's *Die Vererbungslehre in der Biologie*, Jena, Gustav Fischer, 1905, p. 74; and into a full-length book: *Die Vererbungslehre in der Biologie und in der Soziologie*, Jena, Gustav Fischer, 1918, pp. 647.

22 Wilhelm Weinberg, 'Ueber den Nachweis der Vererbung beim Menschen', *Jahreshefte des Vereins für vaterlandische Naturkunde in Württemberg*, Stuttgart, 1908, 64: 368–82; trans. in Boyer, op. cit. (n. 13), p. 9. For Weinberg's study of the inheritance of tuberculosis, see his *Die Kinder der Tuberkulosen*, Leipzig, 1913.

23 A. Hirsch, *Handbook of Geographical and Historical Pathology*, 3 vols, London, New Sydenham Society, 1884–6, Vol. III, p. 228 on phthisis; Vol. II, pp. 635–6 on scrofula.

24 W. W. Stead *et al.*, 'Racial differences in susceptibility to infection by *Mycobacterium tuberculosis*', *New England Journal of Medicine*, 1990, 322: 422–7.

25 J. L. H. Down, 'Observations of an ethnic classification of idiots', *Clinical Lectures*

and Reports of the London Hospitals, 1866, 3: 25; cited in Josef Warkany, *Congenital Malformations, Notes and Comments*, Chicago, IL, 1971, p. 312. See also Lilian Zihni, 'The history of the relationship between the concept and treatment of people with Down's syndrome in Britain and America from 1866 to 1967', unpublished Ph.D. thesis, University of London, 1989.

26 Paul Weindling, *Health, Race, and German Politics between National Unification and Nazism, 1870–1945*, Cambridge and New York, Cambridge University Press, 1989.

27 T. H. Morgan, 'The relation of genetics to physiology and medicine', *Nobel Lectures, Physiology and Medicine 1922–1941*, Amsterdam, Elsevier, 1965, pp. 313–28, see p. 315.

28 J. H. Tjio and A. Levan, 'The chromosome number of man,' *Hereditas*, 1956, 42: 1–6; reprinted in Boyer, op. cit. (n. 13), pp. 232–8, see p. 237. See also M. J. Kottler, 'From 48 to 46: cytological technique, preconception, and the counting of human chromosomes', *Bulletin of the History of Medicine*, 1974, 48: 467–71.

29 P. A. Jacobs and J. A. Strong, 'A case of human intersexuality having a possible XXY sex-determining mechanism', *Nature*, 1959, 183: 302–3. See also D. J. Kevles, *In the Name of Eugenics. Genetics and the Uses of Human Heredity*, Berkeley and Los Angeles, University of California Press, 1985, ch. 16.

30 J. D. Watson and F. H. C. Crick, 'Molecular structure of nucleic acids. A structure for deoxyribose nucleic acid', *Nature*, 1953, 171: 737–8; and 'Genetical implications of the structure of deoxyribonucleic acid', *Nature*, 1953, 171: 64–7.

31 V. M. Ingram, 'A specific chemical difference between the globins of normal human and sickle-cell anaemia haemoglobin', *Nature*, 1956, 178: 792–4.

32 D. Botstein, R. L. White, M. Skolnick and R. W. Davis, 'Construction of a genetic linkage map in man using restriction fragment polymorphisms', *American Journal of Human Genetics*, 1980, 32: 314–31. See also J. E. Bishop and M. Waldholz, *Genome*, New York, Simon & Schuster, 1990, ch. 2.

33 A. G. Motulsky, 'Presidential address. Human and medical genetics: past, present, and future', *Proceedings of the 7th International Congress of Human Genetics*, (Berlin, 1986) Berlin, etc., 1987, pp. 3–13, see p. 13.

34 Ibid., 'Foreword', p. 5. See also F. Vogel, 'Human genetics and the responsibility of the medical doctor', ibid., pp. 44–53.

FURTHER READING

Ackerknecht, Erwin H., 'Diathesis: the word and the concept in medical history', *Bulletin of the History of Medicine*, 1982, 56: 317–25.
Bauer, Julius, *Constitution and Disease*, 2nd edn, New York, Grune & Stratton, 1947.
Bynum, W. F., 'Darwin and the doctors: evolution, diathesis, and germs in nineteenth century Britain', *Gesnerus*, 1983, 40: 43–53.
Ciocco, Antonio, 'The historical background of the modern study of constitution', *Bulletin of the Institute of the History of Medicine*, 1936, 4: 23–38.
Dowbiggin, Ian, 'Degeneration and hereditarianism in French mental medicine, 1840–90: psychiatric theory as ideological adaptation', in W. F. Bynum, Roy Porter and Michael Shepherd (eds), *The Anatomy of Madness, Essays in the History of Psychiatry*, Vol. I: *People and Ideas*, London, Tavistock, 1985, pp. 188–232.

López-Beltrán, Carlos, 'Human heredity 1750–1870; the construction of a domain', unpublished Ph.D. thesis, King's College, London, 1992.

Olby, Robert, 'The emergence of genetics', in Olby, G. N. Cantor, M. J. S. Hodge and J. R. R. Christie (eds), *Companion to the History of Modern Science*, London and New York, Routledge, 1990, pp. 521–36.

Pearl, Raymond, *Constitution and Health*, London, Kegan Paul, Trench, Trubner, 1933.

Pick, Daniel, *Faces of Degeneration. A European Disorder, c.1848-c.1918*, Cambridge, Cambridge University Press, 1989.

Stern, Curt, 'Wilhelm Weinberg 1862–1937', *Genetics*, 1962, 47: 1–5. Also see Stern, 'Wilhelm Weinberg', in C. C. Gillispie (ed.), *Dictionary of Scientific Biography*, New York, Charles Scribner's Sons, 1976, Vol. XIV, pp. 230–1.

Temkin, Owsei, *The Double Face of Janus and Other Essays in the History of Medicine*, Baltimore, MD, and London, Johns Hopkins University Press, 1977.

Weindling, Paul, *Health, Race, and German Politics between National Unification and Nazism, 1870–1945*, Cambridge and New York, Cambridge University Press, 1989.

Wills, Christopher, *Exons, Introns, and Talking Genes*, New York, Basic Books, 1991.

21

MENTAL DISEASES

Theodore M. Brown

From Hippocratic times to the present, the dominant pattern of aetiological thinking in Western medicine has been somatic or biological-reductionist. In antiquity, humours, anatomical configurations, and the state of the vessels and pores were most commonly introduced to explain clinical phenomena, and in more recent times, microstructural defects, sub-visible invading organisms, and biochemical abnormalities have been typically relied on. But while the specific biological and chemical terms have changed dramatically over time, the prevailing explanatory strategy in Western medicine has remained remarkably consistent through the centuries. When confronting the phenomena of disease – whether somatic, psychiatric, or mixed – physicians have regularly appealed to materialist and reductionist explanations in accounting for their clinical observations. (➤ Ch. 2 What is specific to Western medicine?)

But another, less obvious theme also runs through the history of Western medical thought. This is the recurrent secondary appeal to mental, that is, non-material, psychological and socio-environmental, factors: 'soul', 'mind', 'grief', 'passions', 'unconscious wish', 'stress', 'life change events', and the like. Indeed, often running just beneath the surface dominated by biological-reductionism has been an undercurrent of alternative or supplementary explanation formulated in rather different terms. The specifics here have also varied considerably over time, but two features are notable when tracing this history. First, the popularity of non-reductionist alternatives has waxed and waned, being more acceptable in certain historical periods than in others; and, second, these alternatives never fully replaced and only occasionally substantially displaced biological theories. It is this long stream of 'mental' explanatory endeavour in Western medical thought that is the focus of this chapter, which is offered as a supplement to the various accounts of biological reductionism contained elsewhere in this *Encyclopedia* (➤ Ch. 12 Concepts of health, illness, and disease; Ch. 13 Ideas of life and death)

Mental or psychological aetiologies have been introduced most frequently in three principal areas of medical thought:

1 in the explanation of aberrant behaviours and bizarre cognitive processes now typically labelled 'psychotic' or 'severely neurotic';
2 in accounting for disorders in which a mix of psychological peculiarities and somatic symptoms regularly occur, the latter frequently being interpreted as expressions of and/or substitutions for the former;
3 in understanding the ways in which upsetting life events and deeply felt emotions either exacerbate already existing somatic disease or help precipitate previously inapparent physical disorders.

In each of these areas, non-material and socio-psychological explanations have had a long, complex, and frequently shifting history.

PSYCHOTIC AND SEVERELY NEUROTIC BEHAVIOURS

Psychotic and severely neurotic behaviours were often noted in classical Greek antiquity, at the very start of the Western medical tradition. The most common labels for these conditions in the Hippocratic Corpus (fifth to third centuries BC) were 'mania' and 'melancholia', the former characterized by excitement, the latter by depression, and both marked by delusional thinking or intense anxiety and peculiar behaviour. Both conditions were understood biologically, usually in terms of black bile, sometimes in interaction with the brain. In the treatise, the 'Sacred Disease' (primarily focused on epilepsy), the Hippocratic author explained that 'those maddened through bile are noisy, evil-doers and restless, always doing something inopportune. . . . But if terrors and fears attack, they are due to a change in the brain.'[1] (➤ Ch. 14 Humoralism)

Even in the unmistakably biological-reductionist Hippocratic Corpus, however, certain mentalistic aetiological elements show through.[2] In one case, a woman began to exhibit fears, depression, incoherent rambling speech, and the uttering of obscenities after suffering from 'a grief with a reason for it'; and another 'without speaking a word . . . would fumble, pluck, scratch, pick hairs, weep and then laugh, but . . . not speak', also 'after a grief'.[3] A case that reads like delusional melancholia, arising from bile collecting in the liver and settling in the head, is also said to be an instance of a disease that 'usually attacks abroad, if a person is travelling a lonely road somewhere, and fear seizes him'.[4] In the 'Sacred Disease', even epilepsy – the paradig-

439

matic example of naturalistic, biological disease in the Corpus – is said in certain circumstances to be 'caused by fear of the mysterious'.[5]

Mental factors continued to play a minor role in the subsequent development of medical thought in later Greek and Roman antiquity. Authors frequently discussed mania and melancholia and, indeed, contributed significant new insights to symptomatic patterns and therapeutic options. With regard to aetiology these authors, most notably Galen (AD 129-c.200/210), continued to rely primarily on biological-reductionism, although a few, Rufus of Ephesus (AD c.98–117), Aretaeus of Cappadocia (AD c.81-c.138), and especially Soranus of Ephesus (AD 98–138), did manage to keep a non-materialist and socio-environmental approach alive.[6]

Soranus devoted a chapter each to mania and melancholia in his treatise on *Chronic Diseases*, preserved in Latin translation by Caelius Aurelianus (*fl.* fifth century AD). He described symptoms in sensitive detail and discussed aetiology with psychological insight. Included among the causes of mania were 'continual sleeplessness, excesses of venery, anger, grief, anxiety, or superstitious fear, a shock or blow, intense straining of the senses and the mind in study, business, or other ambitious pursuits'.[7]

Despite Soranus's efforts, in the long medieval period from Greek antiquity to the European Renaissance the dominant aetiological style remained the biological-reductionist one incorporated in Galen's works and then codified in the treatises of the Arabic and Latin writers who followed him. Not all medieval writers blended the ancient explanatory components in quite the same proportions, however. Paul of Aegina (AD c.625–90), Avicenna (AD 980–1037), and Bernard of Gordon (*fl.* 1305) seem to have been among the most biological-reductionist, whereas Ishaq ibn Imran (*fl.* 900), Constantinus Africanus (c. 1020–87), and Bartholomaeus Anglicus (*fl.* 1260) were among the most mental. Ishaq, in fact, is said to have brought 'psychical factors into a position of unusual prominence'.[8] Nevertheless, during Middle Ages the biological orientation remained ascendant.

The psychiatric literature of the Renaissance and early modern periods continued to rely not only on ancient nosological categories, but on classical aetiological presumptions. As in the medieval period, individual authors varied in their selection and blend of inherited elements and in the relative weight they assigned to biological versus psychological factors. Felix Platter (1536–1614), André du Laurens (c.1560–1609), and Richard Napier (1559–1634) all included both biological and socio-environmental causal factors in their textbooks and case records, but each combined them in somewhat different proportions.[9] Probably the most comprehensive writer in this period was Robert Burton (1557–1640), whose *The Anatomy of Melancholy* (1621) included the following possible causes of melancholy (in addition to the classic distemperature of the spleen, brain, bile, and blood): 'idleness, solitariness, overmuch study, passions, perturbations, discontents, cares, miseries, vehement desires, ambitions, etc.'[10]

Psychiatric discussion first began to shift from reworked classical formulations during the second half of the seventeenth and first half of the eighteenth centuries. Leading medical writers like Thomas Sydenham (1624–89), Thomas Willis (1621–75), Friedrich Hoffmann (1660–1742), Hermann Boerhaave (1668–1738), and Richard Mead (1673–1754) abandoned ancient humoural explanations for iatrochemical, iatromechanical and neurocentric alternatives. But what also characterized this period was the continued adherence to long-familiar aetiological and therapeutic relationships, even as theoretical concepts changed to ostensibly more 'modern' ones.[11] Thus Boerhaave, after explaining that melancholy resulted from the 'dissipation' (evaporation) of the most mobile parts of the blood and the thickening of the 'black, fat and earthy' residue, listed a familiar mix of biological and non-biological factors leading to dissipation. Psychological and socio-environmental factors included the conventional list: violent exercise of the mind, joy or sorrow, frightful accidents, love, solitude, and fear.[12]

The psychiatric literature of the later eighteenth century was sharply different from that of all preceding periods. Works devoted to madness multiplied, lengthened, specialized, and occasionally softened in tone.[13] In Great Britain, France, Germany, and other European countries, as well as in the United States, essays, monographs, and multi-volume treatises chronicled, catalogued, analysed and attempted to comprehend varieties of insanity, in unprecedented detail and often in rather new ways.[14] In general, these works departed from long-standing neo-classical formulations and tried out a variety of new somatic approaches, often based on some 'doctrine of the nerves'. They also frequently tried to incorporate new 'psychological' theories made popular by John Locke (1632–1704), Etienne Bonnot de Condillac (1715–80), David Hartley (1705–57), and other 'association' theorists.[15]

Most original was the reformulation of insanity by William Cullen (1710–90), who defined it ('vesania') as a type of dynamic nervous disorder (generically 'neurosis', according to Cullen).[16] Symptomatologically, insanity was an 'unusual and commonly hurried association of ideas' leading to 'false judgment' and producing 'disproportionate emotions'. Aetiologically, it arose in the 'common origin of the nerves ... the Brain' and occurred neurophysiologically when there was 'some inequality in the excitement of the brain', for when this happened, 'recollection cannot properly take place, while at the same time other parts of the brain, more excited and excitable, may give false perceptions, associations, and judgments'.[17]

This formulation allowed Cullen to assert that though insanity was clearly grounded in the malfunctioning of the brain, its specific cerebral traces could not always be discovered anatomically. For it had never been possible to 'perceive that any particular part of the brain has more concern in the operations of our intellect than any other'.[18] Cullen's critical contribution was thus to define insanity as mental disorder grounded in dynamic neurophysiology, but not necessarily detectable corporeally. It was understandable, then, that Alexander Crichton (1763–1856), one of his former students, in 1798 devoted an extensive two-volume treatise, *Inquiry into the Nature and Origin of Mental Derangement*, to a detailed analysis and attempted reconciliation of 'corporal' and 'moral or mental' factors in the causation of insanity.

An even more dramatic shift to mentalistic or psychological approaches occurred at the turn of the nineteenth century. This new development was closely connected with the rise of 'moral therapy', a European and American movement beginning in the late eighteenth century associated with trends toward the humane management of asylum patients.[19] *Moral* therapy contrasted to pre-existing *medical* therapy, and meant the lessening of physical coercion and of harsh medical procedures such as drugging, vomiting, and bloodletting. (➤ Ch. 40 Physical methods) Moral therapy also drew from association psychology, postulating that the faulty mental associations of insanity could be carefully re-educated in the humane and orderly regime of a reformed asylum.[20]

Philippe Pinel (1745–1826), who was also influenced by Cullen, was the most famous advocate of the new approach.[21] Although himself a physician, he condemned harsh and indiscriminate medical therapies. Instead of focusing on somatic treatment, Pinel directed attention to the patient's 'story', hoping to derive from it clues to precipitating emotional circumstances as well as ideas for possible behavioural interventions. His specific strategies varied with the individual case, but in all instances he relied on close observation, knowledge of the patient, and carefully planned interaction between asylum personnel and the inmate. By contrast, physical treatment would prove as useless as it was severe because it rested on a fundamentally false premise: 'It is a general and very natural opinion, that derangement of the functions of the understanding consists in a change or lesion of some part of the head. . . . [But] numerous results of dissection . . . have shewn no organic lesion of the head.'[22]

In the wake of Pinel's joining sceptical anatomy to psychological theory and therapeutic management, the moral alternative advanced rapidly. In France, England, the United States, and elsewhere both lay people and physicians promoted Pinel's behavioural methods while playing down medical interventions and somatic theories.[23] Even the American physician Benjamin Rush (1745–1813), though primarily a somatic therapist and theorist, explicitly followed Pinel in claiming that in the majority of cases, 'derangement is more common from mental, than corporeal causes'.[24]

By about 1815–25, biologically oriented physicians struck back. Worried about challenges to their authority and influenced by recent achievements in cerebral patho-anatomy and the rise of phrenology, they aggressively reasserted the principles of somatic psychiatry.[25] Although Anglo-American alienists pragmatically manoeuvred to eclectic positions, French physicians who had previously supported Pinel now became genuinely ambivalent about the relative weights of somatic versus psychological factors.[26] By the 1830s and 1840s, strict proponents of the moral approach were typically either professional philosophers or clerics eager to establish their responsibility for the insane.[27] Only rare physicians were still willing to attack somatic theories and promote moral methods almost exclusively.[28]

Tensions between psychological and somatic approaches were expressed in most extreme form in early nineteenth-century Germany.[29] Members of the mentalistic or psychological school were labelled '*Psychikers*'. Influenced by Pinel, they also drew on eighteenth-century currents of medical animism that were traceable, ultimately, to the philosophical formulation of mind-body dualism by René Descartes (1596–1650) and to the construction of a vitalistic medical system on those metaphysical foundations by G. E. Stahl (1660–1734). German *psychisch* physicians drew inspiration as well from late eighteenth-century German philosophical currents. They insisted on the fundamental aetiological and therapeutic significance of the immaterial soul in both somatic and mental disease.[30] As J. C. A. Heinroth (1773–1843) wrote in 1818: 'in the great majority of cases it is not the body but the soul itself from which mental disturbances directly and primarily originate'.[31]

By the 1820s and 1830s, '*Somatikers*' actively countered the *Psychikers* and challenged them for dominance of German psychiatric thought. Leaders of this organicist school were Maximilian Jacobi (1775–1858), Friedrich Nasse (1778–1851), and Johannes Friedreich (1796–1862). Jacobi, in 1830, insisted that 'there is no disease of the mind existing as such, but ... insanity exists solely as the consequence of disease ... in some part of the bodily system.'[32]

In 1845, Wilhelm Griesinger (1817–68) published *Die Pathologie und Therapie der psychischen Krankheiten* (expanded edition in 1861), which offered an impressive synthesis that attempted to transcend what he regarded as a fruitless dispute. He drew from the patho-anatomical tradition, but also from more recent physiological work and from contemporary ego psychology.[33] He started with the fundamental materialist notion that normal and abnormal mental states exist only as consequences of cerebral activity, or as he put it, 'Every mental disease proceeds from an affection of the brain.'[34] But he quickly made it apparent that not all pathological mental states were actually accompanied by detectable cerebral lesions. Mental disease was typically progressive, moving from depressive states to more behaviourally and cognitively disruptive conditions over what could be a considerable period of time. The underlying somatic abnormality usually started with a patho-physiological condition of excessive but visually undetectable cerebral irritation, and only later progressed to chronic, irreversible, patho-anatomical brain degeneration. As the pathological physical process advanced, so did aberrant thought and behaviour, culminating in the disintegration of the ego common in chronic mania and dementia.[35] (➤ Ch. 9 The pathological tradition)

Griesinger's programmatic statements baldly defining mental disease as brain disease were thus qualified by significant portions of his complex and subtle text. His aetiology was unmistakably multifactorial. Among predisposing conditions and precipitating causes of mental disease, he mentioned heredity, inflammatory processes in the brain, anaemia or hyperaemia, head injury, and acute febrile disease. But he also discussed 'psychical causes', which he said were the 'most frequent' and might operate either indirectly, by disturbing such functions as circulation, respiration, and digestion (which secondarily disturbed cerebral function), or directly, by causing 'a state of intensive irritation of the brain'.[36] As Ackerknecht astutely observed, Griesinger 'showed a full understanding of psychological causes. No psychiatrist before him so consistently stressed the transitions from normal to pathological psychic processes.'[37] Ackerknecht also observed that Griesinger 'turned against both the psychicists and the somaticists, whose contradictory theories he tried to reconcile . . . [and] presents us with a systematic synthesis of the anatomical, physiological, psychological, and clinical points of view'. (➤ Ch. 56 Psychiatry)

Mid-century psychiatrists in other countries moved in essentially the same synthetic direction. Thus in France, J. R. Falret (1794–1870) disavowed his earlier, stricter somaticism, progressively incorporated additional psychological elements in his psychiatry, and eventually arrived at a Griesinger-like position, which he capped in 1865 by writing an introduction to the French translation of Griesinger's textbook.[38] In England, John Charles Bucknill (1817–97) and Daniel Hack Tuke (1827–95) co-authored *A Manual of Psychological Medicine* (1858), 'the first of the modern textbooks'.[39] They blended somatic principles and psychological exploration in an impressive and influential synthesis.[40] In the United States, a variety of mid-century alienists also struggled for a flexible, Griesinger-like combination of psychological and somatic elements.[41] The exact blend may have been a bit different from Griesinger's, but more noteworthy was the parallel American effort to arrive at a middle aetiological position without worrying unduly about departing from a strict somaticism.

Since the mid-nineteenth century, psychiatric theory in both Europe and America has passed through many, often-confusing departures from equilibrium position. In the late nineteenth century, the balance tilted sharply in the somatic direction. Organic neuropsychiatry, hereditarian theory, (➤ Ch. 20 Constitutional and hereditary disorders) and, especially, the 'brain pathology' of Theodor Meynert (1833–92) were the primary forms of the new somaticism.[42]

By the turn of the twentieth century, however, a rebellion against 'brain mythology' was led by clinicians such as Richard Krafft-Ebing (1840–1902), Emil Kraepelin (1856–1926), and Adolf Meyer (1866–1950).[43] They turned from the laboratory to the bedside and to the elucidation of the natural histories or life-courses of mental disorders. Even more dramatic was the release of powerful new psychogenic forces by the psychoanalytic revolution of Sigmund Freud (1856–1939). By the 1910s and 1920s, psychiatrists in both Europe and America had begun to employ Freudian notions of repressed unconscious conflict, symbolism, dream-like condensation, and wish-fulfilment to decode the hidden psychological meaning of the psychoses.[44] (➤ Ch. 43 Psychotherapy)

From the 1930s to the 1950s, American and European psychiatry diverged significantly as the United States accelerated its drift in the psycho-dynamic direction while Europe reverted to a stricter somaticism. America's extra-ordinary enthusiasm for psychoanalysis during these years – even for *émigré* European analysts – accounted for a large part of this divergence.[45] But since the 1950s, American psychiatry has swung dramatically back once again to a biological position. By the 1960s, psychoanalytic psychiatry was in rapid decline and a new style based on the biochemical investigation of psychotropic drug action, a 'renaissance' of genetic studies, and the exploration of brain cytology and neurochemistry was in ascent.[46] (➤ Ch. 8 The biochemical tradition; Ch. 39 Drug therapies) In the 1970s and 1980s, these biological enthusiasms became the increasingly widely disseminated items of a new psychiatric faith, and little time or attention was reserved for constructing a sober, judicious, Griesinger-like synthesis of mental (*psychisch*) and biological (*somatisch*) elements.

THE FUNCTIONAL NEUROSES

At the very time that mid-nineteenth-century psychiatrists were carefully blending psychological with biological factors in their understanding of overt mental disorders, other physicians were actively exploring the 'functional neuroses'. These disorders, such as hysteria, appeared to be somatic but seemed to occur without detectable underlying organic pathology. They were also marked by a mixture of non-psychotic behavioural and cognitive peculiarities and an astonishing array of somatic symptoms. Functional neuroses were defined in the widely read *Treatise on the Principles and Practice of Medicine* by Austin Flint (1812–86) as affections 'peculiar to the nervous system ... which occur without inflammation or any appreciable morbid changes in the nervous structure'.[47] They might occur symptomatically as pain, paralysis, anaesthesia, convulsive movement, or 'a morbid susceptibility to emotions and a defective power of the will to restrain their manifestations'.[48] Among onset conditions could be 'overtasking of mind and body, mental anxiety or grief... violent anger, jealousy, and other kinds of strong mental excitement'.[49] Functional neuroses, in other words, constituted an important yet puzzling category of blended somatic and psychological illnesses that, seen in retrospect, closely resemble the 'somatoform' disorders of current classification.[50] Beginning in the 1820s and 1830s, they attracted a great deal of explicit clinical attention, which continued throughout the nineteenth century and well into the twentieth.[51]

Conditions very much like those labelled functional neuroses in the nineteenth century had actually been identified quite early in the history of medicine. Galen reported the case of a young woman who seemed to exhibit the signs of physical illness but who, upon closer examination, revealed no organic pathology. After eliminating any possible somatic aetiology Galen identified the psychological cause of her somatic signs: a hidden love interest.[52] Other instances of this kind were reported in ancient, medieval, Renaissance and early modern medical literature, and were usually offered as examples of 'love sickness'.[53]

Still other early instances of what would later be identified as instances of functional disturbance were related to intensive imaginative experiences. In these cases, physical symptoms were specifically linked with disembodied images or ideas intensely imagined and then tangibly 'somaticized'. Thus, Avicenna claimed that 'if one were to gaze intently at something red, one could cause the sanguineous humour to move. That is why one must not let a person suffering from nose-bleeding see a brilliant red colour.'[54] During the Renaissance and early modern periods, the causal role of the imagination was even more broadly understood.[55] In the later seventeenth century, Friedrich Hoffman stated: 'In those who are so disposed, terror of a particular disease may readily induce a similar disease in the body.'[56] As a leading physician summarized these aetiological beliefs a half-century later, 'Many Diseases arise from a perverted Imagination; and some of them are cured by affecting the Imagination only.'[57]

Hysteria was also long known in medicine, but not until the seventeenth century was it seriously associated with any sort of nervous or mental aetiology. Until that time, it was regarded as a paroxysmal disorder of uterine origin, as its name implies.[58] The hysteric syndrome was originally thought to be akin to epilepsy, both in certain of its symptoms and in its fundamentally somatic causation. Principal manifestations included respiratory distress, palpitations, vomiting or belching, faint pulse, and cold skin; often present were headache, convulsions, loss of speech, temporary blindness, unconsciousness, anxiety, and confusion. In the seventeenth century, Thomas Willis thought that hysterical disorders were 'primarily convulsive' consequences of 'the brain and nervous stock being affected'.[59] Finally, Sydenham said that the disorder was caused by 'irregular motions of the animal spirits', which were frequently precipitated psychologically by 'some great commotion of mind, occasioned by some sudden fit, either of anger, grief, terror or like passions'.[60]

In the eighteenth century, the clinical and aetiological trends to which Willis and Sydenham contributed resulted in a major new focus on 'nervous diseases'. These disorders were the symptomatic composite of hysteria merged with hypochondriac melancholy (a secondary form of melancholia recognized since antiquity) plus some gastro-intestinal and neurological odds and ends, all neurogenically explicated.[61] They became the subject of a great deal of lay and medical attention, not least from Robert Whytt (1714–66), Professor of Medicine at the University of Edinburgh.[62] In his treatise, *Observations on the Nature, Causes and Cure of those Disease which are Commonly Called Nervous, Hypochondriac or Hysteric* (1764), Whytt acknowledged that these disorders may mimic almost any common somatic condition in a 'chameleon'-like or 'protean' fashion, and may even be precipitated by intense 'imagination', as when a patient falls into convulsive fits upon seeing someone in an epileptic seizure. The nervous diseases are strongly influenced by the emotions and are quite frequently triggered mentally, as by 'doleful or moving stories, horrible or unexpected sights, great grief, anger, terror, and other passions'.[63] (➤ Ch. 67 Pain and suffering)

This emphasis on nervous diseases was continued by Whytt's colleague and successor at Edinburgh, William Cullen. Cullen, in fact, built 'nervous diseases' into the very structure of medical nosology by making all diseases the general product of excess or deficient 'nervous force' and by incorporating specific neurological disorders as one of the four fundamental categories of disease.[64] The class 'Neuroses' contained four orders; hysteria was listed among the Spasmodic Affections and was said to be 'readily excited by the passions of the mind, and by every considerable emotion'.[65] Since neuroses were characterized by generalized disruptions in function and not by specific local abnormalities marked by particular patho-anatomical lesions, hysteria, as Cullen treated it, was soon grouped among the puzzling 'functional' disorders. (➤ Ch. 17 Nosology)

In the first half of the nineteenth century, hysteria was widely considered in medical textbooks, and by the 1840s and 1850s, in separate, often massively detailed monographs.[66] Most remarkable of these was the 800-page *Traité clinique et thérapeutique de l'hystérie* published in 1859 by Pierre Briquet (1796–1881).[67] He presented data derived from 430 hysterical patients observed at the Hôpital de la Charité in Paris over a ten-year period. His treatise brought the study of hysteria to a new level of clinical sophistication.

Another major nineteenth-century development was the employment of hypnotic techniques in experiments with the induction and remission of hysterical symptoms. Originally discovered in the 1770s by the Viennese physician Anton Mesmer (1734–1815), these techniques were modernized in the 1840s by the English surgeon James Braid (1795–1860).[68] Braid hypothesized that hypnotic phenomena resulted from a neurophysiological modification, and claimed that when the nervous system was in the hypnotic state it was 'rendered eminently available in the cure of certain disorders'.[69]

Ideas like Braid's were advocated in the 1880s by Jean Martin Charcot (1825–93), famous for his elucidation of organic neurological syndromes.[70] By the 1870s, he had turned his attention to hysteria and followed the lead of Briquet in studying hundreds of hospital patients in an attempt to specify its precise symptomatology and clinical course. In 1876, his attention was drawn to the therapeutic and diagnostic uses of hypnotism with hysterical patients.[71] From this time, Charcot carefully explored hypnotic manifestations in hysterics, ultimately defining three stages of *grand hypnotisme* as well as several lesser stages.[72]

In the 1880s, Charcot explored the peculiar features of traumatic injuries such as railway accidents. He found that accident victims sometimes seemed to suffer serious somatic consequences although no organic pathology could be discovered. Rather than deliberately dissembling, Charcot hypothesized, these patients suffered a 'nervous' shock at the time of their accident, were thrown thereby into a temporary hypnoid state, in which they became susceptible to the suggestive idea of the physical injury they later manifested. Traumatic accident victims, in other words, were analogous to hysterical patients subject to hypnotic suggestion: when they slipped beyond normal consciousness the special physiological state of their nervous systems predisposed them to psychogenic, ideational influence.[73]

Young Sigmund Freud studied with Charcot in Paris during the winter of 1885–6 and was deeply impressed by his ideas.[74] Freud had already been alerted to linkages between hypnosis and hysteria by the Viennese physician Josef Breuer (1842–1925). Breuer had told Freud about a patient (Anna O.) whose strange hysterical symptoms he treated in 1880–2 by inducing hypnotic states during periods of 'absence' (dissociation) and systematically leading her back to the onset of each symptom. Once the patient re-experienced the precipitating circumstances with a display of emotion, the corresponding hysterical symptom disappeared. Freud's study with Charcot gave him a theoretical frame to understand what Breuer had told him. When he returned to Vienna, he and Breuer began a close collaboration that resulted in 1895 in the publication of their joint *Studies on Hysteria*, in which they hypothesized that hysterical symptoms derive from 'memories' connected to 'psychical traumas which have not been disposed of by abreaction or by associative thought-activity'.[75] These memories originated when the nervous system was in special physiological condition or 'hypnoid state'; they then remained cut off from normal consciousness. Hysterical symptoms resulted from the 'intrusion of this second state into the somatic innervation', a process Freud and Breuer called 'conversion'.

Tensions and differences steadily separated Freud from Breuer.[76] Breuer tended to physiological hypotheses and the continued use of hypnotic techniques. Freud moved more in the direction of psychological mechanisms and the abandonment of hypnosis. As his ideas further matured, he developed a novel set of theories and techniques that he called 'psychoanalysis'. He stressed revolutionary theoretical concepts such as 'unconscious' mental states and their energetic 'repression', the widespread occurrence of infantile sexuality, and the symbolic encoding of psychological meaning in dreams and hysterical symptoms. Freud also stressed the investigative techniques of 'free association' and dream interpretation, two methods for overcoming 'resistance' and uncovering hidden unconscious wishes without resorting to hypnosis.

The strong psychogenetic explanation of hysterical symptoms remained a key feature of Freud's mature work and of later psychoanalysis. In his *Introductory Lectures* of 1916/17, he promoted the notion of conversion as a 'puzzling leap from the mental to the physical' and continued to describe hysterical symptoms as symbolic representations of unconscious conflicts.[77] During the First World War, Freud's ideas about the psychogenesis of hysterical symptoms were often applied to shell-shock and other 'war neuroses'. Soldiers displaying such somatic symptoms as paralysis, muscular contracture, and loss of sight, speech, and hearing for which no organic bases could be found came to be widely regarded as suffering from forms of conversion hysteria.[78] In these cases, sexual aetiology was significantly downplayed and psychogenic explanation usually limited to unconscious conflicts between 'fear' and 'duty' with a resulting 'flight into illness'. (➤ Ch. 66 War and modern medicine)

In the 1920s and 1930s, conversion hysteria gained popularity as a general medical notion, in both fully sexualized and substantially desexualized form. Mainstream psychoanalysts thought in broadly sexual terms, whereas other physicians inclined to more general, even if unconscious, conflicts as the root causes of conversion symptoms.[79] The widespread popularity of conversion aetiology continued into the 1940s, reinforced by the Second World War and the return of shell-shock and its variants.[80] By the late 1940s, conversion hysteria was so common a concept, not only in psychiatry but in medicine generally, that Henry A. Christian (1876–1951) included a section on it in his introductory chapter to the sixteenth (1947) edition of *The Principles and Practice of Medicine* by Osler.[81]

Within the next two decades, however, the concept of conversion hysteria was subject to major assault and substantial revision. Carried along in large part by the psychoanalytically sceptical and biologically tinged wave that began sweeping over Anglo-American psychiatry in the 1950s and 1960s, several important critics started picking at what they judged the loose and unreflective consensus that had come to surround symbolically interpreted hysteria. The most influential of these threw considerable doubt on the putative 'conversion' diagnosis, at least in its orthodox psychoanalytic form. One critic in a widely noted paper published in 1965 called the diagnosis of conversion hysteria 'a disguise for ignorance and a fertile source of clinical error'.[82]

Hysterical conversion continued in retreat during the 1970s and into the 1980s. Perhaps the clearest indication of its downward slide was the account of 'Conversion disorder' in the third edition of the American Psychiatric Association's *Diagnostic and Statistical Manual,* which questioned the clinical importance and psychological significance of conversion by noting that the disorder 'apparently common several decades ago ... is now rarely encountered'.[83] It also reported findings that indicated that in some instances 'the original diagnosis of conversion symptom was incorrect and represented a missed diagnosis of true organic pathology'. Third and perhaps most important, its discussion of conversion several times referred to 'apparent' as opposed to unquestioned mental aetiology, and took pains to define in non-psychoanalytic terms the basis for this causal presumption.[84]

Before conversion hysteria began its decline, however, it contributed significantly to another area of mental aetiology, the last that will be considered here. That area has been called 'psychosomatic' for a good part of the twentieth century. In the 1990s, the label officially preferred by the American Psychiatric Association is 'Psychological Factors Affecting Physical Condition', although the World Health Organization's *International Classification of Diseases* calls the same category of conditions 'Physiological Malfunction Arising From Mental Factors'.[85] The critical events that helped give birth to this important area of clinical study took place in the 1920s and 1930s, when psychoanalytically interpreted hysteria was still growing in medical popularity.

THE ROLE OF EMOTIONAL FACTORS IN SOMATIC DISEASE

In the 1920s, psychoanalysts tried to carve a medical niche for themselves by offering their psychological expertise to internist colleagues who were struggling to specify the 'emotional element in the production of organic diseases'.[86] Interest in the ways in which emotional factors contributed to somatic-disease onset or exacerbation can, in fact, be traced from antiquity through the nineteenth century.[87] Even at the turn of the twentieth century – as medical scientists embraced new reductionist aetiological views derived from cellular pathology, physiology, biochemistry, and microbiology – leading clinicians like Adolf Strumpell (1853–1925) continued to investigate the ways in which the patient's state of mind or personal circumstances caused, complicated, or contributed to the relief of somatic disease.[88]

The longest-standing tradition of mind–body (that is, psychosomatic) speculation in Western medicine is the 'passions' tradition whose roots can be found in Galen's works.[89] According to this tradition, six 'non-natural' factors (including among them the 'passions or perturbations of the soul') are critical for the physician to manage when attempting to conserve or restore health. The influence of strong emotions on physical health and illness was thus a central tenet of classical medical belief which, if it changed at all, grew stronger in the medieval, Renaissance and early modern periods. As Moses Maimonides (1135–1204) expressed it: 'It is known . . . that passions of the psyche produce changes in the body that are great, evident and manifest to all. On this account . . . the movements of the psyche . . . should be kept in balance . . . and no other regimen should be given precedence.'[90]

The doctrine of the passions continued in the seventeenth and eighteenth centuries. Often, detailed discussion was embedded in standard textbook accounts of the non-naturals, sometimes in general treatises on the factors affecting health and well-being, occasionally in idiosyncratic but widely read works such as Robert Burton's *Anatomy of Melancholy* (1621), and, by the later eighteenth century, increasingly in extensive essays or specialized monographs on emotional states and their impact on somatic health and disease.[91] Examples of the latter include *De Regimine Mentis* (1747 and 1763) by Jerome Gaub (1705–80) and *The Influence of the Passions on the Disorders of the Body* (1788) by William Falconer (1744–1824).

Even in the nineteenth century, physicians stressed the mind–body relationships made commonplace by the passions tradition. Indeed, leading scientific physicians in France, Germany, and elsewhere carefully underscored the role of emotion in disease at the very time that they pushed in increasingly reductionist directions. Armand Trousseau (1801–67), for example, a patho-anatomically based Paris clinician, described psychological factors in such diseases as hyperthyroidism, angina pectoris, and asthma, and Carl Wunderlich (1815–77), who pioneered quantitative thermometry, identified them in heart disease, peptic ulcer, and diabetes.[92]

In the early decades of the twentieth century, a marked tendency towards ever more refined scientific reductionism was balanced by continuing attention to mind–body relationships. Internists in Germany and Austria were particularly active, stimulated perhaps not only by Strumpell's example, but also by developments in endocrinology and physiology, controversies with psychiatrists, neurologists, and general practitioners, and competition from lay healers with psychotherapeutic interests.[93] Among the important books published at that time were Gustave Heyer's *Das körperlich-seelische Zusammenwirken in den Lebensvorgangen*, Fritz Mohr's *Psychophysische Behandlungsmetho-*

den, and Oswald Schwarz's encyclopaedic *Psychogenese und Psychotherapie körperlicher Symptome*.

Attracted by this high level of international interest and feeling that they could add depth to the contemporary understanding of emotional factors in somatic disease, psychoanalysts joined the discussion. Contributions were offered by the Austrian Felix Deutsch (1884–1964); the American Smith Ely Jelliffe (1866–1945) and, most provocatively, by the German Georg Groddeck (1866–1934).[94] Groddeck was an especially forceful proponent of the view that the psychological mechanism for hysterical conversion reaction could be generalized to the entire range of somatic disease. With little attention to physiology, endocrinology, or any of the other modern scientific disciplines, he argued that organic symptoms in any physical disorder could be interpreted as the symbolic expression of the id working through primary process on the plastic body.[95]

The *émigré* psychoanalyst Franz Alexander (1891–1964), a physiologist and biochemist from around 1910 until the early 1920s, when he became an analyst, tried to work out a compromise between contemporary physiology and Freudian theory.[96] Soon after his arrival in the United States in the early 1930s, he repudiated the approach taken by Groddeck and like-minded analysts and carefully distinguished between classic conversion hysteria (where symbolic processes are operative) and those disturbances of organic function controlled physiologically by the autonomic nervous system (where they are not). According to Alexander, Groddeck *et al.* had erased a boundary that needed to be carefully redrawn. They had ignored the step-wise, symbolically and psychologically innocent mechanisms that, as Harvard physiologist W. B. Cannon (1871–1945) had demonstrated, controlled the expression of emotion as the body responded to stressful stimuli. (➤ Ch. 7 The physiological tradition) But still faithful to the psychoanalytic tradition, Alexander also identified specific configurations of unconscious wishes and infantile cathexes (for example, the unconscious wish to be fed) in the 'psychic stimuli' that he said precipitated specific chains of physiological response and, ultimately, of specific somatic disease.[97]

Alexander's theoretical formulations helped stimulate serious research in the United States. He organized a group of investigators from various medical backgrounds at the Chicago Institute of Psychoanalysis, and additional groups soon developed elsewhere. Prominent among them was the group of Stanley Cobb (1887–1968) at the Massachusetts General Hospital, and that of Harold Wolff (1898–1962) at the Cornell Medical Center.[98] Cobb and Wolff were more physiologically oriented in their research styles, but all the active groups tried to incorporate psychoanalytic perspectives and, at least initially, took Alexander's 'specificity' formulations seriously. In addition, Helen Flanders Dunbar (1902–59) at the Columbia Presbyterian Medical Center produced a pioneering monograph, *Emotions and Bodily Changes: a Survey of Literature on Psychosomatic Interrelationships*, which synthesized recent research findings and in its subtitle gave the growing American movement a name. In 1939, *Psychosomatic Medicine* was founded, the first medical journal devoted specifically to publishing research in this expanding area of investigation.[99]

From the early 1940s through the 1950s, psychosomatic medicine flourished in North America; research papers and monographs multiplied rapidly; and medical schools and residency programmes institutionalized psychosomatic instruction in graduate and postgraduate education. Alexander supplemented his numerous professional writings with a popular general treatise that was widely read in non-medical as well as medical circles; and Dunbar even published what amounted to a psychosomatic bestseller.[100]

By the late 1950s, however, all was not well. With the vast expansion of activity and interest, conceptual approaches and research styles proliferated wildly. Alexander, Cobb, and Wolff remained important and active figures, but they were now joined by several dozen others who developed a variety of psychoanalytic, physiological, adaptational, ecological, and eclectic explanatory models. Alexander's 'specificity' approach was subject to serious questioning, but no obvious alternative arose to replace it. Some noticed that fissures were developing between research schools, between psychiatrist researchers and others, and between research workers and practitioners. In 1960, Eric Wittkower (1899–1983), in his presidential address to the American Psychosomatic Society, declared the field in crisis.[101]

By the 1960s, the divisions, rifts, and sense of crisis spread to Europe, which had lagged behind North America in the development of psychosomatic research and then in the sense of crisis. Although traces of psychosomatic investigation had been apparent in the 1930s and grew stronger in the 1940s, it was not until the 1950s that energetic European activity really began.[102] The major centres were Great Britain, the Netherlands and Germany, but serious work was also undertaken in Scandinavia, Belgium, Italy, Switzerland, Austria, and, eventually, France.[103] A signal event was the founding in 1956 of the *Journal of Psychosomatic Research* as a forum for the publication of European research, modelled closely on Wolff's laboratory studies of physiological adaptation to consciously perceived 'stress'.[104] Yet psychoanalytically grounded psychosomatics was also represented in Europe in both Groddeck's and Alexander's varieties.[105]

In the last three decades preceding the 1990s, major changes have overtaken psychosomatic medicine. While first apparent in North America, they were soon evident in Europe as well. The most fundamental changes have been a dramatic disavowal of psychoanalytically based studies, a refocusing of clinical attention on the role of social and ecological 'stressors', and the extraordinary development of neurobiological and biochemical investigation.[106]

Today, 'Psychoneuroimmunology' is the latest – avowedly non-reductionist but increasingly molecular – enthusiasm in the field.[107] Medical commentators outside the field have also charted the steady rise of neurobiology and the irreversible decline not only of Alexandrian specificity theory, but of less rigid and once highly regarded psychodynamic alternatives.[108] The rapid change in fortune of psychoanalytic psychosomatics from glorious novelty to embarrassing relic was clearly parallel and closely related to the precipitous decline of psychoanalysis and the concurrent rise of biological psychiatry discussed on p. 453.

As modern psychosomatics has been transformed into a more conventional field of specialized medical research, several of its intellectual leaders, as a kind of compensation, have developed synthetic philosophies that they promote with a missionary zeal reminiscent of the earlier stages of the psychosomatic movement.[109] Thus, George Engel (b. 1913), long loyal to psychoanalysis, moved in the 1970s from his psychoanalytically informed exploration of disease onset conditions in terms of 'object loss' and the 'affect of hopelessness' to an all-encompassing 'bio-psycho-social' approach.[110] Engel argued that the physician must look beyond the narrow strictures of the reigning biomedical model, which in its linear reductionism has become a cultural imperative and a dogma, and recognize the fundamental 'psychobiological unity' of humans. Without sacrificing the advantages of the biomedical approach, physicians must learn to 'span the social, psychological, and biological'. In the 1980s, Engel expounded the 'general systems theory' as a conceptual framework within which he vividly illustrated the clinical application of the bio-psycho-social model.[111] In similar fashion, Z. J. Lipowski (b. 1924) and others strongly urged the adoption of a holistic-medical model and a multifactorial approach to aetiology.[112] These authorities, once internationally recognized as at the centre of psychosomatic medicine, have clearly moved towards some version of global holistic theory that postulates that all human disease is in some sense both biologically grounded and psycho-socially conditioned. That is, not just classic psychosomatic disorders, but *every* disease, must be understood as the complex product of biological, psychological, and ecological factors.[113] This is a modern version of the doctrine of the passions in disease onset and exacerbation, an aetiological nexus to which psychosomatic medicine now seems to have returned after its affair with psychoanalysis.

It is also interesting to note that, while the majority of their medical colleagues do not seem to have been very deeply impressed by Engel's or Lipowski's philosophical efforts, bio-psycho-social language and its variants have become quite popular in modern medical parlance. Professional and lay publications now enthusiastically employ this vocabulary, and since 1977 *Index Medicus* has been using the category 'Life Change Events' to capture the multiplying number of bio-psycho-social studies in its reference grid. Closely related publications continue to be classified under 'Psychophysiologic Disorders', 'Emotions', 'Adaptation', 'Stress, psychological', 'Psychosomatic Disorder', and a half-dozen other rubrics. All of this is striking evidence that, despite recent changes, a strong mentalist undercurrent continues to flow in contemporary medicine, in this instance connecting somatic disease with emotional events in a larger holistic context.

NOTES

1 W. H. S. Jones, E. T. Withington and Paul Potter (ed. and trans.), *Hippocrates, Works*, 6 vols, London, Loeb Classical Library/Heinemann, 1923–88, Vol. II, p. 177.

2 Giuseppe Roccatagliata, *A History of Ancient Psychiatry*, Westport, CT, Greenwood Press, 1986.

3 *Hippocrates*, op. cit. (n. 1), Vol. I, p. 283.

4 *Hippocrates*, op. cit. (n. 1), Vol. VI, p. 235.

5 *Hippocrates*, op. cit. (n. 1), Vol. II, p. 167.

6 Stanley Jackson, *Melancholia and Depression From Hippocratic Times to Modern Times*, New Haven, Yale University Press, 1986, pp. 34–41.

7 Caelius Aurelianus, *On Acute Diseases and on Chronic Diseases*, ed. and trans. by I. E. Drabkin, Chicago, IL, University of Chicago Press, 1950, p. 537.

8 Jackson, op. cit. (n. 6), p. 58. Cf. Manfred Ullmann, *Islamic Medicine*, Edinburgh, Edinburgh University Press, 1978, pp. 73–6.

9 Oskar Diethelm and Thomas F. Heffernan, 'Felix Platter and psychiatry', *Journal of the History of the Behavioral Sciences*, 1965, 1: 10–23; Diethelm, *Medical Dissertations of Psychiatric Interest Printed before 1750*, Basle, Karger, 1971; Michael MacDonald, *Mystical Bedlam: Madness, Anxiety, and Healing in Seventeenth-Century England*, Cambridge, Cambridge University Press, 1983.

10 Robert Burton, *The Anatomy of Melancholy*, ed. by Floyd Dell and Paul Jordan-Smith, New York, Tudor, 1948, pp. 110–11.

11 T. H. Jobe, 'Medical theories of melancholia in the seventeenth and early eighteenth centuries', *Clio Medica*, 1976, 11: 217–31.

12 Hermann Boerhaave, *Aphorisms*, London, W. Innys, 1742, pp. 313, 321.

13 Roy Porter, *Mind-Forg'd Manacles*, Cambridge, MA, Harvard University Press, 1987; Eric T. Carlson and Norman Dain, 'The psychotherapy that was moral treatment', *American Journal of Psychiatry*, 1960, 117: 519–24; Andrew T. Scull, 'From madness to mental illness', *European Journal of Sociology*, 1975, 16: 218–61; William F. Bynum, 'Rationales for therapy in British psychiatry: 1780–1835', *Medical History*, 1974, 18: 317–34.

14 Max Neuburger, 'British and German psychiatry in the second half of the eighteenth and the early nineteenth century', *Bulletin of the History of Medicine*, 1945, 18: 121–45; Norman Dain, *Concepts of Insanity in the United States, 1789–1865*, New Brunswick, NJ, Rutgers University Press, 1964; Kathleen Grange, 'Pinel and eighteenth-century psychiatry', *Bulletin of the History of Medicine*, 1961, 35: 442–3; Raymond de Saussure, 'Philippe Pinel and the

reform of insane asylums', *Ciba Symposia*, 1950, 11: 1222–52; Ida Macalpine and Richard Hunter, *George III and the Mad Business*, New York, Pantheon Books, 1969.

15 Porter, op. cit. (n. 13); Robert Hoeldtke, 'The history of association and British medical psychology', *Medical History*, 1967, 11: 46–65.

16 Eric T. Carlson and R. Bruce McFadden, 'Dr William Cullen on mania', *American Journal of Psychiatry*, 1960, 117: 463–5.

17 William Cullen, *First Lines of the Practice of Physic*, 4 vols, Edinburgh, C. Elliot & T. Cadell, 1784, Vol. I, pp. 117–21, 126.

18 Ibid., Vol. IV, p. 122.

19 Porter, op. cit. (n. 13), pp. 206–28; Anne Digby, 'Moral treatment at the retreat', in W. F. Bynum, R. Porter and M. Shepherd (eds), *The Anatomy of Madness*, London, Tavistock, 1985, Vol. II, pp. 52–72.

20 Jan Goldstein, *Console and Classify: the French Psychiatric Profession in the Nineteenth Century*, Cambridge, Cambridge University Press, 1987, pp. 77, 90–101, 109.

21 Ibid., pp. 64–119, esp. pp. 80–9. Cf. Dora R. Weiner, 'Health and mental hygiene in the thought of Philippe Pinel', in Charles E. Rosenberg (ed.), *Healing and History: Essays for George Rosen*, New York, Science History Publications, 1979, pp. 59–85; Evelyn A. Woods and Eric T. Carlson, 'The psychiatry of Philippe Pinel', *Bulletin of the History of Medicine*, 1961, 35: 14–25.

22 Philippe Pinel, *A Treatise on Insanity*, trans. by D. D. Davis, Sheffield, W. Todd, 1806, pp. 110–11.

23 Dain, op. cit. (n. 14), pp. 12, 22, 26, 214 n. 30.

24 Benjamin Rush, *Medical Inquiries and Observations upon the Diseases of the Mind*, Philadelphia, PA, Kimber & Richardson, 1812, pp. 46–7.

25 Bynum, op. cit. (n. 13); Roger Cooter, 'Phrenology and British alienists, ca. 1825–45', in Andrew Scull (ed.), *Madhouses, Mad-Doctors, and Madmen*, Philadelphia, PA, University of Pennsylvania Press, 1981; Scull, op. cit. (n. 13), pp. 254–7.

26 Goldstein, op. cit. (n. 20), pp. 251–3, Cf. Ian Dowbiggin, *Inheriting Madness: Professionalization and Psychiatric Knowledge in Nineteenth Century France*, Berkeley, University of California Press, 1991, pp. 41–2.

27 Dowbiggin, op. cit. (n. 26), pp. 34, 36, 38.

28 Dowbiggin, op. cit. (n. 26), pp. 39–53.

29 Erwin H. Ackerknecht, *A Short History of Psychiatry*, New York, Hafner, 1959. p. 46.

30 Neuburger, op. cit. (n. 14), pp. 123–4, 131–3, 137; Otto M. Marx, 'A re-evaluation of the mentalists in early nineteenth century German psychiatry', *American Journal of Psychiatry*, 1965, 121: 752–60.

31 Johann Christian August Heinroth, *Textbook of Disturbances of Mental Life*, trans. by T. Schmorak, 2 vols, Baltimore, MD, Johns Hopkins University Press, 1975, Vol. I, p. 23.

32 Neuburger, op. cit. (n. 14), p. 137.

33 Otto M. Marx, 'Wilhelm Griesinger and the history of psychiatry: a reassessment', *Bulletin of the History of Medicine*, 1972, 46: 519–44.

34 Wilhelm Griesinger, *Mental Pathology and Therapeutics*, trans. by C. Lockhart

Robertson and James Rutherford, London, New Sydenham Society, 1867, pp. 3, 7. Cf. Otto M. Marx, 'Nineteenth century medical psychology', *Isis*, 1970, 61: 358–61.

35 Griesinger, op. cit. (n. 34), pp. 207–8.

36 Griesinger, op. cit. (n. 34), pp. 164–7.

37 Ackerknecht, op. cit. (n. 29), p. 63.

38 Goldstein, op. cit. (n. 20), p. 262; Dowbiggin, op. cit. (n. 26), pp. 26–27, 180 n. 77.

39 Richard Hunter and Ida Macalpine, *Three Hundred Years of Psychiatry, 1535–1860*, London, Oxford University Press, 1963, p. 1069.

40 Jackson, op. cit. (n. 6), pp. 166–70.

41 Dain, op. cit. (n. 14), pp. 86–7, 233–4 n. 7.

42 Michael J. Clark, 'The rejection of psychological approaches to mental disorder in late nineteenth-century British psychiatry', in Scull (ed.), op. cit. (n. 25) pp. 271–312; Dowbiggin, op. cit. (n. 26), pp. 54–75, 116–43; Annamaria Tagliavini, 'Aspects of the history of psychiatry in Italy in the second half of the nineteenth century', in Bynum, Porter and Shepherd, op. cit. (n. 19), Vol. II, pp. 175–96; W. F. Bynum, 'Theory and practice in British psychiatry from J. C. Prichard to Henry Maudsley', in Teizo Ogawa (ed.), *History of Psychiatry*, Osaka, Taniguchi Foundation, 1982, pp. 196–216; Otto M. Marx, 'Psychiatry on a neuropathological basis', *Clio Medica*, 1971, 6: 139–58; Kenneth Levin, *Freud's Early Psychology of the Neuroses*, Pittsburgh, University of Pittsburgh Press, 1978, pp. 23–9; Stanley Jackson, 'Introduction', in Theodor Meynert, *Psychiatry: a Clinical Treatise on Diseases of the Fore-brain*, trans. by B. Sachs (1885), New York, Hafner, 1968.

43 Levin, op. cit. (n. 42), pp. 36–9; Jackson, op. cit. (n. 6), pp. 173–4, 188; Ackerknecht, op. cit. (n. 29), pp. 67–70.

44 Eugen Bleuler, *Textbook of Psychiatry*, trans. by A. A. Brill, New York, Macmillan, 1924; and Edward J. Kempf, *Psychopathology*, St Louis, MO, C. V. Mosby, 1920. Cf. Sander Gilman, 'Psychotherapy', Ch. 43 this volume; Hannah S. Decker, *Freud in Germany: Revolution and Reaction in Science, 1893–1907*, Psychological Issues Monograph 41, New York, International Universities Press, 1977; Nathan G. Hale, *Freud and the Americans: the Beginnings of Psychoanalysis in the United States, 1876–1917*, New York, Oxford University Press, 1971; John C. Burnham, *Psychoanalysis and American Medicine, 1894–1918*, Psychological Issues Monograph 20, New York, International Universities Press, 1967; Henri F. Ellenberger, *The Discovery of the Unconscious*, New York, Basic Books, 1970; John G. Howells (ed.), *World History of Psychiatry*, New York, Brunner/Mazel, 1975; Steven R. Hirsch and Michael Shepherd (eds), *Themes and Variations in European Psychiatry*, Bristol, John Wright, 1974.

45 Nathan G. Hale, 'From Berggasse XIX to Central Park West: the Americanization of psychoanalysis, 1919–40', *Journal of the History of the Behavioral Sciences*, 1978, 14: 299–315; Laura Fermi, *Illustrious Immigrants*, Chicago, IL, University of Chicago Press, 1968, pp. 139–73; Leopold Bellak (ed.), *Contemporary European Psychiatry*, New York, Grove Press, 1961; Geoffrey Cocks, *Psychotherapy in the Third Reich*, New York, Oxford University Press, 1985; Jacques M. Quen and Eric T. Carlson (eds), *American Psychoanalysis: Origins and Development*,

New York, Brunner/Mazel, 1978; George E. Gifford (ed.), *Psychoanalysis, Psychotherapy and the New England Medical Scene, 1894–1944*, New York, Science History Publications, 1978; Lawrence J. Friedman, *Menninger*, New York, Knopf, 1990; Henry Alden Bunker, 'American psychiatry as a speciality', in American Psychiatric Association, *One Hundred Years of American Psychiatry*, New York, Columbia University Press, 1944, pp. 479–506.

46 George Mora, 'Recent psychiatric developments (since 1939)', in Silvano Arieti (ed.), *American Handbook of Psychiatry*, New York, Basic Books, 1974, Vol. I, pp. 43–114; Mora, 'Historical and theoretical trends in psychiatry,' in Harold I. Kaplan, Alfred M. Freedman and Benjamin J. Sadock (eds), *Comprehensive Textbook of Psychiatry/III*, Baltimore, MD, Williams & Wilkins, 1980, Vol. I, pp. 4–98; Garfield Tourney, 'History of biological psychiatry in America', *American Journal of Psychiatry*, 1969, 126: 29–42; George Kriegman, Robert D. Gardner and D. Wilfred Abse (eds), *American Psychiatry: Past, Present, and Future*, Charlottesville, University Press of Virginia, 1975; Elliot S. Valenstein, *Great and Desperate Cures*, New York, Basic Books, 1986; Jack D. Pressman, 'Sufficient promise: John F. Fulton and the origins of psychosurgery', *Bulletin of the History of Medicine*, 1988, 62: 1–22.

47 Austin Flint, *Treatise on the Principles and Practice of Medicine*, 3rd edn, Philadelphia, PA, Henry C. Lea, 1868, p. 680.

48 Ibid., 697 ff; see p. 717.

49 Flint, op. cit. (n. 47), p. 724.

50 American Psychiatric Association, *Diagnostic and Statistical Manual*, 3rd edn., Washington, DC, 1980 (DSMIII), 'Somatoform disorders', pp. 241–52; cf. Kaplan, Freedman and Sadock (eds), op. cit. (n. 46), ch. 21.2, 'Somatoform disorders'.

51 See, for example, John Elliotson, *The Principles and Practice of Medicine*, Philadelphia, PA, Carey & Hart, 1844, p. 36; cf. Richard Quain, *A Dictionary of Medicine*, London, Longmans, Green, 1882, p. 389.

52 Stanley Jackson, 'Galen – on mental disorders', *Journal of the History of the Behavioral Sciences*, 1969, 5: 366.

53 Marek-Marsel Mesulam and Jon Perry, 'The diagnosis of love-sickness', *Psychophysiology*, 1972, 9: 546–51.

54 O. Cameron Gruner, *A Treatise on the Canon of Medicine of Avicenna, Incorporating a Translation of the First Book*, London, Luzac, 1930, p. 92.

55 C. E. McMahon, 'The role of imagination in the disease process: pre-Cartesian history', *Psychological Medicine*, 1976, 6: 179–84.

56 Friedrich Hoffmann, *Fundamenta Medicina*, trans. by Lester S. King, London, MacDonald, 1971, p. 55.

57 Peter Shaw, quoted in Stanley Jackson, 'The imagination and psychological healing', *Journal of the History of the Behavioral Sciences*, 1990, 26: 350. Cf. Esther Fischer-Homberger, 'On the medical history of the doctrine of imagination', *Psychological Medicine*, 1979, 9: 619–28.

58 Ilza Veith, *Hysteria, the History of a Disease*, Chicago, University of Chicago Press, 1965; Etienne Trillat, *Histoire de l'hystérie*, Paris, Seghers, 1986; Mark S. Micale, 'Hysteria and its historiography', *History of Science*, 1989, 27: 223–61,

319–51; Micale, 'Hysteria and its historiography: the future perspective', *History of Psychiatry*, 1990, 1: 33–124.

59 Jeffrey M. N. Boss, 'The seventeenth-century transformation of the hysteric affection', *Psychological Medicine*, 1979, 9: 221–34.

60 Veith, op. cit. (n. 58), pp. 140–4.

61 Porter, op. cit. (n. 13), pp. 47–54; cf. Jackson, op. cit. (n. 6), pp. 281–301.

62 R. K. French, *Robert Whytt, the Soul, and Medicine*, London, Wellcome Institute, 1969.

63 Veith, op. cit. (n. 58), pp. 162–3.

64 William F. Knoff, 'A history of the concept of neurosis, with a memoir of William Cullen', *American Journal of Psychiatry*, 1970, 127: 80–4; cf. Lester S. King, *The Medical World of the Eighteenth Century*, Chicago, IL, University of Chicago Press, 1958, pp. 214–19.

65 William Cullen, *First Lines of the Practice of Physic*, with suppl. notes by Peter Reid, Brookfield E. Merriam, 1807, pp. 530–5; cf. Guenter B. Risse, 'Hysteria at the Edinburgh Infirmary', *Medical History*, 1988, 32: 1–22.

66 Veith, op. cit. (n. 58), pp. 184–210; Alison Kane and Eric T. Carlson, 'A different drummer: Robert B. Carter and nineteenth century hysteria', *Bulletin of the New York Academy of Medicine*, 1982, 58: 519–34.

67 François Mai and Harold Merskey, 'Briquet's *Treatise on Hysteria*', *Archives of General Psychiatry*, 1980, 37: 1401–5; Mai and Merskey, 'Briquet's concept of hysteria: an historical perspective', *Canadian Journal of Psychiatry*, 1981, 26: 57–63.

68 Veith, op. cit. (n. 58), pp. 225–8.

69 Hunter and Macalpine, op. cit. (n. 39), p. 906.

70 Micale, op. cit. (n. 58), 1989, pp. 331–8; Micale, op. cit. (n. 58), 1990, pp. 42–3, 62–3, 67–70.

71 Anne Harrington, 'Metals and magnets in medicine: hysteria, hypnosis and medical culture in *fin-de-siècle* Paris', *Psychological Medicine*, 1988, 18: 21–38; Harrington, 'Hysteria, hypnosis, and the lure of the invisible', in Bynum, Porter and Shepherd, op. cit. (n. 42), Vol. III, pp. 226–46.

72 Micale, op. cit. (n. 58), 1990, p. 80.

73 Levin, op. cit. (n. 42), p. 46.

74 Sigmund Freud, *Standard Edition of the Complete Psychological Works of Sigmund Freud*, ed. and trans. by J. Strachey, A. Freud, A. Strachey and A. Tyson, 24 vols, London, Hogarth, 1955–74, Vol. I. pp. 160–72.

75 Ibid., Vol. II, p. 15.

76 Freud, op. cit. (n. 74), Vol. XIV, pp. 7–24.

77 Freud, op. cit. (n. 74), Vol. XVI, pp. 258, 301.

78 Martin Stone, 'Shellshock and the psychologists', in Bynum, Porter and Shepherd, op. cit. (n. 42), Vol. II, pp. 242–71.

79 Elaine Showalter, *The Female Malady: Women, Madness and English Culture, 1830–1980*, New York, Penguin Books, 1985, pp. 167–94.

80 Roy R. Grinker and John P. Spiegel, *Men under Stress*, Philadelphia, PA, Blakiston, 1945, pp. 103–7.

81 Henry A. Christian, *The Principles and Practice of Medicine*, 16th ed., New York, D. Appleton-Century, 1947, pp. 13–24.

82 Eliot Slater, 'Diagnosis of "hysteria" ', *British Medical Journal*, 1965, 1: 1399; cf. Paul D. Gatfield and Samuel B. Guze, 'Prognosis and differential diagnosis of conversion reactions', *Diseases of the Nervous System*, 1962, 23: 623–31.

83 American Psychiatric Association, *Diagnostic and Statistical Manual of Mental Disorders*, 3rd edn, rev., Washington, DC, 1987 (DSM IIIR), p. 258.

84 Ibid., p. 259.

85 American Psychiatric Association, op. cit. (n. 83), pp 333–4; cf. Harold I. Kaplan, 'History of psychosomatic medicine', in Kaplan and Benjamin J. Sadock (eds), *Comprehensive Textbook of Psychiatry*, 4th edn, London, Williams & Wilkins, 1985, p. 1106.

86 Charles P. Emerson, 'The emotional element in the production of organic diseases', *Transactions of the Association of American Physicians*, 1927, 42: 346–55.

87 Edward L. Margetts, 'Historical notes on psychosomatic medicine', in Eric D. Wittkower and R. A. Cleghorn (eds), *Recent Developments in Psychosomatic Medicine*, Philadelphia, PA, Lippincott, 1954, pp. 41–68; Edward Stainbrook, 'Psychosomatic medicine in the nineteenth century', *Psychosomatic Medicine*, 1952, 14: 211–27.

88 Erwin H. Ackerknecht, 'The history of psychosomatic medicine', *Psychological Medicine*, 1982, 12: 17–24, see p. 21.

89 Saul Jarcho, 'Galen's six non-naturals', *Bulletin of the History of Medicine*, 1970, 44: 372–7; L. J. Rather, 'The "six things non-natural" ', *Clio Medica*, 1968, 3: 337–47; Jerome J. Bylebyl, 'Galen on the non-natural causes of variation in the pulse', *Bulletin of the History of Medicine*, 1971, 45: 482–5.

90 Ariel Bar-Sela, Hebbel E. Hoff and Elias Faris, 'Moses Maimonides' two treatises on the regimen of health', *Transactions of the American Philosophical Society*, 1964 (NS), 54 (part 4).

91 Stanley W. Jackson, 'The use of the passions in psychological healing', *Journal of the History of Medicine and Allied Sciences*, 1990, 45: 150–75; cf. Leland J. Rather, *Mind and Body in Eighteenth-Century Medicine*, Berkeley, University of California Press, 1965.

92 Ackerknecht, op. cit. (n. 88), pp. 20–1.

93 For important hints of these influences, see Walter B. Cannon, 'The mechanism of emotional disturbance of bodily functions', *New England Journal of Medicine*, 1928, 198: 877–84; Cannon, 'The role of emotion in disease', *Annals of Internal Medicine*, 1936, 9: 1453–65.

94 Harold I. Kaplan and Helen S. Kaplan, 'An historical survey of psychosomatic medicine', *Journal of Nervous and Mental Diseases*, 1956, 124: 546–68; cf. John C. Burnham, *Jelliffe: American Psychoanalyst and Physician*, Chicago, IL, University of Chicago Press, 1983, pp. 130–8.

95 George Groddeck, 'Traumarbeit und Arbeit des organischen Symptoms', *Internationale Zeitschrift für Psychoanalyse*, 1926, 12: 504–12; cf. Martin Grotjahn, 'George Groddeck and his teaching about man's innate need for symbolization', *Psychoanalytic Review*, 1945, 32: 9–24.

96 Theodore Brown, 'Alan Gregg and the Rockefeller Foundation's support of Franz Alexander's psychosomatic research', *Bulletin of the History of Medicine*, 1987, 61: 168, 170–5.

97 Ibid., cf. Dieter Wyss, *Psychoanalytic Schools From the Beginning to the Present*,

trans. by Gerald Onn, New York, Jason Aronson, 1973, pp. 237–44; and Franz Alexander, 'General principles, objectives, and preliminary results', *Psychoanalytic Quarterly*, 1934, 3: 501–39.

98 Kaplan and Kaplan, op. cit. (n. 94); Bernard Raginsky, 'Psychosomatic medicine', *American Journal of Medicine*, 1948, 5: 857–78; Chase P. Kimball, 'Conceptual developments in psychosomatic medicine: 1939–69', *Annals of Internal Medicine*, 1970, 73: 307–16; Benjamin V. White, *Stanley Cobb: a Builder of the Modern Neurosciences*, Boston, MA, Francis A. Countway Library of Medicine, 1984, pp. 212, 245–6.

99 H. F. Dunbar, 1935, *Emotions and Bodily Changes: a Survey of Literature on Psychosomatic Interrelationships*, 1935; Robert C. Powell, 'Healing and Wholeness: Helen Flanders Dunbar and an extra-medical origin of the American psychosomatic movement, 1906–36', unpublished Ph.D. thesis, Duke University, 1974; *Psychosomatic Medicine*.

100 G. L. Engel, W. A. Greene, F. Reichsman, A. H. Schmale, N. Ashenberg, 'A graduate and undergraduate teaching program on the psychological aspects of medicine', *Journal of Medical Education*, 1957, 32: 859–72; Franz Alexander, *Psychosomatic Medicine*, New York, W. W. Norton, 1950; Flanders Dunbar, *Mind and Body: Psychosomatic Medicine*, New York, Random House, 1948.

101 Eric D. Wittkower, 'Twenty years of North American psychosomatic medicine', *Psychosomatic Medicine*, 1960, 22: 308–16.

102 Noel Harris, 'The relation of psychological medicine to general medicine (psychosomatic medicine)', in N. G. Harris (ed.), *Modern Trends in Psychological Medicine*, London, Paul B. Hoeber, 1948, pp. 1–18; Desmond O'Neill (ed.), *Modern Trends in Psychosomatic Medicine*, London, Whitefriars Press, 1955; James L. Halliday, *Psychosocial Medicine*, New York, Norton, 1948; J. Groen, 'Some notes regarding the origin and development of the psychosomatic research group attached to the second medical service and the department of neuropsychiatry in the Wilhelmina-Gasthuis, Amsterdam', *Journal of Psychosomatic Research*, 1957, 2: 82–4, 147–9; Manfred Pflanz and Thure von Uexküll, 'Guide to psychosomatic literature in Germany since 1945', *Journal of Psychosomatic Research*, 1958, 3: 56–71.

103 Edith Kurzweil, *The Freudians*, New Haven, CT, Yale University Press, 1989, pp. 105–26; C. E. McMahon and Simmon Koppes, 'The development of psychosomatic medicine: an analysis of growth of professional societies', *Psychosomatics*, 1976, 17: 185–7; *Journal of Psychosomatic Research*, 1956, 1: 167–74.

104 'Editorial', *Journal of Psychosomatic Research*, 1956, 1: 1–2.

105 A. Mitscherlich, 'Methods and principles of research on psychosomatic fundamentals (the contribution of psychoanalysis to psychosomatic medicine)', in Arthur Jores and Hellmuth Freyberger (eds), *Advances in Psychosomatic Medicine*, New York, Robert Brunner, 1961, pp. 31–45.

106 E. D. Wittkower and Z. J. Lipowski, 'Recent developments in psychosomatic medicine', *Psychosomatic Medicine*, 1966, 28: 722–37; Lipowski, 'Psychosomatic medicine: an overview', in Oscar Hill (ed.), *Modern Trends in Psychosomatic Medicine*, London, Butterworth, 1976, 1–20; Lipowski (ed.), 'Current trends in psychosomatic medicine', *International Journal of Psychiatry in Medicine*, 1974, 5:

303–610; Louis A. Gottschalk, 'Psychosomatic medicine – past, present, and future', *Psychiatry*, 1975, 38: 334–45.

107 Robert Ader, 'Psychosomatic and psychoimmunologic research', *Psychosomatic Medicine*, 1980, 42: 307–21. Cf. Robert Ader (eds), *Psychoneuroimmunology*, New York, Academic Press, 1981; 2nd edn, San Diego, CA, Academic Press, 1991.

108 Gerald Weissmann, *They All Laughed at Christopher Columbus*, New York, Times Books, 1987, pp. 147–60; Robert Aronowitz and Howard Spiro, 'The rise and fall of the psychosomatic hypothesis in ulcerative colitis', *Journal of Clinical Gastroenterology*, 1988, 10: 298–305.

109 Wittkower and Lipowski, op. cit. (n. 106), p. 724.

110 George L. Engel, 'The need for a new medical model: a challenge for biomedicine', *Science*, 1977, 196: 129–36; cf. Engel, *Psychological Development in Health and Disease*, Philadelphia, Saunders, 1962; and Robert Ader and Arthur H. Schmale, 'George Libman Engel on the occasion of his retirement', *Psychosomatic Medicine*, 1980, 42 (suppl.): 79–101.

111 G. L. Engel, 'The clinical application of the biopsychosocial model', *American Journal of Psychiatry*, 1980, 137: 535–44.

112 Z. J. Lipowski, *Psychosomatic Medicine and Liaison Psychiatry*, New York, Plenum, 1985, esp. pp. 91–117.

113 Herbert Weiner, 'The illusion of simplicity: the medical model revisited', *American Journal of Psychiatry*, 1978, 135 (suppl.): 27–33; Weiner, 'The prospects for psychosomatic medicine: selected topics', *Psychosomatic Medicine*, 1982, 44: 491–517.

FURTHER READING

Ackerknecht, Erwin H., *A Short History of Psychiatry*, New York, Hafner, 1959.

——, 'A history of psychosomatic medicine', *Psychological Medicine*, 1982, 12: 17–24.

Alexander, Franz, *Psychosomatic Medicine*, New York, W. W. Norton, 1950.

Alexander, Franz, and Selesnick, Sheldon T., *The History of Psychiatry*, New York, Harper & Row, 1966.

Bellak, Leopold (ed.), *Contemporary European Psychiatry*, New York, Grove Press, 1961.

Engel, George L., *Psychological Development in Health and Disease*, Philadelphia, PA, Saunders, 1962.

Hale, Nathan G., *Freud and the Americans: the Beginnings of Psychoanalysis in the United States, 1876–1917*, New York, Oxford University Press, 1977.

Jackson, Stanley, *Melancholia and Depression from Hippocratic Times to Modern Times*, New Haven, CT, Yale University Press, 1986.

Lain Entralgo, Pedro, *The Therapy of the Word in Classical Antiquity*, ed. and trans. by L. J. Rather and John Sharp, New Haven, CT, Yale University Press, 1970.

Levin, Kenneth, *Freud's Early Psychology of the Neuroses*, Pittsburgh, PA, University of Pittsburgh Press, 1978.

Lipowski, Z. J., *Psychosomatic Medicine and Liaison Psychiatry*, New York, Plenum, 1985.

Micale, Mark S., 'Hysteria and its historiography', *History of Science*, 1989, 27: 223–61, 319–51.

Porter, Roy, *Mind-Forg'd Manacles*, Cambridge, MA, Harvard University Press, 1987.

Rather, Leland J., *Mind and Body in Eighteenth-Century Medicine*, London, Wellcome Institute, and Berkeley, University of California Press, 1965.

Shorter, Edward, *From Paralysis to Fatigue: a History of Psychosomatic Illness in the Modern Era*, New York, Free Press, 1991.

Valenstein, Elliot S., *Great and Desperate Cures*, New York, Basic Books, 1986.

Weiner, Herbert, *Psychobiology and Human Disease*, New York, Elsevier, 1977.

22

NUTRITIONAL DISEASES

Kenneth J. Carpenter

Perhaps the most striking observation from a general survey of human nutrition is how well different peoples have evolved diets that allowed them all to live and reproduce in very different environments. Thus many Eskimo groups thrived without fruit or vegetables, the Chinese and others without milk, and many Indian communities without meat or fish. (➤ Ch. 18 The ecology of disease; Ch. 15 Environment and miasmata)

With hindsight, we can see that problems commonly arose when people were forced to give up a part of their traditional diet – sometimes because of war and/or expulsion from their former territory and hunting grounds, sometimes because they set out on expeditions on which they could carry only limited supplies. The second important general cause was that a group would adopt a new or modified staple food. This could be a new crop (such as maize or cassava), which gave greater yields than the previous staple or was more convenient in terms of the labour involved, or the ability to store it. It could also be simply a modified form of a traditional crop with a change in processing to make it more palatable (for example, white rice in place of brown) without its being appreciated that some of the nutritional value of the food had been lost. Finally, the introduction of new religious ideas or a new way of life to a community can restrict the range of diets by making people eliminate some foods as being impure or degrading. A modern example is the extreme form of the Zen macrobiotic diet, consisting of nothing but brown rice and sesame seeds, which must be lethal if persisted in because it contains no vitamin C. The availability of store-bought foods to a previously isolated community can be another source of trouble. The great reduction in necessary physical activity (with its accompanying increased metabolism of fats and carbohydrate) for the last four to five generations in the wealthier countries, where it is not accompanied by compensating reductions in food intake, is also apparently leading to 'diseases of affluence' that are nutrition related.

FAMINE

Sheer lack of food in sufficient quantity has, of course, always been the most important cause of nutritional disease. Extreme weather, either in the form of drought or flooding, has been responsible for the death by famine of at least 10 million people in Asia in some years of previous centuries. Even in 1943, the Bengal famine probably caused 2 million deaths. These tragedies have usually come in areas where population growth was already straining resources in years with normal harvests.

Other causes of famine have been the consumption of crops by locusts in Africa, or the destruction of a crop by the spread of an infection, as in the Irish famine of 1845–8, where successive potato crops were rotted by a fungus. Human activities have also been directly responsible for famines – commonly as a result of fighting, making crop production impossible, or a blockade being imposed in order to starve a population into surrender. Accidents have involved smaller numbers of people, with sailing ships becalmed for long periods, or ships being wrecked on an inhospitable shore.

Death usually comes when people have lost 30–40 per cent of their original body weight. Most look like 'living skeletons' but some show oedema, with accumulated fluid swelling their legs and lower body. Most have intractable diarrhoea. Observers have noticed characteristic psychological changes in victims – selfishness, general indifference, and disorientation. The condition of starvation in infants, as a result of mothers' inadequate production of breast milk and inability to provide substitutes, is known as 'marasmus'. (➤ Ch. 45 Childhood)

Epidemic infections have often broken out in starving communities: in Ireland, typhus fever transmitted by lice was a major cause of death. This is explained in part by a reduction in the body's defences; in part by groups wandering from place to place in search of food and unable to practise normal hygiene, or being herded together in large feeding camps. Famine has never been the subject of medical controversy or study because the cause and the remedy both seem obvious. However, if its importance is forgotten, projects such as breeding crops for increased vitamin content may receive undue priority over the need to have high levels of production of strains with maximum resistance to drought and disease.

EARLY IDEAS ON DIET AND HEALTH

From the writings of Aristotle (384–322 BC), and others in the classical Greek tradition, it is clear that correct diet was considered of great importance in the maintenance of health. Food was needed for replacing worn-out tissues and as the fuel for the production of 'innate heat'. The useful parts of foods had first somehow to be converted by stages into 'blood'. The process of 'coction' began in the stomach and was completed in the heart and lungs. An excess of food was particularly damaging to health.

The Greeks, and later the European medical writers c.1550–1750, were also concerned as to the role of food in keeping people in balance, or harmony. The ideal was to be neither unduly wet nor too dry; and neither too hot nor too cold. Most people tended to be out of balance in a particular direction; for example, people with the characteristic, or humour, of being phlegmatic were classed as cold and wet. The foods thought suitable to bring them back into balance included strong wines and spicy foods with garlic and onions. Meals were considered in relation to their positive qualities in producing short-term effects and eliciting particular moods. (➤ Ch. 14 Humoralism)

It was thought that, given sufficient 'coction', there was really no limit to the power of the heart to convert any digestible food into blood. It was only with the chemical revolution led by Antoine Lavoisier (1743–94) in the late eighteenth century that it came to be realized that the elements, carbon, hydrogen, nitrogen, etc., were not interconvertible. Then with the further development of organic chemistry in the nineteenth century by many chemists (of whom Jakob Berzelius (1779–1848) and Justus von Liebig (1803–73) are among the best remembered), it was possible for those doing nutritional studies to begin to express requirements in chemical terms. (➤ Ch. 8 The biochemical tradition)

SPECIFIC DEFICIENCY DISEASES

Diseases which we regard as being due primarily to deficiency in the diet of some particular trace nturient can nowadays be considered as a class. However, before the concept of 'accessory food factors' was developed, each disease was considered on its own and the cause was a matter of continuing debate. For almost every one, for example, papers were published in the medical literature in the last part of the nineteenth century that claimed the isolation of the micro-organism responsible.

It was only in the first two decades of the present century that animal models were developed, and the basic similarities in the causes of the separate diseases began to be understood. I shall therefore first review ideas about three individual diseases in the earlier period, before considering the later, general developments.

SCURVY UP TO 1900

Of the conditions that we would now categorize as deficiency diseases, the first to be recognized as a major problem for Europeans was scurvy. Once seamen had the ships and skills to venture on voyages out of sight of land for periods of months rather than weeks (that is, from 1490 on), this disease began to appear in a familiar pattern. A typical account has been given by a priest, Antonio de la Ascension, on a Spanish expedition that attempted in 1602 to sail from the Pacific coast of Mexico to establish settlements in what is now California. They were delayed by adverse winds, and the crew members began to develop an alarming condition:

> The first symptom they notice is a pain in the whole body which makes it so sensitive to touch. . . . After this, all the body, especially from the waist down, becomes covered with purple spots larger than great mustard seeds. Then . . . some strips or bands come behind the knee joints, two fingers and more wide like weals. . . . These become as hard as stones, and the legs and thighs become so straight and stiff . . . that they cannot be extended or drawn up a degree more than the state in which they were when attached. . . . [T]he upper and lower gums of the mouth in the inside of the mouth and outside the teeth become swollen to such a size that neither the teeth nor the molars can be brought together. The teeth become so loose and without support that they move while moving the head. . . . With this they cannot eat anything but food in liquid form or drinks, . . . they come to be so weakened in this condition that their natural vigor fails them, and they die all of a sudden, while talking.[1]

The writer commented that the disease broke out in this case in exactly the area where the Spanish treasure ship, coming back from the Philippines to Mexico each year, encountered the problem. He noted that, in this area, 'a very sharp, subtle and cold wind blows' and concluded that: 'It must carry with it much pestilence, and if in itself the air is not bad, it produces with its subtlety and coolness some corruption of bad humors, especially in persons worn out and fatigued with the hardships of the navigation.'

They turned back and landed at Mazatlan, where there occurred what the narrator considered to be a miracle sent in response to their prayers to the Virgin Mary of Monte Carmelo. One member of a burial party had an impulse to taste a fruit abundant there on the cactus plants. It seemed to help him; quantities were then harvested, and even those on board who had lost all hope quickly had their health restored.

Essentially the same story recurs over and over – sickness and death at sea, or in wintry coastal settlements – followed by amazingly quick recoveries on eating turnips (in Newfoundland), oranges and lemons (in East Africa), sour plums (in Brazil), or green leafy materials in Canada and elsewhere. In some instances, sailors with symptoms of scurvy also showed nyctalopia. This was also called moon-blindness (nowadays night-blindness), meaning that the affected person did not have the usual degree of sight in dim light. Some observers thought it to be one more sign of scurvy, but most concluded that, since it could also occur in the complete absence of scurvy, it was a different disease.

Since neither lemons nor lemon juice could be stored for long periods without going mouldy, and it was already accepted that dried herbs and seeds were inactive, the College of Physicians advised the British Admiralty in the mid–1600s to provide their ships' surgeons with flavoured sulphuric acid as an alternative treatment for scurvy. This was based on a classification of diseases as resulting from bodies becoming either too 'acid' (cold) or too 'alkaline' (hot). (➤ Ch. 17 Nosology) Since acid (cold) fruits were an effective treatment, it followed that scurvy must be an alkaline disease and that any acid would be an equally effective treatment. It was taken for granted, it seems, that such a train of logical reasoning needed no experimental confirmation. When it was pointed out that a few people living on land had also developed all the symptoms of scurvy, and been cured with 'hot' materials such as watercress, the physicians simply replied that land scurvy must be a different disease.

Sulphuric acid remained the surgeon's standard treatment for sea scurvy for one hundred years. James Lind (1716–94), a young assistant surgeon with no college education, finally tested it in a controlled clinical trial of six different treatments in 1747, and found it to be useless. To modern readers, this experiment has seemed to be an important step forward, but it appeared to make little or no impression at the time. Lemons, or lemon juice, did become a standard issue some fifty years later, but only as the result of further practical experience. I have not seen any reference to the experiment itself in literature published between 1750 and 1900.

Lind went on to Edinburgh University to qualify as a physician, and wrote a scholarly treatise on scurvy that his university re-published as part of a bicentennial celebration in 1953. However, he did not regard the condition as a deficiency disease. Antiscorbutic fruits were simply sources of drugs that cured the disease in a way that was analogous to the treatment of malaria with extracts of Jesuit's bark. He believed that scurvy was always associated with moist air, and that it operated by blocking normal perspiration, which was the route by which the body eliminated the toxins produced during the normal turnover of worn-out parts that were being replaced by newly digested food. Lemon juice acted as a kind of detergent, which further divided the toxic particles so that they could then slip through the constricted perspiration pores to the skin.

Lind knew that a Dutch physician, Friedrich Bachstrom (1686–1742), had already argued that the environment had nothing to do with the disease and that its only cause was long-term lack of fresh vegetable food in the diet. However, Lind felt that this could not be true because people in the High-lands of Scotland went without fruit or green vegetables for six months each year without coming to any harm. Unfortunately, in the large literature review prepared for his treatise, he had missed the report from Newfoundland that turnips were an effective treatment, and had thought only of green leafy material as being 'fresh vegetables'.

The effectiveness of lemons in keeping sailors in good health for record periods at sea was demonstrated by Admiral Nelson (1758–1805) during the Napoleonic Wars, when the British Navy consumed over a million gallons of juice. Indeed, French writers have claimed recently that their navy was not defeated as a result of British skill or bravery, but by their lemons.

With increasing recognition that scurvy could occur on land and, in particu-lar, after a serious outbreak of the disease in a London prison when potatoes were omitted from the diet, it came to be generally accepted that the universal cause was a deficiency of the diet. In 1830, John Elliotson (1791–1868), a lecturer in a London hospital and subsequently Professor of Medicine at London University, gave the following explanation:

> Scurvy is a purely *chemical* disease.... [E]ach part of the system is ready to perform all its functions but one of the external things necessary for its doing so is taken away. This is very different from some other diseases ... in the case of diabetes it is not that the body is overloaded with an excessive supply of sugar ... but that the functions of the body which form urine are diseased.... Give the man with scurvy fresh greens twice a day and he at once becomes well.[2]

Twelve years later, George Budd (1808–82), a professor at King's College, London, gave a series of lectures on 'Disorders arising from defective nutri-ment'. He said:

> It is astonishing that scurvy should still prevail in our prisons, where it might be prevented with certainty by any of the cheapest and most abundant of our succulent vegetables.... The history of our navy abounds with instances that scurvy is not produced by the use of salt, by cold, or by the various other influences to which it has been vaguely ascribed, but simply by prolonged abstinence from succulent vegetables and fruits.[3]

He went on to provide an alternative to Lind's theory that wet weather had been responsible for sailors developing scurvy more quickly on cruises that began in early spring than on those beginning at the end of summer.

The element, whatever it may be, which the vegetable juices furnish, and which is the true preventive of scurvy, is expended slowly. The better a person has been supplied with it, the longer he can subsist without it. We have an analogous fact in the prolonged abstinence from food that animals which have much fat can maintain. . . . The disease [scurvy] shows itself earlier in the voyages undertaken in Spring . . . than at the end of Summer when vegetables and fruits have been for some time abundant.

These ideas seem almost incontrovertible to a modern reader, but in fact they were to be disregarded and fifty years later were replaced by a totally different view of the disease. Reginald Koettlitz (1860–1916), the senior surgeon on the expedition led by Scott (1868–1912) expedition that set out for the Antarctic in 1902, wrote:

Scurvy is chronic ptomaine poisoning. . . . The benefit of the so-called anti-scorbutics is a delusion, as is the idea that some anti-scorbutic property has been removed from foods in the process of preservation. . . . [T]hat goods are scurvy-producing by being . . . tainted is practically certain.[4]

This volte-face was stimulated by two series of observations. First, there had been a number of Arctic expeditions since 1850 where the use of lime juice had failed to prevent outbreaks of scurvy. (It was also in about 1850 that the Navy had begun to use West Indian limes instead of Mediterranean lemons for the production of citrus juice without realizing that their antiscorbutic value was less than that of lemons.) Second, it was known that Eskimos, who were living in areas with no fruit or vegetables, remained free from the disease, and that some British explorers stranded in the Far North had also survived for long periods eating only freshly killed raw meat. There was also the pervasive influence by this time of the successful explanation of other diseases as being caused by bacterial action. In fact, the men on Scott's first expedition suffered severely from scurvy, and they had to revise their ideas as to how to prevent it. The failure of lime juice was to be re-investigated in the next decade using new techniques, which are considered on p. 474.

Another problem that arose during the Victorian period was infantile scurvy. It was found to occur almost entirely among infants who were being fed on either the new proprietary foods being marketed as substitutes for breast milk, or on sterilized, or condensed, cow's milk. The affected children obviously found it painful to be touched, had swollen legs and also swollen gums when teeth erupted. When children died and autopsies were carried out, extensive haemorrhage was seen round the long bones and into the deep muscles. At first it was called Barlow's disease, and some paediatricians, in France and Germany particularly, classified it as a form of acute rickets, but there was gradual agreement after 1900 that it was the infantile form of scurvy.

PELLAGRA UP TO 1920

In 1755, François Thiérry (b. 1719), who had spent some time in Spain, published an account of an apparently new disease there, shown to him by Gaspar Casal (1679–1759), who had first seen it in 1720. It was characterized by dermatitis ('a horrible crust, dry, scabby . . . crossed with cracks'), and by dementia ('a maniacal melancholia'), and flared up each spring. When the disease later spread to Italy, it was called 'pellagra', and a third characteristic, diarrhoea, was added to physicians' descriptions. Casal had said that the victims were always poor people: maize meal was their staple food and they had very little meat or milk. The same was true in Italy, where the disease was first seen in the second half of the eighteenth century, and was becoming a serious problem in the first half of the nineteenth century.

As always, there were a variety of theories as to the cause of the new disease, but the dominant one was that it was somehow related to the consumption of maize. Maize was a New World plant that had been brought back to Spain by Columbus (1451–1506), and had only gradually been adopted in Italy as a major food crop from the middle of the eighteenth century. This coincided with the time of first appearance of the disease in Italy. In Spain, both the use of maize and the appearance of the disease had come earlier, and in countries where maize was not used the disease also was unknown.

A French physician, Théophile Roussel (1816–1903), writing in 1845, had said that the 'efficient cause' of the disease was damaged maize (*mais altéré*) and that the 'predisposing cause' was a diet that contained too little of animal substances. In 1865, a Mexican doctor, Ismael Salas, wrote his MD thesis on this subject, pointing out that pellagra was not a problem in his country despite maize having been their staple food for a millennium, and despite their peasants' very low intake of meat or dairy products. He attributed this to the national habit of soaking maize in a solution of calcium hydroxide (lime water) before cooking. This, he thought, had a disinfectant effect, whereas the baking of corn mush to polenta in the European style would leave it still contaminated with moulds and the toxins that they had produced.

It was accepted in Northern Italy that peasants could not afford a better diet with more animal products. The government's concern was therefore to try to ensure that the corn crop was well dried after being harvested, and inspected for mould before being stored. As the standard of living in Italy improved at the end of the century, the disease gradually disappeared, presumably because people could then afford a more varied diet.

In 1905, pellagra appeared as a new disease in the southern half of the USA, again amongst people who were eating maize meal, though usually their diet also included a roughly equal amount of wheat flour. Again, the sufferers had little animal food except for pork 'fat back', which was virtually all lard with a very small proportion of lean. This was a period when malaria and yellow fever were being shown to result from insect-borne infections, and at first this was also the dominant explanation for pellagra. (➤ Ch. 24 Tropical diseases) This hypothesis was apparently supported by a study showing that pellagra cases in a southern city were concentrated in areas where the houses had outdoor privies which were not efficiently screened against the entry of insects. (➤ Ch. 53 History of personal hygiene) J. F. Siler and his co-authors concluded that flies were carrying infectious material from the faeces of pellagrins and transferring it to the food of future victims.[5] (With hindsight, we can see that really all the investigators found was that the disease was associated with the part of town where there was poverty and all that went with it.)

Joseph Goldberger (1874–1929) and fellow US Public Health Service officers noticed that staff were never affected at orphanages or mental asylums where the inmates suffered. Then, where extra eggs and milk were supplied, the incidence of the disease greatly diminished. After a failure of the officers to infect themselves in some heroic experiments, and the production of scrotal dermatitis in convict volunteers put on a diet based on maize meal but no milk or meat, Goldberger concluded that the disease was due to lack of one or more unknown dietary factors.

BERIBERI UP TO 1910

This was described as 'the national disease of Japan', but became an increasing problem in many parts of South-East Asia in the second half of the nineteenth century. In adults, the disease was characterized by peripheral neuritis with particular weakness and loss of feeling in the legs, a weakening of the cardiac muscles that could lead to heart failure and, in some cases ('wet beriberi'), only a general oedema of the lower half of the body. In infants suckling from afflicted mothers, there was commonly sudden death from heart failure.

In 1882, a Japanese naval vessel was sent on a long training cruise for midshipmen. Of the 275 men aboard, over 60 per cent developed beriberi, and twenty-five died. Kanehiro Takaki (1849–1915), a naval surgeon who had been in Germany for post-doctoral training, noted how far the protein content of their diet had been below the German standard for servicemen. He proposed that the nitrogen-to-carbon ratio of the diet should be increased from 1:28 to 1:16. (In more modern terms, this corresponds to increasing the protein contribution from 10 per cent to 17.5 per cent of the total calories.) The authorities agreed to there being a duplicate voyage the following year, and the diet was modified by replacing part of the rice with barley, and the addition of beef, condensed milk, and tofu (soybean curd). This voyage was a great success, with no deaths, and the 3 per cent who did show signs of the disease admitted that they had not been consuming the full diet. Takaki believed that he had proved that the cause of beriberi was deficiency of protein in the diet. With hindsight, we can see that he had been misled by the contemporary lack of knowledge of the complexity of human nutritional requirements. To quote René Dubos (1901–82): 'Logic is an unrealiable instrument for the discovery of the truth, for its use implies knowledge of all the components of an argument – in most cases an unjustified assumption.'

Nevertheless, the problem in the Japanese army and navy was much reduced by the general adoption of modified diets, even though civilian doctors were not persuaded by Takaki's work. Indeed, further progress was to come from the Dutch colonies in Indonesia, where beriberi was endemic and a novel challenge for the European physicians there.

As with pellagra, it was first thought that the disease was due to infection by a bacterium, and specialists were sent from Holland to try to identify it. These bacteriologists tried to transfer the condition to a flock of chickens by inoculation. By good fortune, Christiaan Eijkman (1858–1930), in 1890, noticing that at one point even some of the uninoculated birds had developed polyneuritis, looked into the possibility of there having been a significant change in their husbandry. He found that the period in which polyneuritis was seen corresponded to the time when they had been fed a surplus from the patients' white rice, instead of the brown rice usually fed to chickens. Eijkman confirmed that this was indeed the significant change. Chickens fed on white rice developed polyneuritis, but recovered when their diet was supplemented with rice polishings (the outer skin removed when whole-grain, brown rice is milled or polished). This evidence was suggestive, but there was still no proof that fowl polyneuritis and beriberi were essentially the same disease and had the same cause. Eijkman could not conduct an experiment with humans that might deliberately induce a disease, but it was known that many prisoners in Java developed beriberi. He therefore persuaded a colleague to distribute a questionnaire to all the eighty-four prisons in Java, asking the incidence of beriberi, the physical characteristics of the buildings, and the type of rice used. The returns showed no relation between the age of the building, adequacy of ventilation or degree of overcrowding and the incidence of beriberi. However, the disease was a serious problem in 71 per cent of the prisons that reported using white rice and in only 3 per cent of those that reported the use of 'rough' (brown) rice.

Eijkman then had to return to Europe because of ill health, but he was convinced that beriberi was caused by a toxin present in white rice, for which nature had provided an antidote in the outer layer of the grain. Gerrit Grijns (1865–1944), Eijkman's successor in Java, went on to show that other foods such as beans could protect chickens from the bad effects of white rice alone, but the efficacy of all such supplements, including rice polishings, was destroyed by long autoclaving. He also demonstrated that a number of food components were *not* capable of providing protection.

Work in Malaysia, then under British control, confirmed the association of beriberi with the consumption of white rice. It also threw up a new finding. Indian workers in that country were essentially free from the disease even though they consumed milled rice. However, this had been produced by a different process, now called parboiling, but in the literature of the period called 'curing.' Essentially, brown rice was soaked for a period of 1–2 hours in water near its boiling point, then removed and steamed for a short period, and left to dry. After this, it was polished in the usual way. The process gelatinized, and thus hardened, the starch in the outer coat of the white rice. This made the polishing easier, with less breakage of grains, and reduced subsequent insect attack that was an important source of loss in hot climates. The processing gave the product a yellowed appearance and changed its flavour to some extent.

Henry Fraser (1873–1930) and A. T. Stanton (1875–1938) carried out a well-controlled experiment in the Kuala Lumpur lunatic asylum in 1905 which confirmed the difference between the two types of material in a randomly divided population. The immediate explanation was that the 'curing' killed or removed micro-organisms that made the white rice toxic. However, they later found that while chickens remained healthy on cured rice, if this material were extracted with hot alcohol, chickens eating the extracted material did develop polyneuritis; furthermore, the alcohol extract cured those on white rice. They reported their findings to an international conference in 1910, and concluded that white rice lacks 'some substance or substances essential for the normal metabolism of nerve tissue.... We believe that the method of estimating diets from the amounts of proteins, fats, carbohydrates and ash contained in them will require reconsideration.'[6]

ANIMAL MODELS AND THE VITAMIN CONCEPT

In 1904, Axel Holst (1861–1931), an experienced Norwegian bacteriologist working in Oslo, set out to study beriberi, which had started to occur in men on Norwegian sailing vessels after recent changes in their rations. He thought that using a mammal as the experimental model might give a picture closer to the human disease than that seen in birds. He chose guinea-pigs, and fed them on different kinds of flours baked into bread. The animals all died after approximately one month. On dissecting them, Holst was surprised to find haemorrhages in the ribs and hind legs. He called in Theodor Frölich (1870–1947), a paediatrician with experience of infantile scurvy, who concluded that they were indeed seeing experimental scurvy. In further trials, it was found that the haemorrhagic changes were prevented by giving supplements of cabbage leaves or lemon juice.

Further developments came quickly. In the next six years, at least three groups reported independently that young rats also failed to grow properly when fed on pure protein, fat, carbohydrates, and minerals, but responded to small supplements of materials such as whole milk or butter, yeast, and cod liver oil. And the prophecy was made by Casimir Funk (1884–1967) that at least four human diseases – scurvy, beriberi, pellagra, and rickets – would prove to be caused by dietary deficiencies of 'vital amines'. There was really no evidence that the organic factors would prove to be amines, so the term 'vitamins' was coined for these still hypothetical materials.

The hunt was then on to isolate the individual vitamins by fractionating the most active supplements and assaying their activity with animals fed on appropriate basic diets. When active crystals had been obtained, they were subjected to chemical analysis and study. Then the final step was for chemists to synthesize what they thought to be the structure of the natural vitamin, and to check the biological activity of the synthetic material.

The leader of one group that had been engaged in the problem of working out the structure of a particular vitamin wrote: 'now that this work is completed, involving the total effort and dedication of a whole group of chemists for 20 years, I suppose that it will all be reduced to one or two lines in a textbook.' And that must be its fate here too. Suffice it to say that within thirty years, eleven different vitamins had been isolated and synthesized. The deficiency diseases could then be seen in a new light.

THE ANTISCORBUTIC FACTOR

The antiscorbutic factor was crystallized from lemon juice, and named 'ascorbic acid' or vitamin C. It was found to be easily destroyed by heat and by contact with metals, particularly copper. This explained why Lind's concentrated syrup, prepared by evaporating lemon juice, had lost its activity. It was also found that fresh lime juice had little more than half the activity of lemon juice, and that the processing used to clarify the juice issued to the navy between 1850 and 1918 destroyed most of the initial activity. This explained the Victorian explorer's loss of faith in the juice.

It was also realized that most animal species, including dogs, rats, and different kinds of ruminants, synthesize their own ascorbic acid, and that raw (or very lightly cooked) meat when eaten in large amounts can supply enough of the vitamin to keep humans free from scurvy. Eskimos regarded seal liver and whale skin as being particularly antiscorbutic, and analyses have confirmed their high content of ascorbic acid. There is no reason now to believe that toxins are involved in the development of the disease.

BERIBERI

The anti-beriberi vitamin proved particularly hard to isolate. It was unstable both when heated and when in contact with alkalis. When finally obtained, it was also found to have a very complex structure, which included a ring made up of carbon, sulphur, and nitrogen atoms, and to be active in very small quantities. We need only about 1 milligram per day, which is equivalent to a total need of only 1 ounce over an average lifetime. Thiamin (or 'thiamine' in older papers), as it was called, was synthesized in 1937.

Chemical analyses for thiamin showed that traditional hand-pounding of rice left a grain that had retained significantly more thiamin than the whiter product obtained by machine milling. The growth of machine milling in the Orient after 1850 therefore explains why the disease became rampant there in the ensuing period. Analyses have also shown that parboiling of rice causes a diffusion of thiamin from the bran to the central endosperm. After subsequent machine milling and ordinary home cooking, it still contains about 1.0 parts per million of dry matter as compared to only one-fifth of that amount in ordinary white rice after cooking.

Nevertheless, the great majority of rice-eaters continue to prefer the flavour and appearance of ordinary, machine-milled white rice. The solution has been to fortify this material with a small proportion of thiamin-rich pills the size of rice grains. This has proved to be a successful public-health measure that has virtually eliminated beriberi in the Philippines and other severely affected countries, without undue expense, and without having to try to persuade people to change their habits.

Wheat-eaters receive rather more thiamin from their grain than do rice-eaters. However, it is now also the practice in most technically advanced countries for white wheat flour to be compulsorily enriched with a powdered mix of several vitamins and minerals to give it a composition more similar to that of whole-wheat flour. This may be unimportant for the majority of people who enjoy a diet based on a variety of foods. However, it has reduced the problems of alcoholics, many of whom do not bother to take regular cooked meals and formerly developed deficiency conditions such as beriberi and pellagra.

Although beriberi, like scurvy, seems now to be entirely a deficiency disease without a toxin playing any role, it would be wrong to go to the other extreme and belittle all 'toxin theories of disease', past or present. Epidemic dropsy, another disease that caused deaths in parts of India, has now been traced to a poison from a weed that can contaminate crops of mustard seed, which is used to provide cooking oil.

PELLAGRA

An animal model was not originally reproduced in rodents, but Goldberger found, in the 1920s, that dogs would develop a condition with at least a resemblance to pellagra. By 1935, it had been discovered that nicotinic acid, an already-known chemical, was a growth factor required by some micro-organisms, and it proved to give a response in dogs, and then also in human pellagrins. The name of the compound was changed to 'niacin' as the public were thought likely to be repulsed by anything apparently related to nicotine.

The full explanation of the distribution of pellagra in time and place is, however, complicated and still controversial. An organic molecule is defined as being a vitamin for a particular species if it needs to have it in its tissues but cannot make it for itself. In the case of niacin, most animal species, including humans, *can* make it – starting from tryptophan, which is a component of nearly all proteins. However, tryptophan has to be abundantly supplied for the conversion to take place to an adequate extent. It is relatively abundant in the proteins of animal foods, and at moderate levels in the proteins of most grains, but is particularly low in maize proteins.

This seems to explain the association between pellagra and a diet of maize with little in the way of animal protein, but not the freedom from the disease in Mexico and Central America. One phenomenon that contributes in these areas is that a compound in coffee beans decomposes to yield niacin when the beans are roasted. Another is that mature maize grain (like other cereal grains) has nearly all its niacin in a bound form that is digestible to only a very limited extent – probably 20–30 per cent. However, the traditional use of lime in the preparation of tortillas in this region makes the corn alkaline enough for the bound material to split to yield free, usable niacin. Anthropologists have noticed that North American Indian groups who traditionally used corn, but have not had access to lime, have used an extract of wood ash instead. This too is alkaline and has been shown to result in the liberation of free, usable niacin.

Finally, the best explanation for the epidemic of pellagra that began in 1905 in the USA is that this coincided with a development in maize milling. A new type of machinery could produce maize meal from which the germ had been removed. This increased the shelf-life of the meal because the ground-up germ fragments in the older type of meal contained most of the fat, and this went rancid. Unfortunately, it also contained most of the tryptophan. Previously, the proportion of wheat flour in the diets of people in the southern states presumably just kept people free from the disease, but the loss of the tryptophan from the maize germ tipped the balance against them.

Lastly, it must be added that a second vitamin, riboflavin, was also apparently present only at sub-optimal levels in most pellagrous diets in the USA, and in cases with some atypical symptoms this shortage was the prime cause of trouble. It was a common experience after the discovery of niacin's activity that a multiple-vitamin source such as yeast was a better long-term supplement for pellagrins than niacin alone.

VITAMIN A DEFICIENCY

The studies with rats by E. V. McCollum (1879–1967) in Wisconsin began in 1908 as an attempt to model a disease seen in cattle fed on restricted diets. He was able to demonstrate that young rats required a fat-soluble substance (called factor A) as well as an unknown water-soluble 'something' (factor B). The former was renamed vitamin A. Fractionation studies and twenty years of work in many countries led to the isolation and identification of the vitamin itself, and also of ß-carotene, which was present in leaves and could be converted to vitamin A by humans and most animals. It was also found that the night-blindness suffered by some sailors in the past was a specific effect of lack of this vitamin, and some of the traditional sailors' diets were certainly deficient in it. The condition was also common in Japan, where eating liver or fish oils, both rich sources of the vitamin, had been folk remedies.

More severe depletion of vitamin A was found to cause drying and ulceration of the cornea, particularly in young children. Often, this was followed by infection and irreversible blindness, and was in fact the most common cause of blindness in the Third World. Vitamin A supplements are cheap, but no more is needed for prevention than regular use of some green leafy food.

RICKETS

This had become an extremely common disease of one- and two-year-old children in northern industrial cities in both Europe and the USA by 1900. Many studies showed at least one-quarter of infants from low-income families had beaded ribs and twisted leg bones. The bones were soft from a lower than normal content of calcium phosphate. It appeared to be a disease associated with particular places rather than particular diets. In some areas, cod liver oil was a commonly used folk medicine. A number of doctors also used it as a solvent for elemental phosphorus, which they believed to be a true curative factor.

Experiments with dogs from 1908 to 1918 showed that puppies could become rachitic if fed on diets that supported growth. There was controversy over the conclusions to be drawn, since one group found that the condition could be prevented by taking the puppies out for exercise with no change in diet, whilst another group reported prevention by supplementing their diet without giving them exercise. Eventually, it was realized that dogs and humans needed to have in their tissues a small amount of a fat-soluble compound, for which cod liver oil was a rich source, and which was named vitamin D. However, it is now clear that the normal source of the substance for human-kind is a chemical reaction that occurs in the skin when it is bared to the ultraviolet rays of the sun. The problem with growing up in Victorian indus-trial cities was that the smoke from burning coal absorbed most of these rays, and that direct solar irradiation of any kind was limited in slums with high buildings and narrow streets. Although dosing with vitamin D is a ready means of prevention, rickets should truly be classified as an 'air pollution' disease rather than a nutritional problem. (➤ Ch. 27 Diseases of civilization)

NUTRITIONAL ANAEMIAS

Anaemia is best decribed as a condition in which the haemoglobin content of the blood is abnormally low. Since haemoglobin is the material carrying oxygen to the tissues, an anaemic person has a reduced capacity for physical activity. The blood is also pale, so that a white-skinned person has less of a pinkish tint to his or her appearance.

Chlorosis (literally 'the green sickness') was described as a disease of young women in many parts of Europe at least by the seventeenth century. It was characterized by loss of colour, lassitude, exhaustion on climbing stairs, palpitation of the heart, and sometimes by failure to menstruate. Thomas Sydenham (1624–89), in 1670, recommended iron filings suspended in wine as a treatment. Later, it was realized that blood contained iron, and that chlorotic blood contained less than normal.

In the second half of the nineteenth century, the condition became quite common in the USA as well as in Europe. It was commonly attributed to constipation and a resulting auto-intoxication from material going putrid in the large intestine. With the development of haematology, it became clear that it was a form of anaemia. Continued experience also confirmed that it responded to treatment with iron salts. R. Stockman (1861–1946) in 1895 reported studies of the condition, and of the iron content of a variety of diets. He concluded that women needed more iron than men because of their need to replace blood lost in menstruation, yet they ate less food and so consumed less iron. Meat was particularly rich in iron, but it was not thought suitable for refined young women to eat very much of it, since popular teaching regarded it as 'too stimulating'.

A recent article has drawn attention to the widespread practice of bloodletting, particularly in the USA in the period from 1850 to 1890, for many vague conditions such as headaches and failure to menstruate. (➤ Ch. 40 Physical methods) This virtually ceased after 1890, and may explain why the disease then became less obvious in the developed countries. There were also social changes that encouraged women to be more physically active, so that they developed larger appetites. However, in the Third World, iron-deficiency anaemia remains one of the most serious nturitional problems affecting not only women, but also children and males, working in the fields or infected with blood-sucking, intestinal parasites.

Deficiencies of folacin and cobalamin, the last two vitamins to be discovered, also lead to anaemia, but of a different type. In 1931, Lucy Wills (1883–1964) reported that the 'tropical anaemia of pregnancy', in which blood cells are macrocytic (that is, abnormally large, in contrast to the small cells seen in iron-deficiency anaemia), would respond to supplements of yeast, but not iron. The condition was limited to women on poor diets, and could be reproduced in monkeys. The active substance in yeast, folacin, was identified in the 1940s.

Another type of macrocytic anaemia has been called 'pernicious anaemia' because from its first characterization in about 1850 until the 1920s there was no effective treatment. It occurred equally in older men and women. It is now understood to be due to the body being deficient in cobalamin, or vitamin B_{12}, which was the last vitamin to be isolated, in 1948. Victims usually had an adequate supply of cobalamin in their diet, but the 'intrinsic factor' needed for its absorption from the gut and normally secreted by the stomach wall was no longer being produced. Before the vitamin was available, concentrated liver extracts, now known to be rich in the vitamin, had been injected directly into the tissues of patients. There can also be a direct dietary deficiency of the vitamin in people who have remained true vegans for long periods.

GOITRE

Another disease once common in Europe and the USA as well as the less developed parts of the earth is goitre, which is characterized by an obvious swelling of the thyroid gland at the front of the neck. It was usually found in areas remote from an ocean. Wherever there was a large incidence of goitre, there was a smaller, but more tragic incidence of cretinism, a condition from childhood of impaired physical and mental development. (➤ Ch. 20 Constitutional and hereditary disorders; Ch. 23 Endocrine diseases) A number of French workers in the 1820s and 1830s believed that goitre could be treated with iodine and that it was due to a deficiency of this element in the local food and water supply; however, the treatment lost favour, and we can now see that this was because of overdosing and its consequent toxic effects. August Hirsch (1817–94), in his encyclopedic *Handbook of Geographical and Historical Pathology*, described the iodine-deficiency theory as 'a short-lived opinion. . . . My further enquiries warrant the conclusion that . . . endemic goitre and cretinism have to be reckoned amongst the infective diseases.'[7]

Nevertheless, work in this century has confirmed that the conditions are caused primarily by a lack of iodine for incorporation into the thyroid's hormones. The fortification of common salt with traces of an iodine compound was begun in the 1920s in the mid-western region of the USA and has now proved to be a very successful preventive measure in many countries, although the problem persists, particularly in areas of Africa, Asia, and South America.

KWASHIORKOR

The World Health Organization has estimated that some 300 million children in the developing countries have growth retardation due principally to a combined dietary deficiency of energy and protein.

A more acute and life-threatening disease was seen by Cicely Williams (1893–1992) in West Africa in 1933. It was characterized by oedema, misery, and blackened patches of skin peeling off in a 'crazy pavement' pattern, leaving a raw, pink surface underneath. The local name 'kwashiorkor' was said to mean 'the sickness the older child gets when the next baby is born'. Typically, the affected child had been weaned early on to a maize gruel. Lives could usually be saved if this were supplemented with milk, so long as the condition were not too advanced. It is now realized that children in very similar conditions were being seen in many parts of the developing world, and that this disease, combined with marasmus, was responsible for a large proportion of deaths in children aged under five years.

In the 1950s, when worldwide attention was focused on the problem, it was thought at first to reflect a simple protein deficiency. Then it came to be recognized as being partly due to weaning foods being too bulky, so that energy intake was also a limiting factor. It also became evident that kwashiorkor often resulted from the stress of an infection superimposed on a condition of chronic undernutrition. Others have suggested that additional deficiencies, of fatty acids and trace minerals, have contributed to the problem.

GENERAL CONCLUSIONS

The great advances in the present century in the understanding of deficiency diseases came from the interacting activities of people in different disciplines: clinicians, epidemiologists, physiologists, biochemists, and chemists. The importance of integrating and advancing knowledge of nutritional problems has also led to the development of university departments and research institutes devoted entirely to these problems.

Although it may be that the individual nutrients required by humans have now been identified, the continual changes in methods of food processing and the addition of various chemicals as preservatives continually pose new questions for the study of food safety. In addition, it is clear that there are more subtle problems associated with affluence. There is good reason to believe that everyone who subsists long enough on a diet lacking vitamin C develops scurvy. Now there is equally good evidence that middle-aged men, and particularly those who smoke and take no regular exercise, are at a higher risk of heart attack and stroke if they also, over many years, have eaten a high-calorie, high-fat diet. Yet many, even a majority, remain healthy. It may be 'prudent' in our present state of knowledge for everyone to give up some of their pleasures, but do only a proportion of the population really need to modify their diets, and can they be identified in advance? Animal models are less useful here than in identifying the substances lacking in deficiency diseases, and further advances seem to require long and expensive human studies. (➤ Ch. 72 Medicine, mortality, and morbidity)

NOTES

1   H. R. Wagner, *Spanish Voyages to the North West Coast of America in the Sixteenth Century*, San Francisco, California Historical Society, 1929, pp. 244–6.

2   J. Elliotson, 'Clinical lecture', *Lancet*, 1830, 1: 649–55.

3   G. Budd, 'Disorders resulting from defective nutriment', *London Medical Gazette*, 1842, 2: 712–16.

4   R. Koettlitz, 'The British Antarctic Expedition: precautions against scurvy in the victualling of the "Discovery"', *British Medical Journal*, 1902, 1: 342–3.

5   J. F. Siler, P. E. Garrison and W. J. MacNeal, *Archives of Internal Medicine*, 1914, 14: 453–74.

6   H. Fraser, and A. T. Stanton, discussion on beriberi at the First Congress of Far Eastern Association of Tropical Medicine, quoted in R. R. Williams, *Towards the Conquest of Beriberi*, Cambridge, MA, Harvard University Press, 1961, p. 48.

7   A. Hirsch, *Handbook of Historical and Geographical Pathology*, London, New Sydenham Society, Vol. II, p. 196.

FURTHER READING

Aykroyd, W. R., *The Conquest of Famine,* London, Chatto & Windus, 1974.

Budd, G., 'Lectures on the disorders resulting from defective nutriment,' *London Medical Gazette,* 1842, 2: 632–6, 712–16, 732–9, 906–15.

Carpenter, K. J. (ed.), *Pellagra,* Stroudsburg, PA, Hutchinson Ross, 1981

——, *The History of Scurvy and Vitamin C,* New York, Cambridge University Press, 1986.

Guggenheim, K. Y., *Nutrition and Nutritional Diseases. The Evolution of Concepts,* Lexington, MA, D. C. Heath, 1981.

Hirsch, A., *Handbook of Historical and Geographical Pathology,* London, New Sydenham Society, Vol. II, 1885.

McCollum, E. V., *A History of Nutrition,* Cambridge, MA, Riverside Press, 1957.

Machlin, L. J. (ed.), *Handbook of Vitamins,* New York, Marcel Dekker, 1984.

O'Hara-May, J., *Elizabethan Dyetary of Health,* Lawrence, KS, Coronado Press, 1977.

Williams, R. R., *Towards the Conquest of Beriberi,* Cambridge, MA, Harvard University Press, 1961.

23

ENDOCRINE DISEASES

R. B. Welbourn

THE ROOTS OF ENDOCRINOLOGY
(Antiquity to 1905)

Endocrinology is the branch of biological science and clinical medicine concerned with hormones and the organs that produce them in health and disease. The crucial events that led to its recognition took place between about 1890 and 1905, in which year the term 'hormone' was coined. Many ideas and discoveries dating from antiquity and apparently unrelated at first contributed to it.

Most of the organs and tissues that form the endocrine system were recognized over one hundred years ago. By about 1600, the gonads, pituitary, and adrenals had been described, and goitres were known to arise in the thyroid. The parathyroids, Leydig cells, islets of Langerhans, intestinal chromaffin cells, and parafollicular cells of the thyroid were discovered in the nineteenth century. Some other endocrine tissues have been recognized more recently. (➤ Ch. 5 The anatomical tradition)

The functions of all these organs remained speculative for centuries. In the eighteenth century, Albrecht von Haller (1708–77) of Berne and Göttingen described the thyroid, the thymus and the spleen as glands without ducts, pouring special substances into the circulation; and Théophile de Bordeu (1722–76) of Paris proposed that all organs of the body discharged 'emanations' into the blood.

INTERNAL SECRETIONS

The first experiments supporting the concept of internal secretions were made on the testicles and the secondary sex characters. The effects of castration in animals and men, known from prehistoric times, were described by Aristotle (384–322 BC). In the eighteenth century, John Hunter (1728–93) of London observed that the secondary sex characters of castrated cockerels could be maintained by implanting the testes at other sites. In the next century, in 1849, Arnold Berthold (1803–61) of Göttingen confirmed Hunter's findings and concluded that the testes controlled the sex characters through the blood.[1] Hunter's and Berthold's work was very pertinent to much that followed, but was strangely overlooked until 1910.

Claude Bernard (1813–78) of Paris first observed internal secretion by an organ when he discovered, in 1855, that glucose was synthesized in the liver and secreted into the portal vein. He described this as internal to distinguish it from bile, which he termed the external secretion of the liver. The idea of internal secretions now had a firm basis.

THE ADRENALS

Also in 1855, Thomas Addison (1793–1860) of London described 'the constitutional and local effects of disease of the supra-renal capsules'.[2] The clinical features included debility and bronzing of the skin. The adrenals were destroyed by tuberculosis, metastatic carcinoma or, in one case, atrophy. Addison's work attracted much attention and the syndrome was named after him. Soon Charles Édouard Brown-Séquard (1817–94) in Paris found that adrenalectomy in animals was fatal and concluded that the adrenals were essential to life. However, adrenal insufficiency was not then accepted as the cause of Addison's disease.

THE THYROID

Goitre and cretinism had been treated with marine products for centuries and had been attributed to iodine deficiency, but nothing definite was known of their causes. (➤ Ch. 22 Nutritional diseases) In 1873, William Gull (1816–90) of London described 'a cretinous state' supervening in adults that was later named myxoedema.[3] Surgeons sometimes needed to remove the whole of the thyroid gland to relieve obstruction of the trachea and oesophagus by goitres. In 1883, Theodor Kocher (1841–1917) of Berne found that most patients so treated had developed 'cachexia strumipriva', which was likened to cretinism in children and to myxoedema in adults.[4] Felix Semon (1848–1921) of London proposed that these states were all associated with absence or degeneration of the thyroid. A myxoedema committee chaired by William Ord (1834–1902) in London investigated reports of many patients and the effects of thyroidectomy in animals. In the 1850s, Moritz Schiff (1823–96) in Switzerland had observed that experimental thyroidectomy caused fatal tetany, and in 1884 he found that death could be prevented by grafting the thyroid into the abdomen. Victor Horsley (1857–1916) of University College London then undertook thyroidectomy in monkeys and observed muscular twitchings and convulsions at first, and myxoedema later. He concluded that the effects of thyroidectomy in patients were due to arrest of thyroid function, endorsing Semon's view, and in 1888 the committee concurred. The parathyroids had been described in humans by Ivar Sandström (1852–89) of Uppsala in 1880, but it was not until they were studied physiologically in the 1890s by Eugène Gley (1857–1930) in Paris, and by others, that the acute effects of thyroidectomy were recognized as due to their simultaneous, inadvertent removal. Tetany sometimes followed thyroidectomy in patients for the same reason. (➤ Ch 42 Surgery (modern))

Excessive thyroid secretion was soon proposed as another cause of disease. Exophthalmic (toxic) goitre had been described by Caleb Parry (1755–1822) of Bath in 1825, and later by Robert Graves (1795–1853) and Carl von Basedow (1799–1854). In 1884, Ludwig Rehn (1849–1930) of Frankfurt-am-Main reported relief of both toxic symptoms and dyspnoea by thyroidectomy, and suggested that overactivity of the thyroid was responsible for the toxicity. In 1893, William Greenfield (1846–1919) of Edinburgh described hyperplasia of the thyroid in this condition, but the idea of hyperthyroidism remained controversial.

ORGANOTHERAPY[5]

In 1889, an extraordinary claim was made by Brown-Séquard, then aged 72 and internationally respected. He had earlier proposed the intravenous injection of sperm to prevent senility, and now claimed that he had rejuvenated himself mentally and physically with injections of canine testicular extracts. This announcement was viewed with contempt by most scientists, but stimulated great interest in internal secretions. In 1893, he claimed that administration of extracts from the testicles and other tissues were beneficial in many serious diseases. Bovine testicular extracts were particularly effective.

Brown-Séquard proposed that lack of secretions caused specific diseases and that important therapeutic effects could be obtained from the products of the appropriate animal organs. This was a valid hypothesis that could have been tested. Instead, it was accepted uncritically by many, and 'organotherapy' was exploited for forty years.

Endocrinology, which began to emerge at this time, was confused with it and, as a result, 'suffered obstetric deformation at its very birth'.[6] Clinical endocrinology took many years to achieve respectability. (➤ Ch. 11 Clinical research)

486

TREATMENT OF MYXOEDEMA

In 1889, treatment of myxoedema by transplantation of thyroid tissue from a sheep was attempted, but without success. Two years later, however, George Murray (1865–1939) of Newcastle upon Tyne injected an extract of sheep thyroid into a woman suffering from myxoedema. He had solid scientific grounds for doing so, but was probably prompted by Brown-Séquard's organotherapy. The patient recovered, and others reported favourably. In 1892, however, oral therapy with sheep thyroid proved equally effective and was adopted widely for the treatment of hypothyroidism.

ADDISON'S DISEASE AND ADRENALINE

In the 1880s and 1890s, atrophy of the adrenal cortex, which left the medulla intact, was recognized in many patients with Addison's disease. It was suggested that the disease, like myxoedema, resulted from deficiency of an internal secretion.

In 1893, George Oliver (1841–1915) of Harrogate prepared extracts of tissues, intending to study them physiologically. He found an adrenal extract that appeared vasoactive by mouth, and hoped that it might prove effective in Addison's disease. Seeking more critical assessment, he took a sample to Edward Schäfer (1850–1935) at University College London, who found (much to his surprise) that, when injected intravenously into dogs, it caused a brisk rise in blood pressure. Oliver and Schäfer found that the extract was derived from the adrenal medulla, which is composed of nervous tissue, and that it caused arteriolar constriction and rapid, forcible beating of the heart. This discovery attracted great interest and, in 1897, an active constituent, named 'adrenaline' in England and 'epinephrine' in the United States, was isolated by John Abel (1857–1938) and Albert Crawford (1869–1921) in Baltimore. Soon it was identified as a catecholamine, and was synthesized. It was the first secretion of a ductless gland to be characterized chemically. Unfortunately, it was ineffective in Addison's disease; however, in 1896, William Osler (1849–1919) relieved one patient with a glycerine extract of adrenals administered by mouth. Transplantation of canine adrenal tissue was ineffective. (➤ Ch. 7 The physiological tradition)

DIABETES MELLITUS AND THE ISLETS OF LANGERHANS

Aretaeus of Cappadocia (AD 81–c.138) described diabetes (Gk, syphon or pipe) as a 'melting down of the flesh and limbs into urine'.[7] Mellitus (L, sweet), was added later because the urine tasted like honey. Diabetes was usually fatal, especially in young people. Diabetes insipidus (another disease) was described in the eighteenth century.

In 1673, the Swiss Johann Brunner (1653–1727) observed that a dog suffered from thirst and polyuria after removal of its pancreas and spleen. A century later, in 1788, Thomas Cawley (*fl.* 1778–88) found pancreatic calculi in a diabetic; and in 1884, Friedrich von Frerichs (1819–85) of Berlin described other pancreatic lesions in some patients. The same year, two Frenchmen, Xavier Arnozan (1852–1928) and Louis Vaillard (1850–1935), found that ligation of the pancreatic ducts led to atrophy of the acinar tissue, while the islets, previously described by Paul Langerhans (1847–88) in Berlin, remained intact. In 1890, Joseph von Mering (1849–1908) and Oskar Minkowski (1858–1931) of Strasbourg found that diabetes followed total pancreatectomy in a dog. Minkowski then prevented the disease by reimplanting a portion of the excised pancreas. In 1893, Édouard Hédon (1863–1933) of Montpellier found that diabetes developed when he removed such a graft, and postulated an internal secretion by the pancreas. The same year, Gustave-Édouard Laguesse (1861–1927) of Lille suggested that it arose from Langerhans' islet cells.[8] He introduced the term 'endocrine' to distinguish their function from that of the exocrine acinar cells, and the hypothesis that lack of an internal secretion from the islets caused diabetes was now widely supported. An attempt to treat a diabetic by transplantation of the pancreas of a sheep was unsuccessful.

GONADECTOMY

At about this time (1870s–1890s), surgical ablation of the gonads was undertaken therapeutically with no firm rational basis, although some effective results were achieved. In 1872, Robert Battey (1828–95) of Augusta, Georgia, removed the ovaries for painful amenorrhoea. The operation was practised irrationally and widely for various other diseases, but fell into disrepute. In 1893, William White (1850–1916) of Philadelphia advocated orchidectomy for prostatic hypertrophy, because the testes promoted growth of the normal prostate. In 1895, George Beatson (1849–1933) in Glasgow undertook oophorectomy for advanced breast cancer, with regression of the growth in one case.[9] (➤ Ch. 25 Cancer)

HORMONES

In the nineteenth century, the nervous system was thought to co-ordinate most bodily functions, and Bernard considered that it maintained *la fixité du milieu intérieur*.[10] Ivan Pavlov (1849–1936) laid stress on nervous reflexes, but at the end of the century, internal secretions were seen to contribute also.

In 1895, Schäfer supported this view.[11] All tissues, he wrote, took up materials from the blood, metabolized them, and returned them to the circulating fluid. Certain glands (liver, pancreas, and kidney), provided with ducts, had important external and internal secretions. Other glands (thyroid, adrenals, pituitary) had internal secretions only. (Schäfer and Oliver had just obtained a vasoactive extract from the pituitary.) Schäfer foretold that internal secretions would prove important therapeutically. He did not mention organotherapy, and stressed that the nervous system mediated the effects of gonadectomy.

In 1902, William Bayliss (1860–1924) and Ernest Starling (1866–1927), Schäfer's successors at University College, made a seminal discovery when they found that acid, introduced into a denervated loop of jejunum, caused a brisk secretion of pancreatic juice. An extract of jejunal mucosa injected intravenously had the same action, but acid similarly injected had no effect. These findings required the operation of a chemical, not a nervous reflex, and Bayliss and Starling proposed the name 'secretin' for the hypothetical chemical messenger.[12] They conceived it as a product of the intestinal mucosa, conveyed by the bloodstream to the pancreas, where it stimulated the exocrine secretion. It represented a new class of substances, not adequately described by the term 'internal secretion'. In 1905, Starling proposed the name 'hormone' (Gk, to excite), and this was adopted generally.[13]

For some years, workers debated the precise nature of hormones and their relations with enzymes, general metabolites, drugs, toxins, antitoxins, and vitamins, all of which had some similar properties. In 1915, Bayliss expressed the view that prevailed eventually. Hormones were produced in particular organs, passed into the blood current, acted as chemical messengers, and influenced cell processes in distant organs. They provided chemical co-ordination of the organism, working side by side with that through the nervous system.[14]

ENDOCRINOLOGY

Bayliss's reference to 'cell processes' reflected the concept of metabolism and the role of enzymes, which had emerged in the previous century, and the recent rapid development of biochemistry. Chemical co-ordination by hormones and the glands that secreted them was the unifying concept of endocrinology, although the term 'endocrine', introduced in 1893, came into general use only about twenty years later. (➤ Ch. 8 The biochemical tradition)

It was now necessary to identify new hormones and their glands or tissues of origin, to study their physiology, pathology, and related clinical syndromes, and to devise methods of investigating and treating them. All these aspects were closely interrelated, and the methods that had proved productive already were employed increasingly. The active principles in extracts were often called 'factors' at first, and were only designated 'hormones' when physiological roles had been assigned to them.

THE GROWTH OF ENDOCRINOLOGY

Much research, at first in Europe and North America and later worldwide, resulted in slow, solid progress, often frustrating, but occasionally illuminated by brilliant highlights. In 1903, Artur Biedl (1869–1933) of Vienna wrote the first book on internal secretions, which was published in English in 1912 with over 1,200 references.[15] Many workers in the field won Nobel prizes, the first being Kocher (1841–1917) in 1909, for his work on the thyroid.

The ease and speed with which progress was made varied greatly for different glands and hormones, and was related to advances in other fields of science. Organic chemistry, biochemistry, physiology, pharmacology, biophysics, microscopy, histochemistry, immunology, cellular and molecular biology, and their application to clinical science contributed most. (➤ Ch. 6 The microscopical tradition; Ch. 10 The immunological tradition)

NORMAL FORM AND FUNCTION

The parathyroids were accepted as endocrine glands when, in 1909, it was found that tetany, after parathyroidectomy, was accompanied by hypocalcaemia, and that both were relieved by injection of parathyroid extract or calcium. The gonads were admitted after 1910, when Hunter's and Berthold's work came to light (see p. 484) and when comparable experiments were undertaken with the ovaries. Gastrin (gastric secretin), which stimulates gastric acid secretion, was obtained from the stomach, while renal extracts were found to raise the blood pressure and to stimulate erythropoiesis. However, these were not accepted as hormones until much later. Apart from the pituitary and the adrenals, both of which had two parts, each gland was long thought to secrete one hormone.

The effects of adrenaline were found to be similar to those of sympathetic nerve stimulation, and the postganglionic nerves were called 'adrenergic'. Then, in 1911, Walter Cannon (1871–1945) described how adrenaline, a hormone, was secreted by the adrenal medulla in response to anger and fear, and prepared the body for 'fight or flight'.[16]

Iodine proved essential to normal thyroid function, and a thyroid hormone, which controlled general metabolism, was purified in 1914. In the 1920s, it was identified as tetraiodothyronine (an amino acid), was synthesized, and was named 'thyroxine' by Charles Harington (1897–1972) of University College London.

In 1921, after many trials and tribulations, insulin was extracted from the beta cells of the islets of Langerhans by Frederick Banting (1892–1941), Charles Best (1899–1978), John MacLeod (1876–1935), and James Collip (1892–1965) in Toronto.[17] Insulin, a peptide hormone which plays the major role in regulating carbohydrate metabolism, revolutionized the treatment of diabetes. Evidence for pancreatic glucagon, an insulin antagonist, was obtained in 1923.

Schäfer's and Oliver's pituitary extract came from the posterior lobe (neurohypophysis) and was later (1928) found to contain two hormones, vasopressin, which is antidiuretic, and oxytocin, which stimulates uterine contractions and the ejection of milk. Total hypophysectomy in animals proved fatal, but subtotal removal caused atrophy and functional impairment of the thyroid, adrenal cortex, and gonads. A growth-promoting extract was obtained from the anterior pituitary by Herbert Evans (1882–1971) at Berkeley in 1921. In the next two decades, this lobe was found to secrete several peptide and protein hormones, and to play a leading role in regulating somatic growth and lactation, by means of growth hormone and prolactin, respectively. Its other hormones stimulated growth and secretions of the thyroid (thyrotrophin), the adrenal cortex (corticotrophin), and the gonads (gonadotrophins). These last were of two types: follicle-stimulating hormone and luteinizing hormone. In the male, the same two hormones promote spermatogenesis and stimulate the interstitial (Leydig) cells of the testes, respectively. In 1931, Langdon Brown (1870–1946), working in London, described the anterior pituitary as 'the leader in the endocrine orchestra'.[18]

The sex hormones, secreted by the gonads, control sexual development and reproduction, and in the 1930s all were identified as steroids, synthesized, and found to restore secondary sex characters in hypogonadism. The Leydig cells secrete an androgen, testosterone. Graafian follicles in the ovaries produce oestradiol and other weaker oestrogens, and the corpora lutea secrete progesterone. The placenta was found to secrete gonadotrophins and female sex hormones.

Adrenocortical extracts were obtained in the 1920s, and the active principle was named 'cortin'. In 1930, a more potent preparation, obtained with lipid solvents, maintained the lives of adrenalectomized animals and of patients in Addisonian crisis. The main function of these hormones, which are steroids also, was thought to be the control of electrolyte metabolism, and a weak mineralocorticoid, deoxycorticosterone, was extracted in the 1930s. The chemical quest was led by Edward Kendall (1886–1972) at the Mayo Clinic and by Tadeus Reichstein (b. 1897) in Switzerland.[19] In the 1940s, however, cortin was found to influence carbohydrate and protein metabolism principally, and to protect the body from stress. In the late 1940s, a potent glucocorticoid, cortisol, and its natural analogue, cortisone, were extracted and synthesized. Cortisone was used clinically in 1948, and revolutionized the treatment of adrenal insufficiency and some other diseases. Small quantities of weak androgens and oestrogens are secreted by the adrenals also.

In 1926, Cannon had coined the term 'homeostasis' to describe the process by which the body maintains its internal stability.[20] He recognized the role of hormones in regulating metabolism, but regarded the autonomic nervous system, which is partly controlled by the hypothalamus, as paramount. The crucial role of hormones became apparent when, in the 1930s and 1940s, a system of negative feedback control was discovered, whereby the trophic hormones of the pituitary are regulated by the main products of its target glands. For example, thyrotrophin is regulated by thyroxine and corticotrophin by cortisol.

The study of metabolism in general was much facilitated by the use of radiosotopes, the first of which, radioiodine, had been introduced in 1938 to investigate thyroid functon. Four important hormones had now been discovered, whose balanced actions control general cellular metabolism. Insulin and cortisol are vital, while thyroxine and growth hormone are essential to health, but not to life. In 1952, a second thyroid hormone, triiodothyronine, was discovered.

Other hormones, working in concert, regulate particular physiological systems. Blood pressure and the metabolism of salt and water are closely interrelated and under the control of at least five hormones:

1 noradrenaline was identified as the adrenergic neurotransmitter by Ule von Euler (b. 1905) of Stockholm in 1946;
2 renin, a renal pressor agent, suspected in 1898, was forgotten and rediscovered in 1932 by Harry Goldblatt (1891–1977) of Cleveland, Ohio;
3 angiotensin (a powerful pressor agent) formulation is stimulated in the blood by renin;
4 aldosterone (found in 1952–55), the secretion of which is stimulated by the adrenals is a strong mineralocorticoid, which acts mainly on the kidneys;
5 vasopressin is controlled by osmoreceptors in the hypothalamus.

Calcium metabolism is controlled by parathyroid hormone, cholecalciferol (vitamin D3), which is synthesized in the skin, and calcitonin. This last, a product of the thyroid parafollicular C cells, was found later (1962–64) and proved less important.

In 1953, in Cambridge, two unrelated, major achievements contributed much to endocrinology. First, Frederick Sanger (b. 1918) analysed insulin; and analysis of many other peptides and proteins soon followed. Some of the smaller peptides were synthesized also, and synthesis of the larger ones began in the 1960s. Second, James Watson (b. 1928) and Francis Crick (b. 1918) described the structure of DNA and gave a great impetus to molecular biology and genetics.

Hormones had long been measured by insensitive bioassays, but chemical methods had recently been introduced for thyroid hormones and for the steroids. In 1959, in New York, Solomon Berson (1918–72) and Rosalyn Yalow (b. 1921) invented a radioimmunoassay for insulin, which made its measurement much simpler and more sensitive. In the 1960s and after, similar assays were developed for other peptides and proteins, and eventually for most hormones. These developments revolutionized endocrine research and clinical endocrinology. An immunoassay, however, does not necessarily reflect biological activity, and sensitive microbioassays were developed for research purposes later.

Control of anterior pituitary secretion was more complicated than at first thought. In the 1930s, secretory cells had been discovered in the hypothalamus, and in the 1950s and 1960s these were found to produce hormones. Two (vasopressin and oxytocin) passed along neurons to the neurohypophysis. Both are small peptides and were synthesized and used clinically in the 1950s. Other regulatory factors are conveyed to the anterior pituitary in a vascular portal system, discovered in the pituitary stalk by Geoffrey Harris (1913–72) of Cambridge. Most of these are stimulatory, or 'releasing', and are regulated in turn by negative feedback mechanisms involving the secretions of the pituitary and of its target glands. Two factors are inhibitory, namely somatostatin and dopamine, which regulate the secretion of growth hormone and prolactin, respectively. Most of these factors were identified as hormones, and were synthesized in the 1970s and 1980s. All but dopamine are small peptides. Several hypothalamic hormones were soon found to have important clinical implications. Higher centres in the brain, especially the limbic system, also control hypothalamic hormones. If the anterior pituitary is the leader, the hypothalamus is the conductor of the endocrine orchestra.[21] It is composed of neurons, but secretes hormones, and forms part of a diffuse neuroendocrine system, whose properties led to extension and modification of the original concepts of hormones and of endocrinology.

Since the discovery of secretin, insulin, and glucagon, evidence had accumulated that the gut contained a diffuse gastro-enteropancreatic endocrine organ, of which the pancreatic islets and the chromaffin and other epithelial cells formed important parts. Many endocrine cells had been found there, and their products – many peptides and a few amines – were identified.[22] About a dozen, including secretin, gastrin, and glucagon, were designated as hormones, although only insulin is vital. The gut emerged as the largest endocrine organ in the body, rivalling only the hypothalamus in complexity. Everson Pearse (b. 1916) of London pointed out in 1966 that its cells had similar properties to those of the anterior pituitary, adrenal medulla, thyroid C cells, and certain other epithelial cells. These, together with the hypothalamus, posterior pituitary, and parathyroids form the neuro-endocrine system.

Many gut hormones were also found elsewhere, especially in the hypothalamus. Some are blood-borne chemical messengers in the original endocrine sense, some are paracrine (local) hormones, acting on neighbouring cells, and others are neurocrine (synaptic) neurotransmitters, like acetylcholine and noradrenaline. Some hormones act in more than one way at different sites and in different circumstances. Somatostatin, for example, first found in the hypothalamus as an endocrine hormone, is paracrine in the gut and elsewhere, inhibiting the release of many peptides and other secretions. Other related chemicals, such as prostaglandins and peptide growth factors, have not yet been integrated within the neuroendocrine complex.

By the 1970s, many newly discovered features of hormonal synthesis, storage, release, transport, and modes of action could be described in general terms. For example, two main modes of action were discovered: peptides, proteins, and catecholamines interact with receptors on the cell membrane, while steroids and thyroid hormones form complexes with receptors in the cytoplasm. With improvements in biotechnology in the 1970s and 1980s, the pace quickened, and developments in molecular genetics led to the synthesis of hormones, including insulin and growth hormone, by recombinant DNA technology, with important clinical applications.

ENDOCRINE DISEASES

Hormones were soon found to influence metabolism. The general metabolic rate, for instance, was increased by adrenaline and varied with thyroid function. Disturbances of endocrine function were recognized, along with nutritional and genetic disorders, as causes of metabolic diseases. These are not mutually exclusive, and other disorders, including renal disease and trauma, were later found to alter both metabolic processes and endocrine function.

MECHANISMS

Three main types of endocrine disturbance were found, namely hypofunction, hyperfunction, and dysfunction, in that order. All glands are affected in at least one of these ways, and some in all three. Diseases of glands that secrete several hormones exhibit many complex combinations of features.

Hypofunction results from failure of glands to secrete their normal products, and numerous causes, both primary and secondary to diseases of other glands, have been identified. In the nineteenth century, destruction of the adrenals by tuberculosis and by tumour was described by Addison, and the effects of thyroidectomy were recognized by Kocher. In the 1900s and 1910s, compression of the pituitary by tumour, its destruction by an infarct, and menopausal degeneration of the ovaries were described. Iodine deficiency was confirmed as the principal cause of goitre and cretinism. Soon after, hypopituitarism was found to cause secondary atrophy and hypofunction of the target glands. Later, hypersecretion by these glands and therapeutic administration of their products were found to inhibit the pituitary and the hypothalamus. In 1956, Deborah Doniach (b. 1912) and Ivan Roitt (b. 1927) in London discovered autoimmune disease as a cause of thyroiditis, and later it was found to be a major cause of other endocrine diseases. In the 1950s and 1960s, enzyme defects, due to inborn errors of metabolism, were recognized as causes of goitrous cretinism and adrenal virilism. Finally, resistance of tissues to hormonal action was identified as a cause of apparent glandular insufficiency.

Hyperfunction is excessive secretion of the normal products of glands. The main lesions were identified as tumours and hyperplasia, although many different names, including struma, were used to describe them at first. Most neoplastic lesions of the endocrine glands were eventually classed as benign adenomas or malignant carcinomas. Hyperplasia may result from overstimulation by a pituitary hormone, a functional response to excessive demand, or genetic causes. Some tumours of endocrine glands are functionless. Functioning tumours usually secrete autonomously, benign adenomas producing normal hormones in excessive amounts. Carcinomas, on the other hand, often secrete hormones in several forms, some normal, some abnormal but with similar functions, and some inactive.

Dysfunction results from hyperplastic or neoplastic lesions secreting hormones that are uncharacteristic of their cells of origin. Dysfunction was found to arise in two main ways: first, the gonads and adrenal cortex, which secrete steroids, give rise to tumours or hyperplastic lesions that produce hormones characteristic of other glands (for example, androgens from the adrenal or ovary); and second, Neuroendocrine tumours may secrete the normal amine or peptide products of any neuroendocrine cell. Corticotrophin or vasopressin, for instance, may arise from epithelial tumours of the bronchus. Noradrenaline and other neurotransmitters may be secreted by tumours as pathological endocrine agents. All these tumours came to be called 'ectopic' or 'paraendocrine', and their secretions 'inappropriate'.

In 1903, Jacob Erdheim of Vienna (1874–1937) described a patient with multiple endocrine disorders. In the 1950s and 1960s two syndromes of multiple endocrine adenopathy (or neoplasia) were recognized in New York, both of which are genetically determined. (➤ Ch. 20 Constitutional and hereditary disorders) The parathyroids are hyperplastic in all cases. In one type, described by Paul Wermer (1898–1978), the islet cells and the pituitary are also affected. The other, described by John Sipple (b. 1930), includes phaeochromocytomas of the adrenal medulla and medullary cancer of the thyroid.

INVESTIGATION

Until about 1930, the diagnosis of endocrine disease was made mainly on clinical grounds, on the basis of clinicopathological correlations and on nonspecific chemical tests, including blood and urinary glucose and calcium. Qualitative analysis gave way to quantitative measurements, and static assays were replaced by dynamic assessments of the effects of stimulating and inhibitory factors. The glucose tolerance test for diabetes was an early example. Measurement of basal metabolic rate, developed in the 1910s, provides an index of thyroid function, and metabolic-balance studies were used to investigate hyperparathyroidism and other metabolic diseases. In 1928, Selmar Ascheim (1878–1979) and Bernhard Zondek (1891–1967) of Berlin developed an important biological assay of urinary gonadotrophins for the diagnosis of pregnancy. Bioassays of other hormones, however, were of little help in early disease, when they were needed most. Radioiodine in 1938 revolutionized the investigation of thyroid disease, and other isotopes were later used for this and other glands.

Chemical measurement of hormones and their metabolites followed. These included thyroid hormones in the 1940s, and adrenal steroids and catecholamines in the 1950s. Electrolytes were measured by flame photometry. Radioimmunoassays and related procedures were adopted for clinical purposes in the 1960s, and have been used increasingly. They improve greatly the diagnosis and management of endocrine disease. Knowledge of the interrelationships of the glands is used to test their functions in response to manipulation of the endocrine environment. X-rays had been used for the anatomical diagnosis of pituitary and thyroid diseases since the 1900s, and before long calcified adrenals were seen in Addison's disease. Many advances in radiographic technique have been applied to the endocrine glands, with great benefit. (➤ Ch. 36 The science of diagnosis: diagnostic technology)

Surgical exploration and biopsy of glands were undertaken often in the early days but have been largely abandoned, except for needle aspiration of the thyroid, as other diagnostic methods have improved.

TREATMENT

By the turn of the century, natural products, surgical operations, drugs and hormone replacement therapy had all been used effectively to treat thyroid disease. Radiotherapy for pituitary tumours soon followed in 1907. All these therapeutic modes continue to be used as alternative or complementary methods for diseases of all the endocrine glands.

Reliable treatment of many deficiency states followed the discovery and synthesis of hormones and the preparation of analogues. The highlights were insulin (1922), sex hormones (1930s), cortisone (1948), and recombinant peptides (1980s). Transplantation of endocrine glands from animals was useless. Human grafts were used later on a small scale, but with little or no benefit, to treat thyroid, adrenal, parathyroid, and gonadal deficiency, and diabetes. All except pancreatic transplantation were abandoned when effective replacement therapy was found.

Treatment of hyperfunction requires surgical operations, radiotherapy, and drugs. Surgery provided the only effective treatment for toxic goitre until the 1940s, and has always played a major part in the treatment of pituitary, islet cell, gonadal, parathyroid, and adrenal lesions. Surgeons who developed special skills in the surgery of these glands obtained the best results. Radio-iodine was first used therapeutically for thyroid diseases in 1942. Drugs which blocked the secretion of hormones, or which antagonized their actions on the tissues, were developed later. (➤ Ch. 39 Drug therapies)

Hormones used pharmacologically were very effective for some non-endocrine diseases, including rheumatoid arthritis (1948), and for contraception (1957). Medical and surgical endocrine therapy have also played important roles in the treatment of cancer of the breast and prostate.

STATUS OF CLINICAL ENDOCRINOLOGY

The prestige of clinical endocrinology depended on the successful treatment of endocrine diseases and on the effective use of hormones for other purposes. The subject was long plagued by confusion with organotherapy, but in 1917 a few endocrinologists in the United States formed the Association for the Study of Internal Secretions and started a journal entitled *Endocrinology*. They did not have an easy time, however, and the 1920s proved critical. In 1923, just after the introduction of insulin, some scientists thought little more of endocrinology than of organotherapy. Starling, however, predicted that endocrinology would provide a growing frontier in medical science, based on biochemistry and genetics.[23] Effective stimuli to hormone production would be found, more deficiency states would be recognized, and other hormones would be extracted, analysed and synthesized, and then used for replacement therapy. Finally, the growth of the secretory cells would be promoted or suppressed.

Within the next few years, hyperparathyroidism, phaeochromocytomas and hyperinsulinism were recognized and cured. The central role of the pituitary also became apparent, and the sex hormones arrived on the scene. In the

1930s, endocrinology was accepted as a reputable discipline. In 1941, a new *Journal of Clinical Endocrinology* was launched in conjuction with *Endocrinology*, which from that time published laboratory work only. By this time also, many endocrine societies and journals had been launched, and books on endocrinology were being published worldwide.

In the 1950s, when radioiodine, antithyroid drugs, and corticosteroids came into general use, successful and life-saving treatment of many endocrine diseases was clear for all to see, and the speciality of clinical endocrinology was firmly established. A few general surgeons soon devoted themselves to endocrine surgery and, in the 1970s and 1980s, formed associations of endocrine surgeons.

Steroids remained at the centre of interest for basic and clinical endocrinologists until the 1960s, when they gave place to amines, peptides, and molecular biology. This latest period has seen great changes in the discipline, widening of its boundaries, and further developments in its therapeutic possibilities. These trends seem likely to continue for some years to come.

CLINICAL SYNDROMES AND THEIR MANAGEMENT

THE THYROID GLAND: (1) SIMPLE GOITRE AND HYPOTHYROIDISM[24]

Deficiency of iodine was confirmed as the principal cause of simple goitre in 1918, when David Marine (1880–1976) in Cleveland, Ohio, used it successfully to prevent goitre. Iodine-deficient goitre is either endemic, mainly in mountainous areas, or sporadic. Deficiency is most marked when the need for thyroid hormones is greatest, especially during puberty, menstruation, pregnancy, and lactation. Deficiency impairs the synthesis of thyroxine, which in turn stimulates the secretion of thyrotrophin, causing compensatory hypertrophy and hyperplasia of the thyroid. When the need for iodine is reduced, or when iodine is restored, the gland undergoes involution. These processes result in simple goitre, although sometimes they cause single nodules or generalized multinodular goitres. Severe iodine deficiency is accompanied by hypothyroidism also. Thyroid nodules were often referred to as adenomas until the 1930s, when they were recognized as manifestations of faulty involution. In the 1940s, chemical goitrogens were identified in some foods and medicines, and found to cause sporadic goitres. In the 1950s, congenital enzyme defects were found as causes of goitrous cretinism.

In the nineteenth century, most goitres were treated with iodine, with benefit in early cases of endemic disease. Thyroid extract was employed similarly from 1895, with comparable results. Large-scale prophylaxis with iodine was introduced effectively in some goitrous areas. Patients who did not respond needed surgical relief and, by the turn of the century, operations by experienced surgeons were safe. Total thyroidectomy was abandoned, and bilateral partial resections were gradually adopted. Thyroid extract for the treatment of hypothyroidism was prepared commercially in the early 1900s. Thyroxine was introduced later, but treatment was uncertain until the 1940s, when reliable preparations were made. Synthetic thyroid hormones came into general use in the 1950s.

THE THYROID GLAND: (2) TOXIC GOITRE

Toxic goitre was named 'hyperthyroidism' by Charles Mayo (1865–1939) at the Mayo Clinic in 1907.[25] It is usually characterized by diffuse goitre, sometimes with exophthalmos, and also by nervous symptoms and tachycardia in young adults. In another form, described by Mayo's colleague, Henry Plummer (1874–1936), the patients are older, often have nodular goitres, are not exophthalmic, and suffer cardiac complications. Thyroidectomy was the first effective treatment, but the operative mortality was much higher than for simple goitre, and recurrence was common. By 1910, Thomas Dunhill (1876–1957) of Melbourne appreciated the need to remove sufficient thyroid tissue, and obtained the best results.

Iodine therapy had been used for toxic goitre, as for simple goitre, but with much less benefit. In 1923, however, Plummer found that, given pre-operatively, it lowered the basal metabolic rate to normal, and greatly reduced the operative mortality. Iodine with subtotal thyroidectomy became the standard treatment for toxic goitre for the next twenty years.

In 1942, radioiodine therapy was introduced, and the next year antithyroid drugs were first used effectively, either alone or as preparation for operation. Within a few years, thyroidectomy, radioiodine, and antithyroid drugs were all used and reduced the mortality of the treated disease almost to zero. Later, a beta-adrenergic blocking drug was found to relieve some acute features of hyperthyroidism very rapidly.

When thyrotrophin was discovered in about 1930, it was assumed that thyrotoxicosis was due to pituitary hyperfunction. However, in 1956, a pathological long-acting thyroid stimulator was found in the blood of thyrotoxic patients by Duncan Adams and Herbert Purves in New Zealand. Soon afterwards, when radioimmunoassay for thyrotrophin became available, levels were found to be low in these subjects, but high in those with hypothyroidism. Thyroid hyperplasia in hyperthyroidism is apparently caused by long-acting stimulating autoantibodies. The orbital lesions in exophthalmic goitre were found to be autoimmune also.

THE THYROID GLAND: (3) OTHER FORMS OF GOITRE

Struma lymphomatosa, one of several forms of thyroiditis, was described by Hakaru Hashimoto (1881–1934) in Japan in 1912. When in 1956 it was found to be an autoimmune disease, it was treated effectively with thyroxine, which suppresses the secretion of thyrotrophin.

Several forms of thyroid cancer have been known since the eighteenth century and were usually fatal. Early diagnosis, especially with fine-needle biopsy, has enabled many patients to be cured. Medullary cancer of the parafollicular C cells was found in 1968 to secrete calcitonin, which has no metabolic effects, but which provides a tumour marker.

THE PITUITARY GLAND: (1) PITUITARY TUMOURS AND SYNDROMES

In 1886 Pierre Marie (1853–1929) of Paris described acromegaly, which he attributed to pituitary insufficiency. It was soon found that acromegaly and giantism were often associated with pituitary tumours, and in about 1900 it was suggested that both were caused by excess of a pituitary growth factor.

In the 1900s, hypopituitarism, associated with pituitary tumours, was described. Children exhibit dwarfism and sexual infantilism, while adults suffer amenorrhoea or anaphrodisia. Large tumours cause headache and blindness. Obesity, an occasional feature, was attributed to hypothalamic disturbance, and diabetes insipidus (polyuria) to disease of the hypothalamus or posterior pituitary. Harvey Cushing (1869–1939) of Baltimore and Boston clarified the relationships between pituitary tumours and syndromes in 1912.[26] Two-thirds of adenomas were apparently functionless chromophobe adenomas, causing pressure effects, including hypopituitarism. One-quarter were chromophil (acidophil) adenomas, causing acromegaly or giantism. About 5 per cent were congenital cysts and caused hypopituitarism. Transcranial (Horsley, 1889) and transsphenoidal (Cushing, 1909) operations and radiotherapy (1907), to reduce pressure, often relieved headache and improved sight, and sometimes partially relieved acromegaly. There were, however, operative complications and deaths. Treatment of pituitary tumours continued to improve, and many acromegalic patients were soon treated for endocrinological reasons. In 1939, analysis of Cushing's large series showed that transcranial hypophysectomy and radiotherapy together provided the best results, and that most of such patients were well five years later.

Until 1932, a tumour secreting growth hormone was the only known manifestation of hyperpituitarism. In that year, however, Cushing proposed a syndrome of pituitary basophilism.[27] Corticotrophin was later found to arise in the basophil cells, and its tumours, which are considered on p. 507, were called corticotrophinomas. In the mid-1960s, some chromophobe adenomas, previously thought to be inactive and to cause hypopituitarism by compression of the normal gland, were found to secrete prolactin, which, in excess, inhibits gonadotrophins, causing hypogonadism and sometimes galactorrhoea. By the 1970s, prolactinomas proved to be the commonest pituitary tumours, and other rare types were recognized also.

Overt disease could be caused by microadenomas (up to 1 cm in diameter). Radioimmunoassay and radiography allowed many to be diagnosed and treated successfully at this stage. Cortisone facilitated great advances in pituitary surgery, and a transsphenoidal, microsurgical technique, developed in Europe and Canada in the late 1950s and 1960s, enabled surgeons to remove some of these tumours completely. Unfortunately, many larger tumours were still found and, although often relieved by operation, few of them were cured. Radiotherapy, however, had progressed also and provided another form of treatment. Drug therapy is sometimes effective for prolactinomas. Successful treatment of tumours restores normal metabolism, arrests disease, and reverses many clinical and pathological features.

THE PITUITARY GLAND: (2) HYPOPITUITARISM

In 1914, Morris Simmonds (1855–1925) of Hamburg described pituitary cachexia (Simmonds' disease) due to infarction of the gland. When hypopituitarism is partial, gonadal function usually fails first. Hypothyroidism was treated with thyroid extract, but hypogonadism could not be relieved until sex hormones were available in the 1930s. In 1939, Harold Sheehan (1900–88) of Glasgow found that postpartum haemorrhage was the commonest cause of pituitary infarction (Sheehan's syndrome). Cortisone provided a great therapeutic advance in the 1950s. Pituitary dwarfism requires growth hormone, but the animal product was ineffective in humans. Human growth hormone was unsatisfactory until the 1980s, when a recombinant form was synthesized and proved very effective.

Curable causes of gonadotrophin failure, due to inhibition by other hormones, include hyperthyroidism, prolactinoma, and Cushing's syndrome, which will be described on pp. 506–7. Fertility was restored in certain other cases by the use of 'fertility drugs'. Human follicle-stimulating hormone was used in Europe in the 1950s, and urinary gonadotrophins were employed later. In the 1960s, synthetic anti-oestrogens, which stimulate the secretion of gonadotrophins, were introduced in the United States and are sometimes effective.

Diabetes insipidus was relieved with posterior lobe extract for many years, and later with pure vasopressin.

DIABETES MELLITUS[28]

Diabetes is the commonest endocrine disease. Until about 1850, treatment was irrational and often harmful, and included doping with opium to dull the despair. Dietetic treatment was based on inadequate knowledge of the disease, and did not help. Some patients were overfed to restore weight and sugar that had been lost in the urine. Others, already emaciated, were starved to withhold the sugar that would be wasted. However, some mild, obese diabetics, who lost weight by reducing their intake of food, fared well.

The metabolic disturbances of diabetes were not understood until after 1921, when the discovery of insulin allowed them to be studied. It then became clear that protein and fat were mobilized and converted into glucose, which could not be burned or stored, with consequent hyperglycaemia, glycosuria, and ketosis, often resulting in coma and death. Insulin, secreted in direct response to the blood glucose level, is an anabolic, fuel-regulating hormone, which promotes storage of glucose as glycogen, increases synthesis of protein, and inhibits lipolysis and gluconeogenesis. In excess, it causes hypoglycaemia. Rational dietetic treatment involves limitation of carbohydrate, provision of sufficient protein, and regulation of fat to restore or maintain the appropriate weight. This often proved impossible until the introduction of insulin therapy by Banting and Best in 1922, when it was produced commercially and restored thousands of diabetics to health. This was the greatest advance in medical therapy since the introduction of antisepsis fifty years earlier.

Insulin is a peptide whose structure differs slightly from one species to another. Animal sources, however, especially bovine and porcine, proved suitable for humans, with few immunological problems. Regular injections, combined with strict diet, correct the metabolic disorder. Many preparations of insulin were developed and improved over the years, some designed for immediate effect and others to mimic the physiological supply. Later (in the 1950s), oral hypoglycaemic drugs were introduced, some of which stimulate the secretion of insulin.

Many causes of diabetes were discovered, but all revealed deficient production of insulin by the islets, its defective utilization by the tissues, inactivation by unknown factors, or increased secretion of antagonistic (diabetogenic) factors.

Two main types of diabetes were recognized, one primary or idiopathic, the other secondary to pancreatic, endocrine, or other diseases. The mechanisms involved in the secondary type were discovered first. The effects of pancreatic disease and pancreatectomy had been known for years. Then, in the 1930s, Bernardo Houssay (1887–1971) of Buenos Aires found that partial hypophysectomy in dogs, rendered diabetic by pancreatectomy, ameliorated their condition (the Houssay phenomenon), and a diabetogenic pituitary factor was postulated for some years. However, several known hormones, including growth hormone, thyroxine, and cortisol (which are secreted or controlled by the pituitary), adrenaline and glucagon, are diabetogenic when secreted in excess. Since diabetes is relieved when their secretion is restored to normal, the idea of a separate pituitary diabetogenic factor was dropped.

Primary diabetes affects two groups of patients: one with juvenile-onset, 'thin', or insulin-dependent diabetes mellitus; the other with maturity-onset, 'obese', or non-insulin-dependent disease. The latter is the milder form and can be controlled well with diet, with or without hypoglycaemic drugs. Insulin-dependent diabetes is the more severe form, and its cause was long obscure. Research in the 1970s and 1980s, however, identified the main lesion as autoimmune destruction of the islets, perhaps triggered by viral infection, in individuals who are genetically predisposed.

As patients lived longer with effective therapy, many with severe disease developed complications, particularly neuropathy, infections, and vascular disease, which cause hypertension, renal lesions, and retinopathy. Ablation of the normal pituitary was used in the 1950s to treat retinopathy, but was later replaced by local forms of therapy. Renal failure is treated by dialysis or transplantation. Regular dialysis is complicated by anaemia, requiring blood transfusions. A renal erythropoietic factor had been suspected in the 1900s, and then forgotten. In the late 1950s, however, a factor which stimulates the production of red blood corpuscles was found in the kidneys and named erythropoietin. Renal failure and nephrectomy lower the blood levels and cause anaemia. Recombinant erythropoietin, a complex glycoprotein, was prepared in the 1980s and used very effectively, obviating the need for blood transfusion.

The serious complications of diabetes are apparently due to inadequate therapy. Good control of the disease may be very difficult, but can be achieved in the highly motivated by continuous infusion of insulin at varying rates, determined by the blood glucose level, and the whole procedure may be automated. Although insulin was synthesized in 1964, human insulin was not available clinically until 1980, when a recombinant preparation was made commercially. It has little practical advantage over animal insulin. Islet cell transplantation and pancreatic grafting, which were reintroduced in the 1960s, when graft rejection was understood, are still imperfect, but hold out hope for the future.

THE PARATHYROID GLANDS[29]

Active parathyroid extracts were prepared in the early 1920s. In excess, they caused resorption of the skeleton and negative calcium balance. Osteitis fibrosa cystica, described in 1891 by Friedrich von Recklinghausen (1833–1910) of Strasbourg, exhibited these same features and was often associated with parathyroid adenomas. Their significance was unknown until 1925, when Felix Mandl (1892–1957) of Vienna removed an enlarged gland from such a patient, with rapid relief. Bone disease, hypercalciuria, high serum calcium, renal stones, and muscular weakness were soon recognized as features of hyperparathyroidism, which could often be cured by parathyroidectomy.

Until 1932, the disease had been diagnosed only in patients with bone disease, when Fuller Albright (1900–69) of Boston began to find hyperparathyroidism among patients presenting with stones. For the next thirty or forty years, many cases were diagnosed in this way, but the disease was still regarded as rare. Most patients responded well to operation, but some died later from renal failure and hypertension.

In the 1960s, routine screening for serum calcium often revealed hypercalcaemia, and many patients with minimal or absent symptoms were diagnosed. By 1965, it was estimated that one in every thousand members of the population suffered from hyperparathyroidism. The differential diagnosis of hypercalcaemia became very important, and sophisticated tests were developed. Radioimmunoassay was of little help until very recently. Most patients have small single adenomas, but in 1958 hyperplasia of all four glands was recognized in some 10 per cent of patients. Some of these have multiple endocrine adenopathy, with hyperfunctioning lesions of other endocrine glands also. Pre-operative localization of the lesions has been attempted by many methods, but experienced surgeons identify them best and cure nearly all patients with one operation.

Secondary hyperparathyroidism, with hyperplasia and severe bone disease, was recognized in azotaemic renal failure in 1934. It was treated with vitamin D or, when this failed, by subtotal parathyroidectomy, which was first used in 1960. Recently, more active analogues of vitamin D have reduced the need for operation.

GASTRO-ENTEROPANCREATIC TUMOURS

The gut secretes many hormones, but it rarely gives rise to functioning endocrine tumours. However, several types have been described, two of which are well known.

(1) *Insulinoma*. Soon after the introduction of insulin, overdosage in diabetics was observed to cause hypoglycaemia. A patient who became hypoglycaemic spontaneously was studied at the Mayo Clinic in 1927 by Russell Wilder (1885–1959), who suspected an insulin-secreting tumour of the pancreas. William Mayo (1861–1939) operated and found an advanced carcinoma, which indeed contained insulin. A benign insulinoma was removed success-

fully in Toronto two years later. Many such tumours have been reported since, most of them benign and curable by operation.

(2) *Zollinger-Ellison syndrome.* In 1955, Robert Zollinger (1903–92) and Edwin Ellison (1918–70) of Columbus, Ohio, reported two patients with recurrent stomal or jejunal ulceration, marked gastric hypersecretion, and non-beta islet cell tumours of the pancreas. Other cases were soon recognized, and the name 'Zollinger-Ellison syndrome' was adopted. The tumours were usually malignant, but grew slowly. In 1960, they were found to be paraendocrine, secreting large amounts of gastrin. Total gastrectomy was the only effective treatment in most patients until antihistamines (H2 antagonists), which inhibit the secretion of acid, were introduced in the 1970s. In the 1980s, benign extrapancreatic microgastrinomas, curable surgically, were found in some patients.

THE GONADS: (1) HYPOGONADISM AND SEX HORMONES

Primary hypogonadism, following castration, and the secondary type, due to pituitary tumours, were recognized early, and many other causes, including autoimmune disease of the gonads, were found later. In women, ovulation and internal secretion nearly always fail together, while in men, defective spermatogenesis is often the only feature.

In the early 1920s, unsupported claims were made that ligation of the vas deferens or transplantation of apes' testicles rejuvenated old men. However, no active testicular extract was found until the late 1920s, when androsterone, a metabolite of testosterone, was used therapeutically; androsterone was replaced by testosterone in 1935. Similarly, oestrone and oestriol, both weak oestrogens, were discovered and used before oestradiol, the principal ovarian hormone, which was introduced in 1936. Progesterone came into use at about the same time. All provide effective replacement therapy in hypogonadism and hypopituitarism, but rarely restore fertility. Progesterone was also used to prevent threatened abortion. In 1938, Edward Dodds (1899–1973) of London discovered stilboestrol, a synthetic, non-steroidal oestrogen, which soon largely replaced oestradiol. Oestrogens are used widely to retard the progress of osteoporosis after the menopause. This is popularly known as 'hormone replacement therapy'.

Androgens were sometimes used to promote protein anabolism, but virilization proved a serious drawback. Less virilizing synthetic anabolic steroids were then prepared and proved useful. They have been used extensively to improve muscular performance in many sports.

Contraception by the administration of hormones was achieved with some success in animals in Austria in the 1920s, and then forgotten. In the 1950s, Gregory Pincus (1903–67) in the United States pursued the subject and, by

1957, managed to suppress ovulation in women for as long as desired; the process was reversible, with oral synthetic oestrogens and progestogens. Within a decade 'the pill' in various forms was used effectively by millions of healthy women to prevent pregnancy.

THE GONADS: (2) SEXUAL ANOMALIES

Anomalies of sexual development, including various forms of hermaphroditism, have been known for centuries, the commonest being congenital virilizing adrenal hyperplasia. Two other anomalous states were recognized in the United States around 1940. Henry Turner (1892–1970) described in 1938 a syndrome in girls, and Harry Klinefelter (b. 1912) reported one in boys in 1942. Many other anomalous states were soon reported. Most of these are caused by abnormalities of the X and Y chromosomes, which result in numerous combinations of anomalies of the gonads and sexual organs.

THE GONADS: (3) BREAST AND PROSTATIC CANCER

Oophorectomy was used widely for a time after Beatson's report on advanced breast cancer, and about one-third of patients obtained worthwhile temporary remissions. Ovarian ablation by radiotherapy, however, introduced early this century in France, had similar effects and largely replaced operation. In the 1930s and 1940s, Charles Huggins (b. 1901) of Chicago discovered that prostatic cancer was stimulated by androgens and depressed by both oestrogens and castration, which often gave great relief for a time. In the 1950s, after the advent of cortisone, adrenalectomy and hypophysectomy were employed in both diseases to reduce additional sources of sex hormones. These were effective in about one-third of patients in whom relapse had followed ablation of the gonads.

In the 1960s, oestrogen and progesterone receptors were identified in the cells of those breast cancers that responded to endocrine therapy, and enabled appropriate treatment to be employed with confidence. From that time also, hormonal manipulation by medical means gradually replaced major surgical operations for advanced mammary and prostatic cancer.

THE ADRENAL CORTEX: (1) SYNDROMES OF HORMONE EXCESS

Carcinoma or hyperplasia of the adrenal cortex, with precocious growth and male sexual development in both sexes, or virilism in adult women, were reported in the eighteenth and nineteenth centuries. Carcinomas were known as hypernephromas. The condition was highlighted in 1905 by William Bullock (1868–1941) and James Sequeira (1865–1948) in London, and was named adrenal virilism or the adrenogenital syndrome. Some children were also obese.

In 1912, Cushing described a patient suffering from a 'polyglandular (or pluriglandular) syndrome', which included central obesity, hirsutism, and amenorrhoea.[30] The causative lesion, he thought, might be in the pituitary, the adrenals, the pineal, or the ovaries. In 1921, Charles Achard (1860–1944) and Joseph Thiers (1885–1960) of Paris described 'diabetes of bearded women', a similar syndrome with hyperplastic or neoplastic adrenals.[31] Tumours, when present, were usually fatal within a few years, but some were cured surgically.

THE ADRENAL CORTEX: (2) CUSHING'S DISEASE AND SYNDROME

In 1932, Cushing described more patients, like the one he had reported in 1912.[32] They were similar to those of Achard and Thiers, but some also had wasted limbs, ecchymoses, osteoporosis, renal stones, and pigmentation. At autopsy, many had small pituitary basophil adenomas, and some had adrenal hyperplasia, but none had adrenal tumours. Cushing boldly postulated that the pituitary lesion caused secondary adrenal hyperplasia. He named the condition 'pituitary basophilism', but it was more commonly known as 'Cushing's disease'. The term 'Cushing's syndrome' was applied later to include this disease and similar states caused in other ways.

The relationship between Cushing's syndrome and adrenal virilism was controversial, and some referred to a single 'suprarenal cortical syndrome'. Many patients with adrenal carcinomas have features of both. Albright, however, was convinced that the two conditions were 'entirely different and opposite'.[33] He attributed Cushing's syndrome to a hypothetical 'sugar hormone' and virilism to a 'nitrogen hormone'. This view was confirmed in the late 1940s, when excess of cortisone, a glucocorticoid, or of corticotrophin was found to cause Cushing's syndrome, but not virilism. Hyperfunction of the adrenal cortex, in which cortisol is secreted in excess, causes Cushing's syndrome, while dysfunctional hypersecretion of androgens causes virilism.

The role of the pituitary in Cushing's disease remained uncertain. It was suggested that the basophil adenomas secreted corticotrophin in excess, but no sensitive assay was then available to measure it. Pituitary irradiation was sometimes helpful, but half of all patients died within five years of the onset of disease. In the 1940s adrenalectomy was attempted for patients with hyperplastic glands, but proved fatal.

In 1949, however, after the advent of cortisone, James Priestley (1903–79) at the Mayo Clinic and others undertook radical adrenalectomy, with good results. Removal of single adrenal adenomas (Cushing's syndrome) was very effective, but most carcinomas were incurable.

Several drugs, which block the synthesis of cortisol, were introduced as definitive treatment of Cushing's syndrome, or as adjuncts to other methods, especially pituitary irradiation. In the late 1960s, corticotrophinomas were confirmed as the essential lesions in Cushing's disease. Most are microadenomas and are treated surgically with good results.

THE ADRENAL CORTEX: (3) CORTISONE REPLACEMENT THERAPY[34]

Treatment of Addison's disease improved somewhat in the 1930s, with the use of cortin, deoxycorticosterone (both parenterally), and sodium chloride; but life was still precarious. The arrival of cortisone (which was active by mouth) in 1948 was spectacular and provided the greatest therapeutic advance in endocrinology since insulin in 1922. Patients with Addison's disease were restored to health, and both adrenalectomy and hypophysectomy were undertaken safely. A few years later, aldosterone and an oral synthetic analogue improved matters still further.

In congenital virilizing adrenal hyperplasia, inborn enzyme defects block cortisol synthesis in various ways. Adrenal deficiency and excessive secretion of corticotrophin follow. The latter, in turn, stimulates alternative synthetic pathways, resulting in excessive secretion of androgens. Treatment with cortisone, first used in the 1950s, corrects the adrenal deficiency, blocks the oversecretion of adrenocorticotrophic hormone (ACTH), and permits normal sexual development.

THE ADRENAL CORTEX: (4) CORTISONE THERAPY FOR GENERAL DISEASE

Cortisone in pharmacological doses was found to be anti-inflammatory, and Philip Hench (1896–1965) at the Mayo Clinic treated patients with rheumatoid arthritis with great benefit. Cortisone is also anti-allergic and anti-fibroblastic, and advantage was taken of these properties to treat many general, non-endocrine diseases. It was described as a modern wonder drug. In large doses, cortisone causes serious complications, but synthetic analogues were developed which overcame some of the problems. Soon, far more patients with common general diseases were being treated effectively with these hormones than were the far fewer patients with endocrine disease. Corticotrophin or a synthetic analogue, instead of corticosteroids, are sometimes administered therapeutically to stimulate the secretion of cortisol.

THE ADRENAL CORTEX: (5) CONN'S SYNDROME

In 1955, Jerome Conn (b. 1907) of Ann Arbor described the syndrome of primary aldosteronism (Conn's syndrome), characterized by hypertension and hypokalaemic alkalosis. The commonest cause is a benign adrenal adenoma, which may be removed surgically, resulting in relief or cure.

THE ADRENAL MEDULLA

Soon after its discovery, adrenaline was used pharmacologically for local haemostasis and for the relief of asthma, allergy, and cardiac arrest. For a time, it was thought that adrenaline maintained the blood pressure and in excess caused essential hypertension.

Adrenaline was well known long before any pathological role was found for it. Tumours of the adrenal medulla and sympathetic ganglia were found in the nineteenth century, and various names were applied to them. Benign ganglioneuromas, usually in adults, were described in 1870. Phaeochromocytomas (paragangliomas) were reported in 1886, and neuroblastomas in 1899. These last, highly malignant tumours of infancy and childhood, were reported with spread to the liver by William Pepper (1874–1947) of Philadelphia in 1901, and with metastases to the skull by Robert Hutchison (1871–1960) of London in 1907.

In the 1920s, phaeochromocytomas were found at autopsy in patients who had suffered paroxysmal hypertension. They were found to secrete adrenaline, and hypertension and other symptoms were attributed to them. Some phaeochromocytomas were diagnosed in life and removed successfully, but the operative mortality remained high for forty years. In 1949, noradrenaline, the main cause of the hypertension, was found in many phaeochromocytomas. The tumours remained lethal, but many began to be diagnosed with the help of the histamine test (1945) and chemical measurements of the hormones and their metabolites (1957). Surgery provided the only hope of cure, but the operative mortality still remained high. In the 1960s and 1970s, however, the use of adrenergic blocking drugs before and during operation, together with blood transfusion, rendered surgery very safe. Some patients, however, still die from unrecognized tumours.

Ganglioneuromas rarely secrete hormones, and most are cured by operation. In the 1960s, however, neuroblastomas were found to secrete catecholamines, which provide tumour markers and allow some to be diagnosed early and cured.

ACKNOWLEDGEMENT

I am grateful to my former colleague, Professor Graham F. Joplin, for his critical review of this chapter.

NOTES

1   C. Barker Jørgensen, 'John Hunter, A. A. Berthold and the origins of endocrinology', *Acta Historica Scientiarum Naturalium et Medicinalium*, Edidit Bibliotheca Universitatis Havniensis, Vol. XXIV, Odense University Press, 1971.

2   Thomas Addison, *On the Constitutional and Local Effects of Disease of the Suprarenal Capsules*, London, Samuel Highley, 1855.

3   William Gull, 'On a cretinoid state supervening in adult life in women', *Transactions of the Clinical Society of London*, 1873, 7: 180–5.

4   Theodor Kocher, 'Ueber Kropfextirpation und ihre Folgen', *Arch. klin. Chir.*, 1883, 29: 254–337.

5   Merriley Borell, 'Organotherapy, British physiology and the discovery of the internal secretions', *Journal of the History of Biology*, 1976, 2: 235–68.

6   Herbert M. Evans, 'Present position of our knowledge of anterior pituitary function', *Journal of the American Medical Association*, 1933, 101: 425–32.

7   *The Extant Works of Aretaeus, the Capadocian*, ed. and trans. by Francis Adams, London, Sydenham Society, 1856, p. 338.

8   Gustave-Édourd Laguesse, 'Sur la formation des îlots de Langerhans dans le pancréas', *Comptes rendus à la Société de Biologie (Paris)*, 29 July 1893, 819–20.

9   George T. Beatson, 'On the treatment of inoperable cases of carcinoma of the mammae', *Lancet* 1896, 2: 104–7.

10 Claude Bernard, *Leçons sur les phénomènes de la vie communs aux animaux et aux végétaux*, Paris, Baillière, 1878/9, Vol. I, p. 113.

11 Edward A. Schäfer, 'Internal secretions', *Lancet*, 1895, 2: 321–4.

12 William M. Bayliss and Ernest H. Starling, 'On the causation of the so-called "peripheral reflex secretion" of the pancreas', *Proceedings of the Royal Society of London*, 1902, 69: 352–3.

13 Ernest H. Starling, 'The Croonian Lectures on the chemical correlation of the functions of the body', *Lancet*, 1905, 2: 339–41.

14 William M. Bayliss, *Principles of General Physiology*, London, Longmans, Green, 1915, pp. 706–34.

15 Artur Biedl, *The Internal Secretory Organs*, trans. by Linda Forster, London, Bale & Danielsson, 1912.

16 Walter B. Cannon and D. de la Paz, 'Emotional stimulation of adrenal secretion', *American Journal of Physiology*, 1911, 28: 64–70.

17 Michael Bliss, *The Discovery of Insulin*, Basingstoke, Macmillan, 1987.

18 Walter L. [Langdon-]Brown, 'Recent observations on the pituitary body', *Practitioner*, 1931, 127: 614–25.

19 Edward C. Kendall, *Cortisone*, New York, Scribner's, 1971.

20 Walter B. Cannon, *The Wisdom of the Body*, New York, Norton, 1932.

21 Walter Langdon-Brown, 'The birth of modern endocrinology', *Proceedings of the Royal Society of Medicine*, 1946, 29: 507–10.

22 Moreton I. Grossman, *A Picture History of Gastrointestinal Hormones*, Los Angeles, CA, VA Wadsworth Hospital Center, 1975.

23 Ernest H. Starling, 'The Harveian oration on "the wisdom of the body" ', *Lancet*, 1923, 2: 865–70.

24 Cecil A. Joll, *Diseases of the Thyroid Gland*, London, Heinemann, 1932; J. Howard Means, *The Thyroid and its Diseases*, Philadelphia, PA, Lippincott, 1948; Franz Merke, *History and Iconography of Endemic Goitre and Cretinism*, Lancaster, Boston, The Hague and Dordrecht, MTP Press, 1984.

25 Charles H. Mayo, 'Goiter with preliminary report of 300 operations', *Journal of the American Medical Association*, 1907, 48: 273–7.

26 Harvey Cushing, *The Pituitary Body and its Disorders*, Philadelphia, PA, and London, Lippincott, 1912.

27 Oliver Cope, 'The story of hyperparathyroidism at the Massachusetts General Hospital', *New England Journal of Medicine*, 1961, 274: 1174–82.

28 Bliss, op. cit. (n. 17).

29 Cope, op. cit. (n. 29).

30 Cushing, op. cit. (n. 28).

31 Charles Achard and T. Thiers, 'Le virilisme pilaire (diabète des femmes à barbe)', *Bulletin de l'académie de la médecine (Paris)*, 1921 (3rd series), 86: 51–6.

32 Harvey Cushing, 'The basophil adenomas of the pituitary body and their clinical manifestations (pituitary basophilism)', *Bulletin of the Johns Hopkins Hospital*, 1932, 50: 137–95.

33 Fuller Albright, 'Cushing's syndrome', *Harvey Lecture Series*, 1942–3, 38: 123–86.

FURTHER READING

Lisser, Hans, 'The Endocrine Society, the first forty years (1917–57)', *Endocrinology*, 1967, 80: 5–28.

McCann, S. M. (ed.), *Endocrinology, People and Ideas*, Bethesda, MD, American Physiological Society, 1988.

Medvei, V. C., *A History of Endocrinology*, Lancaster, Boston and The Hague, MTP Press, 1982.

Rolleston, Humphrey Davy, *The Endocrine Organs in Health and Disease with an Historical Review*, London, Oxford University Press, 1936.

Thorn, George W., 'Metabolism and endocrinology', Bowers, John Z., Purcell Elizabeth F. (eds), *Advances in American Medicine: Essays at the Bicentennial*, New York, Josiah Macy Jr Foundation, Vol. I, 1976.

Vague, Jean, 'Histoire de l'endocrinologie', in *Histoire de la médecine, de la pharmacie, de l'art dentaire et de l'art vétérinaire*, Paris, Société Française d'Éditions Professionnelles, Médicales et Scientifiques, Albin Michel/Laffont/Tchou, Vol. VII, 1980.

Welbourn, Richard B., *The History of Endocrine Surgery*, New York, Westport, CT, and London, Praeger, 1990.

——, 'The emergence of endocrinology', *Gesnerus*, 1992, 49: 137–50.

24

TROPICAL DISEASES

Michael Worboys

In the introduction to his manual of *Tropical Diseases*, first published in 1898, the British physician Patrick Manson (1844–1922) acknowledged that the term tropical diseases was 'more convenient than accurate' and noted that a volume on diseases peculiar to the tropics would only occupy six pages or so. None the less, he produced a volume of several hundred pages and in so doing effectively defined the content of the new specialism of tropical medicine. This concentrated on a limited number of diseases, most of which were vector-borne parasitic infections: malaria, yellow fever, trypanosomiasis (sleeping sickness), schistosomiasis (Bilharzia). Other diseases have featured to a lesser extent: leprosy, cholera, smallpox, plague, amoebic dysentery, yaws, dengue, leishmaniasis, filariasis, and beriberi and other nutritional diseases. These diseases were, in fact, those facing medical practitioners in tropical colonies which were not well covered in the European medical curriculum. In other words, tropical medicine was a residual category, synonymous with the additional requirements of imperial medical practice. As with every other specialism, the institutionalization of tropical medicine and the category of tropical diseases was the product of contingent medical and social factors. However, and again as with other areas of medicine, classifications of disease have come to be assumed to have been given by nature rather than history. (➤ Ch. 17 Nosology)

Until recently, historians also regarded tropical diseases as unproblematic, and followed tropical medicine in focusing on a narrow group of specific diseases and their control. While it is certainly true that the incidence of diseases like malaria and yellow fever have recently been confined to tropical latitudes, historically they were prevalent in temperate regions. It has been suggested that many so-called tropical diseases are, in fact, diseases of poverty, malnutrition, and insanitary conditions.[1] It has been argued further that the term 'tropical' has served an ideological function in associating the causes of these diseases with natural rather than social, economic, or political factors.[2] (➤ Ch. 15 Environment and miasmata; Ch. 18 The ecology of disease)

The dominant tradition in the history of tropical diseases has been to celebrate the discoveries of the aetiologies of the classic group of vector-borne parasitic diseases in the period 1870–1920. Little has been written about earlier periods, as these have been assumed to be characterized by ignorance and misunderstanding. This progressive and heroic genre had its origins in the legitimation of the emergent specialism of tropical medicine and has been sustained in autobiographies and biographies of leading figures during this century. A characteristic and revealing feature of this writing has been the predominance of military metaphors. Tropical medicine has been said to 'march' on in 'triumph', as its practitioners had to 'fight' and 'struggle' in a 'war' against 'foes' and 'enemies' of humankind.[3] The key generals in this campaign, and the enemies successfully engaged, are well known (Table 1). From the identification of causal agents and their modes of transmission, most histories move on to consider the application of discoveries in prevention, control, or therapy. There were many successful campaigns and many millions of lives were saved. Initially, efforts concentrated on protecting European colonists, and only later moved to protect the indigenous populations of tropical countries. These interventions by modern medical science and technology have often been portrayed as major benefits of imperial rule and, more recently, of technical assistance to the Third World. However, historians and other commentators have recently been less sanguine about the achievements of tropical medicine and disease-control programmes in tropical countries.[4] Many control campaigns were only successful in limited areas, and achievements were fragile and often had other costs. (➤ Ch. 58 Medicine and colonialism)

The concentration on disease-specific control or 'vertical' programmes in developing countries has now been questioned.[5] Greater priority is now being given to the broader development of health policies and medical services, or 'horizontal' programmes. While not in any way underestimating the importance of major tropical diseases, like malaria and schistosomiasis, it is now recognized that the disease burden of the tropics was and is much broader than just vector-borne parasitic diseases.[6] Recent estimates show malaria to be only the eighth largest cause of mortality in developing countries. In fact, there was and is a rapidly changing pattern of disease, in part due to the social and environmental changes wrought by imperialism and subsequent socio-economic and environmental changes. An important aspect of the history of tropical diseases is, then, that it forms a large part of the twentieth-century medical history of Third World countries; in other words, the medical history of most of humankind. (➤ Ch. 72 Medicine, mortality, and morbidity)

Table 1 Dates and discoverers of the pathogens and vectors of major 'tropical' diseases

Date	Discoverer	Parasite or vector identified
1872	T. Lewis (1841–86)	*Filaria sanguinis hominis*
1874	Hansen (1841–1912)	Leprosy bacillus
1875	Lösch (1840–1903)	*Entamoeba histolytica*
1876	Bancroft (1860–1933)	*Filaria bancrofti*
1879	Manson (1844–1922)	Mosquito vector of filariasis
1880	Laveran (1845–1922)	Malaria parasite
1897	Ross (1857–1932)	Mosquito vector of malaria
1899	Grassi (1854–1925)	Mosquito vector of human malaria
1900	Reed (1851–1902) and Finlay (1833–1905)	Vector and virus of yellow fever
1903	Bruce (1855–1931)	Protozoan and vector of trypanosomiasis
1905	Leishman (1865–1926) and Donovan (1863–1951)	Organism and vector of kala-azar
1915	Leiper (1881–1969)	Vector of schistosomiasis

The questioning of tropical medicine has also been inspired by changes in the history of science and the development of socio-historical approaches in the history of medicine. (➤ Ch. 70 Medical sociology) Thus, it is now routine to regard the notion of tropical diseases as the construction of a particular time and place, and to view tropical medicine as the institutionalization of a metropolitan medical perspective. The British, who had by far the largest tropical empire, pioneered and dominated both tropical medicine and its history. The bias towards the British and other European empires, and their colonies in Africa, Asia, and Latin America, means that the disease problems of large areas of South America, the Far East, and the Pacific are understudied. This is not because their problems were less serious, but because these countries did not have metropolitan interests defining their medical categories and later writing their medical history. In fact, the notion of tropical diseases came to the Americas from Europe, not from its own tropical regions.

The history of tropical diseases can be divided into three phases and these are considered in turn in this chapter. The first section deals with the period up to the beginning of the twentieth century, that is, before the notion of 'tropical diseases'. Recent work has shown that this should no longer be regarded as a dark age, but rather one where medical endeavour was structured in terms of medical geography and the notion of 'diseases in the tropics'. The second section looks at the decades around the turn of the century, which saw the elucidation of the aetiologies of the classical tropical diseases and the institutionalization of tropical medicine. The final section discusses the measures subsequently taken to control tropical diseases, which have to be taken in a wide context because of the interdependence of medical, social, and political factors. Indeed, the impact of these programmes was not just on pathogens and vectors, but on colonial and post-colonial states and society.

DISEASES IN THE TROPICS

Until the last decade of the nineteenth century, there were no tropical diseases, there were just 'diseases in the tropics'. This notion implied that the diseases experienced in warm climates were basically those found elsewhere in the world, but that they exhibited special characteristics due to climate and other variables. This was supported by dominant medical systems, in which few diseases were seen to be specific and most were the product of an interaction between mind, body, and the environment. The special diseases found in the tropics were explained in terms of the effects of climatic extremes, specific locations, and other variables on the forms and intensities of diseases, especially fevers. (➤ Ch. 19 Fevers) Thus, doctors practised their ordinary medicine in extraordinary tropical conditions, rather than, as later, tropical medicine as a special subject. The differences between diseases across the world were thought to be of degree, not kind. Voyages of exploration, the growth of trade, and population movements had themselves brought about a global exchange of diseases and a convergence of disease patterns across the world.[7]

From the fifteenth century, all European explorations and settlements in new worlds had been accompanied by a high incidence of fevers and high mortality. A common belief was that migrants experienced 'seasoning' as part of the body's initial process of adaptation to a new environment. Many of the non-European peoples came off worse in the exchange, with the best-known example being North America, where the Amerindian population was decimated by diseases carried by settlers from Europe and slaves from Africa. Indeed, until the late eighteenth century, North America was a relatively malign environment for both indigenes and immigrants; mortality rates amongst settlers remained significantly higher than European levels.[8] Mortality in the northern United States fell from the first half of the nineteenth century, but higher levels persisted in the southern states, producing a gradient of mortality from Canada to the West Indies. Also, there were no clear breaks in patterns of disease, with fevers and malaria major causes of death, and with all areas prone to yellow fever epidemics. Similar epidemiological gradients, both in space and time, were evident in North Africa, Southern Africa, and Australia. Only when a decline in mortality levels in both Europe and North America was experienced during the nineteenth century did any marked discontinuity or unique disease situation in the tropics emerge.[9] This was magnified by the growing number of Europeans in the region due to increased mercantile activity and imperial expansion. (➤ Ch. 52 Epidemiology)

Eighteenth-century medical discourses on diseases in the tropics were not about the tropics as such, but about the diseases of particular geographical locations. General manuals and advice only emerged in the second half of the eighteenth century, and even then were based mainly on experiences of one region. For example, James Lind in 1768 published (1716–94) *Essay on Disease Incident to Europeans in Hot Climates*, which was largely derived from West Indian experience. This became the standard English-language work and went through six editions, the last in 1808. It was replaced from 1812 by the work by James Johnson (1777–1845), *The Influence of Tropical Climates on European Constitutions*, which was based on Indian experience and also went through many editions. The main emphasis in these texts and in medical practice was on individual preventive, constitutional, and therapeutic measures; there was little interest in sanitation or the health of communities. (➤ Ch. 51 Public health)

During the eighteenth and most of the nineteenth centuries, fluctuating and high temperatures, humidity, and the sun were seen to be the main factors that weakened the constitutions of European races and increased their vulnerability to disease. In the eighteenth century, such conditions were said to unbalance the humours of the white races, with sweating, 'prickly heat', and leg ulcers being due to the blood throwing off 'fiery and acrid' elements. (➤ Ch. 14 Humoralism) From the mid-nineteenth century, similar symptoms were explained in physiological terms, with excessive heat said to disrupt normal circulation and nutrition, diminishing the metabolism of internal organs, especially the stomach and liver.[10] Given the abnormal, delicately balanced and weakened state of the constitution, much medical advice centred on avoiding shocks to the system and excesses of all kinds; essentially, a whole way of life was being set out, with regulations for clothing, diet, exercise, and 'the passions'.[11] (➤ Ch. 53 History of personal hygiene) There were also variations to standard treatments and precautions, especially bloodletting and the use of quinine as a specific against intermittent fever and malaria, the latter being advocated by an increasing number of practitioners.

The influence of the tropical climate on European constitutions was an issue at two levels: first, immediate practical advice on how best to survive; and second, human acclimatization and the future of imperialism – Could the white races colonize the tropics? From the 1840s, a number of views on the possibilities of tropical acclimatization were evident in medical circles.[12] These ranged from the view of Robert Knox (1791–1862) that each race belonged to a specific region and would degenerate elsewhere, to those who believed that there were no geographical limits to settlement. Further work is needed on the periodization and distribution of these views, but it seems that during the nineteenth century there was growing acceptance of the possibility of human adaptation to climate, place, and disease. This gained impetus from sanitarianism and its emphasis on control of the environment, and was advanced by doctors with tropical experience, although it was tempered by the growing belief that susceptibility to certain diseases was racially determined. The evident ability of Europeans to acclimatize helped illustrate and sustain notions of their racial superiority.

While the health of individuals remained the primary concern, from the mid-nineteenth century more attention was given to the health of European communities in the tropics. In this sphere, there was a direct transfer of the ideas and practices of European sanitary reformers to the tropics. Indeed, many regions of 'darkest' Africa and 'teeming' Asia seemed as malign as the working-class districts of industrial cities. (➤ Ch. 27 Diseases of civilization) The initial context of the transfer was the growing European military presence in tropical territories; this led to problems being approached, not as exotic or tropical, but in terms of military hygiene.[13] The Royal Commission on the Sanitary State of the Indian Army in 1859 concluded that high mortality was caused by poor drainage, housing, and ventilation, inadequate and impure water supplies, and the effects of nuisances, sewage, and animal wastes: exactly the causes of poor health in the Crimea, or in London, Paris, Berlin, or New York. Cholera was very important to this sanitary perspective: it was a disease endemic to India that had spread across the world, thriving in insanitary conditions at every latitude. Arnold has argued that the main differences between Europe and India regarding sanitary reform were cultural and political, not environmental. Political and logistic factors, not uncertainties over the disease environment and its management, inhibited state medicine in nineteenth-century India.[14]

While the main aim of medical and sanitary endeavours was to protect the health of Europeans, in some areas the concerns of the imperial rulers periodically extended to the indigenous population. For example, the Indian authorities waged campaigns against smallpox and cholera, with technologies imported from Europe, though adapted to local cultural circumstances. The environmentalism and anticontagionism of sanitarianism implied that targeting measures on European enclaves would be ineffective. However, in practice, this was all that could be managed; the sheer scale of the problem of 'cleaning up' India or Africa made anything grander unthinkable. Also, anticontagionism was tempered by racism and fear of 'the natives' and their diseases: social and physical separation was often justified on medical grounds.[15] The contrast was, of course, between clean Europeans, increasingly in control of their environment, and 'dirty natives' at the mercy of theirs. In fact, colonialists had little or no knowledge of health and disease amongst indigenous peoples. Views were based on prejudice and a limited picture derived from missions, mines, and plantations, and from the emergency measures taken during epidemics.

Towards the end of the nineteenth century, Europeans were increasingly confident that the tropics would soon cease to be 'the white man's grave'. This view was born of a recognition that European mortality rates had fallen, an achievement for which doctors claimed the main credit. However, medical understanding of diseases in the tropics was being increasingly recognized as weak, especially relative to the recent developments in aetiology and pathology associated with germ theories of disease. Tropical fevers were not well differentiated or managed; malaria had been identified as the main cause of European mortality in the tropics and was the most-feared affliction, although not feared sufficiently to ensure everyone used quinine prophylaxis. Sanitarianism remained strong amongst medical practitioners in India and other colonies, and there were few opportunities or incentives for clinical and pathological investigations in colonial medical practice.[16] At this time of perceived success of European medicine, the mortality rates of the indigenous population in many African and Indian colonies were actually increasing. It seems, moreover, that this was largely due to the accelerating rate of economic, social, and environmental change produced by imperial expansion.[17]

TROPICAL MEDICINE AND TROPICAL DISEASES

Patrick Manson, who invented the idea of tropical diseases as a distinct group of afflictions, was a British physician with experience in China who, in the 1890s, became the leading metropolitan authority on colonial medical practice and its problems.[18] His new category was adopted and sustained in the 1900s by the professionalizing activities of doctors associated with colonial medical practice and parasitology across Europe and North America. This group built the specialism of tropical medicine by linking the ideas, practices, and promises of germ theories of disease with the policies, agencies, and ideologies of late nineteenth-century 'constructive imperialism'.[19] (➤ Ch. 16 Contagion/germ theory/specificity)

In the 1870s, germ theories began to erode geographical and other divisions in pathology and aetiology, as unified concepts of disease and ideas of specificity gained ground. Medical understanding of fevers and infections was recast. Many fevers that had previously been defined in symptomatic or geographic terms were given a specific cause, and those that could not be so accommodated gradually faded from the medical canon. The whole concept of aetiology changed from being concerned with multiple causes to dealing with a single, or at least principal, exciting cause. For many years, the term 'germ' had no precise meaning; it implied anything from a protean life-form to a parasitic worm. Most of the published histories of germs and diseases deal with the evolution of ideas in disciplines like virology, bacteriology, mycology, parasitology, and immunology, and tend to assume that these subjects were given by nature, or emerged as clearly defined areas of knowledge and practice.[20] This is particularly misleading for the biomedical sciences, where work on germs and their effects dissolved old categories and created new ones. In the crucial period of transition, from 1870 to 1890, biomedical science was essentially undifferentiated, and there were various ways in which knowledge and practice might have been divided. Specialization was then the result of contingent factors, a situation exemplified by tropical medicine.

In the last quarter of the nineteenth century, many medical practitioners spoke as if all diseases, everywhere, were caused by germs and would be controllable by killing germs directly, or preventing their transmission. In the 1890s, Manson very much concurred with this view. Fifteen years earlier, he had shown that a filarial worm was the cause of elephantiasis (filariasis), and that the worm was transmitted by the bite of a mosquito. These findings fitted disease models in entozoology, a subject that dealt with the worm and fluke infections, and in subsequent years were interpreted as an example of an infectious germ theory. In the 1870s and 1880s, worm and germ theories were closely linked; for example, when Adolphe Laveran (1845–1922), a French military doctor, identified a protozoan as the parasite producing malaria in 1880, his finding was quickly assimilated into Pasteurian microbiology.[21]

The ideas and techniques of germ theories were quickly transferred and deployed outside Europe. The French colonial empire was rapidly incorporated into the Pasteur Institute network, with laboratories in Saigon (1891), Tunis (1893), Algiers (1894), and Nha Trang (1895). Similarly, the German bacteriologist Robert Koch (1843–1910) saw the world as his province, working in Egypt, India, South Africa, German and British East Africa, and the Dutch East Indies, not to mention a visit to Italy to investigate malaria. Germ theories and practices inspired the search for agents of disease and modes of infection in Latin and South America, Japan, Africa, India, and elsewhere.[22]

An important target and eventual success for germ theorists was the successful incorporation of malaria. Malaria had been an important example of anticontagionism, the name literally meaning 'bad air'. From the 1850s, symptomatic descriptions of the disease had been supplemented by pathological criteria. However, its aetiology remained a mystery and a battle-ground for anticontagionists and contagionists. In 1879, a malarial bacillus was reported, a finding quickly displaced by Laveran's protozoan and a definition of the disease in terms of the presence of parasites in the blood. Interest then focused on the mode and route of transmission, with air, water, and soil all suspected, but investigators could find neither parasites nor their 'spores' in any medium. In the 1890s, Manson offered insect-vector transmission as a way out of the impasse. He was not the first to propose this, but it was his suggestion that led Ronald Ross (1857–1932), an Indian Army surgeon, to start on his classic studies which resulted in the demonstration of the *Anopheles* mosquito-borne transmission of malaria in birds in 1897. This model was confirmed for human malaria by G. B. Grassi (1854–1925), in Italy, the following year. It was interpreted as another triumph for germ theories and one that also supported growing evidence for the role of insects and other arthropods in the transmission of infections.[23]

After 1900, a clear divide developed between germ and worm theories, which put bacteriology and parasitology on separate trajectories.[24] In 1899, Manson produced the first definition of a distinct category of tropical diseases as those caused by protozoan or more complex organisms, which were truly parasitic and whose transmission depended upon the completion of a life-cycle in a vector, or some other factor limited geographically to the tropics.[25] Manson stressed the difference between chance dissemination of germs in the environment or by contaminated organisms, and the role of insect-vectors as specific secondary hosts, in which developmental stages of organisms (mainly protozoa and helminths) occurred. This seemed to many observers an artificial distinction, as parasitic and geographically limited diseases were found at all latitudes, and bacterial diseases were very prevalent in the tropics. For example, malaria had been endemic in Europe, and in 1900 was still a serious problem in many of the countries of southern Europe.[26] Cholera and other diarrhoeal diseases, in which bacteria were implicated, were major problems in the tropics. Manson had moved from a position where all diseases in the tropics would turn out to be caused by germs and for which climate was irrelevant, to one where most important diseases there were climatically limited parasitic diseases.

Manson's characterization of the field was readily accepted as it became linked to post-graduate education, colonial medical policy, and research

Table 2 Major institutions of tropical medicine founded 1899–1914

Institution	Date
Liverpool School of Tropical Medicine, UK	1899
London School of Tropical Medicine, UK	1899
Chair of General Pathology and Tropical Diseases, Harvard University, USA	1900
Institut für Schiffs- und Tropenkrankheiten, Hamburg, Germany	1901
Institut de Médecine Coloniale, Paris, France	1901
Chair of Clinical Therapeutics and Tropical Medicine, University of New Orleans, USA	1902
Wellcome Research Laboratories, Khartoum, Sudan	1904
Robert Koch Institut, Berlin, Germany	1905
School of Tropical Medicine, Brussels	1906
Department of Tropical Hygiene, University of Amsterdam, The Netherlands	1912
School of Tropical Medicine, University of Tulane, USA	1913

opportunities. From the late 1890s, all the major imperial powers gave consideration to special training and research to improve the numbers and efficiency of colonial medical practitioners (Table 2). Special institutions were first established in Britain, at Liverpool in April 1899 and London in the following October. The London School of Tropical Medicine was established with state backing to provide postgraduate medical training for colonial medical officers, and the school became imperial government's centre for advice and research. The Liverpool School was backed by West African trading interests; it too offered courses, but concentrated more on promoting disease-prevention programmes and sanitary reforms in the colonies themselves. Other nations followed the British lead, and certain medical practitioners seized upon the opportunities of a politically important area of medical enterprise. In a number of countries, tropical medicine was developed within medical faculties or infectious-disease institutes. In Britain, which had the largest number of medical practitioners in tropical countries, the subject developed in a separate setting. This was largely because the patronage and new resources brought by the imperial connection allowed separate development when new appointments were resisted by medical schools. Thus, from being just a supplementary postgraduate subject, tropical medicine quickly became a separate and prestigious medical specialism in its own right. Its main constituencies were British colonial interests and the emerging international medical-science community. Indeed, this was one area of laboratory medicine where Britain was not laggardly.

Around the turn of the century the new tropical medicine was an important element in the ideology of progressive imperialism. The practical promise of the new specialism became incorporated into state policies and programmes and into the wider goals of 'constructive imperialism'.[27] The spectre of the 'white man's grave' had diminished, but it still haunted certain areas, especially West Africa, and governments and colonial interests continued to regard disease as a factor inhibiting colonial investment and trade. The mosquito–malaria theory was promoted as having great economic and political potential. It suggested new possibilities for the prevention and control of malaria, principally by eradicating mosquitoes or breaking human contact with them. This was seized upon as the key to making the tropics even safer for 'the white races' and, more importantly facilitating European mass settlement in tropical colonies. Thus, Manson could claim in 1897 that the study of tropical diseases 'strikes, and strikes effectively, at the root of the principal difficulty of most of these Colonies – disease. It will cheapen government and make it more efficient. It will encourage and cheapen commercial enterprise. It will conciliate and foster the native.'[28] In France, Émile Roux (1853–1933) observed in 1912 that, 'Thanks to [researchers in tropical diseases], lands that malaria forbade to the Europeans are opened up to civilization. It is thus that the work of a scientist may have consequences for mankind that go well beyond those of the conceptions of great statesmen.'[29] The political importance of the subject was evident in the number and intensity of the priority disputes over credit for particular discoveries, in what may be termed the 'scramble for Africa's diseases'.[30]

The new specialism continued to produce discoveries of the causes and aetiologies of important diseases. The insect-vector model, as Table 3 shows, brought rich rewards.

Table 3 The successes of the insect-vector model, 1900–20

Disease	Causal organism	Vector organism
yellow fever	virus	*Aedes* mosquito
sleeping sickness	protozoan	tsetse fly
Chagas' disease	protozoan	*Reduviid* bug
plague	bacillus	rat flea
relapsing fever	virus	body louse
schistosomiasis	helminth	snail

Major tropical scourges, like diarrhoeal diseases, which did not fit this model were ignored. The leaders of the new specialism quickly moved from a research orientation to the promotion of military-style campaigns aimed at destroying parasites and vectors, or breaking cycles of transmission. This developed from a metropolitan view of the tropics as a laboratory for experiments in disease eradication and regions to be taken over and secured. From Europe and elsewhere, these 'vertical', single-disease, control programmes were attractive and seemed feasible, though with hindsight, it is clear that few medical planners grasped the scale of the problems or the cultural diversity of the tropics. The term 'tropical' suggested a uniform 'natural' environment in which scientific expertise could be readily deployed and transferred. In many ways, the indigenous population was seen as part of that environment, so there was rarely any specific consideration of peoples and their socio-cultural circumstances.

Those European doctors actually practising in the colonies had a rather different conception of the diseases they encountered. Their knowledge and practice were structured around clinical and hygienic concerns, not with advanced science and technology. Colonial medical practice before 1914 dealt largely with Europeans and was often hospital based, while sanitary activity was still a limited venture, which received periodic boosts from epidemic threats.[31] Many doctors in the colonies continued to practise 'medicine in the tropics', rather than 'tropical medicine'. For example, Leonard Rogers (1868–1962), researching in India in the 1900s, continued to work from the symptom complex, not the parasite or vector.[32] In 1908, he published a volume with the pre-Mansonian title of *Fevers in the Tropics*, and as late as 1921 produced a volume on *Bowel Disease in the Tropics*. With respect to sanitary activity, colonial practitioners seem to have been initially less impressed with bacteriology than their metropolitan counterparts. However, after 1900, germ theories gave new impetus to contagionist measures and brought medical personnel into conflict with colonial political authorities who were reluctant even to consider intervention. In many colonies, the new contagionism firmly tied disease to 'tropical people', leading to the stricter segregation of towns. As noted earlier, these actions were not based upon detailed knowledge of the health of the local people, nor for that matter of their health-care systems and preventive practices. The only reason to take notice of indigenous medical practice was to dismiss it as primitive, super-stitious, and dangerous. (➤ Ch. 60 Medicine and anthropology)

The fortunes of the specialism of tropical medicine fell with the decline of 'constructive imperialism' after the first decade of this century. The problems encountered in tropical theatres during the First World War sustained activity in a number of countries, most notably the United States, where military personnel played a central role in tropical medicine.[33] (➤ Ch. 66 War and modern medicine) The economic crisis of the inter-war years and changed colonial relations had a marked effect. Metropolitan schools continued to train colonial medical personnel, but graduates now went off to serve in the colonial bureaucracy, not to push back the frontiers of knowledge and empire.

During the 1920s, the main orientation of local and metropolitan colonial authorities in tropical regions gradually switched from the health of Europeans to that of the indigenous population. This followed new policies of trusteeship and development. The first and necessarily partial picture of the disease problems of the indigenous populations began to emerge. In West Africa, for example, the diseases affecting the local people, in order of importance, were shown to be: malaria, hookworm, yaws, gonorrhoea, dysentery, pneumonia, tuberculosis, and tropical ulcer. Similar patterns were found else-where. The mismatch between the parasite-vector diseases favoured by metropolitan tropical medicine and incidence of disease at the periphery was striking. Also, many doctors and scientists began to explore the links between disease, nutrition, and other socio-economic factors.[34] (➤ Ch. 22 Nutritional diseases) One consequence of the new concern for the indigenous population was that medical services no longer enjoyed the special priority they had when European health was under threat, and medical departments had to take their place amongst the competing problems and resources of colonial states.[35]

World economic problems and the growing devolution of power to colonies led tropical medical institutions to become ever more marginal.[36] Yet after

1918, many were sustained by an important new sponsor of research and preventive programmes: the Rockefeller Foundation. The future of the London School was only assured in 1929 when it became part of the Rockefeller-supported London School of Hygiene in 1929.[37] During the 1920s, Rockefeller funds were especially important in yellow fever and malaria work, and provided, mainly through support of the School of Hygiene at Johns Hopkins University, the basis for the development of tropical diseases expertise in the United States.[38] (➤ Ch. 63 Medical philanthropy after 1850) Renewed impetus was given to tropical medicine during the Second World War by the problems met by troops stationed in tropical regions. The post-war development programmes of the colonial powers, the activities of the World Health Organization and other aid agencies, and the potential of new chemical insecticides continued this wartime impetus into the second half of the century.[39] (➤ Ch. 59 Internationalism in medicine and public health)

THE PREVENTION AND CONTROL OF TROPICAL DISEASES

In the early and middle decades of this century, tropical medical agencies mounted a number of control programmes against specific tropical diseases. Indeed, these 'vertical' programmes became a defining feature of metropolitan medical endeavour in and for tropical countries. They demonstrated the continuing influence of a vector-based construction of tropical diseases and the extent to which parasites and vectors loomed larger than people and general health in medical planning. Only comparatively recently have 'horizontal' programmes aimed at promoting health and protecting against a wide range of diseases found much support amongst tropical medical specialists.

MALARIA[40]

For most of the twentieth century, malaria has been the 'model' tropical disease. In 1900, it was the major cause of European mortality in the tropics, while in the inter-war period, its toll amongst indigenous peoples became only too evident. No other tropical disease has received as much investment in prevention and control measures.[41]

The basic model for all 'vertical' policies was that drawn up at the turn of the century by Ross for the extirpation of mosquitoes and the eradication of malaria. The plan was to prevent mosquitoes breeding by attacking their aquatic larval stage, either directly with chemicals or indirectly by denying them access to open water. The title of one of Ross's books – *Mosquito Brigades* – nicely illustrates the military assumptions underlying his proposed 'campaigns'. In practice, such measures were very similar to the kind of environmental improvements which had been advocated by sanitary reformers for decades, as they involved nuisance removal, street improvements, and piped water supply, alongside specific larvicidal and drainage schemes. Indeed, Ross noted that such 'vertical' programmes would have 'horizontal' effects. When mosquito control was planned for European settlements, it was backed up by individual preventive measures, such as quinine prophylaxis and the use of nets, screens, and other barriers.[42]

Despite the scientific prestige and imperial rhetoric associated with anti-malarial measures, metropolitan governments gave few resources and no lead in the matter, leaving it to local authorities. In many colonies, the lack of expertise, logistical difficulties, and likely expense meant that anti-malarial programmes were only adopted in the main towns where Europeans were threatened. A number of local campaigns did bring reductions in mortality and morbidity to Europeans and local people. British and American programmes tended to see malaria as a mosquito problem, whereas the French and Germans concentrated on attacking the parasite with quinine. Robert Koch initiated projects in New Guinea and German East Africa involving mass medication, although administrative problems eventually led the local medical authorities to work on the more tractable mosquito.[43] Beginning in 1901, the Indian government undertook an experimental project to see if attacking mosquito larvae would eradicate malaria from the notoriously unhealthy Mian Mir cantonment. This project was given a high profile and considerable investment, but failure was admitted in 1909. If malaria could not be eradicated from a single area, what hope was there for the whole of India? Alongside the fact that the programmes in no way matched the scale of the problem, there was a growing awareness of the complexity of malaria's epidemiology. What caused the disease to wax and wane was not clear, though with hindsight, it seems that the economic and social changes produced by imperialism were altering the human and physical ecology of areas, often to conditions more favourable for mosquitoes and the transmission of malaria.

The Rockefeller Foundation's malaria work began in the 1920s in the southern United States, Latin America, and southern Europe, and was later extended worldwide.[44] The programmes had two main consequences. The first was to aid the establishment of malaria research institutes and to promote the emerging specialism of malariology. The second was to reinforce the Anglo-American policy of mosquito eradication against the growing claims of quinine prophylaxis and treatment. Mosquito control in the 1930s was still primarily through 'campaigns' directed at larvae, although adult mosquitoes were increasingly being attacked with new insecticides, like pyrethrum.

Mosquito control seemed to become a definite practical possibility in the 1940s, with the invention of a new weapon against adult mosquitoes, the persistent insecticide dichloro-diphenyl-trichloro-ethane (DDT). This was marketed by the Swiss company Geigy as a delousing powder, though its wide-spectrum powers were quickly recognized, and both Britain and the USA began large-scale production. Hailed as one of the 'allies of mankind', DDT offered to banish all insect pest problems, improving both health and food supply globally. In the post-war years, DDT spraying was promoted as the single answer to the problem of malaria. Indeed, such was the confidence that in 1957 the World Health Organization adopted malaria eradication as one of its goals.[45] (➤ Ch. 39 Drug therapies)

Within a decade it was clear that such hopes were premature. There had been several successes – for example, in Sri Lanka – but the 1960s saw a resurgence of the disease, even in those places where eradication had been claimed.[46] The development of mosquito resistance to DDT, not to mention growing restrictions on its use because of environmental and health dangers, and the development of resistance in the parasites to anti-malarial drugs, led to a reassessment. The result was a recognition that only the 'control' of malaria was immediately possible and that this would require a number of strategies, amongst which must be measures to raise the social, economic, and environmental conditions of Third World countries. In other words, the fight against malaria must be undertaken as part of 'horizontal' social, health, and medical programmes. In this context, the evidence of historical studies of malaria in Europe are very pertinent as they suggest that long-term decline was due to a range of factors, 'improved agricultural techniques, soil drainage, improvement of soci-economic conditions, and a wider acceptance of medical and sanitary measures'.[47]

YELLOW FEVER[48]

Like malaria, yellow fever came to be regarded as an exotic, tropical disease only in this century. It was placed in this category in the early 1900s, when it both threatened US imperial interests and was shown to be transmitted by the bite of the *Aedes* mosquito. The latter finding was made in Havana in 1901 by a team from the US Army led by Walter Reed (1851–1902). Cuba had passed from Spanish to American control, and a serious problem for the new rulers was the insanitary state of the capital, highlighted by a yellow fever outbreak in 1899. The chief military medical officer responsible for sanitation was William Gorgas (1854–1920) who, together with Reed, devised a control programme.[49] They decided to concentrate on the isolation of sufferers and mosquito eradication, which Gorgas pursued with military authority and vigour. Within a year, success was evident and Gorgas became an international medical celebrity. In 1904, he was invited to Panama, where the construction of the Canal was threatened by yellow fever and malaria. Another successful military-style operation was planned and implemented, and Gorgas became the man who made the Panama Canal possible. These experiences were tremendously important for medical and sanitary authorities worldwide who were trying to control vector-borne diseases, for they demonstrated that campaigns directed against a single disease could work, and provided models for future action.

Control operations at this time were planned without the identification of a causal microbial agent. A number of workers claimed to have identified a bacterium, but none was confirmed. Again, Reed was a key figure in the work which identified the agent as an ultramicroscopic, filterable virus – now recognized as the first virus confirmed as the cause of a human disease. However, difficulties with techniques meant many years passed before the viral agent was accepted, other organisms being canvassed as late as the 1920s. The main approach to the control of disease remained vector eradication, targeted at key centres of infection. Further campaigns of this nature were mounted in urban centres in Cuba and Brazil. In 1913, the Rockefeller Foundation supported the establishment of a Yellow Fever Commission to advise on eradication programmes and to undertake research.[50] Further successes followed in Latin America, and in the 1920s the Commission confidently extended its operations to Africa.

The Rockefeller Center in West Africa soon found that yellow fever was communicable between humans and monkeys, implying that existing eradication schemes would not work in rural areas where there was a reservoir of parasites in wild animals. This problem and the final acceptance of a virus as the cause made a vaccine an attractive solution, and this was set as a target for research in the late 1920s. In an example of successful mission-oriented medical research, the highly effective 17D vaccine had been both created and manufactured by 1937. Mass vaccination of the whole population in affected areas became technically possible, but depended on political will and effective health care delivery, conditions which were uncommon, to say the least, in colonial territories. The value of the vaccine was demonstrated in the Second World War, when it effectively protected the US military in tropical theatres. Since 1945, yellow fever has been effectively controlled in urban areas by a combination of methods, although it has remained a problem in rural areas. Control programmes aimed at rural populations have come increasingly to be based on vaccination, but the problem of creating and sustaining agencies able to deliver the vaccine persists.

TRYPANOSOMIASIS (SLEEPING SICKNESS)[51]

A serious epidemic of sleeping sickness in East and Central Africa in the early years of this century became an important test case for the new specialism of tropical medicine. Colonial authorities were faced with a novel disease, demanding urgent action because of its social and political effects. The disease, previously been known as 'Negro lethargy', was thought to be endemic in certain areas and racially specific. The initial epidemic was in the British colony of Uganda, and a Commission from the Royal Society of London was first in the field. The parasite-vector model was immediately successful, the disease being attributed to a protozoan (*Trypanosoma* spp.) and transmitted by the tsetse fly. As the epidemic spread to other colonies, a number of imperial powers organized research and control ventures. Robert Koch was brought in by the German state, while King Leopold of Belgium employed experts from the Liverpool School of Tropical Medicine.

Work across Africa soon showed that trypanosomiasis was an extremely complex disease. There were many species of the parasite affecting different animals; some could have multiple hosts, including humans and game. The main West and Central African species was identified as *T. gambiense*, which had caused the epidemic in Uganda, but was usually a chronic disease. Later *T. rhodesiense*, which proved to be more common in East Africa, was recognized; this produced a more acute and fatal form of the disease. While this picture was emerging, in Brazil, Carlos Chagas (1879–1934) found a trypanosome in the reduviid bug and in the blood of a child, which led him to identify an associated disease syndrome.[52] In this case, the parasite-vector model identified a pathogen and its mode of transmission before the disease syndrome was described clinically; yet further proof of the power of the model.

The control options were similar to those against malaria and yellow fever, except that unlike the ubiquitous mosquito, the tsetse fly seemed to be limited to specific belts of land. In Uganda, the governor tried to take advantage of tsetse fly ecology by ordering the forced evacuation of villages in fly belts to prevent fly contact with humans. In most British colonies, subsequent policy dealt with sleeping sickness as a tsetse fly problem, with control policy and programmes dominated by entomologists. Other colonial powers made greater use of medical and public-health measures. In German East Africa, the control programme devised by Koch in 1906 was again aimed at the parasite and involved clinical and laboratory screening, followed by isolation and drug treatment. In French colonies, the main approach, developed in the 1920s, was a medical one, involving drugs such as tryparsamide and suramin. Different colonial powers adopted different views of the disease and distinct control policies, which were rooted in different medical approaches and colonial structures.[53] The British attacked the tsetse fly, the Germans and French used chemotherapy against the parasite, while in the Belgian Congo (now Zaire), the authorities favoured social engineering.

The major control programme in the Belgian Congo followed two lines: the medical and the biological.[54] The former involved training, screening programmes, hospitals and clinics, treatment and research; the latter, and initially dominant approach, involved the administration of *cordons sanitaires* and isolation. Lyons's detailed study of trypanosomiasis in the northern Congo shows how the disease and control programmes were so wide-ranging that they shaped the form of the colonial state. However, sleeping sickness policy was not always determinant, with growing conflicts between the political, medical, and sleeping sickness administrations after 1920. Lyons argues that outbreaks of trypanosomiasis were linked to the social dislocation brought about by colonialism, which thus helped create the epidemic. Means of control were then devised, which could be said to be one of the benefits of colonialism. In all these senses, the claim that trypanosomiasis should be regarded as 'a colonial disease' seems well founded.[55]

Assessments of the impact of control efforts mounted under colonial rule, and indeed of subsequent programmes for that matter, have not been very favourable. In the view of John Ford, a leading British expert, trypanosomiasis or tsetse control schemes on their own have not worked and will not work.[56] His view is that control has to be part of broader policies of development and land use. Of course, such schemes depend on social and political stability, economic development, and effective and comprehensive medical and public-health services in affected areas.

SCHISTOSOMIASIS (BILHARZIA)[57]

In terms of level of incidence and current medical efforts, schistosomiasis ranks second only to malaria in importance amongst the 'classic' tropical diseases. Yet, as noted by Farley, it did not feature at all in the comprehensive *History of Tropical Medicine*, by H. H. Scott (1874–1956) and published in 1939. Its relative neglect before the 1940s seems to have been due to the fact that schistosomiasis did not affect Europeans and produced only chronic illness amongst indigenous populations. The disease did not become recognized as a major tropical disease until the Second World War, when it caused problems amongst United States troops in the Pacific. After 1945, as priorities in colonial development and medical aid shifted further towards the health of the peoples of Third World countries, a large and previously submerged public-health problem was revealed.

The disease and associated helminth parasite was first identified in Egypt in the 1850s by T. M. Bilharz (1825–62). In the 1890s and the first decade of the nineteenth century, with greater British involvement in Egypt and the threat of the disease to troops, new investigations were undertaken. Arthur Looss (1881–1923) of the Cairo Medical School proposed that the worm was transmitted directly from human to human through contaminated water, although this was contrary to what was emerging about the role of snail hosts in other worm and fluke infestations. However, much of this knowledge came from Japan, particularly the work of K. Miyairi (1865–1946), and was not that well known in Europe.[58]

British authorities in Egypt maintained an interest in the disease, and in 1912 approached metropolitan experts for further help as scepticism towards Looss's ideas grew. In 1913, the British Colonial Office sent Robert Leiper (1881–1969) and Edward Atkinson (1882–1929) to China to pursue experimental studies of schistosomiasis japonica. Their initial work was unsuccessful, but when they visited Japan, they learnt directly of work on the snail-vector theory.[59] The model was confirmed by the British team on their return to China, and a report critical of the Looss theory was produced. Soon after the outbreak of the First World War, Leiper was sent to Egypt to investigate schistosomiasis haematobia and schistosomiasis mansoni, where the detailed life-cycle and the role of snail vectors was demonstrated.

In Egypt and in many other countries, the disease was ignored as a public-health problem until the 1950s. However, it was taken seriously in South Africa and Zimbabwe due to the threat to whites from blacks carrying the disease, and due to its economic effects on 'native labour'. Control options were similar to those for other vector-borne infections, but in southern Africa, control campaigns were structured by racism and focused on educating and treating the whites most at risk. New scientific research programmes again developed out of the work of the Rockefeller Foundation, specifically its hookworm control programmes. These had begun in the southern United States, but expanded first to other countries and then to other helminthic infections. However, the real turning-point for schistosomiasis was the Second World War. Indeed, after 1945, helminthology became the basis for the institutional development of the specialism of tropical medicine in the United States. Farley has recently argued that this led schistosomiasis to become 'another westernized disease' subject to academic research and high-tech solutions, while 'the very real problems of poverty and malnutrition, with which bilharzia and other tropical diseases are intimately linked, have become essentially buried.'[60]

LEPROSY[61]

Leprosy is another disease now regarded as tropical that was once prevalent across the world. In fact, the causal bacillus was identified by G. H. A. Hansen (1841–1912), in 1874 in decidedly untropical Norway. Leprosy still evokes fear and revulsion, as it is thought to be highly contagious and associated with gross deformations. Lepers were referred to in both the Old and New Testaments and in European medieval literature. Indeed, there would seem to be a continuous history of a disease entity from biblical times to the modern tropics. However, there are major difficulties in showing that the biblical and medieval leper suffered from the same disease identified clinically and pathologically as leprosy today. Recently, Gussow has argued that there was a major discontinuity in the history of leprosy in the late nineteenth century, when the disease was reconstructed in the context of germ theories, colonial expansion, racial fears, and missionary activity.[62]

Although Hansen identified *Mycobacterium leprae* in 1873, he had great difficulty in proving the disease was contagious, let alone showing how it was transmitted. Nevertheless, he followed accepted practice and recommended the isolation of sufferers. His discovery and support for contagion coincided with a new concern over the disease in India and Hawaii, when medical missionaries developed a particular interest in it because of its biblical associations. This concern was also associated with fears that 'natives' might be harbouring the disease and could introduce it into European stock. Contagious-germ theories gave scientific backing to popular fears of the disease and of 'natives'. This potent mixture of racism, Christian charity, and contagionism redefined leprosy as a tropical disease; indeed, an insect vector or carrier was inevitably suspected. According to Gussow, this new conception of leprosy has coloured readings of the Bible and historical documents. Although quite unjustified historically or medically, this racial construction was ideologically useful and has defined attitudes and policies towards leprosy during the twentieth century. In fact, the incidence of the disease in tropical colonies was never that high, and much of the work of leper missions was in fact on tuberculosis. Leprosy's importance was symbolic, a situation evident in the fact that it was targeted by missionaries and metropolitan charities, not colonial medical services. (➤ Ch. 61 Religion and medicine)

DISEASES IN THE TROPICS REVISITED

There is relatively little historical discussion of tropical diseases outside the group of classic parasitic vector-borne infections. A number of diseases could be added to those discussed above – amoebiasis,[63] cholera,[64] dengue,[65] filariasis, leishmaniasis,[66] onchoceriasis (river blindness),[67] plague,[68] and yaws.[69] However, major killers in tropical latitudes – such as dysentery and diarrhoeal diseases, measles, pneumonias, and tuberculosis – have barely been considered by historians in the context of colonialism and tropical health. Historians have followed the agenda of metropolitan tropical medical specialists, not the incidence of disease in tropical areas, nor, for that matter, medical and public-health practice. Important and pioneering exceptions to this have been Patterson's study of health in colonial Ghana, the collection of essays edited by Patterson and Hartwig, and Denoon's history of public health in Papua New Guinea.[70] When historians in 'tropical' countries construct their own agendas for medical history and the history of diseases, it is unlikely that they will organize their enterprise in terms of tropical diseases or tropical medicine. Rather, they will deal with 'medicine in the tropics' and 'disease in the tropics', or, more likely still, medicine and disease in specific cultural and physical environments. Future encyclopedias of the history of medicine will then be unlikely to have chapters on tropical diseases; instead, they will have to carry entries on disease and medicine in particular areas of Africa, Asia, and the Americas, in which the history of tropical diseases and tropical medicine will be an important, but curious interlude.

ACKNOWLEDGEMENTS

I would like to thank Mark Harrison, Helen Power, and colleagues at the Wellcome Unit for the History of Medicine, University of Manchester, for comments on earlier drafts of this chapter.

NOTES

1   M. Turshen, *The Political Ecology of Disease in Tanzania*, New Brunswick, NJ, Rutgers University Press, 1985; D. J. Bradley, 'Tropical medicine', in J. N. Walton *et al* (eds), *The Oxford Companion to Medicine*, Oxford University Press, 1986, Vol. II, pp. 1393–9.

2   Denoon, *Public Health in Papua New Guinea, Medical Possibility and Social Constraint, 1884–1984*, Cambridge, Cambridge University Press, 1989, pp. 20–4.

3   P. Manson-Bahr, 'The march of tropical medicine during the last fifty years', *Transactions of the Royal Society of Tropical Medicine and Hygiene*, 1958, 52: 483–99; R. W. Cilento and C. Lack, *Triumph in the Tropics: an Historical Sketch of Queensland*, Brisbane, Smith & Paterson, 1959; A. Balfour, *War Against Tropical Disease*, London, Baillière, 1920; M. Gelfand, *Tropical Victory: an Account of the Influence of Medicine on the History of Southern Rhodesia*, Cape Town, Juta Press, 1953.

4   O. Ransford, *'Bid the sickness cease': Disease in the History of Black Africa*, London, John Murray, 1983.

5   J. Bryant, *Health in the Developing World*, Ithaca, NY, Cornell University Press, 1969.

6   K. S. Warren, 'Tropical medicine or tropical health', *Review of Infectious Diseases*, 1990, 12: 142–56; J. A. Cook, 'Tropical medicine and health in the developing world', *American Journal of Tropical Medicine and Hygiene*, 1988, 38: 459–65.

7   A. W. Crosby, *The Columbian Exchange: the Biological and Cultural Consequences of 1492*, Westport, CT, Greenwood, 1972.

8   M. J. Dobson, 'Mortality gradients and disease exchanges: comparisons from Old England and Colonial America', *Social History of Medicine*, 1989, 2: 287–97.

9   On North America, see T. Savitt and J. Harvey Young (eds), *Disease and Distinctiveness in the American South*, Knoxville, University of Tennessee Press, 1988.

10 A. Davidson (ed.), *Hygiene and Disease of Warm Climates*, Edinburgh, Young J. Pentland, 1893, pp. 1–24.

11 W. J. Moore, *Health in the Tropics; or the Sanitary Art Applied to Europeans in India*, London, John Churchill, 1862.

12 D. N. Livingstone, 'Human acclimatization: perspectives on a contested field of inquiry in science, medicine and geography', *History of Science*, 1987, 25: 359–94.

13 P. D. Curtin, *Death by Migration: Europe's Encounter with the Tropical World in the Nineteenth Century*, Cambridge, Cambridge University Press, 1989.

14 D. Arnold, 'Medical priorities and practice in nineteenth century British India', *South Asia Research*, 1985, 5, 167–83; Arnold, 'Cholera and colonialism in British India', *Past and Present*, 1986, 113: 118–51; Arnold, 'Smallpox and colonial medicine in India', in Arnold (ed.), *Indigenous Peoples and Imperial Medicine*, Manchester, Manchester University Press, 1988, pp. 45–65.

15 P. D. Curtin, 'Medical knowledge and urban planning in tropical Africa', *American Historical Review*, 1985, 90: 594–613; J. W. Cell, 'Anglo-Indian medical theory and the origins of segregation in West Africa', *American Historical Review*, 1986, 91: 307–35.

16 M. Harrison, 'Public Health and Medical Research in India, c. 1860–1914', Oxford University D. Phil. thesis, 1992.

17 C. A. Bentley, *Report of an Investigation into the Causes of Malaria in Bombay*, Bombay, 1911; I. Klein, 'Death in India, 1871–1921', *Journal of Asian Studies*, 1973, 32: 639 ff; G. W. Hartwig and K. D. Patterson, *Disease in African History: an Introductory Survey and Case Studies*, Durham, NC, Duke University Press, 1978.

18 P. Manson-Bahr, *Patrick Manson: the Founder of Tropical Medicine*, London, Nelson, 1962.

19 M. Worboys, 'The emergence of tropical medicine', in G. Lemaine *et al.* (eds), *Perspectives on the Emergence of Scientific Disciplines*, The Hague, Mouton, 1976, pp. 75–98.

20 W. D. Foster, *A History of Parasitology*, Edinburgh, E. & S. Livingstone, 1965.

21 B. Latour, *The Pasteurization of France*, Cambridge, MA, Harvard University Press, 1988, pp. 140–5.

22 I. Lowy, 'Yellow fever in Rio de Janeiro and the Pasteur Institute mission (1901–1905): the transfer of science to the periphery', *Medical History*, 1990, 34: 144–63.

23 V. A. Harden, 'Rocky Mountain Spotted Fever and the development of the insect vector theory, 1900–1930', *Bulletin of the History of Medicine*, 1985, 59: 449–66; N. Rogers, 'Germs with legs: flies, disease and the new public health', *Bulletin of the History of Medicine*, 1990, 63: 599–617.

24 J. Farley, 'Parasites and the germ theory of disease', *Milbank Quarterly*, 1989, 67 (suppl. 1): 50–68; M. Worboys, 'The origins and early history of parasitology', in K. S. Warren and J. Z. Bowers (eds), *Parasitology: a Global Perspective*, New York, Springer Verlag, 1983, pp. 1–18.

25 P. Manson, 'The need for special training in tropical diseases', *Journal of Tropical Medicine*, 1899, 2: 57–62.

26 L. J. Bruce-Chwatt and J. de Zulueta, *The Rise and Fall of Malaria in Europe*, Oxford, Oxford University Press, 1980.

27 M. Worboys, 'Manson, Ross and colonial medical policy; tropical medicine in London and Liverpool, 1899–1914', in R. MacLeod and M. Lewis (eds), *Disease, Medicine and Empire*, London, Routledge, 1988.

28 Quoted in P. Manson-Bahr and A. Alcock, *The Life and Work of Sir Patrick Manson*, London, Cassell, 1927, p. 217.

29 Quoted in Latour, op. cit. (n. 21), p. 142.

30 J. S. K. Boyd, 'Sleeping sickness: the Castellani-Bruce controversy', *Notes and Records of the Royal Society of London*, 1973, 28: 93–110; cf. N. Stepan, 'The interplay between socio-economic factors and medical science: yellow fever research, Cuba and the United States', *Social Studies of Science*, 1978, 8: 397–423.

31 K. D. Patterson, *Health in Colonial Ghana: Disease, Medicine and Socio-economic Change, 1900–1955*, Waltham, MA, Crossroad, 1981, pp. 16–21; D. Scott, *Epidemic Disease in Ghana, 1900–1961*, London, Oxford University Press, 1965.

32 H. Power, 'Medicine in the tropics: the life and work of Sir Leonard Rogers', unpublished Ph.D. thesis, University of London, in preparation.

33 C. M. White, *Ambassadors in White: the Story of American Tropical Medicine*, Port Washington, NY, Kennikat Press, 1972.

34 M. Worboys, 'The discovery of colonial malnutrition', in Arnold, *Indigenous Peoples*, op. cit. (n. 14), pp. 208–25.

35 See C. Baker, 'The government medical service in Malawi: an administrative history, 1891–1974', *Medical History*, 1976, 20: 296–311.

36 J. Beinart, 'The inner world of imperial sickness', in J. Austoker and L. Bryder (eds), *Historical Perspectives on the Medical Research Council*, Oxford, Oxford University Press, 1989, pp. 109–35.

37 D. Fisher, 'Rockefeller philanthropy and the British Empire: the creation of the London School of Hygiene and Tropical Medicine', *History of Education*, 1978, 7: 129–43.

38 E. Fee, *Disease and Discovery: a History of the Johns Hopkins School of Hygiene and Public Health, 1916–1939*, Baltimore, MD, Johns Hopkins University Press, 1987, pp. 96–111, 219–22; E. R. Brown, 'Public health and imperialism in the early Rockefeller programs at home and abroad', *American Journal of Public Health*, 1976, 66: 897–903.

39 Denoon, op. cit. (n. 2), pp. 67–92.

40 H. H. Scott, *A History of Tropical Medicine*, 2 vols, London, Edward Arnold, Vol. I, pp. 113–251; L. J. Bruce-Chwatt, 'The history of malaria from prehistory to eradication', in W. H. Wernsdorfer and I. MacGregor (eds), *Malaria: Principles and Practice of Malariology*, London, Churchill Livingstone, 1988, pp. 1–59.

41 P. F. Russell, *Man's Mastery of Malaria*, London, Oxford University Press, 1963; G. Harrison, *Mosquitoes, Malaria and Man: a History of Hostilities since 1880*, London, John Murray, 1978.

42 R. E. Dumett, 'The campaign against malaria and the extension of scientific medical services in British West Africa', *African Historical Studies*, 1968, 1: 153–97.

43 A. Beck, 'Medicine and society in Tanganyika, 1890–1930', *Transactions of the American Philosophical Society*, 1977, 67 (3): 13–17.

44 H. Evans, 'European malaria policy in the 1920s and 1930s', *Isis*, 1989, 80: 40–59.

45 J. A. Nazera, 'Malaria and the work of WHO', *Bulletin of the WHO*, 1989, 67: 229–43.

46 M. B. Wickramasingha, 'Malaria and its control in Sri Lanka', *Ceylon Medical Journal*, 1981, 26: 107–15.

47 Bruce-Chwatt and Zulueta, op. cit. (n. 26), p. 147.

48 Scott, op. cit. (n. 40), pp. 279–454; P. A. Brès, 'A century of progress in combating yellow fever', *Bulletin of the WHO*, 1986, 64: 775–86.

49 M. D. Gorgas and B. J. Hendrick, *William Crawford Gorgas – His Life and Work*, New York, Doubleday, Page, 1924.

50 J. Z. Bowers and E. E. King, 'The conquest of yellow fever: the Rockefeller Foundation', *Journal of the Medical Society of New York*, 1981, 78: 539–41; J. Ford, *The Role of Trypanosomiases in African Ecology*, Oxford, Clarendon Press, 1971.

51 Scott, op. cit. (n. 40), pp. 454–547; J. J. McKelvey, *Man Against Tsetse: Struggle for Africa*, Ithaca, NY, Cornell University Press, 1973.

52 B. H. Kean, 'Carlos Chagas and Chagas' disease', *American Journal of Tropical Medicine and Hygiene*, 1977, 26: 1084–7.

53 M. Worboys, 'British colonial medicine and tropical imperialism: a comparative perspective', in G. M. van Heteren, A. de Knecht-van Eekelen and M. J. D. Poulissen (eds), *Dutch Medicine in the Malay Archipelago, 1816–1942*, Amsterdam, Rodopi, 1989, pp. 153–67.

54 M. Lyons, 'Sleeping sickness epidemics and public health in the Belgian Congo', in Arnold, *Indigenous Peoples*, op. cit. (n. 14), pp. 106–7; Lyons, 'The colonial disease: sleeping sickness in the social history of northern Zaire, 1903–30', unpublished Ph.D. thesis, University of California, 1987, p. 401.

55 Cf. L. Vail, 'Ecology and history: the example of Eastern Zambia', *Journal of Southern Africa Studies*, 1977, 3: 129–55.

56 J. Ford, 'Ideas which have influenced attempts to solve the problem of African trypanosomiasis', *Social Science and Medicine*, 1979, 13B: 269–75.

57 J. Farley, *Bilharzia. The History of Imperial Tropical Medicine*, Cambridge, Cambridge University Press, 1991.

58 M. Sasa, 'A historical review of early Japanese contributions to the knowledge of schistosomiasis japonica', in M. Yokogawa (ed.), *Research in Filariasis and Schistosomiasis*, Baltimore, MD, University Park Press, 1972, pp. 235–60.

59 G. S. Nelson, 'A milestone on the road to the discovery of the life-cycles of human schistosomes', *American Journal of Tropical Medicine and Hygiene*, 1977, 26: 1093–100.

60 J. Farley, 'Bilharzia: a problem of "native health", 1900–1950', in Arnold, *Indigenous Peoples*, op. cit. (n. 14), p. 203.

61 M. Vaughan, *Curing their Ills: Colonial Power and African Illness*, Cambridge, Polity Press, 1991, pp. 77–99.

62 G. Gussow, *Leprosy, Racism and Public Health*, Boulder, CO, Westview Press, 1989.

63 Scott, op. cit. (n. 40), pp. 820–39.

64 J. Christie, *Cholera Epidemics in East Africa*, London, Macmillan, 1876 (reprinted 1970); R. Sullivan, 'Cholera and colonialism in the Philippines, 1899–1903', in MacLeod and Lewis, op. cit. (n. 27), pp. 284–300.

65 Scott, op. cit. (n. 40), pp. 808–19.
66 M. Gibson, 'The identification of kala azar and the discovery of leishmaniasis', *Medical History*, 1983, 27: 203–13; Gibson, 'Leishmaniasis: the first century, 1885–1985', *Journal of the Royal Army Medical Corps*, 1986, 132: 127–52.
67 K. D. Patterson, 'River blindness in Northern Ghana, 1900–50', in Hartwig and Patterson, op. cit. (n. 17), pp. 88–117.
68 M. W. Swanson, 'The sanitation syndrome: bubonic plague and urban native policy in the Cape Colony, 1900–09', *Journal of African History*, 1977, 18: 387–410; I. J. Catanach, 'Plague and the tensions of empire: India, 1896–1918', in Arnold, *Indigenous Peoples*, op. cit. (n. 14), pp. 149–71.
69 C. J. Hackett, 'Yaws', in E. E. Sabben-Clare, D. J. Bradley and K. Kirkwood (eds), *Health in Tropical Africa during the Colonial Period*, Oxford, Clarendon Press, 1980, pp. 82–95; M. Dawson, 'The 1920s anti-yaws campaigns and colonial medical policy in Kenya', *International Journal of African Historical Studies*, 1987, 20: 417–35.
70 Patterson, op. cit. (n. 31); Patterson and Hartwig, op. cit. (n. 17); Denoon, op. cit. (n. 2).

FURTHER READING

Arnold, D. (ed.), *Indigenous Peoples and Imperial Medicine*, Manchester, Manchester University Press, 1988.

Denoon, D., *Public Health in Papua New Guinea: Medical Possibility and Social Constraint, 1884–1984*, Cambridge, Cambridge University Press, 1989.

Farley, J., *Bilharzia: the History of Imperial Tropical Medicine*, Cambridge, Cambridge University Press, 1991.

Hartwig, G. W. and Patterson, K. D., *Disease in African History: an Introductory Survey and Case Studies*, Durham, NC, Duke University Press, 1978.

Kean, B. H., Mott, K. E. and Russell, A. J. (eds), *Tropical Medicine and Parasitology: Classical Investigations*, 2 vols, Ithaca, NY, Cornell University Press, 1978.

Lyons, M. I., *The Colonial Disease: a Social History of Sleeping Sickness in Northern Zaire, 1900–1940*, Cambridge, Cambridge University Press, 1992.

MacLeod, R. and Lewis, M. (eds), *Disease, Medicine and Empire*, London, Routledge, 1988.

Patterson, K. D., *Health in Colonial Ghana: Disease, Medicine and Socio-economic Change, 1900–1955*, Waltham, MA, Crossroad, 1981.

Scott, H. H., *A History of Tropical Medicine*, 2 vols, London, Edward Arnold, 1939–42.

Vaughan, M., *Curing their Ills: Colonial Power and African Illness*, Cambridge, Polity Press, 1991.

25

CANCER

David Cantor

INTRODUCTION AND HISTORIOGRAPHY

Two themes dominate much of the historiography of cancer: the increasing visibility of this group of diseases since the late eighteenth and early nineteenth centuries, and the ways in which cancer has become a focus of various power struggles. The term 'visibility' is rarely used by historians of cancer, but it captures two broad strands in the historiography of the disease. In the case of internalist historians, the visibility of cancer refers to the ways in which medical science has illuminated the complex nature of this group of diseases. Such historians focus on intellectual history often to the neglect of social, cultural, or economic context. Crudely put, in this view cancer is more visible simply because it is better understood by scientists today than in the past.

The second meaning of visibility refers to increasing concern about cancer, especially in Western societies, since the nineteenth century. There are numerous indicators of this historical visibility. Specialist hospitals and research institutes, professional societies and specialities, philanthropic bodies, and government legislation are all predominantly products of the nineteenth and twentieth centuries. Furthermore, epidemiologists have highlighted the growing mortality from this group of diseases since the nineteenth century. Today in the USA, about one person in every three contracts one of the various forms of the disease. Small wonder that cancer has excited considerable public anxiety, especially as medicine seems unable to stem the carnage. Even according to official statistics, the survival rates for the major cancers (lung, breast, and bowel) have improved little over the past thirty-five years despite vast increases in research funding. And cancer has become visible in yet another way. Whereas at the start of the century the stigma of cancer was such that few in the USA would admit to having it, today that silence has to some extent been eroded.

As cancer has become increasingly visible in Western societies, it has also become the focus for various power struggles. For internalists, such struggles have predominantly been intellectual debates – for example, between those favouring localist explanations of cancer genesis versus those preferring constitutional explanations, or viral versus hereditarian explanations of aetiology. Regrettably, the social mechanisms of such debates are rarely explicated. Power, in this view, is invested in ideas rather than the social groups or individuals who hold them.

For political and social historians, interest in power struggles focuses predominantly on issues of professional authority and control of philanthropic and government organizations concerned with cancer. In part, this emphasis was a response to traditional accounts, which treated medical divisions of labour as relatively uncontentious. But the process of division has often been bitterly disputed, and varied in different countries. For example, American cancer specialists have embraced chemotherapy much more readily than their British counterparts.

But power struggles around cancer have not been simply about intra-professional disputes within medicine. Philanthropic and governmental interest in the disease has attracted and been the product of substantial lay and political support. (The most famous instance was perhaps Richard Nixon's attempt to use the creation of the 1971 American Cancer Act to win the 1972 presidential election.) At least part of the way in which cancer specialists have created a niche for themselves is through developing political alliances with lay philanthropists or political lobby groups. As such, the history of cancer is also the history of broader social and political power struggles, and at times the medical division of labour around cancer has been little more than a by-product of these struggles. As yet, we know little about how such struggles have shaped medical knowledge and practice.[1] Nor has sufficient historical attention yet been paid to the ways in which attitudes to race, class, and gender structure medical and scientific knowledge and practice, or the multitude of ways in which people have responded to and resisted science's and medicine's interpretations of cancer.[2]

At the root of many of the power struggles around cancer has been scientific knowledge and expertise, but historians have been divided on how to treat these key topics. Whereas at the first half of the twentieth century, historians such as Jacob Woolf, Henry Sigerist, and Richard Shryock would look to science to solve the problems of cancer,[3] since the 1970s – and especially the 1971 American Cancer Act – it has become less clear if such an orientation is desirable. A number of historical studies by Strickland, Rettig, and Studer and Chubin showed how science had failed to deliver on earlier claims that, given more resources, it could find a cure.[4] The message was that, in a crude effort to boost funding, scientists and their sponsors had exaggerated the ability of science to find the cause of cancer and had consequently undermined the credibility of science itself. Yet while such accounts were critical of scientific experts, they were often uncritical of scientific knowledge (an exception is the account of Studer and Chubin). An underlying assumption was that social and economic forces had merely corrupted scientific knowledge.

Ironically, this was a position broadly shared by historians more favourable to the cancer crusade. William Yarumchuck's and Michael Shimkin's accounts of cancer researchers and of the National Cancer Institute, and Walter Ross's history of the American Cancer Society assumed that the politics of funding could speed up or slow down the rate of scientific discovery, or at worst take research in unproductive directions.[5] But such perspectives often measured rate of discovery or direction of research against modern scientific understandings of cancer. For internalist historians such as Victor Triolo, Sigismund Peller, and Lelland Rather, cognitive or technical factors served a similar function to such institutional factors, speeding up or slowing down research or taking it in either fruitful or fruitless directions.[6] All such accounts were infused with a progressivism, as their narratives edged towards modern scientific understandings of the disease, measuring past knowledge in terms of the present.

Susan Sontag's warning against some of the war-like imagery associated with the cancer 'crusade' shared this realist perspective on scientific knowledge. While calling for a way of talking of cancer stripped of its metaphorical load, Sontag assumed that somehow such images distracted from the real scientific account of the disease.[7] Similarly, James T. Patterson's sociocultural history of the disease in twentieth-century America treats the representations of cancer in film, television, and political journalism as epiphenomena of the 'real' experience of disease, rather than as integral factors in the medical and popular understandings of cancer.[8]

Finally, this realist perspective was also shared by most epidemiologists working on long-term cancer mortality trends. Most accounts do not reflect on the social construction of disease, but argue within a positivistic framework about the reliability of sources and the mix of factors promoting disease.

Historians such as Robert Bud, Russell Maulitz, and Evelleen Richards have challenged such assumptions.[9] They argue that social, institutional, and economic forces do not so much corrupt cancer research as routinely shape medical and scientific theories and practices. The limited number of case studies makes generalization from such accounts problematic, but because cancer is such a politically sensitive area, the lesson extends to history itself. Willingly or not, historians have been drawn into contemporary disputes, becoming participants in the fierce fight to construct reality, as Richards and her colleagues put it. She shows how the controversy over vitamin C and cancer shaped her access to primary sources, and how her publications were taken up in ways she did not intend by participants in the controversy.[10]

In fact, historians of cancer have often been a part – albeit a small part – of the history they write about. Wolff's monumental history of cancer was part of attempts to reform and rationalize cancer research in the laboratory at the turn of the century.[11] He and other reformers saw his book as a research tool, a reference work for cancer researchers. In the 1970s and 1980s, historians such as Rettig, Strickland, Shimkin and Ross, and Studer and Chubin saw themselves as contributing to policy debates around the 1971 American Cancer Act.[12]

In view of the different political and historiographic approaches, there is no single history of cancer to relate. In what follows there are essentially two stories. The first is the internalist history of ideas about cancer since antiquity, the history of science's illumination of the complexity of cancer. The second is the history of growing concern about cancer since the nineteenth century. The separation is regrettable, but the two histories are not yet reconcilable.

INTERNALIST HISTORIES

EARLY HUMORAL THEORIES OF CANCER

Until the middle of the nineteenth century, the history of cancer was part of a broader history of inflammation. The word comes from Hippocrates (c.450–370 BC), who likened the long, distended veins radiating from lumps in the breast to a crab – *karkinoma* in Greek, *cancer* in Latin. The term *karkinos* included benign tumours, inflammatory growths, and what we would now think of as neoplastic tumours. And it was Hippocrates who first described the cause of cancer as an excess of black bile, a view elaborated by Galen (AD 129–c.200/210) that was to dominate Western medical thinking for over a thousand years. For Galen, cancers were classified as among tumours contrary to nature, which included a wide range of disorders including phlegmonic inflammations, sinuses, ulcers, fistulas, gangrene and carbuncles, erysipelas and oedema. According to Galenic theory, a cancer could be formed in one of two ways. First, a flux of black bile gave rise to scirrhus, one form of which was related to or capable of converting into cancer. Second, a flux of black bile unmixed with blood gave rise to cancer forthwith, most often in the female breast. (➤ Ch. 14 Humoralism)

By the end of the seventeenth century, iatrochemists replaced black bile as the material cause of tumours with various corrosive acids and ferments. Paracelsus (1493–1541) and Jean Baptista van Helmont (1579–1644) rejected the notion that disease was a function of an imbalance of the body's humours, arguing instead that it was the product of the excess or deficiency of certain fluids. Although Paracelsus was a controversial figure in his lifetime, learned medicine came to accommodate iatrochemistry and humoralism. For example, Daniel Sennert (1572–1637), Professor of Medicine at Wittenberg, argued that no one unskilled in chemistry could lay claim to the name of a finished physician. However, his account of the genesis of tumours was hardly distinguishable from orthodox Galenic accounts – black bile was still the culprit, accompanied by iatrochemical acridities. Another example of accommodation of different schools of thought can be seen in the views of Hermann Boerhaave (1668–1738) on cancer causation. For Boerhaave, blood was the key to life, and if any stasis occurred in the circulation, inflammation would ensue, which might lead to cancer depending on local structure and chemistry. (➤ Ch. 9 The pathological tradition)

Following the posthumous publication in 1628 of the discovery by Gaspare Aselli (1581–1625) of the lymphatic system, attention began to focus on the lymph and lymph nodes as possible causes of cancer. For Georg Ernst Stahl (1660–1734), Friedrich Hoffmann (1660–1742), and John Hunter (1728–93), cancer was simply the most unfavourable outcome of inflammation. Stahl said the bile of the ancients was a composite of salty serum and gelatinous lymph mixed with a small amount of true blood. Trapped in the solid parts of the body, and undergoing further breakdown, this noxious fluid constituted a cancer. The seed of cancer was a ferment, and like other ferments (in bread and wine, for instance) it could reproduce itself.

Similarly, Hunter felt that inflammation was a healthy reaction to injury, but where it did not accomplish a salutary purpose, it did mischief. He argued that cancer was the outcome of what he called 'coagulable lymph', a component of the circulating blood capable of organizing into solid substances. For Hunter, the solid transformations of fluid lymph accounted for all growth, restitution, repair, and maintenance of the body's solid parts. Cancer was merely a corrupt form of these processes: the same process that made normal tissues also made abnormal tissues.

PATHOLOGICAL ANATOMY

The turning-point away from humoral theories of cancer came in the late eighteenth and early nineteenth centuries with the emergence of a range of theories that sought to explain structure in terms of solids, and which favoured localistic notions of disease formation. Marie François Xavier Bichat (1771–1802) located all morbid processes of the body in twenty-one subtypes of tissues, which were the basic units of life. Thus different parts of the body might experience similar disease processes if they were made up of the same tissues; the seat of cancer was 'cellular' tissue. Bichat argued that cellular tissue had the ability to throw out a kind of vegetation, to elongate, and to reproduce itself, and that tumour development depended on this reproductive activity.

Bichat's histopathology was rapidly taken up by the medical establishment in post-revolutionary France, and was elaborated by Bichat's student, René Laënnec (1781–1826). Laënnec rejected anatomical classifications of disease based purely on organs or tissues in favour of one of his own that incorporated structure and function. He made a distinction between inflammation (such as gangrene) and cancer, which was an accidental tissue. Accidental tissues might be either analogous with nature or unlike other natural tissues. This last category was of particular importance to practitioners, since it included the deadly cancerous formations: tubercle, scirrhus, melanosis, and encephaloid. Thus Laënnec took Bichat's division of the body into tissues and made it into a classification of disease. (➤ Ch. 17 Nosology) Disease processes were both local (the products of textural alterations or other processes) and general (similar tissues underwent similar processes). (➤ Ch. 5 The anatomical tradition)

CELLULAR PATHOLOGY

The pathological anatomy of cancers remained at the gross level until the 1830s, and the application by Johannes Müller (1801–58) of the microscope and Schwannian cell theory to the study of tumours. (➤ Ch. 6 The microscopical tradition) Whereas Bichat had believed that cells were little more than pores within the cellular tissue, Theodor Schwann (1810–82), a student of Müller's, believed that the cell was the unit of structure, and its nucleus the reproductive organ. Schwann supported this view by tracing the genesis of tissues to their embryonic beginnings. To Müller, both normal and pathological cells were structured aggregates of transformed cells, developed for the most part *de novo* from an amorphous cytoblastema ultimately derived from circulating blood. Thus Müller effectively integrated cell theory into a general view of the spontaneous generation of neoplasms. The cell theory promoted debates over the mechanism of metastasis: did secondary lesions arise from some *seminium morbi*, as Müller argued, or from displaced cancer cells, as Jacob Henle (1809–85) believed, or by a transferred dyscrasis, as Karl von Rokitansky (1804–78) maintained? Such deliberations indicate that cancer theories were part of broader contemporary cytological and physiological theories of life. (➤ Ch. 7 The physiological tradition)

By the 1850s, Schwannian theory gave way to a belief in cell continuity: '*omne cellula a cellula*', as Rudolf Virchow (1821–1902) summed it up. Virchow believed that tumour cells developed from 'embryonic' cells, scattered throughout the omnipresent connective tissue. Subsequently, opinion shifted away from Virchow's connective-tissue theory of the origin of cancers. In 1867, Wilhelm Waldeyer (1837–1921) reviewed the available evidence in *Virchow's Archiv* to argue for the purely epithelial origin of epithelial cancers. According to Waldeyer, normal epithelium was the sole source of epithelial cells contained in a given carcinoma. The sole mechanism of local spread was the active or passive movement of cancer cells into adjacent tissues, while the sole mechanism of metastatic spread was through the transport of cancer cells to the metastatic sites via the blood, lymph, or other body fluids.

Thus by the end of the nineteenth century, much of the framework of twentieth-century oncology had been laid. 'True' neoplasms were distinguished from inflammatory lesions, cysts, tubercles, and the many other swellings with which they had been grouped for over two thousand years. Pathologists treated tumours as having a cellular nature: they originated in normal cells and tissues of corresponding types; they retained many of the features of their originating structures; they comprised essentially tumour cells that multiplied mainly by mitotic division. In this view, tumours were supported in most instances by a stroma of blood vessels and connective tissues, and nourished by the blood of the host organism. They could either be 'malignant' or 'benign'. Waldeyer identified malignant neoplasms by the way tumour cells thrust themselves into the surrounding normal tissues to form projective growths (invasive growth), or colonized distant body sites after being transported in the blood and lymph (metastasis). In contrast to malignant neoplasms, pathologists saw benign tumours as local, circumscribed growths derived from epithelial or connective tissue but which failed either to invade or to metastasize. They also classified both malignant and benign tumours according to their derivation from the three embryonic germ layers (ectoderm, mesoderm, and endoderm) or from the epithelial and non-epithelial cells (either 'endothelial' cells when they were the flattened cells that line the blood and lymph vessels, or 'mesothelial' when they were the similar cells that lined the body cavities). The malignant epithelial neoplasms were termed 'carcinomas', and their non-epithelial analogues 'sarcomas' or 'carcinosarcomas'. The benign neoplasms were given names such as 'lipomas', 'chondromas', and 'myomas' according to their histological derivation, in these cases from fat, cartilage, and muscle respectively.

More controversially, leukaemias and lymphomas joined the list of malignant neoplastic diseases in the nineteenth century. Leukaemia was described in 1845 by John Hughes Bennett (1812–75) and Virchow, and named by Virchow. For Bennett, the blood's light colour indicated general pyaemia; for Virchow, it indicated a new pathological entity created by an increase in the number of colourless blood corpuscles. But in 1855, certain Paris physicians contended that leukaemia did not exist as a distinct malady; it had no special causes, anatomical lesions, or specific treatments. The dispute continued well into the twentieth century. Lymphomas – the term was the general name given to any neoplastic disease derived from the cellular components of the immune system – were also a problematic introduction. Hodgkin's disease, described in 1832 by Thomas Hodgkin (1798–1866) and named in 1856 by Samuel Wilks (1824–1911), is a case in point. For Wilks, the disease appeared to be somewhere between a cancer and a tubercle, while W. S. Greenfield (1846–1919) saw it as being a local disease that subsequently developing into a lymphatic cancer. As with leukaemia, the dispute continued into the twentieth century. (➤ Ch. 35 The art of diagnosis: medicine and the five senses)

So what was the impact of pathology on practical clinical work? Although Shimkin and others have argued that histopathology was the final arbiter of the diagnosis, histogenesis, and prognosis of cancer by the end of the nineteenth century, Stephen Jacyna has shown that into the early twentieth century the impact was probably more limited.[13] Thus at the Glasgow Royal Infirmary between 1875 and 1910, clinicians rarely saw the pathologist as an integral part of diagnosis of cases of breast cancer. This was not because they discarded science, but rather that they ascribed it only a limited role in practical medicine, essentially as a confirmation or correction of clinical diagnosis *after* surgery had been undertaken. (➤ Ch. 36 The science of diagnosis: diagnostic technology) Pathology would remain a *post facto* commentary on clinical decisions until well into the twentieth century. For their part, some pathologists and other laboratory scientists would increasingly attempt to distance themselves from clinical control, arguing that clinicians knew too little about laboratory research to determine the nature of experimental laboratory research. (➤ Ch. 11 Clinical research)

TWENTIETH-CENTURY CANCER RESEARCH

Much twentieth-century research on the aetiology of cancer has shifted between two polarities: explanations favouring the action of exogenous factors such as viruses, parasites, environmental chemicals, or physical agents such as radiation; and those favouring endogenous factors such as genetic mutation. Late nineteenth-century exogenous approaches included attempts to discover some parasitic or infectious organism as the cause of cancer and to develop vaccines against it. Much interest focused on possible bacterial causes, but in 1907 Amédée Borrel (1897–1936) argued for a viral aetiology of cancer. The following year, two Danish pathologists, Vilhelm Ellermann (1871–1924) and Oluf Bang (1881–1937), reported that a chicken leukaemia could be transmitted from a diseased to a healthy chicken by means of a cell-free filtrate. Since the type of filters used precluded the passage of organisms as large as bacteria, Ellermann and Bang postulated that the disease was caused by a virus. Then in 1911, an American researcher, Peyton Rous (1879–1970) reported the cell-free transmission of a chicken sarcoma.

However, by the end of the first decade of the twentieth century, the search for an infectious agent had lost some momentum. Part of the reason for this came from studies of endogenous factors such as host resistance. Animal transplanation studies (perhaps the principal experimental tool in cancer research by 1905) indicated that viable cells were necessary for successful grafts, and that transplanted cancer cells did not infect surrounding cells. Most transplantation studies focused on the fact that animals implanted with tumours were resistent to further implants if the original tumours regressed or if the tumour was excised. But attempts artificially to stimulate resistance to cancer – for example, with low doses of radiation – faded during the late 1920s and 1930s. Clinical results were disappointing, and laboratory workers felt that what was called resistance was not resistance to a disease, but against the introduced cells of another individual or of a different genetic make-up. (➤ Ch. 10 The immunological tradition)

Another challenge to infectious theories of the aetiology of cancer was the 1914 somatic mutation theory of Theodor Boveri (1862–1915), which stated that all cancers were caused by chromosomal abnormalities or by the agents or events that produced them. (➤ Ch. 20 Constitutional and hereditary disorders) This view was given added weight when in 1927 H. J. Muller (1890–1967) demonstrated the mutagenic properties of X-rays, suggesting that radiation could both change the cell's genetic information, leading to a loss of control over cell growth, and be passed on to following generations of cells. By explaining how such exogenous factors affected the internal structure of the cell, somatic mutation theory also challenged theories that explained cancer production in terms of chemical reactivity. The latter explanation gained credence after the identification of polycyclic aromatic hydrocarbons, such as 1, 2, 5, 6–dibenzanthracene, as the cancer-causative agents of coal tar in the late 1920s and early 1930s. Crudely put, chemists argued that a relationship existed between the capacity to produce cancer and either the chemical structure of, or the chemical reactivity of, an established double-bond in polycyclic hydrocarbons. This theory, however, focused only on the relationship between the cell and its environment, and treated the inside of the cell as a 'black box'. From the 1940s and 1950s, other work showed that carcinogenic chemicals could also produce mutations in bacterial or animal systems.

During the 1950s, viral theories began to attract attention again, especially following the excitement over the identification of the polio virus and the development of techniques for breeding viruses in tissue culture and viewing virus particles by electron microscopy. The roots of this revival went back before the Second World War to a series of discoveries of viruses capable of producing tumours in animals: skin tumours in rabbits (1933), breast tumours in mice (1936), kidney tumours in frogs (1938), and leukaemia in newborn mice (1951). In the 1950s, studies of the induction of a wide spectrum of tumours into several species by a mouse virus (polyoma) grown in tissue culture challenged beliefs in tumour and species specificity derived from work on previous oncoviruses. Researchers showed that viruses of both DNA and RNA types caused a number of cancers in animals, especially neoplasms of the leukaemia-lymphoma complex in chickens, cats, and cattle. In chickens and cats, some forms of the disease behaved as a classic infection with horizontal case-to-case transmission rather than vertical transmission from one generation to the next.

By 1960, interest in tumour immunity had also revived after the discovery of tumour transplantation antigens, suggesting that some tumours produced specific antigens that elicited a cellular type of reaction. The potentials of such work included the possible identification of specific tumour antigens and the enhancement of effects in therapy. Between 1967 and 1970, a vaccine was developed for Marek's disease, a form of chicken lymphoma caused by a herpes virus.

Research on oncogenic viruses included the discovery of enzymes that split the molecules at specific sites. In 1970, David Baltimore (b. 1938) and Howard Temin (b. 1934) simultaneously published a report of the discovery of an enzyme, reverse transcriptase. This enzyme was found in retroviruses, a class of viruses responsible for many types of animal tumours including at least two rare forms of human leukaemia-lymphoma. The genetic core of a retrovirus was built of RNA rather than the more usual DNA, but RNA was not what made the pathogen so singular. Temin and Baltimore announced that once a retrovirus had infected a cell, it employed its reverse transcriptase enzyme to work backwards, turning its RNA core into a strand of DNA. The point was important because it defied one of the central tenets of molecular biology, that DNA made RNA, and not the reverse. Temin and Baltimore showed that information in biological systems can flow into as well as out of DNA.

Two major hypotheses have been put forward to explain the mechanism of viral carcinogenesis. Temin's protovirus theory – a modern restatement of Borrel's viral-infestation theory – postulated that the oncogenic virus acts through a provirus mechanism in which the viral genome is incorporated into the nucleic acid of the cells by virion-RNA-directed polymerase. Any mechanism that disrupted the unstable provirus could induce neoplasia. In contrast, the viral oncogene theory postulated by Robert Huebner (b. 1914) and George Todaro (b. 1937) – the modern parallel to Boveri's earlier theory of chromosomal changes – stated that in the course of evolution, a type of RNA virus became incorporated in the genome and existed there as a silent infection prior to birth. The transmitted oncogene would normally be suppressed but might be activated by the many carcinogens. Thus by the end of the century, cancer could be described as an infectious gene or a viral genetic infection.

EXTERNAL HISTORIES

INSTITUTIONAL VISIBILITY

One of the most striking ways in which cancer has become socially and culturally visible has been the profusion of specialist institutions established since the nineteenth century. The first cancer hospital was set up in Rheims in the mid-1700s, but was forced to close in 1778 due to public fears that cancer might be contagious. In Britain in 1792, the Middlesex Hospital opened the first specialist cancer wards; and in 1802, the Society for Investigating the Nature and Cure of Cancer was established. From the 1850s, the numbers of specialist hospitals multiplied, with the London Cancer Hospital and cancer hospitals in Leeds, Liverpool, Manchester, and Glasgow. Like most specialist hospitals of the nineteenth century, these were set up by medical practitioners often aiming to circumvent blocked career ladders in the general hospitals; they did not provide the stimulus to the creation of a speciality of cancer treatment in Britain. The medical profession regarded many of them as little more than quack emporia and, with the exception of the London Cancer Hospital (renamed the Royal Marsden after its founder, William Marsden (1796–1867)) and the Christie Hospital in Manchester, by the time of the First World War they had all failed. (➤ Ch. 49 The hospital; Ch. 47 History of the medical profession)

Abroad, a similar flurry of cancer-hospital building also occurred during the nineteenth century in France and the USA, where, like Britain, advanced cancer ordinarily disqualified patients from the voluntary or general hospitals. In France, 'Oeuvres du Calvaire' were set up to care for women with cancer in Lyons (1850), Paris (1874), Saint-Etienne (1874), Marseilles (1881), Rouen (1891), and Bordeaux (1909). Inspired by the gift of a philanthropic Lyons widow, Jeanne Garnier-Chabot (1811–53) the staff were themselves widows, and were therefore prepared, according to Garnier-Chabot, for dealing with suffering. In the 1880s they expanded, setting up in Brussels in 1886 and New York in 1899. American cancer-hospital building took off slightly later than that in England or France. The first, the New York Cancer Hospital, was set up in 1884, followed by the St Rose Free House for Incurable Cancer in 1899, and others at Buffalo (1898), Philadelphia (1904), and St Louis (1905). Some of these American institutions embodied a new form of philanthropy that looked optimistically to science and to the laboratory for cures of the disease, rather than to the care of dying patients. And in

Britain too, a similar shift can be discerned. Plans for *Friedenheims* – 'homes of peace' for the dying – at the Manchester, London, and Glasgow cancer hospitals were shelved as a new optimism about treatment and research took over at the end of the century.

As philanthropy shifted towards science and the laboratory at the end of the nineteenth century, cancer researchers created a whole new range of specialist research institutions and the beginnings of professional organization. The first specialist journal, the *Revue des maladies cancéreuses*, appeared in France in 1896, though it lasted only six years. It was followed by the German *Zeitschrift für Krebsforschung* (1904), the Japanese *Gann* (1907), the Italian *Tumouri* (1911), the French *Bulletin de l'Association Français pour l'Étude du Cancer* (1911), and the American *Journal of Cancer Research* (1916). Three international congresses were held before the First World War at Heidelberg (1906), Paris (1910), and Brussels (1913). Following the Heidelberg Congress, national research associations were formed in France (1906), the USA (1907), and Japan (1908). Preceding most of these in Britain were the Middlesex Cancer Research Laboratories (1900) and the Imperial Cancer Research Fund (ICRF; 1902); in Germany, the Central Committee for Cancer Research (1900); and in the USA the unorthodox, Chicago-based American Cancer Research Society set up at the turn of the century.

Thus by the First World War a wide variety of national and international cancer organizations had come into being. What distinguished this new interest from the mid-nineteenth-century phase of hospital building was its emphasis on laboratory research (especially in the study of the infectious nature of cancer and of tumour transplantation) and a growing enthusiasm for X-rays (discovered in 1895) and radium (1898) as possible alternatives or supplements to surgery. By 1914, virtually every European capital had a radium institute, the first being proposed in Paris around 1906. However, both phases of institution building were inspired by fears of rising cancer mortality, increasingly expressed in statistics. In the 1850s, William Marsden publicized a threefold increase in cancer deaths in London between 1839 and 1850 to attract subscribers to his cancer hospital, while a similar concern about rising mortality statistics formed the backdrop to the creation of the French Association for the Study of Cancer and proposals for the Paris Radium Institute, both in 1906. In that year, the statistician Adolphe Louise Jacques Bertillon (1851–1922) showed that Parisian cancer mortality, stable until 1875, had been growing ever since – the eighth cause of death in 1876 and the fifth thirty years later – although it was still way below that of tuberculosis. (➤ Ch. 72 Medicine, mortality, and morbidity)

By 1910, rising cancer mortality attracted the attention of the American insurance industry. In 1912, the chief statistician of the Prudential Insurance Company, Frederick Hoffman (1865–1946), found that the total cost of deaths from cancer to the Metropolitan Life Insurance Company was $717,000 – 4.9 per cent of male and 9.8 per cent of female policy-holders. Cancer, he believed, tended to hit the middle and upper classes, those who could afford insurance, and Hoffman became a key figure in the American Society for the Control of Cancer (ASCC) founded the following year. The ASCC's goal was to educate the public about the dangers of cancer and to break down the silence that surrounded the disease, rather than engaging in research.

The First World War stimulated further institutional initiatives. In France, the incidence of cancer among the older age-groups recruited into the army during the war prompted the Secretary of Health to create cancer treatment centres attached to hospitals in Paris, Lyons, and Montpellier. The advisers to the Secretary of Health were subsequently prominent in establishing the French Anti-Cancer League in Paris in 1918, a public education group advocating increased research, public health, and clinical treatment programmes for cancer. But, unlike its American equivalent, the league was also important in establishing a nationwide network of cancer treatment centres, especially using radium and X-rays. (➤ Ch. 66 War and modern medicine)

In Britain also, cancer statistics and enthusiasm for radium and X-rays would provide a major stimulus to both state and philanthropic initiatives after the war. Thus in 1919, the state-financed Medical Research Council (MRC) established a nationwide research scheme into medical uses of radium (especially for cancer) using war-surplus radium. In 1922, the Ministry of Health (founded in 1919) noted that cancer mortality in England and Wales had trebled in the space of two generations from 0.33 (per 100 people) in 1851–60, to 0.97 in 1911–20, to 1.01 in 1921. Prompted in part by such figures and by dissatisfaction with the laboratory emphasis of ICRF, leading clinicians founded the British Empire Cancer Campaign (BECC) in 1923. Their initial goal was to develop what they called a frontal assault on cancer, aimed at finding its cause. Such an approach worried the MRC, which feared that the basic sciences (pathology, physiology, and biochemistry) could not hope to solve the problem, and that a frontal attack on the disease would damage the credibility of science in the long term. (➤ Ch. 8 The biochemical tradition) Of particular concern to the MRC was the way in which successful Harley Street clinicians were able to manipulate public philanthropy by means denied to basic scientists locked behind laboratory walls. In the end, the MRC forced the founders of the BECC to accept an MRC-dominated majority on its scientific advisory committee. (➤ Ch. 50 The medical institutions and the state)

By the end of the 1920s, the demand for radium had become so great in Britain that in 1929 the government created the National Radium Trust and Commission (1929–48). Financed by a combination of public and private funds, the Trust became the largest purchaser of radium in the world during the 1930s. Radium bought by the Trust was given to the Commission, which (together with the King Edward's Hospital Fund for London) organized a nationwide network of radium treatment centres, based partly on the earlier French scheme as well as one in Sweden. The Radium Commission would become the focus for the specialization of radiotherapy in Britain during the 1930s and 1940s. It encouraged the separation of X-ray therapy from X-ray diagnosis, the merger of the hitherto separate specialities of radium and X-ray therapy, and organized the training of the new radiotherapists. The 1939 Cancer Act promised to provide even more resources for both X-ray and radium therapy, but the Second World War put paid to the scheme. In 1948, the Radium Commission was wound up, its function taken over by the National Health Service (NHS), under which cancer hospitals lost their 'special' designation, and were gradually integrated into large general hospitals. Radiotherapy was available at only one site – usually a general teaching hospital – within each region of the new health service. At the same time, a new cancer charity, the Marie Curie Cancer Relief Fund was created in 1948 to support home care for the terminally ill – a revival of some of the ideals of the earlier and ill-fated *Freidenheims*. Research into control of terminal-cancer pain started at St Luke's Hospital in 1948, and was developed at St Joseph's Hospice between 1958 and 1965 by Cicely Saunders (b. 1918). (➤ Ch. 67 Pain and suffering)

After the Second World War, the focus of cancer research shifted to the USA. Between 1944 and 1946, the ASCC was transformed from an organization devoted principally to education and the provision of treatment facilities to a research organization. The moving figure behind this change was Mary Lasker, the wife of a wealthy advertising tycoon, Albert Davis Lasker (1880–1952), who was himself to die of cancer. The story goes that one day in 1943, Mary Lasker walked into the office of Clarence C. Little, the Managing Director of the ASCC, and demanded to know how much the society was spending on research. Lasker was astonished to find that the answer was nothing. With Little's co-operation Lasker brought leading business people on to the board, and in 1944, personally placed articles on the early detection of cancer in the *Reader's Digest*, inviting readers to send donations to the renamed American Cancer Society (ACS). These articles alone raised $120,000 – more than the ASCC's entire budget two years earlier – and by 1948, the ACS had raised around $14 million. (➤ Ch. 63 Medical philanthropy after 1850)

After revolutionizing the ACS, Lasker turned her attention to Congress. Together with Surgeon-General Thomas Parran Jr (1892–1968), James Shannon (head of the National Institutes of Health), and Congressman Frank Keefe, among others, she lobbied successfully for an increased allocation of federal funds for cancer research. As a result of this and other pressures, the budget of the National Cancer Institute (NCI; founded in 1937) jumped from $1.75 million in 1946 to $14 million in 1947, and the rise continued: in 1961, its budget was $110 million. This funding bonanza was made possible in part by the unparalleled affluence of the USA after 1945, which gave added weight to demands for good health and fears of premature death, especially when set against Congress's relatively small allocations to social-welfare programmes. As a result, despite historical doubts about the role of the state, Americans now had perhaps the most highly centralized and publicly financed research apparatus against cancer in the world. Not only had industrialists taken over the ACS, and provided a powerful lobby for the NCI, they had also provided a model of research at major cancer research laboratories. Laboratories such as the Sloan Kettering Institute and the Institute for Cancer Research organized their research in conscious imitation of industrial laboratories such as those of General Motors and Bell Telephones.

In the late 1960s, Lasker and her associates were behind another effort to push for a federal war on cancer. The term 'war' was well chosen. It took place against the background of Vietnam which, Lasker pointed out, had killed some 41,000 Americans in four years, a tiny figure compared with the estimated 323,000 people who died from cancer in a single year. Yet federal spending on cancer was minute compared to that on defence: as a former Secretary of Defense put it, $410 per person for national defence, 89 cents per person for cancer. President Nixon's National Cancer Act of 1971 resulted in an NCI appropriation of $400 million in 1973, rising to $1 billion by the 1980s.

Such an increase, however, eventually drew attention to the small pay-off in cures and prevention that seemed to result, and to the waste of tax dollars. Enthusiasm for the Cancer Act had been fired in part by the revival of viral theories of cancer, and by the search for a vaccine, but critics argued that it was unclear whether viruses played an aetiological role in more than a handful of cancers. With American defeat in South-East Asia, the metaphors of war began to turn against the proponents of the Act. 'By comparison with the fight against polio', claimed a fomer FDA commissioner in 1978, 'the war on cancer is a medical Vietnam.'[14]

Foreign responses to the US cancer programme were mixed. In Britain, the 1972 Zuckerman report on cancer research cautioned that money alone would not result in new ideas. Despite criticism from some cancer researchers that funding was woefully inadequate in Britain, the Zuckerman report constituted part of a long-term shift of funding away from the state. Since the 1950s, the ICRF and BECC (later the Cancer Research Campaign) have taken on an increasing share of British cancer research. In 1952, they provided 29 per cent of the total funding (£296,220), but this jumped to 79 per cent by 1985 (£46,270,660). In 1988, these two charities ranked third and fourth, respectively, in terms of fund-raising among all charities in Britain. (➤ Ch. 57 Health economics)

THERAPEUTICS

Cancer has also become increasingly visible because of the hopes and fears surrounding treatments. Until the nineteenth century, the bulk of treatments had been conservative. Hippocrates and Galen both cautioned against the treatment of hidden cancers, arguing that treatment more often than not hastened death. Galen advocated the use of purging, bleeding, proper diet, and limited local use of poisons and caustics in breast cancers, claiming that such methods were particularly successful when the atrabiliary of the humour was not too thick. (➤ Ch. 40 Physical methods) Until the eighteenth century, treatment therefore was a combination of crude surgery, cauterization, a variety of salves containing scar-forming corrosive agents such as arsenic, bloodletting and purging, and herbal and magical preparations. Cancers of the lip, skin, and female breast were probably treated surgically, as they were the most accessible. (➤ Ch. 41 Surgery (traditional))

Even the most optimistic statistics on cancer surgery were not encouraging. Although the Viennese surgeon Theodor Billroth (1829–94), argued that cancer could be cured with the knife, in a review of the outcome of 170 operations he had performed for breast cancer between 1867 and 1876, only 4.7 per cent of the women were alive three years later. Surgery itself evoked considerable fears. The prospect of a long, painful, and highly mutilating operation that offered no sure cure was a grim alternative to the pain, disfigurement, and probable death from the disease itself. While radical surgery was by no means the norm, the list of radical treatments grew substantially at the end of the nineteenth century; Halsted's Mastectomy (1891), Wertheim's hysterectomy for cancer of the cervix (1898), Billroth's subtotal gastrectomy (1881), and Schlatter's total gastrectomy (1897) are but a few. The justification for many of these operations was that the total removal of the affected part would reduce the likelihood of recurrence. Yet the fears these operations inspired were at least as great as any hope they may have offered. Indeed, surgery would at times itself be blamed for the increase in mortality. 'Fresh surgical "triumphs" ', wrote one British critic in the 1920s, 'had been attended by rapid rises in the death rates of the organs concerned.'[15] Yet it did not stop the desire among some surgeons for even more radical operations. In the 1940s and 1950s came a fresh wave of new radical procedures: the hemicorporectomy, hemipelvectomy, super-radical mastectomy, complete pelvic exenteration, and the wide resection of head and neck tumours. But again, by the end of the 1950s survival figures showed at the best marginal improvements in cure rates and severe decline in the quality of life. Although a trend away from super-radical operations was evident in the 1960s and 1970s, patients were still often not given the choice between radical and conservative surgery. In a recent British controversy, women with breast cancer were given radical mastectomy and were not informed of an alternative conservative lumpectomy. (➤ Ch. 42 Surgery (modern))

Against such fears, it is hardly surprising that the discovery that X-rays could cure some cancers was greeted with enthusiasm. Discovered in 1895, by the end of the century the new rays were used to treat surface cancers, and from 1903, deep-seated ones. It seemed at last as if a cure might be in sight, and without the need for the knife. Before-and-after photographs regularly showed 'cured' patients without the disfiguring scars of surgery. As French investigators J. A. Bergonie (1857–1925) and L. Tribondeau (1872–1914) showed in 1906, the key seemed to be that rapidly proliferating cells were the most sensitive to X-rays. X-rays thus promised a more sensitive means of treating cancer than surgery, and did not risk dislodging cancer cells that might metastasize.

Yet with hope came fear, and the dangers around this new treatment added to the visibility of cancer. First, between 1897 and 1900 came concern about X-ray burns; and then in 1903, the shocking revelation that one of the assistants to Thomas Edison (1847–1931) had developed cancer after working with X-rays. After successive amputations the assistant died in 1904, the first of many similar cases. Even before this publicity, concern about the dangers of X-ray burns had led to a series of court cases in Germany against physicians, culminating in 1902 in a suit for damages of 36,000 marks against one physician following a criminal judgment of 'negligent bodily damage'. (➤ Ch. 69 Medicine and the law) In subsequent years, the concern about cancer, the harrowing accounts by X-ray patients of their injuries, the risk of sterility, the mounting death toll, and the threats of government intervention and of spiralling insurance costs led in 1916 to protection recommendations issued by the British Roentgen Society following a precedent by the German Roentgen Society prior to the First World War. Despite such concerns, the trend in X-ray therapy was towards more and more powerful machines. Higher voltages made deep-therapy more feasible. The 1913 Coolidge X-ray tube made possible the production of X-rays up to 140,000 volts, and by the end of the 1930s, machines of several million volts were in use. (➤ Ch. 68 Medical technologies: social contexts and consequences)

The other major alternative to surgery was radium. Discovered in 1898, it became a serious alternative to surgery only after the First World War, in part because of its limited quantities and high price. Most radium (or its gas, radon) was initially contained in needles or tubes – in the case of radon, called 'seeds' – which would be inserted surgically into the body or placed in natural cavities such as the mouth, anus, or vagina. When supplies of radium increased (and costs dropped) in the 1920s and 1930s, a new form of therapy developed. Radium-beam therapy employed a large quantity of radium to produce a beam of (often gamma) radiation at a distance from the body in a manner akin to the use of X-rays. As in X-ray therapy, the appeal of this method was often cure without disfigurement. By the 1940s, cobalt began to replace radium in beam therapy, and slightly earlier in the 1930s research began on machines such as the cyclotron which, it was hoped, would provide neutrons for therapy and radioisotopes that could be injected into the body for radiotherapeutic purposes. The first hospital-based cyclotron began operation at the Hammersmith Hospital, London, in 1955.

In the 1940s and 1950s radiotherapy was joined by chemotherapy in the medical arsenal against cancer. Beginning with the trials of the cytotoxic properties of the mustard gases that began after the Second World War, extensive programmes to synthesize and deploy chemicals as specific weapons against cancers were carried out mainly in the USA. The early trials of cytotoxic drugs focused particularly on childhood leukaemias, Hodgkin's disease, and lymphomas, which were almost invariably rapidly fatal. Following some successes with childhood leukaemias, Congress began to invest heavily in chemotherapy, providing the NCI with $3 million in 1954. The following year, the NCI established a Cancer Chemotherapy National Service Centre, and by 1957 the chemotherapy programme absorbed almost half of the NCI's budget. Much of the work involved testing chemicals for their potential value in cancer treatment; by 1970, some 400,000 drugs had been tested. (➤ Ch. 39 Drug therapies)

Overall, American oncologists have been more enthusiastic about chemotherapy than their British counterparts. But even in America, voices have been raised against the potential harmful effects of treatment and have questioned their efficacy. As in the case of radiotherapy, such uncertainties have helped to maintain the profile of the disease. It was as difficult to target cancer cells without damaging normal cells in chemotherapy as in radiotherapy, and both therapies could cause vomiting, loss of hair, fatigue, depression, and even cancer itself. Worst of all, critics contended that chemotherapy was little or no use against many common cancers, including cancers of the gastro-intestinal and respiratory tracts. All the publicity for this treatment had sustained hopes of a cure, but had left people as frustrated and anxious as ever about the disease and its treatments.

In addition to surgery, radiotherapy, and chemotherapy, in the 1970s and 1980s hopes were raised again by the publicity around biotechnology and immunotherapy, especially interferon, which had been discovered in the late 1950s. However, the laborious production process required the culturing of human cells and resulted in the extraction of only minute quantities of the substance. Then, in 1979, the successful cloning of a human interferon gene using recombinant DNA techniques altered the time, quality, quantity, and cost dimensions of it production. As a consequence, recently formed genetic engineering and established pharmaceutical companies in the newly emergent biotechnology field raced each other to exploit its market potential. But as with radium, X-rays, and chemotherapy, the early enthusiasm soon evaporated. The anti-cancer properties of interferon remained more elusive than expected, and the drug had some dangerous side-effects. In the 1990s, it is no longer touted as a cure, although it is used in combination with surgery, radiotherapy, and chemotherapy.

While orthodox medicine and its allies were criticized for over-enthusiastic reporting of therapies from surgery to interferon, so medicine criticized unorthodox practitioners for the same. Yet the growth of alternative treatments for cancer was another indicator of its growing visibility. In part, the reaction of doctors to the unorthodox medicine was tied up with the politics of specialization. In early modern England, practitioners such as the Miss Plunkett who practised surgery, especially the excision of cancers, in the south-west in the 1770s, plied their trade alongside more orthodox practitioners. The latter associated specialization with 'quackery', and (as noted on p. 546) labelled the specialist cancer hospitals of the mid- to late nineteenth century as little more than quack emporia. Specialists and quacks alike threatened the pockets and status of generalist physicians and surgeons. (➤ Ch. 28 Unorthodox medical theories)

During the late nineteenth and twentieth centuries, orthodox medicine attacked cancer quacks for their use of secret remedies. A court case against the cancer quack 'Dr' A. O. Johnson prompted the US Supreme Court to outlaw false and misleading labelling of contents of quack nostrums in 1911, and subsequently, the American Medical Association (AMA) attempted to put numerous alternative practitioners out of business. The conflict came to a head in the USA in the late 1970s. An increasing number of vocal critics attacked orthodox cancer research through organizations such as the International Association of Cancer Victims and Friends (1966) and the Committee for Freedom of Choice in Cancer Therapy (1972), an offshoot of the right-wing John Birch Society, which took up the cause of laetrile (an extract of apricot pits).

Laetrile had been isolated by a Californian pharmacist and physician, Ernest Krebs in 1951, who claimed that it targeted malignant cells while bypassing healthy tissue. In the early 1960s, the Food and Drug Administration (FDA) and others attacked laetrile, claiming the clinical trials had failed to prove its effectiveness. At that point Andrew Robert MacNaughton, a Canadian entrepreneur, took over the laetrile movement, establishing treatment centres in Canada, and campaigned widely in the USA on behalf of the remedy. In the early 1970s, the John Birch Society argued that the FDA's campaign against laetrile was a perfect example of bureaucratic tyranny, and argued for free choice in treatment selection for cancer patients. Its offshoot society claimed that orthodox physicians rejected unorthodox treatments for fear of doing themselves out of a job.

In another widely publicized case in the 1970s, the Nobel laureate Linus Pauling (b. 1901), and Ewen Cameron, a Scottish surgeon, revived 1930s hopes that vitamin C might be a treatment for cancer. But the potential of this therapy became controversial, in part because the medical establishment resented what they saw as the intrusion of Pauling (a non-physician) into therapy and increasingly marginalized him; for example, his position at Stanford University became untenable when he was unable to obtain funding for laboratory space, and he set up an independent institute in 1973. Although forced into the alternative medicine camp, Pauling was nevertheless able to force the Mayo clinic to carry out two clinical trials. Both were negative, but Pauling and Cameron continued to defend their claims for vitamin C, and strongly criticized the design of both the Mayo Clinic's trials.

CARCINOGENS

Cancer has also become increasingly visible in the publicity surrounding various carcinogens. The history of carcinogens is usually traced back to the identification by Percivall Pott (1714–88) of scrotal cancer among chimneysweeps in 1775. By the end of the nineteenth century, shale oil, coal distillates, and petroleum products were added to soot as causes of skin cancer. Lung cancer among Black Forest miners was reported in 1879, and urinary bladder cancer among aniline dye workers in 1895. In 1900 came reports from India of cancer of the abdominal wall among the Kangri, who held warming-pans of charcoal next to their bodies. Such work suggested that chronic, local irritation might be a cause of cancer, and the search began for specific irritants. In 1915, Katsusaburo Yamagiwa (1863–1930) and Koichi Ichikawa (1888–1948) produced cancers of the ears of rabbits by painting them with coal tar. They did not know which specific chemical caused the cancer, but in the late 1920s and early 1930s a London research group under E. L. Kennaway (1881–1958) identified the active chemicals as polycyclic hydrocarbons.

Subsequently, thousands of chemicals were added to the list. By 1951, 1,339 compounds had been tested, of which 322 were reported as having carcinogenic activity. Such data prompted concern over environmental issues such as the discharge of carcinogenic wastes by industry. However, suggestions that preventive measures, such as inspection and licensing of factories, could reduce the exposure to carcinogens got nowhere in the 1950s. Arguments for prevention met opposition from industrialists, and secured little popular support for regulation or social reform. To many American scientists, the principal cause of cancer was not the environment, but individual susceptibility, and that meant studying the inherent imperfections in cells.

Similar concerns also challenged other environmental factors, such as radiation. As noted, the carcinogenic action of radiation had been known since the early twentieth century, but until the 1940s its dangers were generally balanced against its value in therapy, though critics complained that hospitals and other employers often ignored the recommendations of protection committees. The situation changed dramatically after 1945, when the atomic explosions at Hiroshima and Nagasaki raised new fears of cancer. Studies of survivors showed that exposure to ionizing radiation produced myelocytic leukaemia and increases in the occurrence of thyroid and other cancers. Such fears were exacerbated by concern over fallout from atomic tests, fears of occupational cancers in the burgeoning nuclear industry, and renewed concern about the hazards of medical radiation. For example, in 1958 Alice Stewart (b. 1906) first called attention to the possible increased risk of leukaemia following low-dose radiation exposures of the foetus. Nevertheless, the dangers of both atomic radiation and the medical uses of radiation on both sides of the Atlantic were played down by a combination of Cold War patriotism, professional self-interest, and deliberate misrepresentation of existing knowledge. In one notorious case of research (begun in 1965) into low-level exposures to radiation among workers at the Hanford Nuclear Reservation in Washington State, the US Atomic Energy Commission (AEC) tried to pressure the researcher, Dr Thomas Mancuso, to contradict claims by Washington State's Department of Social and Health Services concerning an excess of cancers among Hanford workers. When Mancuso refused, his contract with the AEC was not renewed.

Resistance to environmental explanations also help explain reactions to the evidence on the carcinogenic effects of tobacco smoking. Tobacco had been cited as a possible carcinogen from the nineteenth century, but in general the medical profession exhibited little concern about it. But by the end of the Second World War, fears of rising mortality from lung cancer began to intensify. In 1900, fewer than 400 cases had been recorded in the USA, but the death toll has escalated ever since: 4,000 in 1935; 11,000 in 1945; 36,000 in 1960. Epidemiological evidence in Britain and America linked this rise to cigarette smoking, which had been growing in popularity over the same period, especially in the 1940s. But as with other carcinogenic agents, a combination of industrial pressure, doubts about the value of epidemiological evidence, and resistance from sections of the medical profession combined to confuse the issue. However, in 1962, the Royal College of Physicians of London officially endorsed the link between smoking and cancer, followed in the USA in 1964 by a report of the Surgeon-General.

In the late 1960s and 1970s, environmentalist issues surfaced again in all the areas mentioned – smoking, radiation, and chemical carcinogens. Other human carcinogenic situations were also defined, such as industrial exposures to asbestos leading to mesothelioma or vinyl chloride producing angiosarcoma of the liver. What fired this new environmentalist initiative was a more general concern about the threat posed by pollution to the planet, fears that industrial growth was itself a danger, and a revived interest in personal health. During the recession of the 1970s, the costs of clearing up and preventing pollution hindered this environmentalist surge, as (in Britain and America) later did the election of conservative administrations determined to reduce state regulation of industry and shift much of the burden of health care on to the individual. In the mid- to late 1980s, worries about Chernobyl, industrial pollution in Eastern Europe, leukaemia in certain radiation workers, the depletion of the ozone layer, and passive smoking, among other concerns, have again placed environmental issues on the agenda. (➤ Ch. 59 Internationalism in medicine and public health)

POPULAR FEARS

Partly as a response to its growing institutional, therapeutic, and environmental visibility, cancer has taken over from tuberculosis as the dominant disease metaphor of the twentieth century. From the late nineteenth century, cancer has become a metaphor for the fate of industrial and urban society. As cancer was characterized by uncontrollable growth, so too industrial and urban society seemed to grow relentlessly, destroying the very populations that nourished its development. Popular and medical opinion in Western societies suggested that industrial and urban growth exacerbated the dangers of cancers. Perhaps it was a product of the emotional stresses and strains of living in industrial society, or a product of environmental pollutants, or a contagious disease exacerbated by cramped living arrangements, or a product of 'degenerate' urban habits. (➤ Ch. 27 Diseases of civilization)

Ironically, at the very time that interest in cancer emerged in the nineteenth century, the disease also disappeared from view. It was rarely mentioned in obituary notices, and so great was the fear of cancer that the New York Cancer Hospital was renamed 'Memorial Hospital' in 1899 because the term 'cancer hospital' was objected to by its patients. This was a marked contrast to the early-modern period where, as the horrific account by Fanny Burney (1752–1840) of her mastectomy suggests, people were willing to admit to having the disease. Perhaps the disappearance of cancer by the late nineteenth century was part of a broader fear of the threat the disease posed to modern society. If cancer was both a product of and danger to industrial and urban society, then individuals who contracted the disease were themselves somehow responsible for the social disorder. Moreover, popular and medical fears that cancer was contagious mitigated against public discussion, as did the suggestion that cancer ran in families.

The silence around the disease has been eroded over the course of the twentieth century, beginning to break down in America in the late 1950s, when the word appeared in newspaper obituaries in place of euphemisms about 'prolonged' or 'serious' illnesses. Contrast the secrecy around the treatment of cancer in President Grover Cleveland (1837–1908) in 1893 with the publicity around President Ronald Reagan's cancers in 1985. Whereas Cleveland's cancer was treated secretly on a boat bobbing off Long Island Sound, when Reagan went into hospital for the treatment of cancer of the colon and the removal of a skin cancer, the cameras followed him almost to the doors of the operating room. Yet for many millions of other people, cancer remains deeply worrying and stigmatizing, its diagnosis bringing the threat of pain and death. Despite Reagan's public endorsement of modern medical science, many remain skeptical of medicine's ability to defeat the dread disease.

NOTES

1   Patrice Pinell's *Naissance d'un fléau. Histoire de la lutte contre le cancer en France (1890–1940)*, Paris, Éditions Métailié, 1992, deals with some of these issues. Unfortunately, it appeared too late to be discussed fully in the text.

2   Cf. James T. Patterson, *The Dread Disease. Cancer and Modern American Culture*, Cambridge, MA, and London, Harvard University Press, 1987.

3   Jacob Wolff, *The Science of Cancerous Disease from Earliest Times to the Present*, New York, Science History Publications, 1989 (orig. pub. as *Die Lehre von der Krebskrankheit von den ältesten Zeiten bis zur Gegenwart*, Jena, Gustav Fischer, 1907); Henry E. Sigerist, 'The historical development of the pathology and therapy of cancer', *Bulletin of the New York Academy of Medicine*, 1932, 8: 642–53; Richard Harrison Shryock, *The Development of Modern Medicine. An Interpretation of the Social and Scientific Factors Involved*, New York, Alfred Knopf, 1947, pp. 439–44.

4   Stephen Strickland, *Politics, Science, and Dread Disease: a Short History of United States Medical Research Policy*, Cambridge, MA, Harvard University Press, 1972; Richard A. Rettig, *Cancer Crusade. The Story of the National Cancer Act of 1971*, Princeton, NJ, Princeton University Press, 1977; Kenneth E. Studer and Daryl E. Chubin, *The Cancer Mission. Social Contexts of Biomedical Research*, Beverley Hills, CA, and London, Sage, 1980.

5   William A. Yarumchuck, 'The origins of the National Cancer Institute', *Journal of the National Cancer Institute*, 1977, 59 (suppl.): 551–8; Michael B. Shimkin, *Contrary to Native*, Washington, DC, National Institutes of Health, 1977; Shimkin, *As Memory Serves. Six Essays on a Personal Involvement with the National Cancer Institute*, Washington, DC, National Institutes of Health, 1978; Walter S.

Ross, *Crusade. The Official History of the American Cancer Society*, New York, Arbor House, 1987.

6 Victor A. Triolo, 'Nineteenth century foundations of cancer research. Origins of experimental research', *Cancer Research*, 1964, 24: 4–27; Triolo, 'Nineteenth century foundations of cancer research. Advances in tumor pathology, nomenclature, and theories of oncogenesis', *Cancer Research*, 1965, 25: 75–106; Sigismund Peller, *Cancer Research Since 1900. An Evaluation*, New York, Philosophical Library, 1979; L. J. Rather, *The Genesis of Cancer. A Study in the History of Ideas*, Baltimore, MD, and London, Johns Hopkins University Press, 1978.

7 Susan Sontag, *Illness as Metaphor*, Harmondsworth, Penguin, 1983; orig. pub. 1978.

8 Patterson, op. cit. (n. 2).

9 R. F. Bud, 'Strategy in American cancer research after World War II: a case study', *Social Studies of Science*, 1978, 8: 425–59; Russell C. Maultiz, 'Rudolf Virchow, Julius Cohnheim and the program of pathology', *Bulletin of the History of Medicine*, 1978, 52: 162–82; Evelleen Richards, *Vitamin C and Cancer: Medicine or Politics?*, Basingstoke and London, Macmillan, 1991.

10 Pam Scott, Evelleen Richards and Brian Martin, 'Captives of controversy: the myth of the neutral social researcher in contemporary scientific controversies', *Science, Technology and Human Values*, 1990, 15: 474–94.

11 Wolff, op. cit. (n. 3).

12 For comments on the politics of recent British cancer historiography, see David Cantor, 'Contracting cancer? The politics of commissioned histories', *Social History of Medicine*, 1992, 5: 131–42.

13 Shimkin, op. cit. (n. 4); S. Jacyna, 'The laboratory and the clinic: the impact of pathology on surgical diagnosis in the Glasgow Western Infirmary, 1875–1910', *Bulletin of the History of Medicine*, 1988, 62: 384–406.

14 Donald Kennedy quoted in James C. Petersen and Gerald E. Markle, 'Expansion of conflict in cancer controversies', in Louis Kriesberg (ed.), *Research in Social Movements, Conflicts and Change*, 1981, 4: 151–69, see p. 152.

15 David Cantor, 'The MRC's support for experimental radiology during the inter-war years', in Joan Anstoker and Linda Bryder (eds), *Historical Perspectives on the Role of the MRC. Essays in the History of the Medical Research Council of the United Kingdom and its Predecessor, the Medical Research Committee, 1913–1953*, Oxford, Oxford University Press, 1989, pp. 181–204, see p. 185.

FURTHER READING

Austoker, Joan, *A History of the Imperial Cancer Research Fund 1902–1986*, Oxford, Oxford University Press, 1988.

Bud, R. F., 'Strategy in American cancer research after World War II: a case study', *Social Studies of Science*, 1978, 8: 425–59.

Cantor, David, 'The MRC's support for experimental radiology during the inter-war years', in Joan Austoker and Linda Bryder (eds), *Historical Perspectives on the Role of the MRC. Essays in the History of the Medical Research Council of the United Kingdom and its Predecessor, the Medical Research Committee, 1913–53*, Oxford, Oxford University Press, 1989, pp. 181–204.

Jacyna, L. S., 'The laboratory and the clinic: the impact of pathology on surgical diagnosis in the Glasgow Western Infirmary, 1875–1910', *Bulletin of the History of Medicine*, 1988, 62: 384–406.

Maulitz, Russell C., 'Rudolf Virchow, Julius Cohnheim and the program of pathology', *Bulletin of the History of Medicine*, 1978, 52: 162–82.

Murphy, Caroline C. S., 'From Friedenheim to hospice: a century of cancer hospitals', in Lindsay Granshaw and Roy Porter (eds), *The Hospital in History*, London and New York, Routledge, 1989, pp. 221–41.

Olson, James S., *The History of Cancer. An Annotated Bibliography*, New York, Greenwood Press, 1989.

Panem, Sandra, *The Interferon Crusade*, Washington, DC, Brookings Institute, 1984.

Patterson, James T., *The Dread Disease. Cancer and Modern American Culture*, Cambridge, MA, and London, Harvard University Press, 1987.

Pinell, Patrice, *Naissance d'un fléau. Histoire de la lutte contre le cancer en France (1890–1940)*, Paris, Éditions Métailié, 1992.

Rather, L. J., *The Genesis of Cancer. A Study in the History of Ideas*, Baltimore, MD, and London, Johns Hopkins University Press, 1978.

Rettig, Richard A., *Cancer Crusade. The Story of the National Cancer Act of 1971*, Princeton, NJ, Princeton University Press, 1977.

Richards, Evelleen, *Vitamin C and Cancer: Medicine or Politics?*, Basingstoke and London, Macmillan, 1991.

Shimkin, Michael B., *Contrary to Nature*, Washington, DC, National Institutes of Health, 1977.

Sontag, Susan, *Illness as Metaphor*, Harmondsworth, Penguin, 1983 orig. pub. 1978.

Young, James Harvey, 'Laetrile in historical perspective', in Gerald E. Markle and James C. Petersen (eds), *Politics, Science and Cancer: the Laetrile Phenomenon*, Boulder, CO, Westview Press, 1980, pp. 11–60.

26

SEXUALLY TRANSMITTED DISEASES

Allan M. Brandt

It is a basic and tragic irony of human life that intimate physical relations sometimes entail the risk of infectious disease. The very nature of sexual contact offers obvious opportunities for the movement of micro-organisms – some of which cause disease – from one individual to another. Infectious communicable diseases, transmitted in the course of sexual relationships, have, in all likelihood, always been present. And many infections, not specifically attributed to sexual relations, may none the less be spread during sexual contact. This chapter focuses upon those infections specifically associated with sexuality; it is their particular and peculiar mode of transmission that draws them together as an entity.

Sexually transmitted diseases (STDs) make explicit the significance vested in particular modes of transmission of infectious organisms. In this sense, the meaning and ultimate epidemiological significance of this set of infections is fundamentally tied to the changing historical nature of human sexual relations. Since sexual ethics and practices vary widely over time and across cultures, the meaning and significance of sexually transmitted diseases have also been highly variable. In addition, these diseases suggest the powerful relationship of biological, medical, and social variables as they affect patterns of disease. Tracing medical theory and practice, as well as broader social attitudes and public policies regarding the STDs, reveals important social and cultural conflicts about medicine, sexuality, and disease.

THE ORIGINS OF SYPHILIS

In the last years of the fifteenth century, a devastating epidemic of infectious syphilis swept western Europe. The intensity of the epidemic, as well as the particular symptoms of the disease, led to considerable speculation among physicians and lay people concerning its origins. It was quickly recognized that the disease, characterized by skin ulcers and eruptions, and often causing systemic illness and death, was spread in sexual contact. The sudden onset of this epidemic led many observers to conclude that this was a new disease, brought back from the Americas by Columbus's crew in 1493. And indeed, there is considerable evidence that this was the case. The virulence of the epidemic, according to this argument, suggests that a new organism had been introduced to which Europeans had no previous exposure and, thus, no immunity. This would account for the intensity of the epidemic, as well as the widespread contemporary assessment that the disease was 'new'. Just as the great discoverers had introduced a number of infectious agents in the Americas, devastating the native populations there, so, it seems, some organisms made the return voyage with radical consequences.[1] Using indications from lesions in fossil remains, palaeopathologists have concluded that there is considerable evidence of treponemal diseases in the Americas prior to 1500, with little or no evidence of such infections in European human fossils.[2] (➤ Ch. 52 Epidemiology; Ch. 18 The ecology of disease)

There was broad consensus in Europe at the end of the fifteenth century that syphilis constituted something new, and certainly many literary texts identify the epidemic as unprecedented. As Joseph Grünpeck (1473–1532), author of a famous autobiographical treatise (1503) on the epidemic wrote:

> In recent times I have seen scourges, horrible sicknesses and many infirmities affect mankind from all corners of the earth. Amongst them has crept in, from the western shores of Gaul, a disease which is so cruel, so distressing, so appalling that until now nothing so horrifying, nothing more terrible or disgusting, has ever been known on this earth.[3]

Others, however, have argued that venereal infections had long been present in Europe prior to this time but had never been distinguished from leprosy, which had similar dermatological symptoms. (➤ Ch. 24 Tropical diseases) According to such theories, most treponemal infections (pinta, yaws, endemic and venereal syphilis) had previously been mild and chronic. Treponemal infections would thus probably have been common childhood infections, spread by casual contact and offering substantial immunity to subsequent infections. With improvements in European standards of living, by the time of Columbus's voyages, treponemes dependent on skin contact had become disadvantaged, replaced by hardier, sexually transmitted strains. Better hygiene, for example, reduced skin-to-skin transmission. (➤ Ch. 53 History of personal hygiene) Because many individuals would then reach sexual maturity without treponemal exposure, transmission would occur primarily through contact of mucous membranes during sexual activity, and the severity of disease was a result of no prior infections.[4]

A related theory concerning the origins of syphilis holds that the spiro-chaete was present in both the old and new worlds prior to the epidemic. Varying social and environmental conditions would account for differences in transmission and symptoms; modes of transmission varied with climate. (➤ Environment and miasmata) Social and political disruptions of the late fifteenth century account for the sudden and dramatic nature of the epidemic: the fundamental dislocations engendered by wars, changing sexual norms, and increased travel, as well as papal bulls abolishing leper houses, may all have contributed to the onset of the epidemic.

While these theories do not settle the question of the origins of syphilis, the debate makes clear that the infection was subject to a wide range of biological, climatic, and socio-cultural variables, all of which could affect its clinical and epidemiological patterns. There is no doubt, for example, that the developing technologies of oceanic travel fundamentally contributed to new patterns of infection. Disease occurs within a complex bio-ecological system, influenced by social, political, and cultured events. The debate about the origins of syphilis has engaged the most sophisticated palaeopathologists, archaeologists, and physical anthropologists, as well as medical historians. (➤ Ch. 60 Medicine and anthropology) Underlying the debate are certain core issues that reflect the very nature and shifting meaning of sexually transmitted diseases over time. At stake in determining the origins of the disease is the desire, so typically associated with STDs, of attributing 'responsibility' for the infections. This theme, then, which begins in the first years of the sixteenth century, would continue to characterize the assessment of STDs through the twentieth century. Implicit was a long-standing recognition that no nations or people wished to claim syphilis as their own: it was a disease – feared and stigmatized – of the 'other'. It came from distant lands and different peoples.[5] The French called it the Italian disease; the Italians called it the French disease. Nevertheless, the descriptions of suffering and pain inflicted were uniformly consistent. Deformity, debility, and death all resulted from sexual contact with an infected individual. (➤ Ch. 67 Pain and suffering) By 1502, the 'Great Pox', as it came to be called, had spread to central Europe. The epidemic soon dissipated in intensity, but it had spread more widely to include Africa, India, and parts of the East. The Verona physician Girolamo Fracastoro (1483–1553) named the disease 'syphilis' in his poem of 1530 describing the plight of an afflicted shepherd; 'pox', however, remained in popular usage until the late eighteenth century.

One aspect implicit in the debate about the origins of syphilis is the difficulty – on both theoretical as well as empirical grounds – of differentiating one disease from another. Syphilis, in some of its dermatologic manifestations, resembled leprosy; individuals could often be infected with more than a single disease, thus manifesting a variety of symptoms. Furthermore, individuals could be infected with more than one sexually transmitted organism, accounting for a mix of physical symptoms. With these variables, even the most sophisticated diagnostician could draw incorrect inferences about the identity and natural course of disease.

EARLY TREATMENTS

Physicians and others quickly recognized the sexual nature of the contagion and counselled caution and abstinence. Cleansing the genitals was frequently advocated as a possible prophylactic measure when abstinence failed. Physicians advised patients and public to avoid sexual liaisons with infected persons, but many consulted them after displaying the characteristic symptoms of infection. Mercury, which had in the past been used as an ointment for other diseases characterized by skin eruptions such as leprosy and scabies, became the drug of choice for syphilis.[6]

Mercury held favour regardless of a particular physician's theoretical perspective. Although there was considerable debate about the mechanism of mercury's cure, there nevertheless was broad consensus that with the salivation and sweat induced by the drug, the poison was expelled from the body. Many physicians contended that the heavy metal would rid the body of the poison causing disease. Applied topically, orally, and through fumigation, mercury caused profuse sweating and copious salivation, all perceived as excellent means for purging the pox 'virus' (that is, poison).[7] In humoral terms, some physicians argued, syphilis indicated an excess of phlegm. (➤ Ch. 14 Humoralism) Therefore, mercury, which generated such extensive drooling, seemed a particularly appropriate intervention. Mercury treatment was generally characterized by the isolation of the patient for periods up to one month, although most hospitals denied admission to those afflicted with the pox.

At times the 'cure' became indistinguishable from the disease. Many mistook the considerable morbidity of mercury treatment for the symptoms of syphilis. Mercury elicited severe side-effects, including gum and palate ulcerations, tooth loss, skeletal deterioration, and gastro-intestinal disturbances. Given the recognized dangers of syphilis, these effects were often favourably portrayed and typically accepted as necessary to combat the disease. And, indeed, smaller doses that did not bring on these effects were often deemed inadequate by both patients and healers. The natural history of syphilis, in which initial symptoms of chancre and rash often disappear, must have convinced many physicians and patients of the effectiveness of whatever therapeutic interventions they employed.

The side-effects of mercury revealed an individual's infection: copious salivation and fetid, metallic breath, as well as the other well-recognized effects of treatment, were more difficult to conceal than the symptoms of disease. The punitive nature of mercury treatment brought together therapeutic ideas with moral norms regarding the causes of syphilis. On the premise that serious disease required serious treatment, mercury certainly met the criteria of both patients and doctors. By the nineteenth century, however, although mercury remained the most popular therapeutic approach, physicians had moderated their dosing. Surgeons, who were prominent among those consulted, often also recommended early excision or cauterization of the genital chancre as the only definitive cure.

Debates persist about the anti-treponemal properties of heavy metals, but it is clear that mercury did not cure syphilis. The state of therapeutics until the early twentieth century explains in part the high estimates of the incidence of infection; most studies suggested that 10 per cent of the population was affected. Although the precise levels of infection cannot be known, even conservative estimates indicated that in the absence of effective treatments, syphilis was endemic, constituting a health problem of enormous dimensions.[8]

In the case of venereal therapeutics, there existed no finite boundary between orthodox practice and lay medicine. Venereal diseases – given their intimate nature and moral significance – attracted a virtual sideshow of medical entrepreneurs claiming curative powers. Although most approaches used mercury in some form, the range and confidence of the claims associated with treatment varied significantly. As the side-effects of mercury came to be more clearly distinguished from the symptoms of infection itself, many lay healers found approaches which, though not affecting the disease process itself, nevertheless spared the patient further iatrogenic harm. Among the most popular alternatives to mercury were decoctions derived from guaiac, a wood imported from the Americas.

Lay approaches to syphilis ranged from legitimate popular remedies to overt frauds, eager to trade upon the fear and stigma that the disease engendered. It was not unusual for venereologists to include their addresses on their publications during the eighteenth century, a sign of the nature and needs of their desired reading audience. Central to such writings were grand claims of cure emphasizing a particular author's special therapeutic attainments. Many claimed secret remedies, which were vigorously promoted through advertising, testimonials, and public demonstration. By the middle of the century, the lines between regular and unorthodox practitioners had become more firmly drawn, as professionals placed greater restrictions on secret remedies and overt commercialism, directing their writings to other colleagues rather than potential consumers.[9] (➤ Ch. 28 Unorthodox medical theories) Given the stigmatized nature of the infection, its effect on familial relations, and the desire to maintain secrecy, patients often sought special counsel regarding their symptoms. In some respects, the world of venereology was a world apart, separate, specialized, and, to a degree, secret; an indication of the powerful moral 'valence' of infection.

THE SPECIFICITY OF GONORRHOEA AND SYPHILIS

From the sixteenth century until well into the nineteenth, most doctors assumed gonorrhoea and syphilis were manifestations of the same disease. According to most expert opinion, gonorrhoea (also known as gleet and clap) was considered but one added symptom of the pox, all the result of inoculation with the same poison or 'virus'. In instances in which there was, in fact, symptomatic specificity, it was merely assumed that infection could be exhibited in a number of ways, or that the disease was progressive with symptoms appearing serially. (➤ Ch. 16 Contagion/germ theory/specificity)

By the mid-eighteenth century, however, a vigorous debate had been generated between dualists arguing for specificity, and unicists claiming a single affliction. A series of gruesome self-experiments were initiated to settle the question. John Hunter (1728–93) reportedly inoculated his own penis with pus from a patient with gonorrhoea. When Hunter developed the typical chancre associated with syphilis, he logically concluded that the two diseases were really one, as had often been presumed. He had not suspected, however, that his patient was infected with both gonorrhoea and syphilis, a not uncommon situation given the common mode of infection. Hunter's research left the question of nosology in confusion for another seventy years.[10] (➤ Ch. 17 Nosology)

In 1837, French venereologist Philippe Ricord (1799–1889) established the specificity of the two infections through a series of experimental inoculations from syphilitic chancres. Ricord was also among the first physicians to differentiate primary, secondary, and late syphilis, the three stages of infection.[11] By the late nineteenth century, the systemic dangers of both syphilis and gonorrhoea had been clarified. Because syphilitic infections appear to resolve after the initial inflammatory reaction, chronic ailments resulting from the disease had long been thought to be distinct clinical entities. Rudolf Virchow (1821–1902) established that the infection could be transferred through the blood to the internal organs and was capable of causing significant pathology. By 1876, cardiovascular syphilis had been clearly documented in the medical literature. If spread to the spinal cord, the infection could lead to muscular incoordination, partial paralysis (tabes, locomotor ataxia, paresis), or eventually to complete paralysis.[12] Ultimately affecting the brain, syphilis also led to blindness and insanity in some cases. By the early twentieth century, mental institutions reported that as many as one-third of all patients could trace their symptoms to syphilitic infection.

(➤ Ch. 21 Mental diseases) The wide variety of syphilitic pathologies led William Osler (1849–1919) to tell his students at the Johns Hopkins Medical School, 'Know syphilis in all its manifestations and relations, and all other things clinical will be added unto you.'[13] On another occasion he called syphilis the 'great imitator', because of its range of pathological implications. (➤ Ch. 9 The pathological tradition)

The gonococcus, the causative organism of gonorrhoea, discovered under the microscope of Albert Neisser (1855–1916) in 1879, was also found to have serious long-term consequences for those infected. The bacterium could cause a wide variety of systemic inflammatory diseases, often leading to sterility in both sexes. Communicated to infants as they passed through the birth canal, gonorrhoeal ophthalmia often caused blindness. Physicians vigorously debated the efficacy of silver nitrate prophylaxis to protect newborns from such infections, as well as the larger social repercussions of familial transmission. (➤ Ch. 20 Constitutional and hereditary disorders)

PUBLIC-HEALTH APPROACHES: THE CONTROL OF PROSTITUTION

By the mid-nineteenth century, as concern about the impact of STDs grew, a concerted search began for bureaucratic interventions to control infection. Such strategies were based upon the rationale that these diseases had powerful deleterious consequences, not only for the wayward individual but for family and society as well. Given the rising concerns about the impact of these diseases in an increasingly ordered and industrialized world, no longer would the state leave those infected to their own designs; the meaning and nature of venereal disease had been transformed. What had previously been private, it was suggested, now had increasing public significance. Venereal diseases became a primary vehicle for expanding and defining police powers of the state in the sphere of public health. (➤ Ch. 27 Diseases of civilization; Ch. 51 Public health)

Most public health approaches to the problem centred attention on the role of prostitution in the spread of disease. With increasing diagnostic confidence, public health officials and clinicians came to advocate the systematic inspection of prostitutes for signs of disease. Depending upon the particular approach, evidence of infection would then lead to incarceration and treatment – sometimes in lock hospitals – as well as failure to be officially licensed for commercial prostitution. Concern about prostitutes received particular emphasis within the military (see pp. 568, 569–70).

The most ambitious administrative interventions were the Contagious Disease Acts (CDAs) of Great Britain. The Acts reflected a generally accepted cultural premise of the 'male sexual necessity', the notion that men – as a result of their biological natures – would, as a matter of course, be compelled to seek sexual relationships outside of marriage. Indeed, some observers suggested that the very nature of prostitution was premised on the notion that a pure woman should not be continually subjected to her husband's base sexual designs; the trade in prostitution protected 'better' women from being continually forced to provide sexual favours in marriage. According to this cultural logic, the division of labour among women – 'pure' and 'fallen' – was the very basis of the sexual order. Therefore, it was argued, the state must intervene to make commercial sexual liaisons free of the dangers of disease. (➤ Ch. 38 Women and medicine)

The CDAs resulted from the growing recognition of extremely high rates of STDs within the military; officials attributed both demoralization and inefficiency to frequent bouts of disease. The experience of the Crimean War (1854–6) had demonstrated the impact of disease on military effectiveness, heightening demands for administrative reforms. Statistical reports of troops returning from India included alarming rates of venereal infection, often approaching one-third of all soldiers; among troops in garrison towns and ports in England, rates of disease were reported to be strikingly high. Although many reformers argued against the regulation of prostitution, military officials and politicians expressed scepticism that environmental or moral reform could adequately affect the problem. Drawing upon rising sentiment for the powers of the state, as well as growing public outrage concerning the 'social evil' of prostitution, Parliament passed the first of three Contagious Disease Acts in 1864.[14]

The Act identified ports and garrisons in England and Ireland where women accused of prostitution could be required to undergo physical examination. If found to be infected with a sexually transmitted disease, the woman could be detained for up to three months, during which she would be compulsorily treated. In 1866 and in 1869, the Acts were extended to include additional districts, as well as regular inspections of 'known prostitutes', by a system of 'medical police'. The CDAs marked the considerable expansion of the state into previously undemarcated social territory by creating new institutions of medical supervision and control.

Organizations opposing the Acts soon formed, allying women's groups, physicians, and civil libertarians. The most prominent of these, the Ladies National Association was led by the feminist-reformer Josephine Butler (1829–1906), who toured England galvanizing popular audiences by protesting the 'instrumental rape' of working-class women as she brandished the vaginal speculum, used to perform internal examinations on prostitutes. In 1886, after more than a decade of protest, the Acts were repealed. They had signalled an official toleration of prostitution and vice that proved unacceptable to reformist sentiment in Victorian England.

The issues implicit in the regulation of prostitution continued, none the less, to characterize the debates about the nature of STDs into the twentieth century. Prostitutes became the cultural symbol of sexual danger and degeneracy in many Western societies; the social policy questions of what created commercialized sex and what to do about prostitution became pivotal, and were heatedly debated by physicians, reformers, feminists, and politicians. Inherent in this debate were fundamental ideas about the nature of human sexuality, gender, and disease. While some reformers suggested that only appropriate sexual morality would solve the problem of STDs, other 'sexual pragmatists' argued for the inevitability of prostitution, suggesting the need to reduce the risks implicit in commercial sexual encounters through instrumentalities such as the condom. In France and Germany, various experiments in regulated prostitution were attempted, typically requiring the periodic inspection and licensing of women.[15]

In the United States, on the other hand, a vigorous approach to the repression of all prostitution was pursued by criminalizing commercial sex. By the early twentieth century, cities in the USA had initiated a massive campaign to end prostitution. By the time of the First World War, concern about prostitution and venereal infections had reached unprecedented heights. The war touched off the most vigorous anti-venereal-disease campaign ever conducted. Although the US military devised a programme of vigorous exercise and explicit sexual education to protect the troops, the campaign centred on the problem of prostitution. Virtually every American city had an active prostitution trade in the early twentieth century; it was now feared that trainee soldiers would visit prostitutes, become infected, and be lost to the war effort. The military viewed these red-light districts as a potentially catastrophic health risk for the troops and the efficiency of the war effort. Posters, films, and other educational materials repeatedly warned the soldiers, 'A German bullet is cleaner than a whore.'[16]

Closing down red-light districts became part of the 'hygienic gospel', comparable to the anti-tuberculosis and anti-yellow fever campaigns waged in these years. As one federal official explained, 'To drain a red-light district and destroy thereby a breeding place of syphilis and gonorrhoea is as logical as it is to drain a swamp and thereby a breeding place of malaria and yellow fever.'[17] As a result, local governments closed down prostitution districts. In 1918, the US Congress took action to support local and state initiatives by enacting the Chamberlain–Kahn Act, establishing a 'civilian quarantine and isolation fund', as part of a comprehensive venereal-disease programme. More than 20,000 women were quarantined during the war with the assistance of federal funds, and thousands more were incarcerated as a result of local programmes.[18] Barbed wire and guards secured many of the institutions. A total of 110 districts such as 'Storyville', New Orleans, and the 'Barbary Coast', San Francisco, were closed down during the war.

Closing down red-light districts in the United States had little bearing on the situation in France, where American troops arrived 'to make the World safe for democracy'. The US Army officially forbade the soldiers from using the French-regulated houses of prostitution. This angered French officials, who believed that American demand for street prostitutes – known as clandestines – would defeat their regulatory system of medical inspections of brothels. Although it was widely recognized that latex condoms, available since the mid-nineteenth century, prevented the transmission of syphilis, the military declined to provide them to the troops. It was assumed that this would merely encourage sexual relationships.

Despite these major efforts in social engineering and public health, rates of disease remained high during the war. The incarceration of prostitutes apparently did not serve as an effective public-health measure. The war effort did reveal, however, the lengths to which the military and public-health officials would go in their attempts to control venereal disease. The war tested the basic assumptions of the social hygiene movement, which emphasized rigorous education to promote sexual abstinence coupled with vigorous repression of prostitution to conquer the problem. The war revealed the limits of this approach. (➤ Ch. 66 War and modern medicine)

THE IMPACT OF STDs ON FAMILIES

By the end of the nineteenth century, the medical profession in western Europe and the USA, eager to assert their increasing authority in sexual matters, organized to fight STDs, expressing considerable alarm about their medical and social impact. The period 1890–1910 was a time of great concern about the status and social well-being of the family in Western societies. The problem of STDs was seen as one dimension of a larger breakdown in values that emphasized the sanctity of the home, the domestic role of women, and the principle of marital sexual fidelity.[19] The writings of French syphilologist Alfred Fournier (1832–1914), concerning syphilis in marriage and its severe pathological impacts, received wide discussion throughout Europe and the USA. Fournier had centred attention on sexual infections as a major cause of infertility and congenital disease.[20]

Physicians focused attention on the impact of sexually transmitted infections on the family, calling them 'innocent infections'. Family tragedy was a frequent cultural theme in these years. In 1913, a play by French playwright Eugéne Brieux, Les Avaries – performed before packed theatres in Paris and New York – told the story of a young man, about to be married, who contracts syphilis from a prostitute. Though warned by his physician not to marry, he disregards this advice only to spread the infection to his wife; soon after, she bears a congenitally infected child. The story was told and retold, and it revealed deep cultural values about science, social responsibility, and the limits of medicine.[21] The knowledge that profligate men visited their sins upon their wives and children led to a dramatic change in professional attitudes. Syphilis was redefined from 'carnal scourge' to 'family poison'. The notion of innocent infections had the effect of dividing victims; some deserved attention, sympathy, and medical support, while others did not. This promoted stigmatization and blaming of those who were considered culpable for the epidemic.

In approaches to syphilis and gonorrhoea, concerns about hygiene, contamination, and contagion were expressed, anxieties that reflected a great deal about the contemporary society and culture. These diseases were viewed as a threat to the entire late-Victorian social and sexual system, which placed great value on discipline, restraint, and homogeneity. The sexual code of this era held that sex should receive social sanction only in marriage. But the concerns about venereal disease also reflected a pervasive fear of the urban masses, the growth of the cities, and the changing nature of familial relationships.[22] As concerns about eugenics and race heightened on both sides of the Atlantic, these diseases were typically associated with so-called 'degenerative racial stocks'. Rates of infection were cited as an index of sexual immorality and a failure to exercise individual control. By the early twentieth century, these infections had become, pre-eminently, a marker of sexual transgression and moral degeneracy.

MODERN ADVANCES IN TREATMENT

In 1909, Nobel laureate immunologist Paul Ehrlich (1854–1915) had announced the discovery of salvarsan (arsphenamine), a chemotherapeutic cure for syphilis. Ehrlich's discovery, based on a combination of serendipity, persistence, and brilliance, marked a fundamental breakthrough in the history of modern medical science; for the first time, a specific chemical compound had been demonstrated to kill a specific micro-organism. Ehrlich called the substance – the 606th arsenical he had synthesized – a 'magic bullet', a drug that would seek out and destroy its mark. He posited that the world of twentieth-century bioscience would be the elucidation of magic bullets to cure disease.[23] (➤ Ch. 39 Drug therapies)

Ehrlich's discovery of salvarsan was merely the *coup de grâce* of a generation of path-breaking research that led to a profound shift in biomedicine. Indeed, the target of Ehrlich's bullet was a micro-organism that had only been identified in May 1905, by two German researchers, Fritz Schaudinn (1871–1906), a protozoologist, and Erich Hoffmann (1868–1959), a syphilologist. Found in syphilitic chancres and other infected tissue, the slender, spiral-like organism proved difficult to stain, thus earning the name *Spiro-chaeta pallida*. Later recognized to be a treponemal organism, it was renamed *Treponema pallidum*.[24]

The discovery of the treponeme was rapidly followed by the development of a diagnostic test for the presence of the organism. August Wassermann (1866–1925) and his colleagues Albert Neisser and Carl Bruck (1879–1944) applied the complement fixation reaction discovered by Jules Bordet (1870–1961) and Octave Genou (1875–1957) to the spirochaete.[25] Syphilis could now be detected in the asymptomatic; moreover, the effect of treatment could now be evaluated. These three major discoveries appeared to fulfil the promise of the biomedical revolution of the late nineteenth century. (➤ Ch. 11 Clinical research; Ch. 8 The biochemical tradition)

Salvarsan, in modified forms (neosalvarsan, 914), remained the treatment of choice for syphilis until the discovery of the effectiveness of penicillin in 1943. Ehrlich's magic bullet had its shortcomings; it was toxic, difficult to administer, and required an extensive regimen of treatment, sometimes for as long as two years. Only 25 per cent of all treated patients apparently received the full complement of injections,[26] but at the time of its discovery it was heralded as the dawn of the modern age of clinical medicine. Physicians throughout the world wrote to Ehrlich eagerly seeking supplies of the drug, and triumphantly reported miraculous recoveries from the greatly feared disease.

The identification of the treponeme, the development of a laboratory diagnostic test for its presence, and the discovery of a chemotherapeutic agent presented an elegant model for modern biomedical science. This triumvirate of specific causality, objective diagnosis, and specific treatment formed the basis of what has come to be known as the 'biomedical model'. This paradigm also had powerful implications for the organization and implementation of public-health measures. But as the history of syphilis and other STDs in the twentieth century indicates, the problem of conquering disease through magic bullets proved more difficult than even Ehrlich might have assumed.

The First World War galvanized the attention of Western nations to the impact of STDs on military efficiency and civilian health. In the years following the war, many countries began to introduce more-aggressive public-health approaches focusing on education, early diagnosis, mandated reporting to civil authorities, contact tracing, and the free provision of treatment. In Great Britain, a Royal Commission on Venereal Disease was created in 1913. Upon completion of recommendations in 1916, Parliament enacted the Venereal Diseases Act, which established free clinics for the treatment of these infections; the government guaranteed 75 per cent of all costs to co-operating local authorities. Under the leadership of Colonel Lawrence Whitaker Harrison (1876–1964), the venereal-disease programme of the Ministry of Health met with considerable success in lowering rates of infection. In Denmark and Sweden, major programmes were also instituted, with the addition of rigorous measures for the identification and tracing of infected individuals. In the United States, under the leadership of Surgeon-General Thomas Parran (1892–1968), a major campaign was initiated during the 1930s to mandate diagnosis and treatment of venereal diseases. Parran decried the moralism that had tolerated a 'Shadow on the Land' of disease while stymying effective medical and public-health approaches. He sought to break through the 'conspiracy of silence' to 'stamp out syphilis'.[27] The culmination of Parran's campaign was the passage of the National Venereal Disease Control Act in 1938, which provided federal grants to the state boards of health to develop anti-venereal-disease programmes. Diagnostic laboratories were expanded, as were epidemiological services and treatment facilities for those who could not afford them. Public-health approaches generally emphasized serological testing and treatment during the early stages of the disease when therapy proved most effective. (➤ Ch. 50 Medical institutions and the state)

The introduction of sulpha drugs and especially antibiotics had a dramatic impact on both the incidence and the social meanings of STDs in the years after the Second World War. In early 1943, Dr John F. Mahoney (1889–1957) of the US Public Health Service, using a strain of penicillin provided by Harold Florey (1898–1968) and Ernst Chain (1906–79) at Oxford, found that the drug was effective in treating syphilitic rabbits. Realizing the potential implications of his discovery, Mahoney moved directly to repeat the experiment with human subjects. By September, he had announced his findings and the massive production of pencillin was under way.[28]

Just as Ehrlich's discovery had constituted a revolution in modern therapeutic approaches to infectious disease, so now penicillin beckoned the era of antibiotics. Penicillin had few of the drawbacks of salvarsan. It was truly a 'wonder drug'. With a single shot, the scourge of disease would be avoided. As incidence fell dramatically – in the last years of the 1950s, rates of infection reached all-time lows – it appeared that the venereal diseases would join the ranks of other infections that had come under the control of modern medicine.[29]

Despite the widespread availability of antibiotics, rates of syphilis and other STDs began to climb again in the nations of western Europe, the United States, and the developing world in the early 1960s. Although many public-health officials and physicians attributed this increase to changes in sexual mores in the wake of the growing availability of contraceptives, the rise also correlates with a substantial fall in funding for public venereal-disease programmes. By the late 1950s, much of the machinery, especially procedures for public education, case-finding, tracing, and diagnostics had been cut back.[30]

The bitter irony of syphilis and the other STDs is that the 'magic bullet' did not eliminate them. Even in the face of highly effective treatments, the infections have endured, marking a crucial paradox of modern medicine. The issue is not merely the development of effective treatments, but the process by which they are deployed; the means by which they move from laboratory to full allocation to those affected. Effective treatments without adequate public education, counselling, and timely provision of clinical services may not affect the relative incidence of disease. And while effective treatments exist for a number of highly prevalent bacterial infections such as syphilis and gonorrhoea, for other viral STDs there are no curative treatments. This explains, in part, the dramatic rise in numbers of cases of herpes simplex virus during the 1970s and 1980s. This worldwide resurgence of STDs is particularly worrisome in the current context because it appears likely that individuals with a history of sexually transmitted infection are at increased risk for infection with the AIDS virus.[31]

AIDS

Acquired Immune Deficiency Syndrome (AIDS), first identified in 1981, is an infectious disease characterized by a failure of the body's immune system. (➤ Ch. 10 The immunological tradition) This failure leaves affected individuals vulnerable to many normally harmless micro-organisms which leads eventually to severe morbidity and high mortality. The infection, spread sexually and through blood, has a fatality rate approaching 100 per cent. AIDS can now be found throughout the world, in Western industrialized countries as well as the developing nations of Africa and Latin America. Although there are no precise epidemiological data, public-health officials throughout the world have focused attention on this pandemic and its potentially catastrophic impact on health, resources, and social structure. Palliative treatments have been developed, but there is currently no cure or vaccine.

Beginning in the late 1970s, physicians in New York and California reported the increasing occurrence of a rare type of cancer, Kaposi's sarcoma, and a variety of infections including *Pneumocystis carinii* pneumonia among previously healthy young homosexual men. Because of the unusual nature of these diseases, which are typically associated with a failure of the immune system, epidemiologists began to search for characteristics that might link these cases. Although AIDS was first formally described in 1981, it now appears that the causative virus must have been silently spreading in a number of populations during the prior decade. Early epidemiological studies suggested that gay men, recipients of blood transfusions and blood products (especially haemophiliacs), and intravenous drug users were all at greatest risk. For this reason, research focused on the search for a common infectious agent that could be transmitted sexually or through blood. This research led to the identification in 1983 in French and American laboratories of a previously undescribed human retrovirus. Officially named HIV-1 (human immunodeficiency virus), this organism is an RNA retrovirus; the AIDS epidemic appears to mark the first time this organism has spread widely in the human population. There is no evidence for casual transmission of HIV.

Following the identification of HIV-1, tests to detect antibodies to the virus were discovered in 1984. Although these tests do not detect the virus itself, they are generally effective in identifying infection, since high levels of antibody are produced in most infected individuals. The enzyme-linked immunosorbant assay (ELISA), followed by Western Blot testing, have made possible the screening of donated blood to protect the blood supply from HIV, as well as testing for epidemiologic and diagnostic purposes.

AIDS can now be found throughout the world. Spread by sexual contact, by infected blood and blood products, and perinatally from mother to infant, it had been reported in 138 countries by 1988, according to the World Health Organization. Since HIV infection precedes the development of AIDS, often by as many as seven to eleven years, the precise parameters of the epidemic have been difficult to define. Estimates suggest that worldwide between 5 and 10 million individuals were infected by the end of 1988; it is projected that by the year 2000, 40 million will be infected. Although the co-factors that may determine the onset of symptoms remain unknown, all current evidence suggests that HIV-infected individuals will eventually develop AIDS.

HIV cripples the body's immune system, making an infected individual vulnerable to other disease-causing agents. The most common of these opportunistic infections in AIDS patients has been *Pneumocystis carinii* pneumonia, an infection previously seen principally among patients receiving immunosuppressive drugs. There is also evidence that infection with HIV makes individuals more vulnerable to tuberculosis, a resurgence of which has been reported in nations with a high incidence of AIDS.

Immunological damage occurs by depletion of a specific type of immune cell, a white blood cell known as a helper T_4 lymphocyte. Destruction of these cells accounts for the vulnerability to many normally harmless infectious agents. In some cases, infection of the central nervous system with HIV may cause damage to the brain and spinal column, resulting in severe cognitive and motor dysfunction. In its late manifestations, AIDS causes severe wasting. Death may occur from infection, functional failure of the central nervous system, or starvation.

HIV infection has a wide spectrum of clinical manifestations and pathological abnormalities. After infection, an individual may remain free of symptoms for up to a decade. Some individuals do experience fever, rash, and malaise at the time of infection when antibodies are first produced. Generally, patients present with general lymphadenopathy, weight loss, diarrhoea, and/or an opportunistic infection. Diagnosis may be confirmed by the presence of antibodies for HIV or a decline in T4 helper cells. Most experts now agree that HIV-infection itself should be considered a disease regardless of symptoms.[32]

Researchers have identified three epidemiological patterns of HIV transmission that roughly follow geographical boundaries. Pattern I includes North America, western Europe, Australia, New Zealand, and many urban centres in Latin America. In these industrial, highly developed areas, transmission has predominantly been among homosexual and bisexual men. Since the introduction of widespread blood screening, transmission via blood now occurs principally among intravenous drug users who share needles. Although there is no evidence of widescale spread among the heterosexual population in these countries, heterosexual transmission of the virus via intravenous drug use has increased, leading to a rise in paediatric cases resulting from perinatal transmission.

Within the United States, in particular, the distribution of AIDS cases has been marked by the disproportionate representation of the poor and minorities. As the principal mode of transmission has shifted to intravenous drug use, AIDS has increasingly become an affliction of the urban underclass, those at greatest risk for drug addiction. Serum surveys reveal that 50 per cent or more of the intravenous drug users in New York City are infected with HIV. Blacks and Hispanics, who comprise 20 per cent of the US population, accounted for more than 40 per cent of all AIDS cases in 1988. Infected women, who account for more than 10 per cent of new AIDS cases, are typically infected by intravenous drug use or sexual contact with a drug user; in 70 per cent of all infected newborns, transmission can be traced to drug use. In 1988 it was expected that between 10,000 and 20,000 children in the USA would have symptomatic HIV infections by 1991.[33]

In Pattern II countries, comprised of sub-Saharan Africa, and increasingly, Latin America, transmission of HIV is predominantly through heterosexual contact. In some urban areas, up to 25 per cent of all sexually active adults are reported to be infected, and a majority of female prostitutes are seropositive. Transfusion continues to be a mode of transmission, since universal screening of blood is not routine. Non-sterile injections and medical procedures may also be responsible. In these areas, perinatal transmission is an important cause, and in some urban centres at least 5 to 15 per cent of pregnant women have been found to be infected.

Pattern III countries, which include North Africa, the Middle East, Eastern

THEORIES OF LIFE, HEALTH, AND DISEASE

Europe, Asia, and the Pacific, by 1992 far experienced less morbidity and mortality from the pandemic. Apparently, HIV–1 was not present in these areas until the mid-1980s; therefore, fewer than 1 per cent of all cases have been found there. Infection has been the result of contact with infected individuals from Pattern I and II countries, or from imported of infected blood. The nature of world travel, however, had diminished the significance of geographical isolation as a means of protecting a population from contact with a pathogen.[34] (➤ Ch 72 Medicine, mortality, and morbidity)

Research efforts to develop effective therapies have centred on antiviral drugs that directly attack HIV, as well as drugs likely to enhance the functioning of the immune system. Because the virus becomes encoded within the genetic material of the host cell and is highly mutable, the problem of finding safe and effective treatments has been extremely difficult, requiring considerable basic science and clinical knowledge. Studies are currently being conducted to determine the anti-HIV properties of many drugs, but the ethical and economic obstacles to clinical trials are formidable. Given the immediacy of the epidemic, it is difficult to structure appropriate randomized clinical trials, which often take a considerable time to assess the safety and efficacy of a drug. At the present time, few drugs have been licensed for the treatment of HIV infection. After the onset of symptoms, expected survival averaged in two years 1988, which may increase with anticipated improvements in antiviral treatments.

In its first decade, AIDS created considerable suffering and generated an ongoing worldwide health crisis. During this brief period, the epidemic was identified and characterized epidemiologically, the basic modes of transmission specified, a causal organism isolated, and effective tests for the presence of infection developed. In spite of this remarkable progress, which required the application of sophisticated epidemiological, clinical, and scientific research, the barriers to controlling AIDS are imposing and relate to the most complex biomedical and political questions. AIDS has already sorely tested the capabilities of research, clinical, and public-health institutions throughout the world.

The epidemic began at a moment of relative complacency, especially in the developed world, concerning epidemic infectious disease. Not since the influenza epidemic of 1918–20 had an epidemic with such devastating potential struck. The Western, developed world had experienced a health transition from the predominance of infectious to chronic disease and had come to focus its resources and attention on systemic, non-infectious diseases. AIDS thus appeared at a historical moment in which there was little social or political experience in confronting a public-health crisis of this dimension. The epidemic fractured a widely held belief in medical security.

Not surprisingly, early socio-political responses were characterized by denial. Early theories, when few cases had been reported, centred on identifying particular aspects of 'fast-track' gay sexual culture that might explain the cases of immunocompromised men. Additional cases among individuals who had received blood transfusions or blood products, however, soon led the US Centers for Disease Control to suspect an infectious agent. Nevertheless, in the earliest years of the epidemic, few wished openly to confront the possibility of spread beyond these specified high-risk groups. During this period, grassroots organizations, especially in the gay community, were created to meet the growing needs for education, counselling, patient services, and in some instances, clinical research. Agencies such as the Gay Men's Health Crisis, founded in New York City in 1982, the Shanti Project, established in San Francisco in 1983, and the Terence Higgins Trust in London, worked to overcome the denial, prejudice, and bureaucratic inertia that limited governmental response.

As the nature and extent of the epidemic became clearer, however, hysteria sometimes replaced denial. Because the disease was so powerfully associated with behaviours characteristically identified as immoral, illegal, or both, the stigma of those infected has been heightened. Echoing earlier assessments of other STDs, victims of HIV disease were often divided into categories: those who became infected through transfusions or perinatally, the 'innocent victims'; and those who engaged in high-risk, morally condemnable behaviours, the 'guilty perpetrators'. There was a tendency to blame those who became infected through drug use or homosexuality, behaviours viewed as 'voluntary'. Some religious groups in the United States, for example, viewed AIDS as proof of a certain moral order.

By 1983, as the potential ramifications of the epidemic became evident, national and international scientific and public-health institutions began to mobilize. The World Health Organization (WHO) established a global programme on AIDS in 1986 to co-ordinate international efforts in epidemiological surveillance, education, prevention, and research. Considerable debate concerning the most effective public-health responses to the epidemic have persisted. Although some nations such as Cuba have experimented with programmes mandating the isolation of HIV-infected individuals, the WHO has lobbied against the use of coercive measures in response to the epidemic. Given the life-long nature of HIV infection, effective isolation would require lifetime incarceration. Traditional public-health approaches to communicable disease, including contact tracing and mandatory treatment, have less potential to control infection since there are currently no means of rendering an infected individual non-infectious.[35] (➤ Ch. 59 Internationalism in medicine and public health)

Since biomedical technologies to prevent transmission appear to be some years off, the principal public-health approaches to controlling the pandemic rest upon education and behaviour modification. Heightened awareness of the dangers of unprotected anal intercourse among gay men, for example, has led to a significant decline in new infections among them. Nevertheless, encouraging the modification of risk behaviours would present no simple task, even in the face of a dread disease.[36]

The burden of AIDS, both in human suffering and its demands on resources, is likely to grow in the years ahead. Assuring quality care to those infected will become even more difficult, especially in the epidemic's epicentres, where those infected are increasingly among the minorities and the poor. In the developing world, AIDS threatens to reverse recent advances in infant and child survival, and is likely to have a substantial impact on demographic patterns. Because the disease principally affects young and middle-aged adults, 20 to 49 years of age, it has already had tragic social and cultural repercussions. Transmitted both horizontally (via sexual contact) and vertically (from mother to infant), the epidemic has the potential to depress the growth rate of human populations, especially in areas of the developing world. Thus, the disease could destabilize the workforce and depress local economies.[37] (➤ Ch. 71 Demography and medicine)

AIDS, like other STDs, has clearly demonstrated the complex relationship of biological and behavioural forces in determining patterns of health and disease. Altering the course of the epidemic by human design has already proved no easy matter. The lifelong infectiousness of carriers; the private, bio-psycho-social nature of sexual behaviour and drug use; the fact that those at greatest risk are already stigmatized: all made effective public policy interventions even more difficult. Finally, the very nature of the virus itself, its complex and mutagenic nature, make a short-term technological breakthrough unlikely.

Just as syphilis revealed basic social conflicts regarding the nature of sexuality and responsibility for disease in earlier historical times, in the last decades of the twentieth century, HIV disease has become the focus of these debates. The AIDS epidemic, appearing suddenly and globally, shattered expectations of a relatively stable world of infectious disease. AIDS, like syphilis in the past, engenders powerful social conflicts about the meaning, nature, and risks of sexuality; the nature and role of the state in protecting and promoting public health; the significance of individual rights in regard to communal good; the nature of the doctor–patient relationship, and social responsibility in times of epidemic disease. (➤ Ch. 37 History of medical ethics; Ch. 34 History of the doctor–patient relationship)

CONCLUSION

Throughout the twentieth century the debate about STDs has swung between two essential approaches to the problem. The first, clearly articulated by the social-hygiene movement, argued for adherence to a sexual ethic that made it impossible to become infected. Essentially, this meant restricting all sexual relationships to marriage. This goal could best be achieved through education to encourage abstinence, and the repression of prostitution, assumed to be the central locus of infection. The alternative view, instrumental in orientation, sought to sever the problem of STDs from any particular sexual ethic. According to this position, represented in most public-health approaches to the STDs, individuals should be provided with means of preventing infection and, if infected, appropriate treatment.

These two long-standing approaches have been widely voiced since the onset of the AIDS epidemic. Adherents of the moral approach argue that the instrumentalists actually encourage infection by unwittingly promoting sexual behaviour – according to this argument good morals and good health go hand-in-hand. In this view, STDs function in the social order by making sexual encounters more dangerous, thus encouraging 'appropriate' behaviours. Advocates of the instrumental orientation counter that the moralists promote infection by restricting access to explicit education and preventive techniques. Both approaches reflect implicit social values about sexuality, medicine, and disease.

The STDs reveal certain limitations of the biomedical model of disease, the search for magic bullets. No doubt, effective treatments for specific diseases are a critical component in their control, but as the history of syphilis indicates, they are not a panacea. Infectious diseases constitute complex bio-ecological problems in which host, parasite, and a range of social and environmental forces interact.[38] No single medical or social intervention can thus adequately address the problem. Just as penicillin did not 'solve' the problem of syphilis, no single treatment or even vaccine is likely to free us from AIDS, at least in the immediate future.

The history of STDs is indicative of the complex relationship of human behaviour to health. Behaviour is subject to a range of influences, biological and cultural, economic and political. As the history of STDs repeatedly demonstrates, the modification of sexual behaviour to reduce risk of disease has rarely responded to fear or moral exhortation. In this fundamental respect, sexual relations are likely to remain a mode for the transmission of infectious diseases. The nature of these diseases, their medical and public meanings, as well as their epidemiological patterns, will necessarily be shaped by their particular historical, social, and cultural contexts. (➤ Ch. 70 Medical sociology)

NOTES

1 Alfred W. Crosby Jr, *The Columbian Exchange: Biological and Cultural Consequences of 1492*, Westport, CT, Greenwood Press, 1972, pp. 122–64.

2 Brenda J. Baker and George J. Armelagos, 'The origin and antiquity of syphilis', *Current Anthropology*, 1988, 29: 703–38.

3 Joseph Grünpeck, quoted in Claude Quétel, *History of Syphilis*, trans. by Bradock and Pike, Baltimore, MD, Johns Hopkins University Press, 1990, p. 17.

4 T. A. Cockburn, 'The origin of the treponematoses', *Bulletin of the World Health Organization*, 1961, 24: 221–8; Ellis Herndon Hudson, 'Christopher Columbus and the history of syphilis', *Acta Tropica*, 1968, 25: 1–16.

5 Owsei Temkin, 'On the history of morality and syphilis', in Temkin, *The Double Face of Janus and Other Essays in the History of Medicine*, Baltimore, MD, Johns Hopkins University Press, 1977, pp. 472–84.

6 J. Johnston Abraham, 'Some account of the history of the treatment of syphilis', *British Journal of Venereal Diseases*, 1948, 24: 156.

7 Owsei Temkin, 'Therapeutic trends and the treatment of syphilis before 1900', in Temkin, op. cit. (n. 5), pp. 518–24.

8 See, for example, Prince A. Morrow, 'Report to the Committee of Seven of the Medical Society of the County of New York on the prophylaxis of venereal disease in New York City', *New York Medical Journal*, 1901, 74: 1146. Additional data on the incidence of venereal infections is contained in military archives: see *Report of the Surgeon General for the United States Army, 1910*, Washington, DC, Government Printing Office, 1911.

9 W. F. Bynum, 'Treating the wages of sin: venereal disease and specialism in eighteenth-century Britain', in Bynum and R. Porter (eds), *Medical Fringe and Medical Orthodoxy, 1750–1850*, London, Croom Helm, 1987, pp. 5–28.

10 Kenneth F. Flegal, 'Changing concepts of the nosology of gonorrhea and syphilis', *Bulletin of the History of Medicine*, 1974, 48: 571–88.

11 J. T. Crissey and L. C. Parish, *The Dermatology and Syphilology of the Nineteenth Century*, New York, Praegar, 1981.

12 W. A. Pusey, *The History and Epidemiology of Syphilis*, Baltimore, MD, Thomas, 1933, pp. 53–61.

13 William Osler, *Aequanimitas*, 3rd edn, Philadelphia, PA, 1932; Osler, 'The campaign against syphilis', *Lancet*, 1917, 1: 789.

14 Judith Walkowitz, *Prostitution and Victorian Society*, Cambridge and New York, Cambridge University Press, 1980; F. B. Smith 'Ethics and disease in the late nineteenth century: the Contagious Diseases Acts', *Historical Studies*, 1971, 115: 118–35.

15 Abraham Flexner, *Prostitution in Europe*, New York, Century, 1914.

16 Colonel Care Poster Series [n.d. 1918?], in American Social Hygiene Association Papers, Folder 113:6, University of Minnesota.

17 US Interdepartmental Social Hygiene Board, *Program of Protective Social Measures*, Washington, DC, Government Printing Office, 1920.

18 *Report of the US Interdepartmental Social Hygiene Board*, Washington, DC, Government Printing Office, 1920; Mary Macey Dietzler, *Detention Houses and Reformatories*, US Interdepartmental Social Hygiene Board, Washington, DC, Government Printing Office, 1922.

19 Allan M. Brandt, *No Magic Bullet: a Social History of Venereal Disease in the United States since 1880*, rev. edn, New York, Oxford University Press, 1987, pp. 7–47; orig. pub. 1985, pp. 7–47.

20 Alfred Fournier, *Syphilis and Marriage*, trans. by Prince A. Morrow, New York, Appleton, 1881; Prince A. Morrow, *Social Diseases and Marriage*, New York, Lea Brothers, 1904.

21 Eugéne Brieux, *Damaged Goods*, trans. by Pollack, New York, Brentano's, 1913; Barabara Gutmann Rosenkrantz, 'Damaged goods: dilemmas of responsibility for risk', *Milbank Quarterly*, 1979, 57: 1–37.

22 Brandt, op. cit. (n. 19), pp. 19–23.

23 Martha Marquardt, *Paul Ehrlich*, New York, Henry Schuman, 1951.

24 W. A. Pusey, *Syphilis as a Modern Problem*, Chicago, IL, American Medical Association, 1915, pp. 31–5.

25 A. Wassermann, A. Neisser, C. Bruck, 'Eine serodiagnostische Reaction bei Syphilis', *Deutsches Medizinische Wochenschrift*, 1906, 32: 745–6.

26 Patricia Spain Ward, 'The American reception of salvarsan', *Journal of the History of Medicine*, 1981, 36: 59–60.

27 Thomas Parran, *Shadow on the Land: Syphilis*, New York, Reynal & Hitchcock, 1937.

28 Harry F. Dowling, *Fighting Infection: Conquests of the Twentieth Century*, Cambridge, MA, Harvard University Press, 1977.

29 William J. Brown, James F. Donohue, Norman W. Axnick, Joseph H. Blount, Oscar G. Jones and Neal H. Ewen, *Syphilis and Other Venereal Diseases*, Cambridge, Harvard University Press, 1970.

30 O. W. Anderson, *Syphilis and Society*, Chicago, IL, Center for Health Administration Studies, 22: 1965.

31 Centers for Disease Control, *Morbidity and Mortality Weekly Report*, 1987, 36: 393.

32 Anthony S. Fauci, 'The Acquired Immune Deficiency Syndrome: the ever broadening clinical syndrome', *Journal of the American Medical Association*, 1980, 249: 2375–6; Fauci, 'The human immunodeficiency virus: infectivity and mechanisms of pathogenesis', *Science*, 1988, 239: 617–22.

33 James W. Curran, Harold W. Jaffe, Anne M. Hardy, W. Meade Morgan, Richard M. Selik and Timothy J. Dondero, 'Epidemiology of HIV infection and AIDS in the United States', *Science*, 1988, 239: 610–16.

34 Jonathan M. Mann, James Chin, Peter Piot and Thomas Quinn, 'The international epidemiology of AIDS', *Scientific American*, 1988, 259: 82–9.

35 Larry O. Gostin, 'The future of communicable disease control: toward a new concept in public health law', *Milbank Quarterly*, 1986, 64: 79–96.

36 Harvey V. Fineberg, 'Education to prevent AIDS: prospects and obstacles', *Science*, 1988, 239: 592–6.

37 Robert M. May, Roy M. Anderson and Sally M. Blower, 'The epidemiology and transmission dynamics of HIV-AIDS', *Daedalus*, 1989, 118: 163–201.

38 L. Eisenberg, 'Human health ecology: the control of disease', paper presented at WHO Meeting on Human Ecology and Health, Greece, 1986.

FURTHER READING

Aral, Sevgi O. and Holmes, King K., 'Sexually transmitted diseases in the AIDS era', *Scientific American*, 1991, 264: 62–9.

Bayer, Ronald, *Private Acts, Social Consequences: AIDS and the Politics of Public Health*, New York, Free Press, 1989.

Brandt, Allan M., *No Magic Bullet: a Social History of Venereal Disease in the United States since 1880*, rev. edn, New York, Oxford University Press, 1987; orig. pub. 1985.

Brown, William, Donohue, James F., Axnick, Norman W., Blount, Joseph H., Jones, Oscar G. and Ewen, Neal H., *Syphilis and Other Venereal Diseases*, Cambridge, MA, Harvard University Press, 1970.

Bulkey, L. Duncan, *Syphilis of the Innocent*, New York, Bailey & Fairchild, 1894.

Connelly, Mark Thomas, *The Response to Prostitution in the Progressive Era*, Chapel Hill, University of North Carolina Press, 1980.

Fee, Elizabeth and Fox, Daniel M. (eds), *AIDS: the Burdens of History*, Berkeley, University of California Press, 1988.

Fleck, Ludwik, *Genesis and Development of a Scientific Fact*, trans. by Trenn, Chicago, IL, University of Chicago Press, 1935; reprinted 1979.

Flexner, Abraham, *Prostitution in Europe*, New York, Century, 1914.

Fournier, Alfred, *Syphilis and Marriage*, trans. by Prince A. Morrow, New York, Appleton, 1881.

Gilman, Sander L., *Difference and Pathology: Stereotypes of Sexuality, Race, and Madness*, Ithaca, NY, Cornell University Press, 1985.

Grmek, Mirko D., *The History of AIDS: Emergence and Origin of a Modern Pandemic*, trans. by Russell Maulitz and Duffin, Princeton, NJ, Princeton University Press, 1991.

Holmes, King K., Mardh P. A., Sparling, P. F. and Wiesner, P. J., *Sexually Transmitted Diseases*, New York, McGraw-Hill, 1990.

Jones, James H., *Bad Blood: the Tuskegee Syphilis Experiment*, New York, Free Press, 1981.

Morrow, Prince A., *Social Diseases and Marriage*, New York, Lea Brothers, 1904.

Parran, Thomas, *Shadow on the Land: Syphilis*, New York, Reynal & Hitchcock, 1937.

Pusey, William A., *The History and Epidemiology of Syphilis*, Springfield, IL, and Baltimore, MD, C. C. Thomas, 1933.

Quétel, Claude, *History of Syphilis*, trans. by Bradock and Pike, Baltimore, MD, Johns Hopkins University Press, 1990.

Rosebury, Theodore, *Microbes and Morals: the Strange Story of Venereal Disease*, New York, Viking, 1971.

Shilts, Randy, *And the Band Played On*, New York, St Martins Press, 1987.

Thomas, Keith, 'The double standard', *Journal of the History of Ideas*, 1959, 20: 199.

Vedder, Edward B., *Syphilis and Public Health*, Philadelphia, PA, Lea & Febiger, 1918.

Walkowitz, Judith, *Prostitution and Victorian Society*, Cambridge and New York, Cambridge University Press, 1980.

27

DISEASES OF CIVILIZATION

Roy Porter

No man is an island, and very few are eremites. Practically all humans live in social groups of some kind, sharing common cultures, habits, and socio-economic organization; and, to that degree, all diseases afflicting humankind may be said, at least trivially, to be diseases of civilization. Infections such as measles need pools of susceptibles to provide continuous chains of hosts in space and time. Other maladies – for example, bovine tuberculosis – are hosted by the domesticated animals that accompany human settlement. Air-borne and droplet-carried infections clearly require crowded habitation patterns, just as typhoid, cholera, and other water-borne diseases need the defective waste-disposal arrangements and hygiene endemic to towns, ports, jails, and camps. In short, as is fully argued in Kenneth Kiple's contribution to this volume, it has been a fact of history – at least until recent times – that disease incidence runs in direct ratio to settlement density. (➤ Ch. 18 The ecology of disease) Palaeopathological evidence confirms the findings of medical anthropologists studying such 'primitives' as the Kalahari bush-people, that, whatever hardships may be entailed by technological backwardness, disease levels tend to be low amongst small, nomadic communities. (➤ Ch. 60 Medicine and anthropology)

THE FACTS OF EPIDEMIOLOGY

Beyond such truisms, can the notion of 'diseases of civilization' be given greater analytic bite, by more selective and specific application? It seems so. It is well established that rising population density, consequent upon the development of specialized, labour-intensive agriculture in the great Asiatic river valleys some 8,000 years ago, upon the founding of centralized military and political empires (the Assyrian, Egyptian, etc.), and above all upon the building of metropolises like Babylon, led, if not to the *appearance* of lethal diseases, then certainly to their attaining epidemic and endemic status. The great Egyptian pestilences dramatically recorded in the Old Testament, the 'plague' that laid Athens low in the fourth century BC (its specification still baffles epidemiologists, though it can surely be no accident that it struck a besieged, refugee-packed city), the well-documented tidal waves of plague and perhaps smallpox within the Roman Empire: these all indicate how demographic densification, the development of overseas commercial markets, communication improvements, and heightened personal mobility provided pathogens with golden opportunities to go forth and multiply. (➤ Ch. 71 Demography and medicine)

The great migrations of peoples and conquerors, and the expansion of trade routes in the High Middle Ages enabled bubonic plague to decimate urbanized regions of Asia and Europe. From the close of the fifteenth century, syphilis spread like the plague, being particularly associated with conurbations like Naples and London, notorious for their traffic in sexual vice. (➤ Ch. 26 Sexually transmitted diseases) From the same time, a clutch of grave airborne infections (a multitude of ill-defined 'fevers', including the lethal but short-lived English 'sweat') brought mortality crises to towns in France, the Low Countries, and England, all subject to the Malthusian scissors-effect of rising population and falling nutritional standards. (➤ Ch. 22 Nutritional diseases)

Smallpox grew in seventeenth-century Europe, and peaked in the eighteenth century, being then, in aggregate terms, the most lethal of the infections. Great cities proved lasting reservoirs of infection, and young migrant workers from the countryside were especially vulnerable, lacking acquired immunity. The seventeenth century also saw the rise to prominence of what were known as 'new diseases', including rickets, commonly associated by contemporaries with deleterious facets of urban life (poverty, deficient diet, poor housing conditions). And, from around the same time, phthisis (consumption, or '*the* consumptions' – revealingly, the plural form was often used to signify a cluster of perceptibly interconnected wasting and debilitating constitutional afflictions) began its three hundred years' rampage. Tuberculosis, the new 'white plague' that replaced the old Black Death, was widely identified as essentially an urban disease, especially tragic because, as Dr Erasmus Darwin (1731–1802) put it, 'like war, it cuts off the young in their prime'. (➤ Ch. 52 Epidemiology)

Naturally, the countryside was not without its dangers. Until the close of the *ancien régime*, famine struck in many regions of Europe: around one-third of the population of Finland may have starved to death in the terrible winter of 1696. Nevertheless, isolated rural enclaves often escaped epidemics. While plague decimated trading towns in the early modern era, their rural hinterlands often remained free. And historical demographers have drawn attention to the remarkably low disease mortalities experienced by rural areas far from the main trade arteries which twinned as the chief channels for microbial transfer. By contrast, the Bills of Mortality and vital statistics carefully tabulated by the physician bureaucrats of the emergent nation states confirmed that city gates were gateways to death; and that within such conurbations, quintessential types of urban institution, harbouring dense population concentrations, created the worst hazards of all. 'Jail fever', 'hospital fever': such phrases, generally indicating outbreaks of typhus, are eloquent of the habitual linkage of town and disease amongst the 'great wens' of Europe and the expanding empires overseas. (➤ Ch. 19 Fevers)

Early modern medicine made the connection between societies and sickness quite explicit. The appalling incidence of syphilis in princely armies and cities in the sixteenth century led to appelations such as the 'Spanish disease', the '*morbus Gallicus*', and the 'Neapolitan bone-ache'. And in the seventeenth century, the maverick British physician Gideon Harvey (*c.*1640–*c.*1700) began to speak of the 'morbus anglicus' (1672), by which he meant consumption, and *The Disease of London* (1675), which, as his subtitle explained, signified *A New Discovery of the Scorvey*. Harvey's perception, shared by many, was that the capital had become the breeding-ground for a throng of constitutional maladies, wasting conditions, skin complaints, tubercular infections, scrofula, scurvy, and probably venereal infections. (➤ Ch. 20 Constitutional and hereditary disorders)

Charting, containing, and curbing town-specific diseases exercised the medical administrators of early modern Europe. Public-health experts in Renaissance Italy promoted and perfected quarantine protocols. In many Mediterranean and Atlantic ports, vessels were detained forty days (hence, the term 'quarantine') after embarkation before being granted a clean bill of health. In times of plague, produce markets were closed, embargoes imposed upon inter-regional commerce, city gates bolted and policed, travellers arrested, and intercity traffic halted. Compulsory house-confinement was common for suspects, and the infected were removed to lazarettos.

With the receding of plague in the generations after 1660 (possibly a testimony to the efficacy of quarantine measures), and with commercial rights and personal liberties being accorded enhanced status, new strategies had to be evolved to counter the perceived correlation between the commercial city and dire morbidity levels; it had grown both impracticable and politically unacceptable to contemplate immobilizing immense populations through house arrest and similar measures in the name of public salubrity. As James Riley has emphasized, renewed efforts were made during the Enlightenment to document disease and plot patterns of incidence against natural and social-environmental factors such as climate, temperature, atmospheric conditions, prevailing winds, soil, standing water, population distribution, occupational structure, building materials, waste disposal, and so forth. (➤ Ch. 15 Environment and miasmata) Pioneer surveys, such as that by John Haygarth (1740–1827) in Chester in the 1770s, were undertaken in the expectation that fuller knowledge of natural and artificial variables would produce practical policies for containment and eradication. The Enlightenment 'medical police' strategy for the *polis* may be seen as the forerunner of 'health and towns' drives in the nineteenth century, and in some sense the distant ancestor of 'garden city' theorists in the twentieth century who denied the habitual linkage of urban life with insalubrity.

It was during the nineteenth century that the correlation between disease and the city appeared most inescapable, not least, to noses, as when 'the Great Stink' emanating in 1852 from the River Thames forced the adjournment of Parliament. The great medical statistician William Farr (1807–83) correlated disease with population density. As Dorothy Porter's essay in this *Encyclopedia* documents more fully, rival aetiological theories were proposed to explain the disproportionately high urban-disease incidence. (➤ Ch. 51 Public health) 'Contagionists' could point to the myriad indiscriminate bodily contacts towns created. 'Miasmatists' like Edwin Chadwick (1800–90) would counter-argue that the new 'shock towns' produced the highest concentrations of garbage, rotting refuse, decaying animal and vegetable remains, faeces, industrial pollution, and so forth, all of which emitted those gaseous effluvia, which were disease in its own right or at least its bearers. Others emphasized the *moral* links between sickness and the city. Idleness, indigence, and ignorance amongst the working classes bred the defective life-styles that, in turn, bred disease. Such evil habits were naturally most conspicuous in inner-city areas that attracted the great unwashed, and seduced by example, especially where gin-palaces and brothels inflamed temptation. Such arguments (focusing upon 'moral contagion') enjoyed great popularity on both sides of the Atlantic during the cholera pandemics of the 1830s and 1840s. (➤ Ch. 16 Contagion/ germ theory/specificity)

A time-honoured, and rather dramatic, repertoire of measures had been used for centuries to protect the health of cities: firing cannon to break up pockets of infected air; lighting vast bonfires to stir ventilation; fumigation; dredging rivers and sewers; and performing religious purifications (within Catholic nations, processions; amongst Protestants, fasts and prayers). These were supplanted in the nineteenth century by the marvels of engineering, creating a subterranean sanitary infrastructure for the industrial city barely applicable to the countryside: the installation of mains drainage and piped water supplies, slum clearance, and widening of thoroughfares, the enforcement of building standards, and the construction of suburban cemeteries to replace noisome churchyards – all measures that paid indirect tribute to the health hazards of urban life.

For reasons complex in nature and still contested by historians, a great transformation was wrought as the nineteenth century passed into the twentieth. For two thousand years, the disgust for urban corruption – 'the whore of Babylon', 'Rome' – so widely voiced by priests and moralizers, had been substantiated by medical evidence that town-dwellers enjoyed poorer life chances than their country cousins. In many parts of the Western world, that had ceased to be so by the twentieth century, or was only locally and class-selectively true. The great killer infections that had so long decimated urban communities – typhoid, typhus, diphtheria, tuberculosis – were in rapid retreat. The affluent city came to be recognized as the site of the most effective health-care delivery system. It was in backwoods rural areas that isolation, poverty, poor services, and antiquated attitudes combined to hamper therapeutic interventions and keep infant and maternal mortality rates dispro-portionately high. In most advanced countries nowadays, 'healthiness' – as measured by morbidity incidence and life expectation – is no more a consist-ently rural phenomenon than it is the privilege of the Third World. It is the First World, urbanized, industrialized, civilized, that enjoys longevity and salubrity at the close of the twentieth century.

DISEASES OF CIVILIZATION AS IDEOLOGY

These primary epidemiological considerations and vital statistics are, however, but part of the story. For, especially over the last couple of centuries, the concept of 'diseases of civilization' has proved a powerful ideological construct in shaping normative relations between nations and classes; between past, present, and future; and between peoples, the medical profession, and govern-ments. The concept of 'diseases of civilization', superimposing the medical and the moral , first became activated during the eighteenth century, serving in many respects as a secularized revamping of the Christian legend of the Fall, wherein Original Sin and the expulsion from Paradise had inaugurated the regime of hard labour, disease, suffering, and death in the temporal world. (➤ Ch. 61 Religion and medicine) Jean-Jacques Rousseau (1712–78) and other pre-Romantic 'primitivists', and such popularizing physicians as the Scot George Cheyne (1673–1743), the Genevan S.-A.-A.-D. Tissot (1728–97), and the naval physician Thomas Trotter (1760–1832), argued that what might be termed 'noble savages', and their sturdy hunter-gatherer and peasant descendants, of necessity pursued healthy life-styles: engaging in physical labour, enjoying abundant exercise in the open air, and dieting frugally on grains, green vegetables, milk, and water. Their disorders were as few as their needs.

The development of town life, commerce, and indoor employment, opu-lence, fashion, and emulation had changed all that. Deleterious habits had set in: over-eating, hard drinking, want of exercise, late rising, tight-lacing, and a love of luxury. Financial speculation, the strict protocols and etiquettes of court and metropolis, the obligations of etiquette – all had begotten anxiety, in turn exhausting and sapping the constitution. Enervated hot-house creatures – and Tissot singled out *gens de lettres* and *gens du monde* – turned to sedatives (opiates, tobacco, and medicaments) to soothe the nerves, and to stimulants (alcohol, ether) to invigorate. These recourses, in turn, became habit-forming, harming bodies and minds equally. In short, the artificial demands of smart, high-pressure high society, and of enlightened living amongst the literati and the glitterati, were creating (so many eighteenth-century medical commentators asserted) a new world of diseases.

Cheyne, Tissot, and their followers offered complementary physiological diagnoses pinpointing the nervous system as the seat of such disorders. Discarding conventional theories of humoral balance, they emphasized that the key to health and happiness lay in correct nervous tone. (➤ Ch. 14 Humoralism) Excessive consumption of fine foods and alcohol, and lack of exercise combined to obstruct the nervous fibres, impeding communications between the brain, the vital organs, and the extremities, and leading to pains, inflammation, stoppages, and habitual sensations of lethargy and lassitude unknown to strapping peasants. Thus the notion of diseases of civilization went hand-in-hand with the increased explanatory importance of the central nervous system, to suggest a psychophysiological doctrine of widespread applicability. 'Nervousness' became a buzz-word of doctors and patients alike. In the 1670s, Thomas Sydenham (1624–89) guessed that about one-third of all disorders in Britain were 'nervous'; by 1800, Trotter was suggesting that their incidence had doubled. As statistics, these are worthless, but what is significant is the perception of an inflamed problem, often linked to depopulation scares, due to the supposed increased incidence of impotence and infertility created by nervous disorders.

Profound but productive ambiguities were contained in the notions of the nervous constitution, and of diseases of civilization. As was widely noted by eighteenth-century observers, the 'nervous disorder' diagnosis was being packaged in ways that imparted a positive appeal. One had to be rich, ingenious, talented, and fashionable to suffer from such conditions. Hence 'nervousness' could, by a ready reversal, be taken as a symptom of success no less than sickness. Cheyne insisted that the poor were too impoverished in natural endowment to succumb to nervous complaints. The same story that was told for nervous complaints equally applied to gout, that notorious status symbol of affluence.

This observation applied not just to individuals but to nations as well. It was kingdoms characterized by commercial success, political and religious liberty, and artistic and intellectual achievement that were cursed, or blessed, with these nervous conditions and such tell-tale accompaniments as high suicide rates. When in 1733, Cheyne deployed the label *The English Malady* as a book-title, it was, perhaps, more an accolade than a stigma.

The medical philosophies of the Enlightenment extended these intriguing possibilities. In particular, many began to emphasize that while illness was typically the product of essentially organic causes – imbalances, infections, toxins, or miasmas – cultural aetiologies could also play important parts. In line with their heightened receptivity to psychology, and their investigations of the enigmas of the association of ideas, Enlightenment physicians explored the intricacies of mind–body circuits, and examined the propensity of imagination, *idées fixes*, and emotional states to disturb the equilibrium of health and illness. Within this psychosomatic paradigm, doctors dismissed those supernatural agents formerly thought to induce illness – Satan, demons, and witches – as figments of the imagination, albeit no less capable of provoking complaints by suggestion and sympathy. Likewise, it became common for physicians to suggest that the key to drunkenness did not lie wholly in the chemistry of alcohol, but in the disposition (constitutional, mental, cultural) of the drinker. Similarly, sexual abnormalities such as nymphomania or satyriasis, traditionally explained largely physiologically, in terms of genital defects, were increasingly reinterpreted as the products of over-stimulated imaginations and bad habits. In particular, Tissot singled out masturbation as a prodigious evil, deeming it to occur not primarily because of the pathological irritability of the genitals, but thanks to an irritation of the mind, imaginative over-stimulus, consequent upon leisure, solitude, and reading titillating novels. (➤ Ch. 21 Mental diseases)

Not least, framed by the notion of diseases of civilization, the eighteenth and nineteenth centuries saw a striking revision in theories of the nature and aetiology of madness itself. The manifestations of insanity had traditionally been understood to be either supernatural in origin (visitations of God or the Devil) or essentially organic, provoked by an excess of black bile (melancholy), or yellow bile (choler), or by some brain defect. Now a socio-pathological account achieved popularity. Madness was increasingly seen as in the mind, a disorder of the imagination or understanding. It was, in other words, psychological, and the realm of the psyche was viewed as being significantly programmed by the ensemble of linguistic, literary, and intellectual signals in cultural circulation (for example Methodism, Romanticism). Hence it became possible to interpret lunacy as sociogenic; spectacularly so, when apparent epidemics of delirium were attributed to the French Revolution, suicide outbreaks to stock-exchange crashes, and depression to the pernicious hell-fire rantings of the religious lunatic fringe. In particular, mild mental afflictions (today's neuroses) became standardly interpreted, at least amongst élite sufferers, as the by-products of stressful life-styles. Leading mad-doctors suggested that insanity, barely known (it was claimed) in primitive socieities, was rampant amongst the most advanced. (➤ Ch. 56 Psychiatry)

Rapid change, and all the paraphernalia of the eighteenth-century civilizing process, forced medical theorists and clinicians alike to pay greater attention to the dialectics of sickness and society. Interest grew in the historical forces of change seemingly producing pathological transformations parallel to 'progress'. The spread of big city life was apparently making populations more vulnerable not merely to 'filth diseases', but to new modes of ailment mid-wived by modernity: hysteria, hypochondria, the vapours, chlorosis, and their nineteenth-century neuropathological successors, like 'spinal irritation', neur-algia, and neurasthenia. (➤ Ch. 67 Pain and suffering)

Indeed, it was in the nineteenth century that the notion of 'diseases of civilization' attained its greatest credibility and its maximum scare-power. There had, after all, been something, if not exactly frivolous, at least eligibly engaging about the notion in the Enlightenment: to sport a disease of civiliz-ation had signified superiority in wit, talent, or style, if not in robustness and longevity. This changed. The idea's dark side was to become dominant.

This was partly because certain disorders that fell under the epithet's umbrella grew more deadly; above all, tuberculosis, which climaxed around the mid-nineteenth century, accounting for up to a quarter of all urban deaths in north-western Europe and the eastern seaboard of the United States, especially those of young adults. In both the weak and strong senses, tuberculosis was a classic disease of civilization. Its incidence was clearly associated with the big city's unwholesome environment: damp, coalfires, smoke, etc.; its mythology furthermore suggested that the brilliant, spiritual, and delicate formed its main harvest. Leading tuberculosis doctors, Thomas Beddoes (1760–1808) for instance, explicitly blamed the menacing curse of the disease upon the effete and aetiolated hot-house life-styles cultivated by the *beau monde*.

This darkening of the vision was also due to a plethora of cultural anxieties maturing after 1850: a growing stress on the role of heredity in spreading sickness down the generations and throughout society; a new sensitivity to supposed diatheses (hereditary constitutional-disease dispositions); the Dar-winian, or, more properly, social Darwinist, view that nations and races were locked in a struggle for survival that would penalize weakness; the related apprehension that traditionally laudable cultural traits (altruism, benevolence, sensitivity, 'politeness') might turn out to be, in the cold light of biomedical evolutionism, maladaptive for racial or national survival. Not least, as class conflict and social strains grew more intense in the age of industrialization and emergent revolutionary Marxism, there was a widespread feeling that the social body itself was sick; sick (according to prophets such as Thomas Carlyle (1795–1881) and F. W. Nietzsche (1844–1900)), perhaps even unto death. Thus the initially rather lightweight notion of 'diseases of civilization' could fuel the deeper dread that civilization itself was diseased, indeed a disease. Drawing upon the age-old *topoi* of the body social and the body politic, viewed as macrocosmic representations of the individual body natural, it was often claimed by ideologues from both ends of the political spectrum that the very premises of *laissez-faire* and possessive individualism must necessarily be pathological, denying as they did the priority of the social organism, and thereby (as etymology itself suggested) the very possibility of social wholeness or health. (➤ Ch. 70 Medical sociology)

Other prophets of doom, echoing Charles Dickens (1812–70) or Gustave Doré (1832–83), pinpointed the frantic acceleration in the pace of living, the mad crush of humanity in the city of dreadful night, the power of the money demon and the cash nexus, the deluge of information and business ('getting and spending we lay waste our powers'), and all the demands these were laying upon stamina: surely, sooner or later, individuals and society at large must collapse of enervation, or explode in some paroxysm of fury? In particular, fears grew that society itself was being crippled by the growing burden of the delinquent and maladapted, the parasites of the ghetto and its subcultures.

The theory orchestrating such fears was known as degenerationism. Originally associated with the French psychiatrist, B.A. Morel (1809–73), and espoused by leading physicians, intellectuals, psychiatrists, moralists, criminologists, and politicians from Vienna to New England in the second half of the nineteenth century, degenerationism argued that the socio-cultural traits of modernity were morbidly self-destructive. The élite were amongst the victims of exhausted nerves. Illustrious American nerve-doctors like George Beard (1839–83) and Silas Weir Mitchell (1829–1914) argued that career strains in the business rat-race devitalized high-flyers: brain-fagged by stress and tension in the cockpit of commerce, they cracked, ending up nervous wrecks, their psychological capital overtaxed. Cerebral circuits suffered overload, mental machinery blew fuses, batteries ran down, brains were bankrupted. But the problems pervaded the whole of society. The factory production-line and its division of labour; the *anomie* accompanying vast towns and the lonely crowd; the dissolution of once-stable household units, employment, rural communities, and organized religion; the vapid and vicarious excitements of Megalopolis, and its accompanying destitution, alcoholism, ubiquitous prostitution, and venereal-disease epidemics – all these were inherently psychopathological manifestations that were spawning a degenerate *classe dangereuse* of drunks, syphilitics, paralytics, defectives, and atavists. Worse still, the interbreeding of misfits and profligates – and it was widely assumed that the degenerate, driven by perverted sexual appetites and lacking self-control, would breed disproportionately – would lead, over the generations, to the swamping of the healthy by the residuum. Society would grow ever more disgenic, eventually distintegrating not, as Karl Marx (1818–83) predicted, through revolutionary class conflict, but through internal psycho-physiological decay.

CIVILIZATION AND ITS DISCONTENTS

Influential physicians and social commentators in the latter part of the nine-teenth century – notably Moreau de Tours (1804–84) in France, Henry Maudsley (1835–1918) in Britian, Cesare Lombroso (1936–1909) in Italy, Max Nordau (1849–1923) in Germany – subscribed to a 'degenerationist' model. The tensions of modern living were eroding basic constitutional stability and sanity. According to eugenists, politico-social arangements (the tax system, Poor Laws, indiscriminate charity) were encouraging the unfit to breed, but dissuading better and more-responsible stock from self-perpetuation. Art and letters were repudiating sense, taste, rationality, and discipline: *fin de siècle* culture – bohemianism, Impressionism, Post-Impressionism, expressionism – was widely diagnosed as symptomatic of inner decay, or at best a vehicle of protest contributory to the problem it exposed. (➤ Ch. 66 Medicine and literature)

Medico-scientific movements aspired to understand, alleviate, or arrest such developments. As pioneered by Lombroso, anthropometry and psychi-atric criminology employed cranial measurement and photography to identify the diseased sectors of civilization, with a view to isolating, treating, or even sterilizing criminal and prostitute types, atavists, and immoralists. The emergence of sociology, social psychology, and social work enabled experts, physicians, and legislators to extend their sights from the patently sick and depraved to encompass *potential* deviants, degenerates, and 'problem people' (a tell-tale coinage of the early twentieth century), and the lumpenproletariat at large.

The invention of eugenism and the growth of the eugenist movement were direct responses to such perceived problems. Eugenism was the child of social Darwinism: after all, Francis Galton (1822–1911), the science's founder, was the cousin of Charles Darwin (1809–82) cousin, and Leonard Darwin (1850–1943), the long-term president of the Eugenics Society in Britain, was one of his sons. Eugenists developed programmes of positive eugenics, to encourage the 'fit' – that is, the professional middle-class élite – to breed, and of negative eugenics, designed to curb the fertility of the 'unfit' (the sick, feeble-minded, effete, and depraved). In Britain, despite the passing of the Aliens Act of 1905, the conviction of extreme enthusiasts that negative eugenics should involve state-sanctioned sterilization of the severely mentally defective was rarely realized. Such gloomy fanatics met with better success elsewhere. In the USA, fears that diseased or inferior stock would swamp the more progressive races led, early in the twentieth century, to restrictions upon immigrants with supposedly hereditary defects (tuberculosis, glaucoma, etc.), and to heightened suspicions against certain ethnic strains (Mediterraneans, Semites, Ashkenazis, Chinese, and other Orientals). Several state legislatures promoted programmes of castration and sterilization, pursued by energetic asylum physicians against feeble-minded recidivist inmates, sex offenders, cretins, and the seriously psychiatrically disturbed. An all-too-predictable and even respectable racism left blacks the prime beneficiaries of these policies, which were upheld by the Supreme Court, with Justice Oliver Wendell Holmes (1809–94) notoriously commenting, 'three generations of imbeciles are enough'.

This eugenist sting in the tail of 'diseases of civilization' spelt out the shape of things to come. For in the Third Reich, Nazi ideology, voiced in the 1920s and implemented following the Nazi seizure of power in 1933, built its programme of race hygiene overtly on the framework of socio-pathology and on the efficient treatment of 'moral sewage'. Some groups (gypsies, for instance) were judged throw-backs, unable to cope with modernity and progress, and therefore in need of a helping hand towards inevitable extinction; others – *par excellence*, Jews – were symptomatic of the sordid evils of money-mad capitalism and sexual corruption, and hence ripe for extermination in the grand 'stocktaking' crusade that would purify the Teutonic homelands and end the decadent obscenities of modernity (schizophrenia, homosexuality, physical impairment, declining birth rate, the flight from motherhood, etc.). Nazi policies were not a personal quirk of Adolf Hitler (1889–1945) nor mere flights of political opportunism; they had their roots in well-established anthropological, evolutionary, racial, and medical discourses, and many high-ranking members of the medico-scientific community earnestly sought their fulfilment, in expectation of the progress of the perfecting of the master race. (➤ Ch. 37 History of medical ethics) The degenerationist cast of mind found logical expression both in the experimental laboratories of the extermination camps (half a million schizophrenics and mental defectives were sterilized or eliminated, apart from the killing of the Jews), and in the Nazi cult of simple, rustic living, rude health, physical fitness, psychic hygiene, radiant motherhood, body-culture, and youth-hostelling.

Related to such trends in exceptionally complicated ways were the views of Sigmund Freud (1856–1939). Hostile, from early in his career, to racial and hereditarian readings of psychiatric disorders, the young Freud none the less concluded (this was the lesson of his psychotherapeutic practice) that the complaints commonly presented by his patients (nervous exhaustion, depression, neurasthenia, anxiety, hysteria, suicidal tendencies, and, above all, sexual frustrations and dysfunctions) could be attributed to the psycho-pathology of everyday life in modern, urban, affluent civilization, specifically in *fin de siècle* Vienna. Bourgeois respectability and prudishness and delayed marriage took a heavy psychological toll. The 'repression' model, developed by Freud to explain the functioning of the unconscious in psychogenic disorders, presumed that certain elemental and biologically healthy drives (above all, the libido) were necessarily suppressed or sublimated to meet the demands of social order (morality, property, justice, the bourgeois, Oedipal family). Civilization's price was therefore an inhibition of instinctual eroticism, which commonly resulted in a florid repertoire of psychological and, by extension, psychosomatic disorders. Such views were elevated to the status of universal truths in the series of speculative anthropologies Freud wrote in later life, above all *Civilization and its Discontents* (1926). In a manner affording parallels to Rousseau, Arthur Schopenhauer (1788–1860), and Nietzsche, he suggested that the phenomenon of civilization is invariably attended by psychopathological manifestations. (➤ Ch. 43 Psychotherapy)

The First World War concentrated Freud's attention on institutionalized aggression as a further symptom of the costs of civilization. Violence derived from the death-wish, which was rooted in individual drives. But, believing, as a lifelong Lamarckian, in the inheritance of acquired characteristics, Freud was also convinced that, down the generations, culture became the carrier of such dispositions; thus violence became socialized. In counting the costs of civilization, Freud shared something with 'primitivist' critics of the late nineteenth and early twentieth centuries, who extolled the superiority of the spontaneous and the unconscious, and often, as with D. H. Lawrence (1885–1930) and Freud's own one-time follower Wilhelm Reich (1897–1957), touted instinctual sexual release as a panacea. Unlike many of these nostrum-mongers, however, Freud had no truck with simplistic schemes to resurrect the 'primeval', or to return to Nature, embracing instead a dignified pessimistic realism.

MODERN TIMES, MODERN PROBLEMS

The more grandiose scenarios for linking disease and civilization, biology and society – be they social Darwinist, degenerationist, Freudian, or Nazi – have become discredited during the past half-century, though attempts to recreate attractively simple solutions surface occasionally, as with sociobiology. Nevertheless, not least because of the phenomenal growth of the social sciences of health and disease, and the extraordinary increase of governmental intervention in health care in post-industrial society, perceptions of interlinkages have grown stronger. (➤ Ch. 50 Medical institutions and the state) In the 1930s and 1940s, 'social medicine' arose on both sides of the Atlantic, championed in particular by Milton Winternitz (1885–1959) at Yale and John Alfred Ryle (1889–1950) at Oxford. Social medicine contended that the development of scientific medicine under the mixed blessing of bacteriology was counterproductively narrow and impoverished. Epidemiology had to move beyond the pathology laboratory and into society as a whole. The movement's proponents claimed that sickness trends were functions of social variables such as class, income, status, occupation (or, commonly, unemployment), family size, housing standards, educational achievement, and so forth. Thanks to their researches and publicity efforts, it became common wisdom that certain sorts of disorders (for instance, duodenal ulcers and postnatal depression) were consequential upon deleterious life-styles and environments (in one case, the pressures upon the business person; in the other, the alienation of the young mother in run-down inner-city accommodation or on the council estate). And what was psycho-socially triggered could not adequately be treated by pharmaceutical or surgical interventions alone. Programmes of the kind recommended by Ryle led to exploration of the social pathology of ulcer and other gastric conditions, heart disease, diabetes, cancer, depression, and, later, smoking-related diseases.

For, since the late-Victorian age, as the airborne and water-borne infections classically associated with high-density living (typhoid, diphtheria, tuberculosis, etc.) have been vanquished, new classes of diseases have gained in prominence, supposedly attributable to pathogenic elements in modern civilization: cardiovascular disorders, degenerative conditions of the nervous system, hypertension, diabetes mellitus, cirrhosis of the liver, the cancers, Alzheimer's disease, and depression. (➤ Ch. 25 Cancer)The Canadian physician Hans Selye (1907–82) developed a prominent theory of the biological effects of environmental stress. Long-term malfunctions build up, leading to ulceration and high blood pressure and a variety of conditions that he called 'diseases of adaptation'. In the late twentieth century, we seemingly have a crop of allergies and other as-yet mysterious conditions, like chronic fatigue syndrome (myalgic encephalomyelitis, or ME). One should also mention iatrogenic disorders, including addictions, so often the side-effects of medical treatment. Pollution, refined sugars, and other highly refined food treated with chemical additives, carcinogens at the workplace, nuclear fallout, atmospheric pollution, and other environmental factors are widely blamed.

But it may be question-begging to seek to fit these disorders too neatly into the 'diseases of civilization' mould. Might not the apparent escalation of these complaints largely be, in reality, an optical illusion? Are not more people dying today of disorders that their forebears never lived long enough to contract? Are not superior diagnostic techniques and more intense screening resulting in the showing-up of a far higher proportion of cancers and degenerative neurological conditions than could have been identified in earlier centuries? (➤ Ch. 36 The science of diagnosis: diagnostic technology) The Victorian 'lunatic' becomes today's parkinsonism sufferer; hardly anyone dies any more of natural causes or old age; today, they are all, following the protocols of medical bureaucracy, victims of a disease.

There is nevertheless widespread agreement that many elements of today's living patterns and environment have contributed to increased incidence of these chronic and often incurable conditions: atmospheric carcinogens, obesity, cigarette smoking, addictions, etc. Yet this dressing-up of the old myth of 'diseases of civilization' in new garb requires careful corroboration against the facts. The cliché image of the obese but hyperactive executive as the archetypal candidate for coronary thrombosis proved to be less fact than fiction. As has been demonstrated by the *Black Report* and other British surveys, heart attacks (contrary to the ingrained Cheyneian expectation) pre-eminently afflict not social groups one and two, but four and five: the poor, deprived, and under-educated. In any case, much in heart disease that has been associated with the amorphous and emotional category 'civilization' may, in truth, be attributable specifically to nicotine.

Moreover, with the spread of health education, with enlightened eating habits, and with the enhanced freedom of choice that affluence commands, it appears likely that today's so-called diseases of civilization are not in any straightforward sense the products of affluence, but rather diseases disproportionately afflicting the less privileged members of advanced societies. In this light, it is highly significant that cancers, heart conditions, respiratory diseases, and so forth are rapidly worsening amongst the masses of the Third World, evidently spread by industrial toxins, dietary dislocation, and by cigarette smoking. It may also be equally pertinent that AIDS – for many moralists, the quintessential disease of modern life-styles, and supposedly the product of sexual promiscuity and drug habits – has mainly devastated the Third World. (➤ Ch. 26 Sexually transmitted diseases)

Ideological indictment of modern life-styles has often been extended to modern medicine. Like modern living, scientific medicine proves pathogenic, argue critics such as Ivan Illich (b. 1926) and advocates of alternative medicine, precisely because it shares the same features: a reliance upon hi-tech fixes, the industrial division of labour, the commodification of cures via the pill or the hyperdermic needle, the depersonalizing prioritization of the technical over the personal, the material over the mental and spiritual. The mechanical age, critics allege, has produced mechanical medicine ('the medical model'). It is widely suggested, furthermore, that such diseases as the cancers have defied scientific research and resisted cure precisely because the methods of science (fixated upon a reductionistic, materialist approach to the body, and the expectation of specific remedies, a 'pill for every ill') are inappropriate for handling systemic and constitutional disorders, from multiple sclerosis to ME, whose aetiology may include an irreducible psychosomatic component and be personality linked. In his *Limits to Medicine* (1977), the hammer of modernity, Ivan Illich, argues that modern medicine is one of the prime diseases of civilization, not only spreading iatrogenic disorders, but orchestrating a disabling 'expropriation of health'. Illich has commended the health and disease cultures of simpler times and peoples.

From such arguments it is clear that much of the allure of modern alternative medicine lies in its ability to link philosophies of sickness to a wider disaffection with, and a critique of, industrial society, nostalgically evoking myths of golden ages of health, and seeking a return to Nature, through herbal remedies, natural cures, spiritualism, jogging, and ginseng. Whatever epidemiological truth lies in the notion of diseases of civilization, civilization-blaming still exercises a powerful Romantic hold, largely over those who are the greatest beneficiaries from the civilizing process itself.

FURTHER READING

Black, Douglas, *The Black Report*, ed. Peter Townsend, Harmondsworth, Penguin, 1982.

Cheyne, George, *The English Malady*, ed. by Roy Porter, London, Routledge, 1990; orig. pub. London, 1733.

Cohen, Mark Nathan, *Health and the Rise of Civilization*, New Haven CT, Yale University Press, 1989.

Coward, Rosalind, *The Whole Truth: the Myth of Alternative Health*, London, Faber & Faber, 1989.

Illich, I., *Limits to Medicine: the Expropriation of Health*, Harmondsworth, Penguin, 1977.

Inglis, B., *The Diseases of Civilisation*, London, Hodder & Stoughton, 1981.

Lobo, Francis M., 'John Haygarth, smallpox and religious dissent in eighteenth-century England', in Andrew Cunningham and Roger French (eds), *The Medical Enlightenment of the Eighteenth Century*, Cambridge, Cambridge University Press, 1990, pp. 217–53.

McKeown, T., *The Role of Medicine: Dream, Mirage or Nemesis?*, Princeton, NJ, Princeton University Press, and Oxford, Blackwell, 1979.

Mercer, Alex, *Disease, Mortality and Population in Transition. Epidemiological-Demographic Change in England since the Eighteenth Century as Part of a Global Phenomenon*, Leicester, Leicester University Press, 1990.

Pick, Daniel, *Faces of Degeneration: Aspects of a European Disorder c.1848–1918*, Cambridge and New York, Cambridge University Press, 1989.

Riley, James C., *The Eighteenth-Century Campaign to Avoid Disease*, Basingstoke, Macmillan, 1987.

——, *Sickness, Recovery and Death: a History and Forecast of Ill Health*, London, Macmillan, 1989.

Stevenson, L., ' "New diseases" in the seventeenth century', *Bulletin of the History of Medicine*, 1965, 39: 1–21.

Tissot, S.-A.-A.-D., *An Essay of Diseases Incidental to Literary and Sedentary Persons*, London, E. & C. Dilly, 1768.

——, *An Essay on the Disorders of People of Fashion*, London, Richardson & Urquhart, 1771.

Trotter, Thomas, *A View of the Nervous Temperament*, London, Longman, Hurst, Rees & Orme, 1807.

Weindling, Paul, *Health, Race and German Politics between National Unification and Nazism, 1870–1945*, Cambridge, Cambridge University Press, 1989.

PART IV

UNDERSTANDING DISEASE

28

UNORTHODOX MEDICAL THEORIES

Norman Gevitz

An unorthodox medical theory is one whose principles of causation and/or practice directly challenge the beliefs, knowledge, and experience of the dominant group of health practitioners in a society. When such theories gain significant public support, produce defections from the ranks of established physicians, or lead to the rise of competing healers, the cultural authority behind the established mode of apprehending and treating illness may be seriously weakened. This real or potential threat usually results in a process of self-definition by regular physicians, a corresponding combating of those practitioners who deviate from established norms, and a determined effort to retain or win back the patronage of the laity. The response of the medical establishment to such theories justifies the preference herein for the use of the term 'unorthodox' as opposed to the more value-neutral expression 'alternative' medicine, which does not sufficiently fix the phenomenon in terms of its contemporary medical repute.

The epistemological questions that may be asked respecting unorthodox medicine are those we would enquire of the principles and practices accepted by regular practitioners. Upon what intellectual sources do these theories draw? What form of evidence is offered? How and why do the theories change over time? In addition, it is essential to consider what impact unorthodox theories have on the thinking of the dominant group of practitioners.

After Paracelsus (1493–1541) challenged the inviolability of Galenic teachings, there developed in Europe competing theoretical systems underlying the practice of medicine. In the seventeenth century, there was the division between so-called iatrochemical and iatrophysical schools, although the differences between physicians with respect to remedies were not significant. Furthermore, each group saw itself as within the orthodox tradition, a perspective that was maintained by the followers of the great systematists of the first half of the eighteenth century. However, in the late eighteenth century and continuing to the present, a number of unorthodox theories have been promulgated in the West that have both rejected standard therapies and offered distinctive substitutes. Their followers have sought to distance themselves from the mainstream.

Some of these unorthodox systems have been more comprehensive than others, providing the opportunity for a more detailed comparison with the theoretical premises underlying orthodox medicine. Given the constraints of space, it would be useful to focus upon a limited number of the broader approaches, particularly those that have had significant and longer-lasting public appeal, while briefly alluding to other systems as they appear relevant. Under the heading of 'Drugging alternatives' I shall look at homoeopathy, Thomsonism, and eclecticism; under 'Natural healing' I shall examine the popular health movement, hydropathy, and naturopathy; and under 'Manipulative medicine', magnetic healing, osteopathy, and chiropractic. Some non-Western systems, including Chinese and āyurvedic medicine, elements of which have achieved some popularity among the laity in Europe and America, are examined elsewhere in this volume. (➤ Ch. 29 Non-Western concepts of disease; Ch. 31 Arab-Islamic medicine; Ch. 32 Chinese medicine; Ch. 33 Indian medicine)

DRUGGING SYSTEMS

Of all the progenitors of irregular systems, none was more articulate or scathing of established ways of thinking about or treating disease than Samuel Hahnemann (1755–1843), founder of homoeopathy, which became the first important sect of the modern era and provided much of the rhetoric for the critique of orthodox medicine for subsequent movements. Hahnemann grew up in Meissen, Germany, where his father eked out a living as a painter of porcelain. Despite his circumstances, he obtained a formal education from a private tutor who, reputedly because of the young boy's considerable intellect, offered to teach him without fee. In 1775, Hahnemann began his medical training at Leipzig, but left after two years to continue his education for some months in Vienna. For financial reasons, he temporarily abandoned his studies to work as a cataloguer in a private library; in 1779, he resumed taking courses, now at the University of Erlangen, where he received his medical degree later that year.

Over the next fifteen years, Hahnemann was unsuccessful in establishing a continuing medical practice. He travelled from one German town to another, his family often living in desperate circumstances. Much of his income was earned from translating English medical works and other treatises. He was also able to carry on a number of chemical experiments, published widely, and was respected both for the breadth of his knowledge and his practical contributions by contemporary German physicians and scientists. This period also provided him with considerable time for contemplating the existing state of the principles and practices of the healing art.[1]

In the eighteenth century, medicine in Europe was characterized by competing forces. On the one hand, there was a long line of theorists, most notably Georg Stahl (1660–1734), Friedrich Hoffmann (1660–1742), William Cullen (1710–90), and John Brown (1735–88), who hypothesized general processes to explain the presence of disease. For Stahl, it was a stasis in the blood vessels; for Hoffmann, it was plethora which acted through the stomach and intestines; for Cullen, fevers were due to a spasm of the arteries; and for Brown, disease represented a deviation from the normal excitability of the organs. On the other hand, there was also a growing effort to eschew theory arrived at by deduction, and instead to ground medicine upon the direct observation and measurement of phenomena, to conduct controlled experiments and to correlate facts. Replicated discoveries in anatomy, chemistry, physiology, and pathology, particularly the relationship of clinical symptoms to lesions, as advanced by Giovanni Morgagni (1682–1771) and systematically pursued by Matthew Baillie (1763–1823), ushered in new understandings of the pathogenesis of disease. (➤ Ch. 9 The pathological tradition) In Germany, the effects of each of these trends was felt, although the Romantic movement, in part reflected by the idealism of the *Naturphilosophie* school, encouraged metaphysical thinking on many fronts including medicine, where it was common for physicians to explain medical phenomena solely on the basis of speculative theorizing, while failing to pursue opportunities for positivistic lines of inquiry.[2]

Looking upon the various systems that had come and gone, and the seeming lack of practical utility to clinicians of the advances in the basic sciences, Hahnemann sought his own answers. His search centred on the basis for medical treatment. Much of the existing materia medica was a hodge-podge of tradition and empiricism. Polypharmacy was rampant, and the use of drugs, as well as bloodletting, marked by great debate and uncertainty. In 1790, he translated William Cullen's *Materia Medica*, wherein he noted the results of his own experiment with cinchona, which was recognized as one of the few drugs that appeared to have a specific effect on a given disease; that is, intermittent fever. (➤ Ch. 19 Fevers) Cullen explained the action of cinchona on the basis of the 'strengthening power it exerts on the stomach'. For Hahnemann, this was a vague speculation. In a footnote, he noted that for several days he took four drachms of the bark, twice daily. After its administration, he felt his feet and fingertips grow cold. He became exhausted and sleepy. Later, he experienced tachychardia and his pulse became hard and rapid; he experienced anxiety, trembling, prostration in all limbs, followed by a throbbing in his head, flushing of the cheeks, and thirst. 'In short all the ordinary symptoms of intermittent fever appeared one after another, but without febrile rigor.' The episode lasted a few hours and was repeated each time he dosed himself. Once he stopped taking cinchona, he resumed his good health.[3] The following year, in a translation of another English work, he offered an explanation for the results of his experiment with the bark: that cinchona 'overpowers and suppresses the intermittent fever chiefly by exciting a fever of short duration of its own'. He noted that other drugs were also able to produce an artificial fever, and 'given shortly before the paroxysm, check intermittent fever quite as specifically, but they cannot be relied on with such certainty'.[4]

The only way drugs could be used with any certainty was if their action on the human body could be known. In 1796, Hahnemann published his 'Essay on a new principle for ascertaining the curative powers of drugs.'[5] He observed that hitherto there was no accepted systematic way of testing medicines and finding specifics. The physician, he argued, needed to determine 'what is the pure action of each by itself on the healthy human body'. Thus, as in his own initial experiment with cinchona, he called for practitioners to engage in 'provings'. Only healthy persons were appropriate for this form of drug testing, since diseases interfered with the understanding of which symptoms were part of the disease and which were produced by the drug. As for ascertaining the effects of a given drug, practitioners were to record all the impressions or symptoms following its ingestion, however seemingly trivial.

There was a great utility in this. From his single experiment with cinchona, he laid down the axiom in this essay that to cure a disease physicians needed to employ a 'medicine which is able to produce another very similar artificial disease'. This he called the principle of *similia similibus curantur* (like cures like). Thus, once the effects of drugs were tested and recorded, physicians could compare the observable symptoms of a given disease with the consciously reported effects of the drugs, and select the most appropriate one, which, Hahnemann would argue, somehow had the effect of both substituting for the natural disease and then disappearing. Not surprisingly, Hahnemann interpreted the introduction of vaccination by Edward Jenner (1749–1823) in 1798 as a confirmation of the law of similars.

The second major aspect of his system was the use of infinitesimal doses. In his essay, he observed that the drug selected should be in a dose just powerful enough to produce a slightly perceptible indication of the expected artificial disease. He also argued for relatively long intervals between dosages. However, the size of his dosages was still relatively moderate. In the next few years, he began to prescribe much smaller dosages of given drugs. In 1801, in treating scarlet fever, he recommended tincture of opium, wherein one part opium was shaken up with 500 parts of alcohol, and a drop from this was to be mixed with another 500 parts of alcohol, the patient being given drop doses. In 1805 he wrote, 'None but the careful observer can have any idea of the height to which the sensitiveness of the human body to medicines is increased in disease.'[6]

After the turn of the century, his fortunes improved. Not only had he already laid out the two major elements of his theoretical system, but his practice in the town of Torgau prospered. There he composed his principal work, the *Organon of Rational Medicine*, first published in 1810 and which went through five editions in his lifetime.[7] The following year, he moved to Leipzig, where he lectured at the university. Meanwhile, he had also brought out the first edition of his *Materia Medica Pura*, which contained the results of his 'provings'.[8]

While his early writings contained critical comments about the practice of medicine, they were relatively mild in comparison to those that would appear in the *Organon*. Two years before this work was published, Hahnemann anonymously wrote, 'It must some time or other be loudly and publicly said ... before the whole world, that our art requires a thorough reform from top to bottom.' Speaking undoubtedly of his forthcoming change in tactics, he noted, 'The evil has come to such a pitch that the well-meant mildness of a John Huss is no longer of any use, but the fiery zeal of a stalwart Martin Luther is required to clear away this monstrous leaven.'[9] The *Organon* proved to be his version of Luther's ninety-five theses, and solidified his standing as an anathema to medical orthodoxy.

Hahnemann attacked medical systems as 'unnatural sophistry'. They dazzled readers with their display of wisdom, but none of them could produce any improvement in the art of healing. 'Mere theories', he called them, 'spun out of a refined imagination ... practically inapplicable at the bedside of the patient, and only fitted for idle disputation.'[10] Basic scientists were also under a delusion in their search for a material cause of disease. In most illnesses, they had confused the pathological changes or effects of disease with its cause. To him, the cause of the disease was immaterial or spiritual and dynamic, and the belief in disease being caused by a thing – the ontological argument – led to faulty thinking with respect to therapeutics. By conceiving disease as 'morbid matter', physicians had administered depleting remedies on the doctrine of *contraria contrariis curantur* to 'disencumber' these from the bloodstream through phlebotomies or from the digestive tract through purging and cathartic medicines, etc. But, Hahnemann declared, if there were morbid matter in the body these were the consequences of the derangement of the 'vital force'. Other physicians might well have agreed with Hahnemann that these bodily changes constituted only the effects of disease but nevertheless justified evacuative treatment on the basis that this approach simply imitated and aided the body's natural ability to repair itself (*vis medicatrix naturae*). (➤ Ch. 40 Physical methods) It was therefore logical, they argued, to stimualte patients' vomiting or haemorrhaging. Hahnemann thought this irrational, arguing that what physicians were doing was imitating a disordered vital force, thus adding to the patient's problems. He called these plans of treatment 'inefficacious, debilitating, and injurious, in ameliorating, and dissipating disease, which arouse another and worse evil to occupy the place of the former. Can we call that healing which rather deserves to be called destroying?'[11] He conceded that some drugs such as morphine, used in the prevailing manner, might have a seemingly beneficial effect in countering pain, but only temporarily. To continue to work, more doses, in greater amounts, would be necessary, and this would only add to the woes of the patient. (➤ Ch. 67 Pain and suffering) Furthermore, physicians prescribed unreasonably, mixing a large number of drugs, the effects of which, singly and especially in combination, they did not understand. To Hahnemann, the sufferer had in the hands of orthodoxy become a medical victim. Although he differentiated the various accepted competing approaches to drug therapy then extant, he gave an all-embracing name to regular practice, calling it 'allopathy'. This term, however imprecise, was employed by his followers and other unorthodox movements to identify the prevailing methods as constituting nothing more than a competing 'school' of medicine, however dominant in terms of number of practitioner proponents and patients. (➤ Ch. 39 Drug therapies)

Hahnemann argued that the homoeopathic approach was 'the only true method'. In his theory, the ultimate cause of the spiritual or dynamic derangement of the vital force can never be known, and there remain the changes of the state of the body and mind,

> felt by the patient himself, remarked by the individuals around him, and observed by the physician. The *ensemble* of these available signs represents, in its full extent, the disease itself – that is, they constitute the true and only form of it which the mind is capable of conceiving.[12]

Where some allopathic physicians might approach disease with a vitalistic outlook, they none the less looked at symptoms in isolation from one another, fruitlessly treating each with separate drugs. Homoeopathy, through its testing and recording of the multiple effects that each pure medicinal substance produced on a healthy person, was able to allow its exponents to proceed systematically and scientifically in choosing the one drug that could combat the greatest number of symptoms in a person suffering from a natural disease.

Hahnemann's theories were beset by a number of difficulties. His vitalistic approach, critics declared, both explained everything and nothing, and was decidedly anti-intellectual. In denying the possibility that science could ever discover a material cause of most disease, he brushed aside, from a clinical standpoint, the utility of these continuing lines of inquiry. Furthermore, by defining disease as solely the aggregate of symptoms that appeared to the consciousness of patients, Hahnemann reduced disease to a purely subjective state. Those processes not resulting in symptoms brought to the mind of the patient were therefore irrelevant.

It is interesting to note that the concept of *similia similibus curantur* drew the least criticism of all Hahnemann's ideas. As he himself observed, other physicians, many distinguished, had in the past put forward the doctrine, and as a theoretical principle, many physician opponents were willing to grant its possible applicability to healing in particular cases. Where many attacked Hahnemann was on his belief that this had to be the 'sole law' of cure, that other principles such as *contraria contraiis curantur* were of no utility; in fact, that physicians acting in any way not consistent with Hahnemann's beliefs were only doing harm to their patients. In Germany, many of his physician contemporaries thought Hahnemann mad for rejecting on theoretical grounds the use of particular remedies which 'experience' had taught were essential, particularly venesection, the absence of which, it was argued, meant certain death in given fevers.[13]

Considerable problems were inherent in Hahnemann's methods of testing drugs, some of which he himself recognized. As this research was based on subjective impressions, he stressed the importance of getting truthful people to report what they experienced. He also knew that there were individual differences between the bodies of people, which meant that one person might be affected by a given drug differently from the way it affected another, but he argued that there would be certain symptoms that would be excited 'in every human being'. However, he uncritically assumed that every symptom that a person experienced after ingesting a particular drug was exclusively a result of the drug's actions. As a consequence, the number of symptoms 'produced' by a particular drug, as recorded in his *Materia Medica Pura*, ran into the hundreds. This posed the obvious difficulty of correlating the symptoms of these medicinally produced 'artificial' diseases with the subjective impressions of patients suffering from 'natural' disorders. Hahnemann conceded to the realities of practice that the selection could be made less onerous by being attentive 'to the symptoms that are striking, singular, extraordinary, and peculiar [characteristic]'.[14]

The use of very small doses of drugs in disease required an extraordinary leap of faith, particularly as Hahnemann's recommended levels became increasingly infinitesimal in later editions of the *Organon*. To prepare the dose, the practitioner would take two drops of equal parts of a mixture of the juice of a medicinal plant and alcohol, and dilute this with ninety-eight drops of alcohol. The vial would then be shaken twice so that 'the medicine become exalted in energy'.[15] This was designated the first potency. One drop from this mixture would be mixed with another ninety-nine drops of 'spirits of wine', the vial shaken again, which produced the second potency. This process would be repeated twenty-eight more times to reach the thirtieth, or what Hahnemann called the 'decillionth development of power'. Drugs in powdered form would be similarly potentized through the process of titration. Thus, if properly diluted and succused, the smaller the 'material' dose, the more active its 'spiritual' medicinal qualities.

This logic would provide much ammunition for orthodox physicians, who constructed humorous descriptive calculations of what would happen if, instead of one drop from each of the dilutions, all of the material from the first dilution on were saved. Oliver Wendell Holmes (1809–94) claimed it would take 'the waters of ten thousand Adriatic Seas' to achieve just a seventeenth dilution.[16] Worthington Hooker (1806–67) similarly estimated that 'if medicine be given in the thirtieth dilution ... and, if all inhabitants of the earth should take from one single grain thus attenuated, three of four doses daily, generation after generation, and if the population of the earth should remain the same that it is now, the grain would not be all gone till the lapse of about a sextillion years.'[17] But, of course, Hahnemann only kept a drop from each dilution except the thirtieth or last, thus having the same quantity of fluid or powder he began with. How much of the original medicinal substance remained with this method? If one assumed that the substance he employed was completely soluble, by only the fourth dilution the ratio of the medicine to the solution would be 1:100,000,000. As Hahnemann had given his readers warnings about the dangerous effects that a thirtieth dilution might produce upon the body, some orthodox physicians, to demonstrate the speciousness of this argument, drank vast quantities of 'potent' homoeopathic medicines and experienced no apparent physiologically damaging changes.

Late in life, Hahnemann enunciated one further principle that laid his system open to considerable ridicule. In 1828, he published a multi-volume tome entitled *The Chronic Diseases*, the outline of which is to be found in the last revised edition of the *Organon*.[18] Hahnemann concluded that except for syphilis and 'sycosis' (that is, the cauliflower-like venereal warts), all chronic complaints were produced by psora – or 'the itch'. Thus, diseases as diverse in their symptomatology as gout, hysteria, paralysis, asthma, and cancer were all due to this one condition. To fight any of these successfully, one had to root out the problem by using anti-psoric medications. Hahnemann, who for decades attacked the nosological efforts which constructed hundreds of diseases, had now responded by reducing the number of ailments *ad absurdiam*. (➤ Ch. 17 Nosology)

Given its theoretical inconsistencies and apparent lack of touch with reality, leading German, English, and American orthodox practitioners all predicted that homoeopathy would constitute nothing more than a passing fad. They were bitterly disappointed. The tenacity of this movement was due in large part to the intellectual accommodation that homoeopathic physicians were able to make with Hahnemann's original doctrines and the external medical and social world. Assuredly, there were cultists or true believers who followed Hahnemann unreflectively and unquestioningly. But it has been too often assumed that all sectarians, whatever their stripe, are narrow dogmatists, a view that presents some real obstacles in understanding the exponents of a particular school of medicine.

Unlike a commune, where patterns of daily living and practice are regulated and deviations from dogma punished, private homoeopathic practice in the nineteenth century was characterized by autonomy and relative intellectual independence with only weak attempts to ensure uniformity of thought and action. In the fifth edition of the *Organon*, Hahnemann complained bitterly about those 'mongrel Homeopaths' who did not follow him in all particulars, but there was nothing that he could do to bring into line those who failed to accept his principles as 'revealed truths'. Holmes noted that the doctrine of the psora 'has met with great neglect and even opposition from very many of his own disciples', yet despite this, he considered American homoeopaths to be credulous and delusional.[19]

On the other hand, homoeopathic physicians argued that they followed a mode of healing surer and better than that of orthodox medicine. They believed that the law of *similia similibus curantur* was proved by experience, namely the results of homoeopathic care as compared with orthodox treatment. During the great cholera epidemics of 1832 and 1848–9, homoeopaths in Europe and America published statistics purportedly demonstrating recovery rates vastly superior to those obtained through the bleedings and purgings of the allopaths. Though the regulars disputed these claims and condemned the logic behind homoeopathic doses, they could not offer compelling evidence that their own therapeutic regimen or the reasoning behind it was any more scientific.[20]

But again, homoeopathic medicine was not a uniform practice, and this became especially pronounced in America, where there were several thousand practitioners, and followers established several medical schools, hospitals, and societies. After the Civil War (1861–5), homoeopaths were divided not only over Hahnemann's theory of chronic diseases, but also over the most appropriate dilutions and even the validity of the law of *similia similibus curantur*. Many believed that they were doctors first and homoeopaths second. This encouraged them to act in whatever manner they thought in the best interests of their patients, which included using orthodox remedies in standard doses for particular diseases, and even bloodletting where indicated. In the 1880s, those homoeopaths who believed the profession was seriously straying from, or even abandoning, Hahnemannian principles left the national organization

– the American Institute of Homeopathy – to form a competing but much smaller group – the International Hahnemannian Association. This schism served to isolate those who opposed change and encouraged a more unrestricted practice for the majority of homoeopaths.

At the time that Hahnemann was writing his *Organon*, a largely self-trained American practitioner, Samuel Thomson (1769–1843), was fashioning his own system of medicine. Born in rural New Hampshire, Thomson as a child was instructed in healing by an old woman who gathered and prepared drugs and attended his family when sick. He learned of the properties of drugs through trial and error, as opposed to books, and soon gained a reputation among his neighbours. Unlike his German counterpart, who wrote for fellow physicians, Thomson sought to make his botanical principles available to the laity to allow them to treat themselves.[21]

Roughly following classical theory (➤ Ch. 14 Humoralism), Thomson noted that health arose from a balance of the four elements (earth, water, fire, and air). When this balance was upset, the body became disordered, whereby there was always a diminution of internal heat, or an increase of the power of cold. 'All disorders', he wrote, 'are caused by obstructed perspiration, which may be produced by a great variety of means; that medicine, therefore, must be administered, that is best calculated to remove obstructions and promote perspiration.' Thomson stressed the role of the stomach, which through the process of digestion provided nourishment and thereby internal heat throughout the body. If a person ate food that was not 'suitable for the best nourishment', indigestion occurred which caused 'the body to lose its heat – then the appetite fails; the bones ache and the man is sick in every part of the whole frame'. Medicine should therefore be directed at clearing the stomach and bowels to restore the digestive powers. 'When this is done, the food will raise the heat again, and nourish the whole man.'[22] Thomson provided a mechanical analogy that both reflected the process of healing and the capacity of any person to direct it.

> As a person knows how to clear a stove and the pipe when clogged with soot, that the fire may burn free, and the whole room be warmed as before. The body, after being cleared of whatever clogs it, will consume double the food, and the food will double the nourishment and heat, that it did before.[23]

Thomson argued that 'fever' was a 'struggle of nature to throw off disease' and that orthodox medicine in its efforts to combat fever with 'their whole train of depletive remedies, such as bleeding, blistering, physicing, starving, with all their refrigeratives; their opium, mercury, arsenic, antimony, nitre, &c. are so many deadly engines, combined with the disease, against the constitution and life of the patient.'[24] In its place, he offered six classes of remedies consisting of botanical drugs and the steam bath, all designed to produce great internal heat forcing out cold, and allowing the body to re-establish its normal balance.

Although Thomson in his *New Guide to Health*, published in 1822, quoted some orthodox medical authorities, particularly in reference to the short-comings of standard medical practice, his theory of medicine represented an elaboration of a folk conception of health and disease and the standardization of a group of remedies that had long been employed in domestic practice (his claim to be the first to use *Lobelia inflata* as an emetic notwithstanding). (➤ Ch. 30 Folk medicine) Furthermore, his distrust of physicians, particularly their efforts to limit the professional practice of medicine to the learned, struck a responsive chord in many Americans imbued with the idealism of the virtues of the common person in Jacksonian America. Obtaining a patent for his system, he charged heads of families twenty dollars for his guide and the privilege of practising his methods. He encouraged his followers to form 'Friendly Societies', which, in turn, successfully lobbied for the repeal of medical practice acts. Thomsonism proved to have great appeal in both the American Midwest and South.[25]

As in the case of homoeopathy, Thomsonians, while agreeing with the founder on certain parts of his practice, were not necessarily content to be bound by his rigid principles. Other leading botanical practitioners proffered remedies other than Thomson's: some combined Thomsonian remedies with orthodox drugs; while still others decried Thomson's rejection of formal education and called for the establishment of botanical schools. Thomsonism flourished in America through the 1840s, and a wave of interest in his methods continued on in England.[26]

By the 1830s, two professionally oriented, botanical groups had been established. One, physio-medicalism, under the leadership of Alva Curtis (1797–1881), followed Thomson's methods more closely and had but a small following until its demise shortly after the turn of the century. More important was the group led by Wooster Beach (1794–1868), which evolved separately from Thomsonism, eventually being called 'Eclectic Medicine'. Beach studied with a botanical practitioner in New Jersey, then went to New York City, where he attended lectures at the College of Physicians, from which he claimed to have received an MD degree. He established a medical infirmary there, treating hundreds of patients along botanical lines, and later won plaudits for his operation of a cholera hospital during the epidemic of 1832. Meanwhile, he had established the Reformed Medical Society, gathered a number of supporters together, and in 1833 issued his three-volume *The American Practice of Medicine*, which disseminated his beliefs to a physician audience. Later, he condensed this work and issued it as a domestic medical guide.[27]

Unlike Hahnemann or Thomson, Beach had no distinctive theoretical principles to guide his practice. He accepted Thomson's belief that fever was due to a loss of internal heat, but otherwise agreed with regular practitioners in terms of the range of remote, proximate, and immediate causes of disease. Beach attacked rigid systems, but, unlike Hahnemann, did not substitute one of his own. Indeed, he accepted as an appropriate therapeutic approach the doctrine of *contraria contrarii curantur*. Like Thomson, however, he attacked the use of bloodletting and mineral drugs, using as evidence of the untoward effects of these remedies the opinions of well-known orthodox European and American writers. On the other hand, he disagreed with Thomson on the latter's criticism of the employment of purgatives and the restriction of the materia medica to a limited number of agents from the vegetable kingdom. Although initially calling his approach the 'American System' or the 'Reformed System' of medicine, he ultimately adopted the term 'Eclectic', first suggested by the botanist Constantin Rafinesque (1783–1840), since his goal was to adopt from whatever source anything that could be demonstrated to be useful therapeutically.[28] Over the years, Beach and his followers established schools around the country. He also visited England several times, where his ideas and methods generated some initial but unsustained enthusiasm. Eclectic physicians trained in the United States also sought to practise in Canada.[29]

One central problem for eclecticism was its inability to establish a separate identity. In many respects, it resembled orthodox medicine in its approach to the patient, and acted on the same principles, merely substituting botanical remedies for mineral ones and eschewing the use of bloodletting. In the 1850s, so-called 'concentrated medicines' were produced and employed by eclectics, which for a time made them distinctive, but these were abandoned when they proved ineffective. Later, 'specific medicines', which achieved some level of popularity were introduced. Eclectic practitioners also discovered and boosted the medicinal virtues of some native plants, a number of which were subsequently incorporated by the regulars. Eclecticism found its greatest support in rural areas of America, where such practitioners often became the only medical practitioners available.[30] Though otherwise quite similar to orthodoxy, eclecticism in challenging the efficacy of venesection and mineral drugs was as antipathetic to orthodoxy as homoeopathy.

On the European continent, in England, and in America, national and state societies did what they could to stamp out these heresies. In some European countries, physicians practising homoeopathy could be imprisoned and lose their licences.[31] In America, and later in England, consultation restrictions were enacted by the respective national medical associations, whereby no orthodox practitioner could have any professional intercourse with an irregular. As a consequence, formerly respected regular physicians who had publicly announced their new beliefs lost their positions in teaching institutions, hospitals, and clinics, and were shunned by their former colleagues. Furthermore, the irregulars' attempts to join the military medical corps, state health commissions, or engage in any public service were frustrated. In response, they attempted to form their own parallel institutions: associations, schools, and hospitals.[32]

Worthington Hooker, in his book *Physician and Patient*, which was the first work by an American devoted to ethics, enunciated five reasons why the Consultation Clause of the American Medical Association (AMA) was appropriate against healers such as homoeopaths and eclectics.[33] He maintained that the belief system of sectarian healers was alien to the accumulated experience of the profession; their practices were dangerous to patients; their education was inferior to that of regular practitioners; their social behaviour did not conform to that expected of gentlemen; and any association with these healers both legitimized the irregular and lowered the status of the regular profession before the public. Not surprisingly, sectarian practitioners had a different view as to the motives of the supporters of the code. They postulated three reasons why the AMA opposed them: first, they were getting better results than the regulars; second, orthodox physicians were dogmatically committed to their own system, which resulted in their branding everything else as quackery; and third, and most important, the regulars wanted to restrict economic competition.[34] (➤ Ch. 47 History of the medical profession)

Hooker was sensitive to the charge that the principal motive of regulars' intolerance to sectarians was to restrain competition. In a footnote to his chapter on homoeopathy, he noted, 'it may be proper to state at the outset, that the author himself suffered no encroachments from homeopathy, and so has no personal feelings to gratify in attacking it.' Other regular physicians argued that if a concern for the business side of practice dominated their behaviour with respect to unorthodox challengers, it would make sense to do nothing to restrain their rivals' activities. The malpractice of the irregulars would produce more illness and thus generate greater business for themselves. Orthodox physicians, however, have always had a difficult time convincing the public that their underlying motive was not economic self-interest.

The professional careers of these sectarian movements have varied widely by country. On the European continent and in England, homoeopathic groups were unable to establish their own schools. Instead, they had to recruit physicians who had obtained their 'allopathic' education. As a result, neither in Germany nor in Britain were there ever many more than four hundred homoeopathic physicians in practice throughout the nineteenth century.[35] In America, where competition between medical groups was encouraged by the absence of licensing laws, sectarians were able to make considerable inroads; by 1900, there were 10,000 homoeopaths and 5,000 eclectics, representing approximately 15 per cent of all physicians in practice.[36]

Whereas in England and Germany, there was no need to moderate the profession's attitude towards such small numbers of heretics, in America the regulars eventually saw the desirability of making some accommodations with their rivals, particularly as their policy of exclusion had the unintended result of generating public sympathy for sectarian groups. In fact, over the latter decades of the nineteenth century, the educational background of many sectarian practitioners, as well as their practice patterns, changed, which made the characterization of the irregular as an unprincipled quack more difficult to apply successfully. Homoeopaths and eclectics, as well as the regulars, were all affected by the growing scientific understanding of the body. Advances in pathology, physiology, and bacteriology changed the way each type of practitioner thought about disease. (➤ Ch. 7 The physiological tradition; Ch. 11 Clinical research) Bloodletting, the symbol of orthodox therapeutics, had long been in eclipse, and even though regulars might still defend its occasional use, the fact that it no longer constituted a principal intervention was interpreted as a victory by the sects.[37] Furthermore, each type of practitioner now used more similar drugs.

With these changes in progress, a growing number of regulars questioned the validity of the consultation restrictions. In 1903, the AMA replaced the old clause with a much milder sounding principle, which allowed licensed homoeopathic and eclectic physicians to join the Association, if they no longer designated their practice as sectarian. In the early twentieth century, fewer students enrolled in these sectarian schools, which either closed or dropped their sectarian designation and became orthodox institutions. Thereafter, homoeopathy and eclecticism faded rapidly in America, both in terms of numbers of practitioners and adherents. Recently, however, the rise of public interest in holistic medicine, New Age, and alternative therapies generally, has stimulated a growing interest in homoeopathy and botanical remedies in North America and Europe.[38]

NATURAL HEALING

In the nineteenth century, the regulars, homoeopaths, and various botanical practitioners all claimed that their respective methods were most in harmony with nature. However, this was disputed by other healers who argued that swallowing 'drugs' was artificial, dangerous, and unhygienic. Healing, they argued, could be improved by using simpler means and by understanding the physiological laws of living. People could 'perfect' themselves by controlling their own health destinies through diet, life-style, and the prophylactic and therapeutic virtues of water. (➤ Ch. 12 The concepts of health, illness, and disease)

In the West, the orthodox medicinal uses of water can be traced to Hippocrates (c.460-c.370 BC).[39] However, when employed in succeeding centuries, it was generally used by physicians as an adjunct to other methods.

In the eighteenth century, a number of publications stimulated interest on the subject. Its most extensive use was promoted by Johann Sigmund Hahn (1664–1742) of Breslau, Silesia, whose volume *On the Power and Effect of Cold Water*, first published in 1738, went through several editions.[40] Nevertheless, despite the considerable successes of these practitioners with water in a variety of ailments, comparatively few physicians sought to integrate this modality as a standard, let alone significant, part of their therapeutic armamentarium. It was instead a self-taught Silesian peasant, Vincenz Priessnitz (1799–1851) who, in the early nineteenth century, was able to create a popular sensation with his 'water cure'. (➤ Ch. 40 Physical methods)

Priessnitz, as a youth, while toiling on his father's farm, was kicked in the face by a horse, throwing him into the path of a cart which rolled over him, breaking two ribs. When a surgeon declared that he would never work again, Priessnitz decided to experiment on himself. He set his own ribs by leaning with his abdomen hard against a table or chair and held his breath to swell out his chest. With the ribs having returned to their proper position, he applied wet cloths to the affected parts, imbibed lots of water, ate little, and did not move in order to allow the ribs to heal. After a week, he was ambulatory, and at the end of a year he was able to return to his usual daily routine. Thereafter, he would occasionally treat his neighbours, and apparently through experience alone, he evolved his own system consisting of a primitive theory of disease and incorporating a variety of water-based remedial techniques. From 1829 until his death, he practised at a spa he established at Gräfenberg, which by the 1840s was accommodating fourteen hundred visitors annually, including numerous members of European royalty.[41]

Priessnitz's theory of disease was based on a folkish understanding of humoral pathology. He argued that all diseases, other than surgical, arose from bad internal juices produced by poor food, the suppression of perspiration, the lack of exercise, unwholesome air, or mental distress. These bad juices, in turn, produced either general derangement of the body, or localized disorders. Accordingly, the object of therapy was to remove any obstructions and expel these noxious or stale fluids, allowing the body to replace them with good or fresh ones. Pure water, so essential for health, constituted the natural and thus ideal medium through which the body might be properly flushed.[42] (➤ Ch. 53 History of personal hygiene)

Water was used both internally and externally. Patients were expected to drink at least twelve glasses a day, which helped clean the bowels and kidneys. Priessnitz placed chief emphasis upon the pores, and thus the bulk of his techniques were designed to be sudorific. All patients at Gräfenberg would daily be placed on a feather bed, 'hermetically enveloped' in a blanket with only the face exposed for up to two hours until they began to sweat, whereupon they might spend another two hours in this state. Patients were allowed to drink a glass of water every half-hour, which was designed to produce more sweating. When the patients were thought to have had enough, they were unwrapped and placed in a cold bath for up to eight minutes. Both practitioner and patient looked for a fine red colour of the skin after the bath, which signalled that the body was expelling the morbid humours. Other methods included the use of wet sheets, a variety of different baths, and water clysters. In no cases were patients to resort to drugs or bloodletting. Priessnitz, like Hahnemann, believed that many of the most inveterate diseases were medicinally produced.[43]

Priessnitz's lack of medical qualifications led Austrian medical officials to create a committee to investigate his activities. The chief inspector, who personally visited Gräfenberg, became convinced that patients were being helped, and that Priessnitz was not violating the law in that he neither gave drugs nor performed surgery. His protection from medical opposition was also ensured by the high status of many of his clients, who helped to open as many as forty to fifty similar establishments in Germany, Hungary, Poland, Russia, and Italy. By the 1840s, water-cure institutions were established in England at Stansteadbury, Sudbrook Park, Moor Park, London Fields, and Malvern, the latter gaining international recognition under the Edinburgh-trained physician James M. Gully (1808–83), who counted Alfred Tennyson, Thomas Carlyle, and Bishop Wilberforce among his clientele.[44] In the United States, hydropathy had a large following, with approximately two hundred water-cure institutions and a number of short-lived medical schools established.[45]

Hydropathy offered a particular appeal to American middle-class women. Many leaders of the movement had a positive vision of woman's potential. They believed in the 'naturalness' of such events as menstruation and childbearing, as well as the ability of women to contribute fully both as wives and mothers and in the external world outside the family. Women were encouraged to become professional hydropathists – approximately one-half of all students were female; many others learned hydropathy through domestic medical guides. In either case, by practising hydropathy, women acquired new skills, gained confidence, and were able to exert greater control over their lives. The water-cure establishments also provided a means of rest from daily social demands, a time for reflection, and an opportunity to meet with others who shared common interests and concerns. A number of these institutions became focuses for advocates of dress reform, greater educational opportunities for females, and other women's rights issues.[46] (➤ Ch. 38 Women and medicine)

Next to water, the most significant modality to be employed by hydropathic practitioners was diet. Priessnitz excluded from his patients' tables those foods he considered sour, heating, and unwholesome. These included all sorts of spices, alcoholic beverages, coffee, tea, chocolate, acids, and salt fish. Otherwise, his dietetic allowances appear traditional. One English follower noted that at dinner, patients were served soup with beef boiled in it. After this one might see pork, veal, beef, ducks, geese, potatoes, sauerkraut, gherkins, cucumbers, and pastry. He further observed that patients tended to overeat, but Priessnitz maintained that patients needed at first to keep their strength up, that the mountain air and exercise as well as their improved health would eventually restrain their appetites, and besides, the great amount of water they were drinking would digest anything. This visitor observed, 'I should say that if more attention were paid to diet, cures would be effected in a much shorter time than they are.'[47] In America, many hydropathic institutions added substantially to Priessnitz's list of prohibited foods, following the recommendations of the prominent lecturer and writer on popular health, Sylvester Graham (1794–1851), who made a considerable impact in the country prior to the introduction of hydropathy.

Graham began his career as a temperance speaker. His belief in the destructive effects of alcohol on the body led him to consider what other unhealthy substances people consumed. He based many of his arguments on the theoretical system of pathology devised by the French physician François Broussais (1772–1838), who had argued that disease resulted from excessive stimulation of the tissues, most notably the digestive tract, and that chronic irritation and inflammation can be transported by the nerves elsewhere in the body. Therefore, Graham believed that any food that caused too much stimulation must be avoided. For him, as well as other American health reformers of the period, this meant all fleshy meats. Graham also used the doctrine of overstimulation to warn of the powerful dangers of too much sexual energy. Eating meat produced a heightened sex drive, which, from whatever cause, was health-destroying. The more excited a person became, whether by engaging in intercourse or even thinking about it, the more likely that physical debilities, such as apoplexy or exhaustion, would appear. While proprietors and clients of hydropathic institutions might argue over the merits of sexual pleasure, they shared Graham's beliefs in the healthiness of vegetarianism.[48]

By the 1860s, greater attention to diet, dress, and later exercise began to erode water's central place in the thinking of leading unorthodox health reformers. Though a number of water-cures in America and Europe continued to attract clients and generate publicity, such as the establishment of Father Sebastian Kniepp (1821–97) in Bavaria, the employment of other modalities eventually led to the renaming of this general approach to healing as either the nature-cure or naturopathy.[49]

Naturopaths in the twentieth century have continued to stress the unhealthiness of particular foods, and have increasingly emphasized the ill effects of employing artificial means such as chemical pesticides and fertilizers to grow fruits and vegetables. While retaining the basic theoretical orientation that disease was primarily the result of unhygienic living, in addition, they argued that many diseases resulted from auto-intoxication, particularly the accumulation of impacted matter in the lower digestive tract. To resolve the problem, or to prevent it occurring, they championed the use of colonic irrigation. Though the theory underlying this proposition was scientifically invalidated early in the century, and the dangers of the therapy chronicled, its popularity continued.[50] Furthermore, one of the characteristics of naturopathy internationally was its incorporation of many 'drugless' modalities, even though the theoretical underpinnings of their respective uses differed considerably. These included vision-strengthening techniques, foot reflexology, homoeopathy, iridology, and psychotherapy.[51] Although originally claimed by naturopaths as part of their movement, chiropractic and osteopathy evolved as more coherent and enduring systems. They succeeded in establishing schools and gaining legal recognition.

MANIPULATIVE MEDICINE

The intellectual progenitor of both osteopathy and chiropractic was magnetic healing. Franz Mesmer (1734–1815), an Austrian physician, postulated that the key to health, particularly in nervous disorders, was a magnetic fluid that flowed throughout the body. As too much or too little in the respective parts would result in disease, treatment aimed to re-establish the natural balance. Mesmer argued this could be accomplished through magnets and hands.[52] Often, he employed a huge indoor tub with extended 'magnetized rods', or treated clients outdoors under 'magnetized' trees or beside 'magnetized' rocks. Patients might be brought to seizure-like states, which Mesmer believed were necessary to achieve catharsis. Forced to leave Vienna, he settled in Paris, where his methods caused a sensation. Two separate commissions, one of which included Benjamin Franklin (1706–90), Jean Sylvan Bailly (1736–93), and Antoine Lavoisier (1743–94), argued that 'animal magnetism' did not exist and that Mesmer's cures were the result of suggestion.[53] Although after the appearance of these reports Mesmer's personal standing declined, he influenced many on the fringe, including Hahnemann, who ended his *Organon* with an endorsement of Mesmer's methods in affecting the 'vital force'. Some of Mesmer's followers abandoned the more sensational aspects of his practice and tried to gain greater legitimacy. Subsequently, they progressed, and a somewhat favourable report on the subject was issued in 1831 by the French Academy of Medicine. Backhanded support later came from the writings of James Braid (1795–1860) on what he called hypnosis.[54]

Magnetic healing spread to America in the 1830s. One of its earliest exponents was Phineas Parkhurst Quimby (1802–65), whose practice consisted of largely verbal suggestions combined with light stroking of the body.[55] Mary Baker Eddy (1821–1910) was a follower of his, and a number of her later doctrines, which were central to her new religion 'Christian Science', bore his influence.[56] Quimby is also regarded as the intellectual fountainhead for other religious movements that flourished in America under the general heading of 'New Thought'.[57] (➤ Ch. 61 Religion and medicine)

The practice of magnetic healing varied in terms of both the methods employed and their rationale. The best-known magnetic healer before the Civil War was Andrew Jackson Davis (1826–1910), who was the leading American exponent of spiritualism. Davis sought to combine both belief systems. Conceiving of the body as a machine, he maintained that health was simply the harmonious interaction of all the body's parts in carrying out their respective functions, due to the free and unobstructed flow of 'spirit'. Any diminution or imbalance of this 'fluid' would cause disease. Davis placed emphasis upon healing with his hands. Of particular interest was his management of asthma, which consisted in part of vigorous rubbing along the spinal column.[58] Later magnetic healers, perhaps influenced by the attention given the spine by such orthodox physicians as Charles Bell (1774–1842), François Magendie (1783–1855), and Marshall Hall (1790–1857), made extensive use of this therapy. One was Warren Felt Evans (1817–89), whose name is most often associated with 'Mind Cure'. He noted, 'the hand of kindness, of purity, of sympathy, applied here by friction combined with gentle pressure, is a singularly effective remedy for a morbid condition of the internal organs. It is a medicine that is always pleasant to take.'[59] Edwin Dwight Babbitt (1828–1905) employed spinal manipulation for convulsions, apoplexy, sunstroke, headache, muscle complaints, common rheumatism, and paralysis.[60] While magnetic healing in America, as in Europe, never gained sectarian status, it nevertheless provided much of the theoretical foundation and practical application of the manipulative systems that followed.

Osteopathy was founded by Andrew Taylor Still (1828–1917), a Midwestern American physician trained through the apprenticeship system. Still's dissatisfaction with orthodox medicine crystallized during an epidemic of spinal meningitis in 1863 which, despite the best efforts of neighbouring physicians, claimed the lives of three of his children. As a self-described Columbus, he explored a variety of alternative movements. In examining the various drug-based sectarian substitutes, he realized that they were less harmful to patients than regular therapy, but just as empirical. The central issue for him was not which drug to use and in what dosage, but whether drugging itself was a scientific form of therapy. Also significant was his moral concern. As a Methodist, Still adhered to the temperance views of his church.

After the Civil War, he asked if drinking was sinful, should drugging be viewed any differently? Still also looked at substitutes. His familiarity with Graham's dietetic notions and hydropathy could be traced to the 1850s, when a utopian colony following a combination of these ideas was established in his vicinity. Still was not impressed with those particular systems, but did come to believe in a drugless approach, eventually embracing a number of the principles and practices of magnetic healing, most notably the metaphor of the body as a machine, health as the harmonious interaction of the body's parts and the unobstructed flow of fluid, and especially the use of spinal manipulation.[61]

His most significant departure from other magnetic healers would be over the nature of the fluid. While for the remainder of his life he spoke obliquely of the physiological role of magnetic energy, it was the free flow of blood that constituted the key to health. He later noted, 'He who wished to successfully solve the problem of disease or deformity of any kind in every case without exception would find one or more obstructions in some artery or vein.'[62] Severing his ties to orthodox medicine in 1874, he was ostracized in his home of Baldwin, Kansas, eventually settling in Kirksville, Missouri, where he was tolerated but for many years achieved little recognition.

Some time during the late 1870s, Still became interested in bone-setting, another form of manipulative practice limited to the field of orthopaedics. On the European continent, and in the United Kingdom as well as America, bone-setters had for centuries enjoyed a relatively unfettered practice among the poor, who could not afford orthodox treatment. However, bone-setters, many of whom were illiterate, could also draw the patronage of the wealthy and royalty, who believed that their talent was a gift or art that transcended book-learning.[63]

Bone-setters not only reduced dislocations, but also manipulated painful and diseased joints under the rationale that they too were caused by bone misplacement. Although physicians and surgeons ridiculed their crude diagnoses and the value of their therapy, many patients with restricted joint mobility, whom regulars had failed to relieve, were happy to provide testimonials for bone-setters' beneficial services. In 1867, Sir James Paget (1814–99) startled his colleagues by declaring his belief that there were joint maladies that bone-setters could cure, and that only through a thorough study of their techniques could the relative value of their methods be appreciated.[64] In 1871, Wharton Hood (1833–1916), a surgical colleague of Paget, published a volume based on his experience as a bone-setter's apprentice. He noted, 'the art of overcoming by sudden flexion or extension, any impediments to the free motion of joints that may be left behind after the subsidence of the early symptoms of disease or injury' could be of use in cases of stiffness, pain, and adhesion following fractures and sprains of one or more of the bones forming a joint; rheumatic and gouty joints; displaced cartilages; subluxations of the bones of the carpus and tarsus; displaced tendons; hysterical joints; and ganglionic swellings. However, he cautioned that bone-setting was successful only where there was mobility in the joints. Hood also noted that patients complaining of back pain were consulting bone-setters: 'these applicants are cured by movements of flexion and extension, coupled with pressure upon any painful spot'. He observed that these techniques often produced a 'popping' or 'clicking' sound emitted by the spinal joints, which convinced the patient that the obstruction to health had been removed.[65]

It is unclear how Still became the 'lightning bonesetter' described in his advertisements throughout the 1880s. He could have come across Hood's book, which was published in America, but it seems more likely that his knowledge was obtained by directly observing another practitioner. One medical author in the mid-1880s observed that in every city of the United States 'may be found individuals claiming mysterious and magical powers of curing disease, setting bones, and relieving pain by the immediate application of their hands.'[66] Still soon made an important discovery, namely that the sudden flexion and extension procedures peculiar to bone-setting had an application to other than orthopaedic problems, and that they constituted a more reliable general means of healing than simply rubbing the spine. Still synthesized some of the major components of magnetic healing and bone-setting into one unified doctrine. The effects of disease, according to the former, were due to the obstruction or imbalance of the fluids, but this, in turn, was caused by misplaced bones, particularly of the spinal column. At this point, Still had evolved his own distinctive system, which he would eventually call osteopathy. By the late 1880s, Still's methods produced a considerable sensation in Missouri. He made Kirksville his permanent base of operations, and in 1892 established a college, the American School of Osteopathy. By the end of the century, graduates had helped establish twelve other osteopathic institutions across the country.

Unlike the erudite Hahnemann, who had immersed himself both in historical and contemporary literature to gather evidence to support his theories, Still made little reference to other medical authors or practices and beliefs that were similar to his own.[67] However, some of his followers, most notably his early faculty at Kirksville, a number of whom were university and medical-school graduates, scrutinized the literature on massage, Swedish movements, spinal irritation, and neurophysiological research to explain their good results not only in musculoskeletal disorders, but in a large variety of chronic complaints. They also reconciled osteopathy to the germ theory, arguing that germs might be the active cause of disease, but spinal displacements, or what were later being called 'osteopathic lesions', could be predisposing causes. If, as they believed, these structural anomalies produced derangement of physiological functions, it would follow that in their presence the body would be put into a state of lowered resistance. Thus, correcting lesions shortly after they occurred lessened the likelihood of germs gaining a foothold. By correcting lesions after infection struck, the body's natural defences could more effectively respond to the invaders. Under these assumptions, osteopathic procedures seemed entirely appropriate.[68] (➤ Ch. 16 Contagion/germ theory/specificity)

As osteopathy was making significant gains in popularity, Daniel David Palmer (1845–1913) launched a manipulative system he would call chiropractic.[69] In 1886, Palmer, who had no medical training, set up as a magnetic healer in Davenport, Iowa. In 1895, a janitor in the office building where Palmer practised told him that he had lost his hearing after experiencing a sharp pain in his back. Palmer examined him, diagnosed a misplaced spinal segment, and forcefully restored it to its proper position, whereupon the patient reported his hearing had returned. This case, as well as another in which a heart condition was improved through spinal manipulation, convinced Palmer that all disease was due to impingement of the nerves passing through the spine. In 1898, he began his own school in Davenport, but within the first five years only fourteen students enrolled. (At this time, there were more than four thousand osteopathic graduates in practice.) After chiropractic began making headway, early osteopaths claimed that it was but another name for their system, which Palmer had crudely copied. On the other hand, one of Still's first graduates, who later studied with Palmer, argued that the latter's principles and practices were independently formulated.[70]

As osteopaths were successful at obtaining their own state licensure acts, many early chiropractors were charged with practising osteopathy without a licence. In court, the chiropractors cited a number of differences between the two systems. Osteopaths commonly adjusted several vertebrae to treat a given disorder: chiropractors invariably adjusted but one. The techniques also varied. Osteopathic manipulations were based on the lever principle: namely, placing pressure on one part of the body to overcome resistance in motion elsewhere. This meant twisting the patient's torso in certain directions while maintaining a firm hold upon the point in structure to be influenced. The most common chiropractic procedure had the client lying prone with little, if any, support below the spine. The operator placed both hands over what the chiropractors called the 'subluxated' segment and administered a quick thrust downward with all possible force. Osteopaths testified that these methods were dangerous and they would not employ them. These statements only worked to the chiropractors' advantage, since they indicated to juries that there were indeed divergences in approach. With respect to the element of danger, the defendants were only too glad to present patients to attest to the safety of such manœuvres. To cement their position further, some chiropractors cleverly managed to obtain and circulate letters signed by officials of recognized osteopathic schools stating that a course in chiropractic was not the same as one in osteopathy. As a result of these tactics, they were generally acquitted. Beginning in 1913, chiropractic began to obtain its own licensure acts.[71]

Osteopathy and chiropractic differed most significantly in their professional outlook. Almost from their inception, osteopathic schools sought to produce general practitioners. Before the turn of the century, these colleges incorporated training in the basic sciences, surgery, obstetrics, some adjuncts like hydrotherapy and diet, and the use of anaesthetics, antiseptics, and antidotes. By 1916, they expanded their training to four years. Although for a few decades there was a hard-fought battle between self-described 'lesion' and 'broad' osteopaths over the scope of practice, those favouring osteopathic physicians having the same rights and privileges as physicians from the regular, homoeopathic, and eclectic schools prevailed. In 1929, the American Osteopathic Association sanctioned a complete course in supplementary therapeutics, including pharmacology, and moved thereafter ever closer to the medical mainstream, with the employment of palpatory diagnosis and manipulative therapy of the spine occupying a decreasing segment of the osteopathic undergraduate curriculum and practice.[72] (➤ Ch. 48 Medical education)

Although osteopaths have conducted controlled basic scientific research on the 'osteopathic lesion' since the early 1940s and have published the results in independent journals, little evidence was presented that showed the significance of the lesion in the aetiology of visceral disease and the effect its elimination through manipulation had on the disease process. While clinical research in distinctive osteopathic procedures made little headway, the value of new 'orthodox' therapies was steadily demonstrated. In addition to antibiotics, a number of analgesics, anti-inflammatory agents, muscle relaxants, tranquilizers, and other classes of drugs were introduced that displaced manipulative procedures from the treatment of many disorders. In addition, by employing these agents, osteopaths sought to appear less 'deviant'.[73] Indeed, problems with their social status and the growing similarity between the two professions led to the willing amalgamation of most Californian Doctors of Osteopathy into the ranks of Californian Doctors of Medicine in the early 1960s. Other efforts, initiated by the AMA to facilitate mergers, have not been successful, though in recent years a large percentage of osteopathic graduates have trained in and affiliated with MD hospitals, which appears to have weakened the position of organized osteopathy.[74]

Most chiropractors, on the other hand, did not seek to replicate the scope of services employed by licensed physicians. However, they too were divided over scope between the so-called 'straights', who adhered to the original Palmer philosophy, and the 'mixers', who incorporated some other drugless modalities as well. For many years a number of chiropractic schools, in addition to awarding Doctor of Chiropractic degrees, also issued naturopathic diplomas.[75] Institutionally, chiropractic made its largest gains as osteopathy increased the length of its curriculum and diluted the significance of spinal mechanotherapeutics. By the 1920s, chiropractic schools, which maintained far lower entry requirements, had ill-equipped facilities and a much shorter curriculum than osteopathic colleges, produced more graduates. And unlike osteopathy, which sought to accommodate its beliefs and practices to expanding scientific knowledge, chiropractic was comparatively slow in doing so.[76] In the last few decades, however, chiropractic education in America has significantly raised its matriculation requirements and the length of its curriculum. There are also greater efforts underway by Doctors of Medicine, Osteopathy, and Chiropractic to investigate both the scientific and clinical bases of spinal manipulative therapy.[77] Although osteopathy and chiropractic are strongest in the United States, each has made headway in Europe, Canada, and Oceania. Where legally or otherwise recognized, chiropractic worldwide roughly reflects the scope of practice as it exists in America. Legal barriers have prevented any osteopathic school outside the United States from producing 'physicians and surgeons', although in the United Kingdom one school offers medical graduates a postdoctoral course in osteopathy.[78]

CONCLUSIONS

At the beginning of this chapter I asked several questions related to the development and progress of unorthodox medical theories. With respect to the intellectual sources of the principal movements described, they represent a culmination or new synthesis of ideas and doctrines already in circulation. The principle of *similia similibus curantur* long predated Hahnemann, and the reliance on botanical remedies as championed by Thomson, Beach, and others has prehistoric origins. The use of water by Priessnitz was not particularly original, nor certainly was his crude humoral theory of disease; the restriction of diet as a principal means to prolong life and avoid illness had many advocates before Graham; and the use of the therapeutic touch or physical manipulation to treat a variety of disorders had been employed for many centuries. While some progenitors of unorthodox medical theories were loath to pay their intellectual debts, all appear to have been influenced by other theories and practices, whether from the orthodox or unorthodox traditions. Nevertheless, the movements covered herein appeared distinctive, at least initially, by the special emphasis they gave certain causative factors, their diagnostic process, and their means of treatment, to the exclusion of those others accepted by orthodoxy.

The proof of each system's worth was in the satisfaction of its clientele.

Quite unabashedly, the founders of these movements claimed that their approach could succeed where allopathy failed. Orthodox medicine, they declared, only created drug dependency, iatrogenesis, and a premature trip to the grave. The irregulars offered different forms of evidence demonstrating their therapeutic superiority. While claiming excellent results in acute cases, it was with chronic diseases that they believed they could achieve most, since many of these patients had already tried allopathic physicians. Each of these systems provided numerous examples of clients who suffered from rheumatism, palsy, failing eyesight, nervous disorders, chronic respiratory problems, joint and muscle dysfunctions, liver and kidney problems, skin diseases, etc., unrelieved by orthodox doctors, who found cure or relief under their ministrations. Such patients were glad to provide testimonials, which were published by the irregulars in their own journals, and used in direct advertising to the public. In addition, many groups of unorthodox practitioners constructed statistical comparisons between orthodoxy and their own approach: to no one's surprise, these numbers consistently showed the superiority of the latter. These healers also publicly challenged their competitors to trials, where, under controlled clinical conditions, the exponents of a particular system would treat one group of patients suffering from a given disease while the regulars would oversee a matched set. The results could then be compared. Orthodox physicians rejected these challenges as publicity stunts. These refusals indicated to the irregulars that their opponents had no confidence in their own methods, and that they were dogmatic and unscientific. If such trials were conducted, they argued, the public would once and for all recognize the danger and absurdity of orthodox treatment.[79]

(➤ Ch. 34 History of the doctor–patient relationship)

Nevertheless, despite the evidence presented for the efficacy of their various treatments, unorthodox movements underwent significant changes in both their theoretical orientation and in their methods of diagnosis and treatment of disease. As in the case of orthodox medicine, most irregular, non-religious-based systems were affected by new scientific and technological knowledge and innovations, which either could not be satisfactorily accounted for by the prevailing theoretical orientation or challenged practitioners' belief in the supremacy of approved procedures. Most progenitors of unorthodox systems began with the premise that their approach represented 'science' and constituted a polar opposite to conventional medicine. Yet, as shown, many unorthodox physicians, while adhering broadly to the philosophy and tools of their sect, were never so dogmatic as to ignore powerful evidence, from whatever source, to support other therapies that would appear to benefit their patients. Nor would they, in a client-driven profession, be able to survive if they resisted the wishes of their patients to integrate certain modalities in their overall management. Homoeopaths, eclectics, and osteopaths, who all sought recognition as fully qualified physicians in the United States, have travelled this road of assimilating all that seemed valuable. In the process, however, they all became less oppositional and less distinct, and weakened both their philosophical justification for remaining separate from orthodoxy and the loyalty of their many followers to their respective sects. Furthermore, the advantages offered by orthodox medicine, both in terms of extending educational and practice opportunities as well as effacing the stigma of deviance, pushed each of these groups toward amalgamation. On the other hand, in those unorthodox movements that did not seek full physician status, there was a less powerful pull on its members toward the mainstream. They were satisfied to specialize in limited types of disorders and a particular form of therapy; for example, chiropractic's emphasis on spinal and other joint manipulation in musculo-skeletal complaints. However, when limited-therapy unorthodox movements, such as Thomsonism, hydropathy, and magnetic healing, did not expand to meet changing needs, they lost both practitioner and client support and died from within.

Historically, what influence have unorthodox movements had upon conventional medicine? Certainly, orthodox physicians contemporaneous with the launch of these systems almost unanimously declared that the theories underlying them were unscientific and their therapeutic approaches posed real or potential dangers to patients, if not by doing physical harm, then by delaying or precluding proper management of their problems. A number of present-day historians, most notably Rothstein, have noted that in criticizing the worst aspects of standard orthodox treatment, by their success in attracting patients, securing the support of some orthodox physicians, and offering, in general, a safer therapeutic regimen, homoeopathy, eclecticism, and hydropathy pushed regular practitioners to abandon their heroic approach.[80] Recently, however, Warner presented statistical evidence that orthodox physicians in America were decreasing their dependence on bloodletting and mercury much earlier in the century than generally believed, and argued that other, more orthodox theoretical currents and innovations accounted for much of the regulars' change in approach. Indeed, he maintains that the principal effect of the irregulars' challenges was to produce on the part of orthodox medical writers vehement symbolic defences of the appropriateness of these depletive tools, despite their eclipse.[81]

Nevertheless, there is considerable evidence that the therapies that unorthodox systems championed helped stimulate public and professional interest in remedies that had previously attracted little attention from regulars but which the latter ultimately incorporated. A number of homoeopathic and eclectic drugs were integrated into the orthodox materia medica; some magnetic healing methods did gain legitimacy as hypnosis; elements of hydropathy were transformed into hydrotherapy; the popular health movement and later naturopathy, despite its extravagances, did stimulate greater interest in dietetics; and recently, spinal and joint manipulation has achieved greater recognition and use by North American and European orthodox physicians. As a consequence, these unorthodox systems, though unappreciated by regular physicians, have left an enduring legacy to the history of medicine. (➤ Ch. 55 The emergence of para-medical professions)

NOTES

1 See Wilhelm Ameke, *History of Homeopathy*, London, E. Gould, 1885, pp. 150–71; Lester S. King, *The Medical World of the Eighteenth Century*, Chicago, IL, University of Chicago Press, 1958, pp. 157–91; Martin Gumpert, *Hahnemann: the Adventurous Career of a Medical Rebel*, New York, L. B. Fischer, 1945.

2 The best general introductory survey of the intellectual issues of the period is King, op. cit. (n. 1).

3 Quoted in Ameke, op. cit. (n. 1), pp. 103–4.

4 King, op. cit. (n. 1), pp. 165–6.

5 Samuel Hahnemann, 'Essay on a new principle for ascertaining the curative powers of drugs', *Hufeland's Journal*, 1796, 2: 391–439, 465–561; trans. in *Lesser Writings*, New York, William Radde, 1852.

6 Quoted in Ameke, op. cit. (n. 1), p. 129.

7 Samuel Hahnemann, *Organon of Homeopathic Medicine*, 3rd American edn, New York, William Radde, 1849.

8 See Samuel Hahnemann, *Materia Medica Pura*, New York, W. Radde, 1846.

9 Ameke, op. cit. (n. 1), p. 98.

10 Hahnemann, op. cit. (n. 7), p. 25.

11 Hahnemann, op. cit. (n. 7), p. 41.

12 Hahnemann, op. cit. (n. 7), p. 96.

13 Ameke, op. cit. (n. 1), pp. 196–9.

14 Hahnemann, op. cit. (n. 7), p. 173.

15 Hahnemann, op. cit. (n. 7), p. 217.

16 Oliver Wendell Holmes, *Homeopathy and its Kindred Delusions*, Boston, MA, W. D. Ticknor, 1842, pp. 37–40.

17 Worthington Hooker, *Homeopathy: an Examination of its Doctrines and Evidences*, New York, C. Scribner, 1852, p. 22. For a British critique, see James Y. Simpson, *Homeopathy: its Tenets and Tendencies*, 3rd edn, Edinburgh, Sutherland & Cox, 1853.

18 Samuel Hahnemann, *The Chronic Diseases*, Philadelphia, PA, Boericke & Tofel, 1896.

19 See discussion in Norman Gevitz, 'Sectarian medicine', *Journal of the American Medical Association*, 1987, 257: 1636–40.

20 See James Cassedy, *American Medicine and Statistical Thinking*, Cambridge, MA, Harvard University Press, 1984, pp. 124–35; Ameke, op. cit. (n. 1), pp. 240–51.

21 See William G. Rothstein, 'The botanical movements and orthodox medicine', in Norman Gevitz (ed.), *Other Healers: Unorthodox Medicine in America*, Baltimore, MD, Johns Hopkins University Press, 1988, pp. 29–51; Alex Berman, 'The

Thomsonian movement and its relation to American pharmacy and medicine', *Bulletin of the History of Medicine*, 1951, 35: 405–28, 518–38.

22 Samuel Thomson, *New Guide to Health*, Columbus, OH, Horton Harvard 1827, p. 8. For a discussion of the religious elements of nineteenth-century unorthodox medical systems, see 'Religion and medicine', ch. 61 of this *Encyclopedia*.

23 Ibid., p. 9.

24 Thomson, op. cit. (n. 22), p. 12.

25 Rothstein, op. cit. (n. 21), p. 45; Berman, op. cit. (n. 21), pp. 520–2.

26 See Ursula Miley and John Pickstone, 'Medical botany around 1850: American medicine in industrial Britain', in Roger Cooter (ed.), *Studies in the History of Alternative Medicine*, Oxford, Macmillan Press, 1988, pp. 139–53.

27 Wooster Beach, *The American Practice Condensed*, Cincinnati, OH, Wilstach, Baldwin, 1879.

28 See Alexander Wilder, *History of Medicine*, New Sharon, ME, New England Eclectic Publishing, 1901, pp. 421–39.

29 J. T. H. Connor, ' "A sort of 'selo-dese'" ': eclecticism, related medical sects, and their decline in Victorian Ontario', *Bulletin of the History of Medicine*.

30 William G. Rothstein, *American Physicians in the Nineteenth Century: From Sects to Science*, Baltimore, MD, Johns Hopkins University Press, 1972, pp. 217–29.

31 Ameke, op. cit. (n. 1), pp. 245–59, 278–87.

32 For England, see Phillip A. Nicholls, *Homeopathy and the Medical Profession*, London, Croom Helm, 1988, pp. 133–64. For the United States, see Martin Kaufman, *Homeopathy in America*, Baltimore, MD, Johns Hopkins University Press, 1971, pp. 48–62.

33 Worthington Hooker, *Physician and Patient; or, a Practical View of the Mutual Duties, Relations and Interests of the Medical Profession and the Community*, New York, Baker & Scribner, 1849.

34 See Norman Gevitz, 'The chiropractors and the AMA: reflections on the history of the consultation clause', *Perspectives in Biology and Medicine*, 1989, 32: 281–99.

35 For homeopathy in England, see Nicholls, op. cit. (n. 32), pp. 186, 215–16; in Germany, see Ameke, op. cit. (n. 1), p. 277.

36 Rothstein, op. cit., (n. 30), p. 345.

37 Gevitz, op. cit. (n. 19), p. 1638.

38 For recent American events, see Martin Kaufman, 'Homeopathy in America: the rise and fall and persistence of a medical heresy', in Gevitz op. cit. (n. 21), pp. 113–23. For Britain, see Nichols, op. cit. (n. 32), pp. 215–87.

39 See G. E. R. Lloyd (ed.), *Hippocratic Writings*, Harmondsworth, Penguin, 1978.

40 See Roy Porter (ed.), *The Medical History of Waters and Spas*, London, Wellcome Institute for the History of Medicine, 1990.

41 See R. T. Claridge, *Hydropathy, or the Cold Water Cure, as Practised by Vincent Priessnitz*, London, James Madden, 1842, pp. 57–72.

42 Ibid., pp. 73–6.

43 Claridge, op. cit. (n. 41), pp. 96–112.

44 See Richard Metcalf, *The Rise and Progress of Hydropathy in England and Scotland*, London, Simpkin, Marshall, Hamilton, Kent, 1906; Kelvin Rees, 'Water as a commodity: hydropathy in Matlock', in Cooter, op. cit. (n. 26), pp. 28–45; R. Price, 'Hydropathy in England 1840–70', *Medical History*, 1981, 25: 269–80.

45 See Joel Shaw, *The Water Cure Manual*, New York, Fowler & Wells, 1849; R. T. Trall, *The Hydropathic Encyclopedia*, New York, Fowler & Wells, 1853; Mary Gove Nichols, *Experience in Water Cure*, New York, Fowler & Wells, 1850.

46 See Jane B. Donegan, *Hydropathic Highway to Health: Women and Water-Cure in Antebellum America*, Westport, CT, Greenwood Press, 1986; and Susan E. Cayleff, *'Wash and Be Healed': the Water-Cure Movement and Women's Health*, Philadelphia, PA, Temple University Press, 1987.

47 Claridge, op. cit. (n. 41), pp. 55–6.

48 See James C. Whorton, *Crusaders for Fitness: the History of American Health Reformers*, Princeton, NJ, Princeton University Press, 1982, pp. 38–91; Stephen Nissenbaum, *Sex, Diet and Debility in Jacksonian America*, Westport, CT, Greenwood Press, 1980.

49 See Sebastian Kniepp, *My Water-Cure*, Edinburgh, William Blackwood, 1891. Some orthodox physicians, on the other hand, incorporated some hydropathic elements into what they called hydrotherapy; see Simon Baruch, *The Principles and Practices of Hydrotherapy*, New York, William Wood, 1903. For an informative biography of Baruch, see Patricia Spain Ward, *Simon Baruch: Rebel in the Ranks of Medicine, 1840–1921*, Tuscaloosa, University of Alabama Press.

50 For a discussion on the relationship between bowel obstruction and disease in late nineteenth-century thinking, see Whorton, op. cit. (n. 48), pp. 201–38.

51 For naturopathy, see Adolf Just, *Return to Nature*, London, Routledge, 1912; Henry Lindlahr, *Philosophy of Natural Therapeutics*, Chicago, IL, [the author], 1924; Harry Benjamin, *Everybody's Guide to Nature Cure*, London Health for All Publishing, 1967.

52 See F. A. Mesmer, *Mesmerism: a Translation of the Original Scientific and Medical Writings of F. A. Mesmer*, trans. by George Bloch, Los Atlas, CA, William Kaufmann, 1980; Vincent Buranelli, *The Wizard from Vienna: Franz Anton Mesmer*, New York, Coward, McCann, & Geoghagen, 1975.

53 *Report of Dr Benjamin Franklin and Other Commissioners charged . . . with the Examination of the Animal Magnetism*, London, printed for L. Johnson, 1785.

54 See *Report of the Magnetical Experiments made by the Commission of the Royal Academy of Paris . . .*, trans. by Charles Poyen, Boston, MA, D. K. Hitchcock, 1836; James Braid, *Neurypnology; or the Rationale of Nervous Sleep: Considered in Relation with Animal Magnetism*, London, J. Churchill, 1843. In America, mesmerism was also combined with phrenology to form phrenomagnetism; see Taylor Stoehr, 'Robert H. Collyer's technology of the soul', in Arthur Wrobel (ed.), *Pseudo-Science and Society in Nineteenth-Century America*, Lexington, University Press of Kentucky, 1987, pp. 21–45.

55 Annetta G. Dresser, *The Philosophy of P. P. Quimby*, Boston, MA, George H. Ellis, 1895; Frank Podmore, *From Mesmerism to Christian Science: a Short History of Mental Healing*, New York, University Books, 1963, pp. 250–99.

56 Mary Baker Eddy, *Science and Health with Key to the Scriptures*, Boston, MA, First Church of Christ Scientist, 1981; Robert Peel, *Mary Baker Eddy: the Years of Discovery, 1821–1875*, New York, Holt, Rinehart & Winston, 1966; Norman Gevitz, 'Christian Science healing and the health care of children', *Perspectives in Biology and Medicine*, 1991, 34: 421–38.

57   See Horatio Dresser, *A History of the New Thought Movement*, New York, T. Y. Crowell, 1919.

58   Andrew Jackson Davis, *The Great Harmonia*, 4 vols, Boston, MA, Benjamin B. Mussey, 1853. See also Robert W. Delp, 'Andrew Jackson Davis: prophet of American spiritualism', *Journal of American History*, 1967, 20: 43–57.

59   Warren Felt Evans, *Mental Medicine*, Boston, MA, H. H. Carter, 1885, p. 109. See also John F. Teahan, 'Warren Felt Evans and mental healing', *Church History*, 1979; 48: 63–80.

60   Edwin Dwight Babbitt, *Vital Magnetism*, New York, [the author], 1874.

61   See Norman Gevitz, *The D.O.'s: Osteopathic Medicine in America*, Baltimore, MD, Johns Hopkins University Press, 1982, pp. 1–18.

62   Andrew Taylor Still, *Autobiography*, Kirksville, MO, [the author], 1908, p. 108.

63   For bone-setting in Britain, see Roger Cooter, 'Bones of contention? Orthodox medicine and the mystery of the bone-setter's craft', in W. F. Bynum and Roy Porter (eds.), *Medical Fringe and Medical Orthodoxy, 1750–1850*, London, Croom Helm, 1987, pp. 158–73. For America, see Robert J. T. Joy, 'The natural bonesetters with special reference to the Sweet family of Rhode Island', *Bulletin of the History of Medicine*, 1965, 28: 416–41.

64   See James Paget, 'Cases that bonesetters cure', *British Medical Journal*, 1867, 1: 1–4.

65   Wharton Hood, *On Bonesetting, So-Called, and its Relation to the Treatment of Joints crippled by Injury*, London, Macmillan, 1871, pp. 4, 26–7.

66   Douglas Graham, *A Practical Treatise on Massage: its History, Mode of Application and Effects*, New York, William Wood, 1884, p. 20.

67   In addition to his autobiography (op. cit. (n. 62)), see Andrew Taylor Still, *Philosophy of Osteopathy*, Kirksville, MO, [the author], 1899.

68   See Gevitz, op. cit. (n. 61), pp. 29–34.

69   See Daniel David Palmer and Bartlett Joseph Palmer, *Science of Chiropractic*, Davenport, IA, Palmer School of Chiropractic, 1906; Daniel David Palmer, *The Chiropractor's Adjuster*, Portland, OR, Portland Printing House, 1910.

70   See Walter Wardwell, 'Chiropractors: evolution to acceptance', in Gevitz, op. cit. (n. 21), pp. 157–91; and Russell Gibbons, 'Physician-chiropractors: medical presence in the evolution of chiropractic', *Bulletin of the History of Medicine*, 1981, 55: 233–45.

71   Gevitz, op. cit. (n. 61), pp. 57–60.

72   Gevitz, op. cit. (n. 61), pp. 61–74.

73   Gevitz, op. cit. (n. 61), pp. 88, 116.

74   op. cit. (n. 21), pp. 117–48.

75   Wardwell, in Gevitz, op. cit. (n. 21), pp. 162 and *passim*.

76   Gevitz, 'AMA and chiropractors', op. cit. (n. 34), pp. 291–7.

77   Murray Goldstein (ed.), *The Research Status of Spinal Manipulative Therapy*, Bethesda, MD, US Department of Health, Education and Welfare, 1975.

78   Hans Baer, 'The drive for professionalization in British osteopathy', *Social Science and Medicine*, 1984, 19: 717–25.

79   See Norman Gevitz, 'Three perspectives on unorthodox medicine', in Gevitz, op. cit. (n. 21), pp. 1–29.

80   Rothstein, op. cit. (n. 30).

81   See John Harley Warner, *The Therapeutic Perspective*, Cambridge, MA, Harvard
     University Press, 1986.

FURTHER READING

Bynum, W. F. and Porter, Roy (eds), *Medical Fringe and Medical Orthodoxy, 1750–1850*,
London, Croom Helm, 1987.

Cayleff, Susan E., *'Wash and be healed': the Water-Cure Movement and Women's Health*,
Philadelphia, PA, Temple University Press, 1987.

Cooter, Roger (ed.) *Studies in the History of Alternative Medicine*, Basingstoke, Macmillan, 1988.

Eddy, Mary Baker, *Science and Health with Key to the Scriptures*, Boston, MA, First
Church of Christ Scientist, 1981.

Gevitz, Norman, *The D.O.'s: Osteopathic Medicine in America*, Baltimore, MD, Johns
Hopkins University Press, 1982.

—— (ed.), *Other Healers: Unorthodox Medicine in America*, Baltimore, MD, Johns
Hopkins University Press, 1988.

Hahnemann, Samuel, *Organon of Homeopathic Medicine*, 3rd American edn, New York,
William Radde, 1849.

Just, Adolf, *Return to Nature*, London, Routledge, 1912.

Kaufman, Martin, *Homeopathy in America: the Rise and Fall of a Medical Heresy*,
Baltimore, MD, Johns Hopkins University Press, 1971.

Mesmer, F. A., *Mesmerism: a Translation of the Original Scientific and Medical Writings
of F. A. Mesmer*, trans. by George Bloch, Los Altas, CA, William Kaufmann, 1980.

Nicholls, Phillip A., *Homeopathy and the Medical Profession*, London, Croom Helm,
1988.

Palmer, Daniel David and Palmer, Bartlett Joseph, *Science of Chiropractic*, Davenport,
IA, Palmer School of Chiropractic, 1906.

Porter, Roy (ed.), *The Medical History of Waters and Spas*, *Medical History* suppl. 10,
London, Wellcome Institute for the History of Medicine, 1990.

Rothstein, William G., *American Physicians in the Nineteenth Century: from Sects to
Science*, Baltimore, MD, Johns Hopkins University Press, 1972.

Still, Andrew Taylor, *Autobiography*, Kirksville, MO, [the author], 1908.

Thomson, Samuel, *New Guide to Health*, Columbus, OH, Horton Howard, 1827.

Whorton, James C., *Crusaders for Fitness: the History of American Health Reformers*,
Princeton, NJ, Princeton University Press, 1982.

29

NON-WESTERN CONCEPTS OF DISEASE

Murray Last

This chapter excludes medical systems that constitute 'great traditions', to use Redfield's classic distinction;[1] Chinese, Indian, Islamic, and Galenic medicine are discussed elsewhere in this *Encyclopedia*. (➤ Ch. 31 Arab-Islamic medicine; Ch. 32 Chinese medicine; Ch. 33 Indian medicine) Excluded too is the generic humoral medicine that not only underlies all these four systems but has also influenced many medical systems of the 'little tradition'. (➤ Ch. 14 Humoralism) By 'little tradition' we mean, first, systems that are purely local and specific to the community (for example, the Gnau as described by G. Lewis[2]); and second, systems that are subordinate to a 'great tradition'. To be subordinate does not necessarily mean being less popular, even perhaps less successful than medicine of the dominant 'great tradition'; it does mean, however, that government resources, formal education, and social status privilege the 'great tradition', thus leaving the 'little tradition' not only as the disparaged alternative but also as a possible means of subverting the cultural hegemony of the political élite. The political uses of a medical system as an ideology have become particularly significant with the advent of European colonialism (a good example is the role of homoeopathy in Brazil). Similar processes of medical change due to other imperialisms (Islamic, Chinese, or Indian, for example) are not so well documented, but have nonetheless shaped, in varying degrees, local systems of medicine. (➤ Ch. 58 Medicine and colonialism)

Into this category of 'non-Western theories' falls potentially a vast range of ideas and practices, from the time of early humans up to the present, in all areas of the globe. Clearly, only a fraction of the history of these ideas is known, and such history as there is has often come to us through the lens of some outside observer to whom the practices seen had to be sufficiently exotic to be of interest to record. This chapter summarizes academic attempts to make sense of this range of ideas, and ends with an outline of some significant variables in non-Western theories of illness. For detailed analysis of any particular system of medicine the reader must turn to a monograph that focuses on that system; there, the complexity and the nuancing inherent in the actual experience of illness in a community will be found, and the subtlety of changes in ideas over time, and that sense of stable continuity that often makes those ideas all the while still seem to be 'right', will be noticed.

Attempts to systematize the ethnographic data worldwide on non-Western medical theories and to construct a general schema have taken two forms. The first, an evolutionary model, divides the history of these theories into stages that match developments in the socio-economic and political components of a culture. The second offers a typology of medical systems using as a criterion concepts about the cause of illness, and shows the distribution of these theories worldwide. (➤ Ch. 60 Medicine and anthropology)

EVOLUTIONARY MODELS

DATA

Evolutionary models draw on two kinds of evidence. Archaeological data are used particularly to demonstrate the shift in the patterns of disease that occurred when communities, ceasing to be small-scale bands gathering and hunting their food supply, became instead sedentary populations with large numbers concentrated in fixed settlements: a shift associated with the 'neolithic revolution' and the invention of agriculture. (➤ Ch. 18 The ecology of disease) Further archaeological evidence for the evolutionary model focuses on the changing patterns of morbidity, mortality, and nutrition. The second body of evidence is drawn from ethnographic accounts of gatherer-hunter societies in the twentieth century, the assumption being that both the way of life of these groups and their ideas have changed little over the last ten thousand or more years, and that these ideas are typical of palaeolithic and mesolithic populations which subsequently either became agriculturalist or died out. Materials from burial and other sites dating to these periods have been adduced as evidence that the choice of medicinal plants, surgical procedures such as trepanning, and ritual equipment have persisted unchanged over millennia. Artefacts, however, yield few clues to the actual theories people held at the time. None the less, in the absence of better evidence, the evolutionary model remains in use.

STAGE I

In the first stage – so the model goes[3] – small egalitarian gatherer-hunter groups managed their health collectively, without ritual experts. An individual's ill health was seen to reflect primarily on the health status of the group, with the cause or causes of the illness located outside the sick person's own body. Treatment was done openly and collectively.

The diseases to which these bands were exposed would not have included the acute infections such as measles, influenza, or polio; nor would there have been a pattern of recovery from infection and subsequent immunity. So long as there was no animal reservoir, populations were too small and scattered to allow for epidemics of this kind. Given the band's mobility, diarrhoea brought about by faecal–oral transmission of micro-organisms would have been largely absent. But infections with a long latency and the possibility of recurrence would have been common, as would diseases (like tuberculosis) that could be transmitted across generations. (➤ Ch. 20 Constitutional and hereditary disorders) Chronic skin infections, it is suggested, would also have been common. Injuries due to hunting and other accidents or to warfare (the extent of which at this period is much debated) would have been a further source of disability and death.

In this model, there is also the general argument that concern over ill health as such may have played a smaller role in people's culture than it did subsequently among sedentary populations. Models for how people behaved towards the sick are drawn from primate behaviour and take mother–child bonding as the primary source of care-giving and -seeking. Calculations of the risk for small bands of looking after the sick and disabled – risks from predators attracted by calls of distress, or from the band's reduced ability to move in search of food – have given rise to theories that infanticide and the premature disposal of the elderly were a significant part of the medical culture of early humans.

There seem to be, for humans as for animals, two contrasting 'sick roles' available: one when the sick person behaves as a 'child' again, to be fed and guarded during the whole period of disability; the other when the sick person either leaves the group to hide away alone until recovery or death ensues, or is simply abandoned by the group. In the latter, the sick are socially dead before they are physically dead; in a sense, they are prematurely aged by illness, and, should they recover, they may be treated as having gained the sort of experience and wisdom that only elders have. Both roles, the 'elderly' and the 'young', are thus available for use as contrasted models or metaphors for the dependency that physical illness imposes on the sick. Which role is chosen by a particular culture as the dominant model for the sick is not necessarily clear; much depends on the context.

STAGE 2

In the second stage of the evolutionary model, when people are sedentary farmers, population numbers rise and settlements are large by comparison. If the initial extra food supply allowed for a growth in the population and for a lowered morbidity, the initial gain was soon offset by a rise in the range of infections to which individuals were exposed, thanks to the ease of transmission and to a larger population pool. Furthermore, epidemics were possible, particularly as trade and other reasons for people moving between settlements exposed hitherto virgin populations to new diseases. Where irrigation was developed, faecal–oral transmission of micro-organisms will also have increased. The implications of these changes are that infant and child mortality, due to acute infections, diarrhoea, and malnutrition, will have become a major feature, whereas adult illness may have lost, relatively speaking, its salience, once adults developed an immunity or resistance to a wide range of infections. (➤ Ch. 52 Epidemiology)

The medical systems and theories that developed in this second stage under these new conditions reflect (it is argued) more the economic and political developments in the society than any environmental changes. In contrast to the egalitarian bands of gatherers and hunters, the communities of the second stage are internally ranked, with some few individuals or groups within the community having greater access to wealth of whatever kind – people, goods, land – and being given greater authority in making decisions for the community as a whole. Most notably, there is a division of labour in which medical expertise, along with religious and other specialisms, are isolated out as the *métier* of particular individuals or families. Whereas previously there was a lay knowledge about illness and how to cope with it – a 'common sense' in which some individuals might be wiser than others through personal interest or their experience as former sufferers – in this second stage open, lay knowledge was competing with potentially arcane, specialist theories of diagnosis and therapy. But it is important to recognize not only the search now for new theories of medicine by the new specialists (whether medical or religious), but also the way that lay knowledge none the less persisted, albeit often within the family, as the first line of defence against illness. (➤ Ch. 12 The concepts of health, illness, and disease)

Two points need to be made: first, that the incidence of new types of illness in this second stage would have discredited much of the 'common sense' knowledge existing at the time; built up over the generations on the basis of experience and experimentation with handling the old range of illnesses, the traditional remedies would have proved ineffective against the new infections. Hence considerable intellectual space would have been opened up for new explanations and solutions to new illnesses, thereby

637

allowing a different style of healer and therapy – more specialized and elaborate – to enter the field. A new, effective 'common sense' to cope with the new diseases would have taken time to develop while incorporating the traditional ways of coping still with the old diseases. Second, the occurrence of epidemics, affecting as never before all the young of the community and killing many, would have posed a new challenge to the new political and social system with its rankings and proto-specialization. In these circumstances, the new religious and medical experts would have had to come up with explanations for a totally novel and devastating phenomenon: social disaster due to illness on a major scale. Obviously, we do not know the psychologies of early communities and cannot reconstruct a people's response to disaster, but we do have to recognize the potential impact such disasters might have on the organization of society and the development of its theories about illness.

Characteristics of the medical systems in this second stage include greater patient-centredness, with care managed by the kin group and with illness treated as a family or private matter. The focusing on the patient allowed for a wider range of therapies and explanations, with supernatural causes being only one type among many possibilities. The new breed of medical specialists would eventually have included diviners, shamans, herbalists, birth-attendants, bone-setters, barber-surgeons, and priests. Alongside them, there remained all the diversity of lay knowledge and the smattering people usually also have of their neighbours' medical expertise. The result is that, for many societies, their medical culture comprised widely disparate interpretations and treatments of illness. Very few societies are so isolated that they have no experience of another culture's ideas; and the internal diversity of a society is often great enough for households and kin groups to have differing bits of lay expertise. Hence a certain pluralism – and with it a certain scepticism – is a feature of these more complex second-stage societies. And as their complexity grew, with new elaborate economies and extensive political systems, so competition for dominance in the provision of medical services increased. It is possible that in polities that were people-short the need for cures was intense, particularly if new environments were being opened up for settlement and cultivation.

Furthermore, as people's labour became more valuable, we assume that earlier practices such as infanticide or the abandonment of the elderly declined except for ritual purposes, and that the 'sick role' that came to predominate was modelled on child care: the patient becoming a 'child' but with the proviso that there was no overt malingering. Conversely, with labour increasingly valuable, the conditions for which an adult could afford to be off sick decreased and consequently the category of legitimate ailments countable as 'illness' contracted at a time when the number of possible infections was on the increase. The physically very demanding labour required of farmers at certain seasons (when usually food supplies were shortest and illness most common) emphasized the need for medicines to give strength and overcome exhaustion, and hence opened up a new field for suppliers of various 'tonics' as well as the usual range of medicines to relieve fevers, stomach aches, and pain. Such tonics would include recipes not just for prolonged hard work but for such social ailments as unpopularity, impotence, and lack of confidence in battle. Finally, with the advent of politically stratified societies, the incidence of illness may have become unequally distributed and hence more problematic politically, both in explanations of illness and in the special treatments required. In some communities, a new king or chief was likely to be among the healthiest of eligible candidates. With access to more and better food and less liable to heavy, debilitating labour, such royal groups were better able than their subordinates to withstand infection. And when illness did strike, royals were able to call upon a range of specialists, both local and alien, to whom commoners normally had no recourse. In so far as differences in rank and status are maintained by different interpretations and treatment of illness, and given the way new therapeutic fashions are apt to trickle down the social hierarchy, social stratification offered fresh scope for enterprising healers. In short, the demand for medicines became considerably more diversified.

Some areas and some groups are richer than others in medically useful resources. Interest and expertise in therapy are not evenly distributed, with some groups gaining great reputations as healers or diviners. The specific reasons may be lost in the past, but there are some potentially relevant environmental factors, at least for gaining a reputation as a herbalist. For example, plant communities in ancient rain forests have a very wide range, exploiting specialized niches and developing in their defence pharmacological properties that are highly toxic to specific predators and rivals; similarly, some predators (such as insects) are able to ingest and then isolate such toxins within some part of themselves without harm. Such forests are a source, then, of several pharmacologically very active medicines – some poisonous, some psychotropic, others bactericidal. Social groups that learnt to exploit the forests' plant communities and to understand the use of available plants were at a considerable advantage. Other groups, in less pharmacologically rich environments (such as lands once affected by ice ages), had a smaller repertoire to draw upon. But the matter is not so simple: that the rain forest, with its catena of distinct ecologies, was always used by its inhabitants as a vast botanical 'library' cannot be taken for granted. At least today, most of the plants used medicinally by people living in or by rainforests are drawn, it seems, from the forest edge or grow wild around areas of settlement; and the actual range of properties required – of poisons in particular – is limited, and the relevant types of plants are available in a wide range of habitats. Both Siberia and the Amazon basin, for example, had plants enabling shamanism to flourish as a therapeutic technique. In general, 'local cures for local ailments' seems the usual principle; the quest for exotic cures from exotic sites is the stuff of folk-tales.

Other groups have specialized in developing rituals and have elaborated the symbolic significance of the therapies they had to offer. Generally speaking, it would seem that expertise in the use of plants as medicines is widespread (being based on experience and experiment) whereas ritual and symbolic expertise, making particular use of the placebo effect by drawing on ideas with great resonance within a specific community, can be retained as the secrets of a specialized group. Whereas it suits such ritual experts to remain more local, capitalizing upon their insight into local social relationships and into the symbols that have a particular significance in the culture, herbalists, by contrast, are apt to travel, offering their expertise in societies where their special reputation can be valued. In part, this is because the plants, minerals or animal-derived substances on offer as medicines are 'tonics' rather than poisons, or, if they are inherently poisonous, are to be taken in such low dosages that they are not dangerous. (Dosages that are appropriate – and safe – for very young sick children pose a real problem for herbalists; they tend to err even more on the safe side, making their treatment in effect a placebo.) There are, however, certain forms of ritual, such as the *ngoma* dances found all over southern Africa, that follow a common pattern and thus permit specifically ritual expertise to travel across social or ecological boundaries.

STAGE 3

In urban and/or industrial society, with the increasing rarity of epidemics and the declining danger of infectious disease, the clinical picture is dominated by the so-called 'diseases of civilization': coronary heart disease, for example, and the various cancers, but also back pain or symptoms associated with stress. (➤ Ch. 27 Diseases of civilization) 'Non-Western' theories, in such societies, offer alternative therapies for chronic, often incurable ailments and malaise; above all, they offer psychotherapy. (➤ Ch. 43 Psychotherapy) Patients using these therapies are not necessarily interested in the theories themselves (any more than patients are interested in always understanding 'Western' theories); and rarely are the theories underlying a therapy elaborated – they are taken as matters of faith. Furthermore, being more practices than theories, these therapies are exempt from the scepticism normal in more tradition-rooted societies. Apparent evidence that they 'work' is sufficient. Non-Western theories of illness, then, in modern urban or industrial societies differ from earlier versions of them in that

1 the legal constraints of modern society inhibit if not prevent certain kinds of 'traditional' medical practice (though the degree of constraint varies from state to state);
2 healers are apt to modify their explanations and their pharmacopoeia to fit local circumstances, especially where their clientele may not share the conceptual matrix out of which has developed the particular therapy on offer;
3 in order to win recognition in an otherwise-fluid urban milieu, healers may form an association that lays down formal rules prescribing the principles and practice of its members, thus professionalizing an expertise that was never so precisely formulated.[4] (By contrast, in a stable rural community, the efficacy of a theory and the therapy derived from it, as well as the credibility of the practitioner, are proven over time; no certificate offers a guarantee as good as long co-residence.)

None the less, non-Western therapies, whatever their underlying theories of illness, offer the patient a rather different sick role, giving greater power to the patient-as-customer while at the same time calling explicitly upon the patient's faith in the treatment. Compared with conventional Western theories, the range of emotions involved can be wider, too, whether it be fear generated by notions of illness as a 'battle against evil forces' or by anxieties of bewitchment or poisoning, or exaltation from acquiring for oneself special mystical powers. But the very fact that there are many non-Western therapies simultaneously on offer within the urban context (both in the developed and in the developing world) potentially reduces the power of any particular theory over its clientele. As a result, patients may pick a particular therapy only for a specific type of malaise, hence negating the wider 'truth' of the theory that underlies it. Since therapies of this kind are empirical practices based only tangentially on any believed-in theory, it is possible for quite contradictory therapies to co-exist in a community without the contradiction at the theoretical level proving a problem.

The evolutionary model summarized here offers only a very generalized account of the contexts in which non-Western theories and practices have developed, with the focus particularly upon the growth of healing as a specialized trade. Missing is an account of the diversity of these theories; missing too is an analysis of why ideas are what they are in any specific instance or of what people do with them.

TYPOLOGIES OF MEDICAL CONCEPTS

The shifts in the social organization of medicine on a time-scale as broad as the evolutionary one just outlined, though they indicate the contexts in which ideas might arise, none the less tell us little about the range of ideas actually in use worldwide. The very diversity of ideas is itself problematic: should we be surprised by the differences in the way people explain illness – or more surprised by how limited is the range of ideas, how constrained is the human imagination? For, broadly speaking, there are, apart from notions of natural causation, only five major traditional theories about the causes of illness: sorcery, soul loss, breach of a taboo, intrusion by a disease object, and intrusion by a spirit.[5] Only two attempts, first by Forrest E. Clements and then by G. P. Murdock and his colleagues using the Human Relations Area Files, have been made in the last sixty years to examine the range of theories about illness worldwide and to see if there is a pattern to their distribution.[6] The relevance of their work to a history of non-Western theories of illness lies in their efforts to match distribution with diffusionist models of the movement of either actual peoples or ideas.[7]

Two points stand out from these surveys. One is the relatively small range of theories about illness; almost all interpret illness as *injury* and hence posit that some form of aggression has taken place: illness is not accidental. The other point is that preferences for one explanation of illness over another are bunched, and regions vary in their apparent preoccupation with one sort of aggressor more than another. It suggests that illness-as-injury is a matter that spans cultural differences even where one culture is not necessarily dominating another. We know how readily and widely such theories as the humoral model of illness have spread; we know too how relatively obscure theories from other cultures can find acceptance in a wholly different milieu. So too, it seems, in smaller-scale societies the problem of coping with illness-injury can transcend cultural boundaries: medicine in all its forms is less culture-constrained than other aspects of a society's behaviour.

There are obvious problems and limitations to these surveys. First, they depend on published literature of variable quality and sensitivity to the subject being surveyed. Monographs that focus on one particular theme need not necessarily be accurate on matters of marginal interest (especially one as marginal to most research projects as medicine). Second, these surveys are, despite their impressive size and the effort involved, none the less relatively small: the number of distinct societies, past and present, is enormous – and we have records only for those that have survived. Third, societies vary in size, from a few hundred members to groups that number ten million plus. Hence some non-Western theories have a vast following, thus giving the operative theories of illness not only a considerable diversity but also great internal resilience. Lastly, I suspect we have presented to us here only the medical 'common sense' rather than the subtler, more idiosyncratic beliefs of groups responding to particular experiences at particular periods; hence this ethnographic mapping proved to be of only limited interest, and was soon replaced by detailed studies of single communities in order to show how medical ideas and practices articulate with other aspects of the social system. None the less, until a systematic exercise of this kind had been done and re-done, global generalizations were only anecdotal and any overview was severely limited.

Theories worldwide can be divided into two major categories. First, there are the theories of natural causation, that locate illness as a result of normal activities that have gone awry; infestation with intestinal worms, or parasites on or in the surface of the skin; dietary mistakes; hunger; the effects of climate, overwork, etc.; common one-off accidents (repeated accidents are more suspicious) and wounds; old age. Often, however, these are only proximate causes; the ultimate cause, why such 'natural' events took place, is not to be found in 'nature' or in chance, but in social or 'super-social' relations of hostility. ('Super-social' here refers to the extension of human society to include another sphere of superhuman beings, namely that of ancestors and patron-spirits; 'supernatural' refers instead to a similar but more-limited extension of natural forces, with their minimal capacity for social relations.)

Second, there are theories that posit a social or a super-social (or supernatural) causation. These theories assume that illness (but not necessarily death) is an injury – whether it is intended or not – inflicted by some human or superhuman agency. Illness is brought upon a victim by other people whether intentionally (as by a sorcerer) through magical devices using words or rituals through which an object can be shot into the victim, or unintentionally because of an innate power for evil (such as witches have). In a number of societies, pollution from another person categorized as unclean is enough to cause illness – most commonly, and especially in Africa, a menstruating woman or her menstrual blood; in north-American societies particularly, by contrast, a corpse is similarly polluting.

Using the data on 1,300 distinct cultures that comprise his *Ethnographic Atlas*, Murdock and his colleagues plotted the distribution of theories of illness by 'cultural province' with a sample of 139 carefully selected societies.[8] The supernatural kinds of illness are reduced to three subcategories:

1 mystical, in which illness is the *automatic* consequence of an act or experience, brought about impersonally;
2 animistic, in which the agent causing illness is a personalized supernatural being;

3 magical, where a malicious human being uses covert, magical means to make a person ill.

Rarely do communities have only a single theory of illness, although one may well be dominant. Which theory is dominant appears to vary more by region than by, say, the type of political system. Overall, Murdock concludes that Africa ranks very high in theories of mystical retribution in which broken taboos, especially involving sex and etiquette, are responsible; and of supernatural beings, ancestors, more in Africa than elsewhere, are the most commonly responsible. East Asia is associated with 'spirit aggression', whereas witchcraft is reportedly almost absent. The Pacific-island societies are also high in spirit aggression, as well as sorcery theories, but despite their reputation, the incidence of theories of taboo-caused illness is below average. North America is high on theories involving sorcery and broken taboos (especially food, ritual, and the senses), but low on those about spirit aggression. By contrast, South America scores high on spirit aggression (especially ghosts), and very low on mystical retribution. Witchcraft, the evil eye, and aggression by gods are particularly commonly used to explain illness in Europe and India, with comparatively little interest in sorcery and broken taboos. (It is important to recognize that there are notable local exceptions to all these generalizations.)

We could interpret the tendency for a marked regional grouping of the various kinds of theories about illness as evidence that people in any community have a certain degree of knowledge about the medical practices of their neighbours and that they find little or no difficulty in using 'alien' interpretations of illness. Furthermore, where a particular explanation is especially frequent, it is liable to act as a stereotype, a catch-all label used to make (often temporary) sense of what would otherwise be an ambiguous ailment, and, if necessary, to bring all further debate to a halt.[9] Such stereotyped illnesses and their explanations may not necessarily be an accurate guide either to the 'real' diagnosis made or to the subsequent therapy; instead, they are cognitive weapons within the politics of illness, and as such are readily accessible to the visiting ethnographer.

Seen in political terms, then, stereotypical theories of illness can also be grouped in the following ways. The first group is those theories that blame *things* for illness – tabooed things, polluting things, dangerous things (like stars) whose influence upon the individual can bring about sickness. In these, it is the environment that is explicitly thought to pose a risk, with or without blame for the illness being laid at the patient's door. But implicitly it is the *rules* that society makes for proper, safe behaviour within that environment that are being given especial emphasis. Hence illness can be interpreted as a means of social control through enforcing obedience to a variety of rules, and through the rituals laid on to cleanse the patient. Otherwise, illness is not being used for inter-personal politics and hence poses less of a threat to the community's stability.

The second group is those theories that blame other *people* for illness – sorcerers, witches, and others who intentionally or not can cause another harm. Commonly, sorcerers have 'shot' into the victim some object that is causing illness, thus enabling healers to 'extract' it in a dramatic healing ritual. Identifying the person responsible is more dramatic still – and disruptive. The hunt for the witch uses divination or mass searches for witches' weapons – with potentially cathartic consequences for the community and certain disaster for the scapegoat. In such conditions, illness is treated as central to a community's political life, liable to destroy it as a social entity and liable too to encourage paranoia as a valuable political asset;[10] it also offers witchfinders a major role in the community. But the effects should not be exaggerated: in some contexts, gossip about suspected witchcraft may be as habitual and as unprovocative as comments about the weather, and equally lead nowhere. But where illness focuses scrutiny on social relations, the politics of illness can take over from the illness itself as the problem requiring solution.

The third group is those theories that focus on *spirits* or *souls*. In these theories, either spirits of the dead or nature spirits are thought to have attacked the ill; or the patient's own soul has grown weak or has gone missing (this may be voluntary, though more commonly it is the result of an attack). The politics involved in this category of explanation are sometimes those of either the first or second groups of theories: that is, it is simply a matter of *indirect* control or attack, with treatment focusing on spirit beings who are credited with powers over (weak) people. But compared with theories of witchcraft, theories of explicitly indirect causation allow for much more convoluted or devious explanations of the social enmities that are thought to cause illness – there need be no simple, single scapegoat. Given the complexities inherent in positing an extra set of unseen forces, the special intimacy of healers with this other, more powerful world and hence their ability to recognize which particular being is currently causing illness provides healers with considerable political capital of a kind usually monopolized by rulers. In this context, then, the political debate over a case of illness may pit healer against chief or against the head of the patient's household; and the debate may then be used to give recognition to other splits in the domestic or communal fabric. Similarly, the idiom of both 'soul loss' and spirit possession can be used indirectly to give voice to the patient's own inner feelings and wishes, in circumstances where direct complaint is disallowed. In short, the indirectness inherent in a spirit theory of illness permits considerable social space to the ill, and yet at the same time allows people, if they wish, to use that space to manœuvre in order to mitigate the social implications of illness and its wider social consequences.

The fourth group is those theories that take *natural* causes or *chance* to be a sufficient and satisfactory explanation of illness – in other words, posit the proximate cause as being also the ultimate one. For these theories of illness to become and then remain so dominant in a particular society at a particular period that they are stereotypes and considered to be 'common sense' depends in part on how effective a monopoly there is of political or religious authority. Monotheist religions and centralized states are commonly promoters of such theories, but signs of failure in either kind of authority provoke a renewed search for a further, ultimate cause of illness; then answers like 'that's the way it is, it's natural', or 'it's just bad luck', 'it's God's will', prove to be no longer an adequate response to the questions 'why us, why me? Why *always* us, why *always* me?' In consequence, the waning of a previously strong political or religious monopoly is apt to find early expression in (initially) tentative theories of illness, to be interpreted by analysts outside as a form of resistance or as the stirrings of intellectual disquiet. And it is in this context that not only notions of a 'political economy of health', but also non-Western theories of disease, are now beginning to gain, or regain, a constituency.

Given the political implications of the various kinds of explanations of illness, recent analysis has sought to focus on how the politics of illness meshes with the wider politics of society, and has done so not by surveying broadly whole regions but by examining particular communities in which to demonstrate the connections between the patient's body and the body politic. We now turn to these studies.

ANALYTICAL MODELS IN WHICH ILLNESS THEORIES ARE SECONDARY

A third approach to the analysis of non-Western theories has been to treat them as a subset of ideas within the broader corpus of a society's thought. The concern here has been to show how one could illuminate indigenous concepts about society and its processes through the refractions of those same concepts to be seen in the context of illness or in everyday ideas about the body and the self. The insights from this quest for the social meaning of health and illness proved very productive. Illness could be analysed for the way it expressed social stress, revealing fault-lines in the otherwise solid façade of communal life.[11] Illness provided the occasion (but rarely the cause) of changes in social systems; the social response to illness varied according to the immediate political context, with some cases scarcely noticed while others became the centre of great concern. From this perspective, the significance of illness and the theories about it lay in the way they articulated with social structure. Thus, just as religious rituals may act as social cement, so illness can 'function' as social dynamite. In a crisis over an illness, the existing hierarchies of local power are called into question: for example, a particular case could give rise to accusations of witchcraft, and these accusations lead to the exile or death of the chief – or more often to the hiving-off of a section of the community to found a new settlement. In this instance, illness could be seen as a motor driving the developmental cycle of a domestic group. The occasion of illness could equally be used to victimize an opponent or to set up a scapegoat; conversely, when manipulated by the powerful, it can reinforce the *status quo*. In large-scale states, epidemics (like other disasters) call into question the legitimacy of the government, if not the entire social hierarchy. Conversely, governing groups may impose diagnostic rules that explicitly exclude them from being implicated in illness.[12] In all these analyses, illness and its explanation are shown as being manipulated for political ends, and consequently, publicly expressed theories of illness are analysed simply as a subset of more general theories of religion or social structure. In these models (and in the fieldwork from which the supporting data are derived) the actual cases of illness and the diagnostic debates and doubts that surrounded them are of secondary interest. This may reflect truly the culture's own relative lack of concern about illness; on the other hand, it may spring from the disciplinary bias of the observer, or indeed the observer's own sense of uncertainty when confronted by medical problems. But there is a certain triteness in explanations of illness solely in terms of the wider political process, whether the bias is towards illness as conflict or towards therapy as communal solidarity-in-action. Not all cases of illness are used as weapons in the political arena, nor, when they are so used, are the outcomes so predictable or the interpretations so uniformly accepted. In short, politics is only one dimension in the analysis of cases structured by non-Western theories of illness.

In analyses that focus on the structure of a people's medical ideas, detailed concepts of illness or subtler notions about the body are subsumed within broader dichotomies such as nature and culture, the raw and the cooked. Here, concepts of the body are seen to reflect those held about the way the body politic is constituted; indeed, the more elaborate ideas about anatomy (for example, its various moral connotations) are shown to be determined by social interests, with anatomy merely a ready source of metaphors.[13] Thus communities with a more rigidly demarcated system of social organization are liable to have the same rigidity expressed in their rules about the body and its functions. A fundamental assumption is that there is an overall unity to people's ideas, with theories about therapy or aetiology being just one field of application for a general underlying principle. A further assumption is that a therapy that conforms to these basic patterns and principles has not just its truth-value confirmed, but its efficacy as a therapy enhanced. Hence the placebo effect of a therapeutic ritual derives, or so it is argued, from the cognitive consistency of the symbolism that informs it.[14] A similar argument is that remaking consensus in a community is in itself therapeutic.[15]

These assumptions have their weaknesses. Since an illness may not necessarily respond to a placebo, or, if it does, the effect may be only temporary, clearly the actual course of illness is always liable to discredit both diagnosis and therapy. But a general faith in the ideas behind a ritual can be actually reinforced by a widespread scepticism about the particular healer or the specific case, as Evans-Pritchard showed in his classic study of the rationality of Zande theories about illness.[16] In short, a 'common sense' that is situated within a society's general structure of ideas is proof against disproof. As a consequence, theories of illness are not so much disproved as discarded. Proof of efficacy is less important than efficacy itself. New ideas can be adopted not because they are logical or even consistent, but because they appear to work. Novelty – or inconsistency – can thus be as efficient a placebo as the accepted, commonsensical therapy. The new treatment may indeed be fitted later into existing ideas, or a rationale for it be made to square with the previous set of concepts; however, that does not necessarily happen. People's tolerance of inconsistency in practical matters is greater perhaps than analysts like to allow.[17] Hence the need to give a certain autonomy to the field of illness and not to allow all the phenomena associated with illness to be subsumed as simply a part of the religious, political, or social system.

ANALYTICAL MODELS IN WHICH ILLNESS THEORIES ARE PRIMARY

A fourth approach to analysing non-Western theories has therefore been to focus on the actual experience of illness in particular groups, and to treat, if only heuristically, the whole culture of health as an autonomous field of enquiry. Interest has shifted towards how individual people come to make sense of their ailments, and away from the society-wide stereotypes about health and the more publicly political interpretations which had been the theme of earlier studies. In the new analyses, it has been necessary not merely to search out retrospectively people's ideas about illness, but to seek a sense of how illness is being perceived at the time of crisis. The assumption here is that others, by not focusing on illness itself but upon the wider social context, have failed to be sensitive to the nuanced variables, the uncertainties, the subtler differences of perception that can create the intellectual space necessary for theories to change without reference to the cultural matrix. In this section, I shall outline some of the variables in the way illness is perceived and diagnosis and therapy managed, in order to emphasize both the flexibility and the complexity of non-Western theories about illness.

DEFINING ILLNESS

A key cultural variable in non-Western theories of illness is the way the category 'illness' itself is demarcated from other kinds of misfortune, such as crop damage, a house burnt down, a spouse who has gone off with another person. All such misfortunes are interpretable as injuries and hence can share a single theory explaining why they occurred when they did. If, however, 'illness' is limited to an injury done to the person and refers only to misfortunes that affect just the body, then a second cultural variable is what is the range of bodily malaise that constitutes the category 'illness'. This, in turn, depends on who is the patient. Not all children's ailments, for example, are defined as illness, any more than are the ailments of old age; similarly, not all women's ailments are illnesses. In short, what is considered normal (and in consequence needs no treatment) varies; there may not even be agreement within the community as to what, in a particular instance, constitutes illness.

A related definitional variable concerns wounds and broken limbs, and other more chronic impairments like deafness; even changes in a person's capacity to behave socially, whether because of mental illness or excessive emotion, may or may not be counted as an injury on a par with other illnesses. If social impairment generally can be considered one important criterion of illness, of equal importance must be the way a community defines health and what it sees as its *needs* for a healthy life. Health and illness are not necessarily two sides of a single coin. Variables such as the quantity, quality, and kind of foods required for health, and the types of shelter and clothing, constitute only one set of needs; another set includes less obvious social needs such as 'a good fate', 'a good character' – shorthand not just for prosperity and contented social relations but also for glory in battle, success in the hunt, and triumph over others. Practically speaking, however, notions of positive health are less accessible than the concepts that cluster around illness; the successful management of illness – or merely coping with it – has been, in consequence, the major theme of analysis.

Even when the definitional boundaries that a community uses for 'illness' can be formally identified, those boundaries are none the less liable to fluctuate. A crisis of one kind can narrow the definition, whereas a widespread scare can expand it rapidly. Symptoms, for example, that are normally disregarded become suspicious when accusations of witchcraft are on the increase; furthermore, a wider range of illnesses is then attributed to witchcraft than would be the case in times of reduced social tension. Similarly, the seasons

649

affect the perceived incidence of illness and the interpretation of symptoms. Ailments perceived to be new are also problematic; some may not count as illness, others have an ambiguous status and attract different labels and attitudes. Finally, some individuals may be notorious as hypochondriacs and their claims to be ill give rise to domestic conflicts over what should truly count as illness. Illness, in short, is not self-evident; it is negotiable, and the rules of negotiation vary.

A third cultural variable is the moral loading given to an illness – a guide to which are the differing 'sick roles' ranging from extreme stigmatization (as sometimes with leprosy) to the patient being regarded as almost sacred. Illness may be a matter of such shame (as reportedly among Hawaiian Japanese) that no 'sick role' is even conceivable. Alternatively, some illnesses are seen as stereotypical of a particular social group, and as a result among members of that group a wide range of nonspecific ailments are included under that one label; it is a more serious matter if a non-member of the group is caught by an 'alien' ailment. Other illnesses are paradigmatic (for example, 'madness') for a range of similar conditions. Such illnesses, whether stereotypes or paradigms, may be used symbolically to express social fears or even to carry privileges: for example, after committing a serious *faux pas* people may prefer to claim 'madness' rather than face shame and ridicule. Nor is it necessary that every instance of a particular illness be considered a misfortune. An illness can be a rite of passage into the status of one of the elect; so too, a childhood illness may be a necessary preliminary to entry into adulthood. Indeed, the diseases of the very young can be welcomed as the strengthening required of every child who is destined to reach maturity: better, some people say, for a baby to die early than to cause greater grief by dying later.

A fourth cultural variable is the way an episode of illness is defined in time and space. Instead of considering ill health as a series of discrete episodes of disease, both acute and chronic illnesses can be counted as a single event spread over time and with multiple symptoms yet having a single cause. An illness can move about the body (much as referred pain does) yet be classified as the same illness. Thus rather than there being a host of potential causes of illness, in practice there may be only one that is considered actually to be affecting a particular patient. In calculating the incidence of illness, then, cultures may be either 'lumpers' (merging illnesses into one) or 'splitters' (forever slicing up experience into smaller units). The merging of illness episodes thus reduces the number of illnesses reported, taken for diagnosis, and treated, and the frequency and the risk of illness appears reduced. Conversely, a community that multiplies episodes of illness can give the outside observer an impression of a sickly society paranoid over matters of health, though, in fact, the multiplicity of incidents may instead have trivialized the experience of sickness. Overall, illness can be likened to a quarrel with a potentially difficult, powerful kinsperson or neighbour: normally relations are amicable over the course of a lifetime, but occasionally they flare into conflict; conflict, however, should not lead to death.

The definition of death is an extreme example of a cultural variable. Illness and death are conceptually distinct processes: why people die may be unconnected with why they are ill; and illness may not necessarily carry with it the fear of death. Only under particular circumstances need death be categorized as a misfortune. Similarly, at what point death is thought to occur is variable: social death can occur – and can be made to occur – at any time, and physical death may or may not immediately follow. Thus 'burial alive', for example, in this context is a contradiction in terms: although victims may be breathing, they are already 'dead' and therefore the act of burial is not killing them, let alone being 'murder'. Conversely, cessation of breathing or heartbeat may be less relevant to defining death than the point of time at which all the flesh on the body has finally rotted: that is, only when the corpse has become a skeleton is the person fully dead. Similarly, the time that elapses between the cessation of life and the departure of the soul or spirit from the dead body is another well-known variable (cf. the Christian convention that puts it at three days). (➤ Ch. 13 Ideas of life and death; Ch. 61 Religion and medicine)

At what point life is said to start – the definition of birth – is a more obvious variable, since the beginning of life outside the womb is clearly an arbitrary point at which to begin an individual's entry into the human condition. From well before birth to long after it, cultures have elaborated the process of entry into full social status; indeed, some persons are permanently excluded from that status, most notably aliens or strangers. 'Humans are not born but made.' The boundary between the categories 'human' and 'non-human' is not self-evident. While our own system currently has a category 'primates' and creates a subcategory from which are excluded all primates other than those we denote as human, other systems divide their categories differently – or appear to do so. For example, white-skinned people were initially regarded in many places as non-human, just as the white-skinned themselves tended to regard as non-human or only semi-human some of the many non-white peoples they 'discovered', and therefore these they decided could be hunted as animals. More significant is the often-hazy dividing line between those diagnostic and therapeutic techniques suited for humans and those applicable to animals; in practice, medicines for both are ordinarily the same, but not the rituals. Babies too may not be counted as fully human, but rather as still belonging in part to the other world whence they came. Twins, in particular, are anomalous beings, but so too may be others, such as those with other 'defects' or even those born after a series of babies have already died in the household. Treatment for such beings can differ from that appropriate for those more truly human.

In all these variables we are not dealing with an either–or dichotomy, rather with a gradient or a process: what is in question is the weighting given to various points on that gradient, and this weighting is itself variable, with different groups in a community (such as women or elders) holding different opinions. Both the meaning given to an event and the action that results are negotiable. The important issue here is that when social analysts use data on illness from another culture to construct a broader picture of society, they are in danger of being far too facile if they fail to examine the kind of variables raised here. Illness is too serious, and too fluid, a category for its definition to be taken simply for granted.

CONCEPTS OF ANATOMY, PHYSIOLOGY, PATHOLOGY

How people conceive of themselves and their bodies is hard to discover, in part because many do not consciously have a ready worked out map of their internal anatomy and its processes. For some, the symbolic meanings that society attaches to particular parts of the body colour all other interpretations of the body. Notions of purity and propriety determine the model of the body, while parts of the body are used as key metaphors in political discourse. But metaphors should not be confused with the meanings people actually give to experience; some metaphors have long been mere clichés, and etymologies ignored or forgotten. Similarly, diagrams and drawings of the body (such as are found, for example, among Indian groups in South America) show definite, elaborate notions of how the body works, but they may yet not represent how people in the course of an illness conceptualize themselves and their pain. Also commonly elaborated are ideas about embryology; again, these are liable to have a formal version that reflects the politico-legal arrangements current in the community. Thus notions of how conception occurs and the role of the uterus can depend on whether inheritance is patrilineal, matrilateral, or bilateral; bone and blood are similarly used to express the complementarity of penis and uterus, of paternal and maternal contributions to a child. Alternatively, the duality of bodily entrances and exits – the windpipe/gullet and urethra/anus – can map either the dual nature of social processes or the differences between a person's outer, fluid social personality and the inner, essential being.

Though these ideas with their symbolic or political resonance are the ideas most readily articulated and therefore accessible to study, it does not mean there is not a parallel if muted series of other ideas based upon, for example, the known anatomy of animals – and it is these that may inform actual therapeutic practice. But the extent of a culture's interest in or knowledge of anatomy varies. In particular, communities that herd livestock tend to have an extensive understanding of internal anatomy, physiology, and pathology, with an interest in the signs of disease: they have used their herds to identify, for example, plants useful against worms and to learn basic surgical skills for use in repairing wounds or extracting an obstructed foetus. (➤ Ch. 5 The anatomical tradition) Hunters, whether of game or of whales (for example, the Eskimo), are often very knowledgeable about the anatomy of their kill, but the question is, how far is this knowledge applied by analogy in treating human beings? For there are often considerable social constraints on what kinds of knowledge it is legitimate to have: for example, if only witches have the X-ray eyesight to see inside another person's body, it is decidedly risky to display an interest in internal anatomy. Indeed, the ambiguities surrounding healers, who are usually seen as having the power both to harm and to heal, and the greatest healers, people say, must have gained their skill by having served first as the most evil of sorcerers, are apt to make the body and its processes themselves ambiguous, and hence limit the development of a technical medical discourse. By comparison, skin ailments and other surface symptoms are usually articulated in more detail.[18] But the exact extent of people's knowledge may be sometimes hard to determine: ethnographers have argued at length over whether the Trobriand islanders 'really' believe only in 'virgin birth', as their kinship system requires.

Different organs of the body notoriously attract differing degrees of attention, whether symbolically or therapeutically. There is usually a hierarchy in which head and/or heart are prominent, but more important may be the liver and the stomach, the sexual organs (linked sometimes with the kidneys), and sometimes, too, the knees. The order in which body parts are enumerated varies – some start with the feet – while the boundaries between parts vary (for example, between hand and arm). Other parts may be paired (for example, the uvula and the clitoris). Similarly with the senses: some systems merge sound and smell and contrast them with sight; some, too, treat the eye as the chief conduit for evil, others emphasize instead potential evil from the mouth. Again, which part of the body is particularly vulnerable, and at what age, varies. Not all orifices are thought to be equally at risk, nor are all organs equally prone to injury by outside forces. Some internal organs are more likely to be transformed: for example, a witch can be distinguished from an ordinary person by the fact that the witch's stomach is ice cold instead of warm. Children may be considered much less at risk from spirits than adults, who are often at their most vulnerable during coition. The emotions, a person's character, popularity even, are inscribed in various parts of the body; but once again, care is needed so as not to confuse metaphors with actual beliefs. The various bodily fluids – including 'dead blood', sweat and other 'salts' from different surfaces within the body, or mucus of various kinds that collects in particular regions – all these suggest complex notions of physiology; and some are elaborated, as in New Guinea, for example, where a male menstruation is induced.[19] Finally, the location of the soul, what it is and how it functions, is very variable, though the concept of the soul is apparently almost universal. (➤ Ch. 7 The physiological tradition)

Much less attention has been paid to people's theories about how food and drink are absorbed, and the way these theories differ, if at all, from those in medicine; or about the pathology associated with illness and how it is transmitted. Generally, it seems that whereas food and drink assuage hunger and thirst, medicine tackles the two dominant sensations of illness: weakness and discomfort (expressed either as pain that is unbearably hot, or as fever that is shiveringly cold). Of these two, weakness can be represented as being due to a powerful, invisible force gripping or draining the patient; hence medicine aims at loosening that grip, either by making the patient so unpleasant that the attacker voluntarily lets go, or by directly driving the attacker off. Access to the parts of the self (such as the mind) where the patient has been caught is through fine, fluid substances such as sounds or smells. The pathology of illness, then, is not described as the breakdown of a system or even as a process of decay or rotting (which are more appropriate to describe ageing). 'Wounds', 'poisons', the abstraction of life force, are the more common notions to depict the mechanism of illness. The exception is where pollution is the dominant idiom of illness, and cleansing the appropriate therapy. Here, transmission of illness from person to person is possible, whereas notions of illness as injury tend to preclude ideas of infection or contagion. In the latter, natural, ecological causes can be called upon to explain the spread of illness. In practice, ill people (especially, for example, those with smallpox) are apt to be isolated to some degree, and places known to be infected abandoned, whatever the theoretical reasoning. (➤ Ch. 9 The pathological tradition)

Such a summary of variables in non-Western theories about the body is unsatisfactory precisely because the data at the mundane, clinical level are thin and of uncertain value; cosmologies offer more complete and more consistent accounts, but represent often the opinions of elders or of experts familiar with formulating complex concepts. Yet the experience of illness is not theirs alone; popular notions formulated in a crisis are as true a representation, if more inchoate.

THE THERAPEUTIC PROCESS

A further set of variables is found in theories underlying diagnostic practice and therapy. First, it needs to be noted that diagnosis and therapy are analytically distinct processes (though they may empirically be one process), just as discovering the cause of a fire is distinct from the task of actually putting the fire out. Diagnosis is concerned with divining the cause of the illness, and therefore works primarily with the past; therapy is concerned with curing the present symptoms. Causal explanations, therefore, are not necessarily an accurate guide to clinical practice, not least because the patient need not be the same person as the victim of the agent causing the patient's illness. For example, a sorcerer intending to harm a powerful opponent may inflict illness upon that opponent's weakest client or kinsperson. Children's illnesses are commonly explained in this way: a child is ill because of some wrongdoing by one of the parents. Hence diagnosis explores the parents' histories; therapy tackles the child's complaint. Subsequent therapy may then treat the parents, too, but from a different theoretical standpoint.

Techniques of diagnosis vary. The essential problem is how to elicit information, in the form of an answer to a question, from invisible beings who either witnessed or should know about the illness-injury when it was in the making, since it was the use of power on their plane of being that enabled the illness to be inflicted. Broadly speaking, two kinds of divination are particularly common. First, there are those that use divining equipment: nuts, shells, bones; a sand table; a grid marked on the ground; shooting at birds; inspecting entrails; poisoning chicks, etc.: after a specific question has been put to the oracle, it is possible to interpret the answer, which has been given apparently automatically. Second, there are those techniques that use possession or trance, and have the answers to questions put to the medium spoken out loud. The first system assumes that the invisible beings can 'speak' to us only through signs; the second assumes that they can take over the speech organs of a human (and talk either a specific oracular language or the standard language of the locality). Although participants can use either system to make public what otherwise could not be openly stated, it is implicit that these beings know, and tell, the truth. They are infallible; error enters only when the medium is imperfect. Disputes over the validity of the information obtained through divination centres on the diviner and not on the technique itself, nor is the existence of these beings called into question. Hence it may be necessary to try out a number of mediums if the diagnosis does not lead to a cure. The fact that there are a number of rival mediums tends to confirm rather than invalidate the credibility of the whole divinatory system; 'they cannot all be wrong'.

The process of therapy may simply involve the sick person hiding away alone, undergoing self-debasement by smearing dirt on the body and waiting for recovery eventually to occur.[20] More active therapies use two main techniques: herbs or other medicines; and rituals. Medicines are either tonics to strengthen the patient, physically or psychologically, or 'poisons' to drive off the aggressor or loosen its hold. Selection of appropriate herbs involves both the symbolic properties of the plant and its more empirical qualities. The more commonly used plants – for fevers or wounds, for expelling parasites, or as emetics – are chosen for their recognized pharmacological properties; so too the active poisons are well known for what they are. But a larger range of plant material and other items is chosen instead for their colour or shape, for their sap or because of their habitat – all attributes that fit into a broader pattern of symbolic meaning to be created ritually.

Medicines, whether rubbed on to the body, inhaled, or drunk, are not necessarily only taken by the patient; being tonics, other participants are likely to partake of them too. The communal nature of therapy is particularly pronounced in the rituals of healing where large numbers may join in.[21] In some instances,[22] it is the community itself that is being cured, with the patient being just the unlucky victim, the most vulnerable in the group. Rituals have been analysed as a rite of passage, with distinct phases of separation and reincorporation; other rituals are shaped like drama, building up to a climax followed by a release of tension through humour. Some are dances that last all night, others are songs; some are very brief, others are repeated night after night. As a rule, the patient, if strong enough, is the active performer, guided or prompted by the healer, and creates his or her own response to the highly charged occasion. Hence, therapy may be in two stages: an initial cure to relieve the immediate symptoms, followed later by initiation into a 'cult of affliction' or a ritual to confirm recovery and to prevent a recurrence.

A further variable centres around whether the patient is being freed from the attentions of unseen forces ('exorcism') or is being prepared for welcoming a spirit into the home as patron and guardian ('adorcism', to use de Heusch's term[23]). Similarly, some rituals wash a person clean and get rid of all pollution; others achieve the same effect by using smoke and inhalations. In general, those communities that regard themselves as weak or use their vulnerability as a political pose tend to welcome spirits as guardians and seek to domesticate them. By contrast, communities who see themselves as leaders are apt to use rituals that drive away all forces that appear to threaten their hegemony. The acceptance of spirits as personal guardians forms the basis of 'cults of affliction' or communities of suffering in which ex-patients are united by their common experience of illness diagnosed in a particular way. Membership of such a cult offers a special status in the community and certain other advantages, along with the costs incurred in serving the spirit. It may also enable members to act as healers of others, affliction being the necessary initiation into a valuable trade.

Yet another variable is who controls the choice of diviner or makes the decision of which healer to call in. Rarely is it the patient who autonomously selects the way back to health, in part because the illness itself prevents the patient from being able to make the selection. The politics of the 'quest for therapy', as Janzen called it[24], has its own constraints, operating partly through the rules of kinship, partly through fears of failure and the accusations that may follow; partly too through, say, the chance arrival in the locality of this or that specialist. Furthermore, local theories about the causal links in illness affect the constitution of the 'therapy management group', which, in turn, affects which particular divinatory technique will be given credence first and therefore at whom the finger is, at least initially, likely to be pointed.

CHANGING SYSTEMS

It is clear from what has been described so far that there is considerable flexibility, at the micro-level, in a community's theories about illness; and that there are fluctuating fashions or rhythms according to which the scope of one diagnosis or therapy expands or contracts, at the expense of another. Furthermore, there is wide scope for scepticism over particulars if not over principles, together with an openness which allows that other cultures may have cures that work better for 'new' illnesses. Given how politically embedded the practice of medicine is in some communities, such openness is strengthened out of political, and not just therapeutic, considerations. In addition, the entrepreneurial nature of the healing trade puts a premium on innovation. Although this openness has obviously been increased in the twentieth century due to colonial and capitalist pressures, inter-societal exchanges of knowledge are not new – pluralism is commonplace on the edges of society.

None the less, major changes, and not mere fluctuations, have affected many non-Western systems. Though a history of local medical systems of the 'little tradition' would require details we may never have, except perhaps for a very few societies, one model explaining the mechanism of change can be summarized as follows. Pre-colonial societies are marked by a high infant mortality due to infectious diseases; those who survive childhood then form an adult population that is largely immune. (➤ Ch. 10 The immunological tradition) Given their inevitable ineffectiveness in preventing childhood infection, traditional medical systems developed treatments mainly to serve this largely immune adult population. Since most adult physical ailments are self-limiting and require social support rather than intervention with herb-based chemotherapy, the most sophisticated techniques developed by traditional medicine have lain particularly in the area of providing therapies for adults whose greatest problem was illness arising from social, not physical, pathology – in short, psychotherapy. This psychotherapy offered, in the form of elaborate rituals, placebo treatments that proved to have a certain efficacy over a wider range of ailments; furthermore, it was able to increase through its placebo effect the efficacy of plant-based medicines whose dosage was kept for reasons of safety so low that they would otherwise have had little effect. Whenever specific rituals and symbols lost their efficacy as placebos (as they inevitably would?), they could be replaced by fresh ones, whether presented as new discoveries or as a revival of the 'true' ancestral forms. Hence, around a powerful ritual and symbolic core, systems of medicine developed which adequately and adaptably managed much of the burden of illness experienced by adults.

The main danger to the health of the adult population served by this traditional, psychotherapy-based medicine was to come from new, imported diseases to which adults were not immune and which thus gave rise to epidemics. These epidemics rapidly killed off that section of the population previously least likely to die young: young adult men and women in their prime. The failure of the existing traditional methods of psychotherapy and placebo-backed medicine to halt an epidemic that destroyed the core of the community discredited utterly the established healers and their rituals. There was space now for new practitioners who offered, in the emergency, fresh rituals and methods that went to extremes of a kind the culture would never normally have sanctioned (such as human sacrifice). As the epidemic waned, these new healers might claim the credit, though they would not gain the reputation of being 'truly traditional' until the older generation died out.

The best-documented crisis of this kind is the series of epidemics c.1920 that started with the influenza pandemic and then involved a variety of more-localized outbreaks of other diseases. It seems that some European stereotypes of non-Western medical systems (particularly the notion of 'witchdoctors' and their fearsome reputation) derive from such periods of crisis, when, of course, it was the Europeans themselves who were responsible for introducing the new diseases to non-immune communities and for thus bringing about the collapse of the traditional medical system. But popular European stereo-types have been reinforced by historians who tend to be incautious in their handling of data derived from epidemics, treating the data as if they could be generalized as true too for more 'normal' times and not simply for the period of acute political, social, and intellectual crisis that accompanies an epidemic. As a consequence, cultures have had attributed to them quite bizarre, atypical ideas, which were, in fact, simply symptoms of panic. (➤ Ch. 30 Folk medicine)

NOTES

1   Robert Redfield, *Peasant Society and Culture*, Chicago, IL, University of Chicago Press, 1956.

2 Gilbert Lewis, *Knowledge of Illness in a Sepik Society*, London, Athlone Press, 1975.

3 For example, P. U. Unschuld, 'Medico-cultural conflicts in Asian settings', *Social Science and Medicine*, 1975, 9: 303–12; Horacio Fabrega, 'Culture, biology and the study of disease', in H. Rothschild (ed.), *Biocultural Aspects of Disease*, New York, Academic Press, 1981; M. N. Cohen and G. J. Armelagos (eds), *Paleopathology at the Origin of Agriculture*, Orlando, FL, Academic Press, 1984.

4 Murray Last and G. L. Chavunduka (eds), *The Professionalisation of African Medicine*, Manchester, Manchester University Press for the International African Institute, 1986.

5 Forrest E. Clements, *Primitive Concepts of Disease*, University of California Publications in American Archeology and Ethnology, 1932, 32 (2): 185–252.

6 Ibid.; G. P. Murdock, S. F. Wilson and V. Frederick, 'World distribution of theories of illness', *Ethnology*, 1978, 17 (4): 449–70.

7 A diffusionist model for the spread of humoral medicine is discussed in ch. 14 ('Humoralism') of this *Encylopedia*.

8 Mudock *et al.*, op. cit. (n. 6).

9 Murray Last, 'Strategies against time', *Sociology of Health and Sickness*, 1979, 1.3: 306–17.

10 Reo Fortune, *The Sorcerers of Dobu*, London, Routledge & Kegan Paul, 1932.

11 M. G. Marwick, 'Witchcraft as a social strain gauge', *Australian Journal of Science*, 1964, 26: 263–8; Alan Harwood, *Witchcraft, Sorcery and Social Categories Among the Safwa*, London, Oxford University Press for the International African Institute, 1970; I. M. Lewis, *Ecstatic Religion*, Harmondsworth, Penguin, 1971.

12 Edward E. Evans-Pritchard, *Witchcraft, Oracles and Magic among the Azande*, Oxford, Clarendon Press, 1937.

13 Mary Douglas, *Purity and Danger*, London, Routledge & Kegan Paul, 1966; Douglas, *Natural Symbols*, London, Routledge & Kegan Paul, 1970.

14 Claude Lévi-Strauss, *Structural Anthropology*, New York, Basic Books, 1963.

15 John M. Janzen, *The Quest for Therapy in Lower Zaire*, Berkeley, University of California Press, 1978.

16 Evans-Pritchard, op. cit. (n. 12).

17 Murray Last, 'The importance of knowing about not knowing', *Social Science and Medicine*, 1981, 15B: 387–92.

18 Charles Frake, 'Diagnosis of disease among the Subanum of Mindanao', *American Anthropologist*, 1961, 63: 113–32.

19 Gilbert Lewis, *Day of Shining Red*, Cambridge, Cambridge University Press, 1980.

20 Lewis, op. cit. (n. 2).

21 Richard Katz, *Boiling Energy*, Cambridge, MA, Harvard University Press, 1982.

22 For example, V. W. Turner, *The Forest of Symbols*, Ithaca, NY, Cornell University Press, 1967.

23 Luc de Heusch, *Pourquoi l'épouser? et autres essais*, Paris, Gallimard, 1971.

24 Janzen, op. cit. (n. 15).

FURTHER READING

Blacking, John (ed.), *The Anthropology of the Body*, London, Academic Press, 1977.

Bloch, M. and Parry, J. (eds), *Death and the Regeneration of Life*, Cambridge, Cambridge University Press, 1982.

Buckley, A., *Yoruba Medicine*, Oxford, Clarendon Press, 1985.

Cohen, Mark Nathan, *Health and the Rise of Civilization*, New Haven, CT, Yale University Press, 1989.

Fabrega, Horacio and Silver, D. B., *Illness and Shamanistic Curing in Zinacantan*, Stanford, CA, Stanford University Press, 1973.

Fraenkel, S., *The Huli Response to Illness*, Cambridge, Cambridge University Press, 1986.

Good, C. M., *Ethnomedical Systems in Africa: Patterns of Traditional Medicine in Urban and Rural Kenya*, New York, Guilford Press, 1987.

Janzen, John M., *Lemba 1650–1930: a Drum of Affliction in Africa and the New World*, New York, Garland, 1982.

Lévi-Strauss, Claude, 'The effectiveness of symbols', and 'The sorceror and his magic', in *Structural Anthropology*, New York, Basic Books, 1963.

Lindenbaum, S., *Kuru Sorcery*, Palo Alto, CA, Mayfield, 1979.

Loudon, J. B. (ed.), *Social Anthropology and Medicine*, London, Academic Press, 1976.

McKeown, Thomas, *The Origins of Human Disease*, Oxford, Basil Blackwell, 1988.

Moerman, D. E., 'Physiology and symbols; the anthropological implications of the placebo effect', in L. Romannuci-Ross, D. E. Moerman and L. Tancredi (eds), *The Anthropology of Medicine*, New York, Praeger, 1983, pp. 156–67.

Ngubane, Harriet, *Body and Mind in Zulu Medicine*, London, Academic Press, 1977.

Prince, R., 'Shamans and endorphins: hypothesis for a synthesis', *Ethos*, 1982, 10: 409–23.

Reichel-Dolmatoff, G., *Amazonian Cosmos: the Sexual and Religious Symbolism of the Tukanao Indians*, Chicago, IL, University of Chicago Press, 1971.

Taussig, Michael T., *Shamanism, Colonialism and the Wild Man: a Study in Terror and Healing*, Chicago, IL, University of Chicago Press, 1987.

Turner, V. W., *Drums of Affliction*, Oxford, Clarendon Press, 1968.

Velimirovic, R., 'Traditional medicine is not primary health care', *Curare*, 1984, 7: 61–79, 85–93.

Zempléni, Andras, 'La dimension thérapeutique du culte des rab, ndöp, tuuru et samp; rites de possession chez les Lébou et les Wolof', *Psychopathologie Africaine*, 1966, 2: 295–439.

30

FOLK MEDICINE

Françoise Loux

The terms 'popular medicine', 'traditional medicine' and 'folk medicine' are often used interchangeably. Although in certain countries, notably the USA and parts of eastern Europe, folk medicine has a very precise status, in France this expression is only used occasionally by researchers, for it has a pejorative and ideological connotation implying an artificial and nostalgic recourse to the past. Furthermore, it designates both a topic (popular medical beliefs and practices), and the researches concerning it.

All these ambiguities mean that it is not easy to present folk medicine in a succinct and general manner. Taking as a point of departure the most current definition, we are interested here in methods of curing, but also in interpretations of sickness and health, transmitted principally by oral means in the popular classes of the industrial or industrializing nations with access to biomedicine. Three elements are important in this definition:

1 the notion of transmission and the notion of tradition associated with it;
2 the intervention of oral culture (it is generally agreed to exclude from folk culture elements that would come within the category of written records); and
3 finally the marginalized situation of folk culture. Folk culture is in a position dominated by its relations with learned or official cultures: that is, biomedicine in the case of folk medicine.

Recent historical and anthropological researches enable us to bring some nuances to this definition and, above all, to shatter too-rigid and narrow categorizations of folk medicine – for instance, the so-called opposition between oral and written records. It would, however, be regrettable if this renewal should sweep away all the earlier works which, provided they are reconsidered, have a real value. In order to consider these works, a historical perspective will prove indispensable. (➤ Ch. 60 Medicine and anthropology)

FROM 'POPULAR' ERRORS TO 'FOLK MEDICINE'

For a long time, beliefs and practices falling outside the category of official medicine were considered as fallacies to be condemned. Thus the first collections of popular-medicine recipes are pamphlets which, from the sixteenth century until modern times, were concerned with these 'popular errors'. One of the first and most famous is that of Laurent Joubert,[1] reissued numerous times. The authors of such works were mainly either physicians who denounced what they considered to be dangerous practices, or clerics such as the Abbé Thiers[2] who condemned 'superstitions', many of which concerned the body and health. The practices that they described with precision are very interesting for the modern researcher: through what was forbidden, but was actually performed, we are able to perceive a living network of popular practices, some of which were still being met with in the nineteenth century. In spite of their non-scientific orientation, it is possible to consider these works as the ancestors of surveys of folk medicine.

Other texts, apparently nearer to folk medicine, have in fact a more ambiguous position. These are the cheap editions of works of popularization and health-advice manuals, which flourished throughout the eighteenth and nineteenth centuries. Among historians, there has been a debate about these, particularly concerning the precise definition of the term 'popular'.[3] Was it a question of literature of learned origin, intended to educate the populace, or rather one of writings reflecting popular thought and practices? Recent researches carried out on these works have enabled us to distinguish several categories of booklets. Certain of them, written by physicians, are aimed at an educated public. Many are described as 'books of charitable medicine', and are addressed to lay people – clergy, housewives, and housekeepers – in order to teach them to cure the poor cheaply. Other works were not written by medical practitioners but by well-meaning persons, sometimes by lay healers. These booklets are often considered as 'witnesses' to folk medicine. A comparison with accounts of popular medicine collected in the field shows, however, some important differences. In these works, the symbolic dimension (the significance of numbers and colours, for example) or ritual gestures (like making the sign of the cross) are less often present. We cannot reconstruct the folk medicine of past centuries from the ensemble of therapeutic procedures that appears throughout these writings. But the influence of 'cultural intermediaries' who utilize these works leads us to question the set image of a folk medicine of uniquely oral transmission, remaining free from all contact with scholarly medicine. The interest of these texts also resides in their prefaces; we see there, at the heart of these commentaries where the authors make themselves known, that the terrain of folk medicine has always been a speculation, a subject of aspirations and conflicts.

It was in the nineteenth century that interest in 'popular errors' was accentuated. Notably with regard to infant welfare, the advice of grand-mothers was violently attacked.[4] In this case it is not even a question of folk medicine, but of 'superstition' and 'ignorance'. It is no longer a question of a list of errors to be denounced, but rather one of combating an entire system. At the same time, however, certain rural notabilities decided, in France as in many other countries, to gather together the traditions that they thought were on the brink of disappearing. This threatened character confer-ring on them the 'beauty of death',[5] resolved for the authors the ambiguity of the collection. In fact, several of these folklorists were physicians who themselves aimed at the disappearance of these methods of cure; they col-lected the different elements of them like stamps or butterflies to be cased and classified. This ambiguity, still present with certain local scholars, gives to these collections both richness and methodological bias. The richness comes from what the folklorists have processed in a meticulous and systematic fashion. They were not isolated, but were linked to an international and global movement concerned principally with the domain of oral literature, one extending to the field of beliefs and of popular medicine. These researchers had journals and meetings; they corresponded with each other, exchanging discussions concerning their methods.[6] What limited the scope of their collections was that they did not consider this medicine as a whole system, but as a set of curious recipes and bizarre superstitions, which they did not seek to relate to a system of beliefs or a social function.

RETHINKING RESEARCH ON FOLK MEDICINE

It would be too limiting, however, to consider the work of the folklorists only from this point of view. Marcelle Bouteiller, whose work holds a pivotal position in France, has tried to show this.[7] In spite of certain formulations inherited from the ideology of the folklorists, many aspects of Bouteiller's work are an advance on her generation. It is regrettable that they have not had a larger audience among anthropologists who, for reasons both theoretical and methodological, have long been much more preoccupied with exotic societies than with their own.

For all these reasons, research on the folk medicine of industrial societies has not really benefited from the impetus that has developed during these last decades for studies in anthropology and the history of medicine. Con-sidered banal and of little importance and accused of ideological bias, folk-medicine studies have been, if not scorned, at least cast aside. Provided, however, that they bring about a theoretical and methodological renewal, they ought to occupy a pivotal position between history and anthropology, essential for the study of complex societies that now preoccupy the latter. They are on the side of history, for, analysing what is transmitted from earlier generations, they are in fact concerned with the popular medicine of the past, but in the way that this healing is perceived by the actual generations. They sail, therefore, between historical and mythical times;[8] so this being, historians have been able, with justification, to reproach them for being situated in a past which has not always been precisely dated. They are also on the side of anthropology, for they attach themselves to an important dimension of popular knowledge: rapport with the past and family transmission; however, but in the way that these traditions have been reported, detached from all context, they appear fixed and of little use to an anthropologist. Especially in France, where debate on this subject has been liveliest, anthropologists insist on the necessity of starting from sickness as it is experienced, in its relations with other dimensions of the social field, without departing from a priori biomedical definitions.[9]

The problem, in fact, is that the three elements of the above definition can lead to enclosing folk medicine in too rigid a categorization. In the first place, tradition has too often been likened to immobility. But in reality, at each level of transmission between the generations, some new elements are retained, others abandoned, and each time a new coherence, a new equilibrium is achieved. This phenomenon cannot be completely understood if one excludes analysis of the elements which do not appear truly traditional. We have thus noted that the role of cultural intermediaries has been to introduce some elements of contemporary official medicine into popular medicine, which, in return, has sometimes influenced scholarly medicine.

In the second place, it would be necessary to discard too narrow a definition, of a kind that would isolate the oral field alone as relevant to folk medicine. On one hand, everything that is oral is not necessarily popular; there is an oral tradition that is scholarly and literary. But above all, on the other hand, there is no pure oral tradition. As much of ancient popular medicine as of present-day popular medicine is composed both of ancient traditions transmitted orally through families (such as prayers for cures or knowledge concerning certain plants) and of elements transmitted by means of books. It would be necessary to make numerous systematic comparisons between manuscript texts of popularization, learned texts, and oral accounts of popular medicine to gain a better understanding of the mechanisms of the interpenetrations between the written and the oral. Such a project has just been undertaken in an exemplary fashion by some researchers in the South of France in respect of a manuscript book of veterinary-medicine recipes.[10]

We thus arrive at the last point of the definition: folk medicine cannot be studied in isolation, but only in its relations with other sectors of the medical field – notably biomedicine. Such an approach is applied with increasing frequency to non-complex, exotic societies (a distinction which, however, is more and more questioned by anthropologists). To this purpose, two stumbling-blocks have been in the way of research into folk medicine. First, for a long time folk medicine was considered as self-contained, detached from scientific medicine, or, in any case, analysed outside of this context. Second, opposed to this conception was the viewpoint of a certain branch of the sociology of the ruling classes, which, insisting on their cultural alienation, considered the healing practices of the lower social classes – popular medicine – as some obsolete manifestations of scholarly medicine or as incoherent practices. From this perspective, speaking in terms of folk medicine has no meaning. But neither can folk medicine be considered as a world completely apart from scholarly medicine. Numerous researchers have, on the contrary, shown that, from the patients' point of view, recourse to both types of medicine is not incompatible. For example, very often the sick go first to the physician for confirmation of their own diagnosis of a malady. If the physician seems to hesitate, they would conclude that the sickness 'belongs to another register' and go in search of a lay healer. Often, after cure, they return to the physician for confirmation. From the patients' point of view, there is a constant passage between the official and the non-official, which has been referred to by various researchers under the term 'therapeutic itinerary'.

Moreover, as certain anthropological studies are beginning to show, biomedicine is not exempt from ritual and symbolic elements, which are generally considered as more of the order of folk medicine. Sometimes, tradition and oral transmission are also found there. (➤ Ch. 29 Non-Western concepts of disease)

HOLISTIC CONCEPTIONS OF THE BODY AND TRADITIONAL THERAPISTS

Rethought in this way, in spite of the problems posed by the ancient researches, folk medicine is far from presenting itself as a disparate collection of recipes. Provided that the materials collected by the folklorists are not examined in isolation but considered as a whole, they richly illuminate the conception of the body in nineteenth-century rural society, to which reference is generally made when considering tradition.

A first point is fundamental: the holistic conception of the body, which sustains all features of this medicine. The different parts of the body are perceived not only as interdependent, but as linked to the whole of nature and the cosmos. Health is conceived as a state of equilibrium, always precarious, between this complex system of relations, and healing often consists of re-establishing this equilibrium, if lost. For example, to soothe a headache, considered as emanating from excessive heat, cold baths to the feet would be recommended; or to cure sciatica, an incision to the ear on the side opposite to the pain would be made.

Another aspect of this holistic conception is the unity of time and place for the body, as observed in traditional societies: the place and time of labour and of leisure, or carnival, are not completely dissociated and interact with each other. This unity of place and time is one of the characteristics of the traditional therapists differentiating them from physicians. In fact, they are not uniquely specialists for the sick body; it is as specialists in other techniques that they are specialists in the sick body as well, even when they have a 'gift' for healing. Thus the village healer may be an artisan or a farmer recognized for possessing professional skills and dexterity. In addition, being of the same social milieu as the patient, everyday language is used to communicate with the patient. Thus by introducing sickness into the everyday social system, the same time, rights and duties to the patient and meaning to the illness are given at the same time. Finally, the healer places the body at the centre of the sickness. In contrast to the doctor, who places it at a distance, the healer addresses the body directly and discusses the symptoms and the pain with the patient. A relationship between all these different elements is thus established.

Another type of healer who alike cannot be understood except in relation to this holistic conception of the body is the charlatan, who is an outsider from the village, and generally comes at the time of the annual fête. The sellers of miracle products or the tooth-drawers occur in the context of the show or fair. They take their place among the series of phenomena and uncommon physical exploits exhibited at fairs: monsters, magicians who transform natural objects, acrobats who defy equilibrium. In all this ritual and theatrical context, the patient becomes an actor and the sensations of pain – for example, in the case of a tooth extraction – are perhaps less severe.

RESEARCH ON EQUILIBRIUM AND PREVENTION

In this traditional medicine, the body is considered as the centre of the universe. A consubstantiality exists between humans and the territory that they inhabit. But in addition to terrestrial nature, they are subject to the weather and the seasons, the signs of the zodiac, and, above all, to the moon, which possesses an influence over everything that grows, reproduces, and moves in the universe. It presides equally at the growing of plants and of hair, or at the birth of children. Linked to the blood, it influences bloodletting and the healing of wounds; it regulates women's menses and determines the time of birth. Such a relationship between the body and the universe goes further than simple influence connections. In fact, the body is considered as a plant in which the sap would represent the humours. (➤ Ch. 14 Humoralism) It is also more than a plant, for it is the focal point of the universe.

The principle of analogy, theorized under the name of 'medicine of the signatures', is met constantly in popular medicine. By their sensible properties – colour, form, smell, heat, humidity, etc. – the elements of nature 'sign' their profound relationship with the human body and indicate the fact that they are either inauspicious or beneficent to it. For example, in most of the traditional medicine systems, red is used to cure disorders connected with blood. Thus, the geranium or oil of St John's wort are used against cuts. On the other hand, yellow calms digestive disorders: for example, celandine is beneficial to that end.

In such systems, health is considered as a state of precarious balance, always being reconstructed, between the human body and, on one hand, the universe, and on the other, society. More important than curing is the necessity of preventing the imbalance from occurring in the first place. In the light of recent researches, we should discuss the assertion that traditional societies did not know anything about prevention. On the contrary, prevention constituted an important element in folk medicine, but it was more a question of preventing death than of preventing specific diseases. Prevention is, in the first place, living in accord with nature, in harmony with the seasons: a concrete, but, at the same time, symbolic harmony. Thus, it is necessary to purge the body in spring to clean it of effervescent humours; in summer, one should not have any activities or foods that are too heating; and in autumn, fragile people need great care: 'at the time when leaves rise and fall, man also rises and falls', says a French proverb.

Another principle of prevention is good diet, which keeps the physician away. By good diet is meant absorbing foods that give strength, but also ingesting those natural products which, resembling the body, are beneficial for it, such as wine and red meat. 'Meat makes flesh and wine makes blood', says another French proverb.

The way to achieve bodily equilibrium is, in fact, to avoid all excess. That is why moderation is generally agreed to be a principle of prevention. This everyday moderation, which allows the husbanding of strength for daily work, does not, however, exclude excess at times of festival.

FLEXIBILITY AND ADAPTABILITY OF TRADITIONAL MEDICINE SYSTEMS

There is often a tendency to confine traditional medicine systems into typologies and categorizations. In the light of actual researches, that appears too limiting, always leaving aside some important aspects, for instance the empiric and symbolic. On this plan, two stumbling-blocks lie in wait for the researcher. The first danger appears conspicuously in the claims of the pharmaceutical industry, but also appears throughout certain ethno-scientific works determined by the early education of their authors (physicians or botanists, for example). It consists of effecting a classification of the recipes, of conserving only what appears efficacious or rational – or at least explicable according to our own rationality – in the utilization of plants, for example; and eliminating or considering as trivial everything that one does not know how to analyse and which appears strange or bizarre. For example, one recipe purporting to restore strength after a fall states, drink a verbena tisane after having made the sign of the cross three times; here, only the plant will be considered of interest to this school of research. An inverse error, but equally reductionist, is to take into consideration only the symbolic dimension and to consign these folk medicines to the category of the strange or the different without taking account of the empirical dimension. This occurs both among folklorists and anthropologists researching universals without first paying attention to the minute observation of cultures and their differences. In fact, the empirical and symbolic dimensions are indissociable. It may be this coexistence that determines folk medicine's strength, permanence, and capacity for change.

Let us take certain procedures which, at first sight, would be able to be integrally ranged beside the symbolic. For example, prayers for cures appear to be of the order of an oral and ritual relation between the patient and the healer. However, in the majority of cases, it is not sufficient to say a prayer; rather, this is often accompanied by a gesture, such as touching the affected region, or breathing upon it. Another example is the utilization of writing in popular medicine. The way one refers to it is sometimes similar to its current use in biomedicine (to verify or to complete information), and sometimes different. In these cases, the book, carried as an amulet or simply carefully conserved, is in itself a depository or a guarantor of power. Thus there exist some minuscule booklets containing prayers to be recited against plague, to facilitate childbirth, and to avoid sudden death. In addition to reciting them regularly, these prayers must be carried on the person. (➤ Ch. 61 Religion and medicine)

An error of the same type would be to want to insert traditional therapeutic indications into a biomedical classification of illnesses. An important characteristic of these traditional medicine systems – and which differentiates them from biomedicine – is the fact that they are more interested in the symptoms than in the diseases. Just as the sensible properties of the elements of nature are the signatures of their internal properties, the symptoms are the signature on the exterior of the body of the fact that an imbalance has been introduced.

It is thus not surprising that sensations of heat and fever are amply treated, or equally that folk medicine accords great importance to pain. Although biomedicine is only beginning to be interested in this, one of the characteristics of folk medicine is that it takes account of pain, asserts power over it, talks about it and talks to it, and, in doing so, gives meaning and perhaps makes the suffering more acceptable. (➤ Ch. 67 Pain and suffering)

One must be wary of making certain a priori classifications when addressing the question of the explanatory principles of the symbolic function of these therapeutics. Thus, people often oppose the therapies that extirpate the malady from the patient, over and against those that restore the body's equilibrium by adjunction of remedies. This distinction would correspond to two different conceptions of the sickness: the exogenous and the endogenous.[11] In fact, a remedy can often correspond simultaneously to an exogenous and an endogenous conception: it can, at the same time, restore the body's equilibrium and also expel the unhealthy humours. After all, for an identical group of symptoms, several remedies belong at the same time to the conceptions exogenous and endogenous. For example, one might drink some tisanes while reciting prayers of exorcism addressed to the illness to make it leave the body.

Rather than seeking to confine folk medicine within these categorizations, it would seem to be more fruitful to concentrate on diversity, to ask how this medicine system has been able to adapt, and to integrate some foreign elements, without thereby losing its coherence.

Another example of these erroneous reductive classifications is the series of distinctions or assimilations between magic and medicine on the one hand, and magic and religion on the other hand. In fact, the most recent studies on folk medicine confirm what the anthropologists working on phenomena of magic and religion have shown: we cannot effect a precise separation between what belongs to religion and what belongs to magic. Such a distinction, made from outside, would risk considering as religion only what we would call, from our point of view, recourse to the supernatural. It is only from within the indigenous culture that a distinction could conveniently be made. From the point of view of folk medicine, this does not seem truly pertinent, all the different levels being inextricably linked. For example, in the practice 'go to church on the day of the patronal fête, take home with you some consecrated bread, and give it at Christmas to the animals to preserve them against rabies', is it possible and significant to separate what belongs to religion from what belongs to magic?

INTERPRETATIONS OF SICKNESS AND THERAPEUTIC MEASURES

The examples that I have given on the contents of traditional medicines highlight the importance of the aggregate, of the unity. This aggregate does not always appear in the recipes of popular medicine that have been collected at other times, and the task of the researchers is to rediscover it and to restore it in comparing those recipes one with another.[12] Thus re-evaluated, researches into folk medicine would have to be at the heart of the problems preoccupying researchers into anthropology and history of disease as much as health professionals. Three points in particular seem highly relevant: the question of interpretation of sickness; that of the importance of domestic medicine; and that of the relationship with the past and with tradition.

Work on the anthropology of disease during recent years has, for the most part, placed the accent on one characteristic of the healers' activities, equally in European and non-European societies: to give meaning to the malady, to make of the illness – always perceived as an 'abnormal' phenomenon, throwing the natural course of life into disorder – an event that takes its meaning in the continuity of life.[13] Doubtless, the role of treatments in this research on interpretation – which is equally research into coherence – has not been analysed sufficiently. By placing rituals of biological rites of passage or rituals of cure in the setting of everyday life, the body is reinserted, in effect, into the familiar culture: the patient, although passive, is an actor in the system of cure. The patient's participation, confidence, and belief are explicitly necessary.

It is not uniquely by the rituals, but more deeply still by the influence given to the perceptible qualities that coherence is achieved for the sufferer. From infancy, children – girls in particular – acquire knowledge relative to the body and to sickness by aiding their grandmothers to cultivate or to collect plants, to find the therapeutic ingredients at the centre of their familiar environment. Thus an entire mental universe evolves, and much of the remembrance of this coherent childhood universe, concerning sickness, probably creates an effect, if not of cure, at least of the relief of pain. That is why it is excessive to affirm, as certain anthropologists have done, that the content of these beliefs has no importance, only the social function of the therapist taking part.[14] Further, if the universal function of the healer is to give meaning to the malady and to relieve it, that cannot be done as an absolute but only in the particular context of each culture. Whence the importance, when working on traditional medicine systems, of analysing at the same time the universals, the constants, and the local and regional particularities. In fact, researches into folk medicine, whether theoretical or applied, occupy an intermediary position between research into universals and into cultural diversity. Their object is in effect the body, in its biological unity and also in the diversity of its cultural contructs. Thus, the importance of blood, the opposition between heat and cold, and the relation between the moon and the human body appear as constants in many cultures, although often expressed in different terms. However, even if the elements of the therapeutics are subject to cultural variations strongly linked to the natural milieu, we can find in this diversity a certain number of constants. Thus, in a current research project comparing French and Quebecois folk-medicine recipes concerning haemorrhage,[15] it has been established that the use of serpent's skin in France and of cod's skin in Quebec, despite the difference, contains a similarity: animals characterized as cold-blooded are used in opposition to the heat of the blood. It is from these common underlying structures, but also by taking account of the diversity of cultures, that the activity of curing in the different cultural contexts must be examined.

Rediscovering the content of each culture before undertaking any health care is the principle followed by a very promising tendency of ethno-psychiatry, including such researchers as Tobie Nathan and Marie Rose Moro in France, and, in Italy, Mariella Pandolfi. Starting from a straight definition of ethno-psychiatry as treating mental troubles, they have arrived at an approach integrating folk medicine. Insisting on the fact that the culture is like a 'second skin', they demonstrate, on the one hand, that there is often a tendency to catalogue as mental trouble a behaviour that is simply culturally different, and, on the other hand, that contempt or rejection of other cultures can lead to mental troubles. (➤ Ch. 21 Mental diseases; Ch. 56 Psychiatry)

DOMESTIC MEDICINE AND FOLK MEDICINE

A problem which constantly crops up is that of the relations between domestic medicine and folk medicine. The American anthropologist Arthur Kleinman has, very rightly, shown the importance of domestic medicine as a centre for prevention, diagnosis, treatment, and convalescence.[16] Folk medicine is an important part of this domestic medicine, but the latter has recourse equally to biomedicine and to parallel systems of medicine, both traditional and modern. Anthropologists and folklorists, emphasizing the spectacular, have always had a tendency to minimize the role of this everyday, predominantly feminine, domestic medicine and to stress that of healers. With the object of giving to domestic medicine the role that it justly merits, Kleinman proposes to reserve the term 'folk medicine' for what has been called elsewhere 'parallel medicine' or 'soft medicine' or 'heteromedicine'; that is, that which is practised by therapists exterior to the family, but which does not belong to biomedicine. Such a definition has the merit of clarifying the three poles of the therapeutic field, but does pose some problems. On one hand, it is always dangerous to limit the meaning of a term that varies from one country to another. On the other hand, in practice, there is a continuum rather than a clean break between family medicine and recourse to lay healers: for example, reciting a healing prayer can be done equally well in the family as with an exterior therapist. Finally, more and more, the parallel medicine systems are not traditional, but the very ambiguous term 'folklore' could lead us to think the contrary. Personally, I prefer not to employ the term 'folk medicine', which is too evocative of diverse ideologies. The term 'heteromedicine' seems (more than 'folk medicine' because it is neutral) to be able to characterize all the medicine systems outside biomedicine, if it is well understood that this other recourse is extremely diverse. The term 'domestic popular medicine' is, without doubt, the best to characterize popular knowledge that is gathered together under the name of 'folk medicine', the term 'traditional' being sometimes added to qualify the knowledge which has been transmitted. Such an option averts the danger of enclosing traditional knowledge in a separate discipline: it allows the domestic and the traditional dimension to be better included in the field of researches into anthropology and the history of disease. (➤ Ch. 2 What is specific to Western medicine?)

The accent placed upon domestic medicine emphasizes the role of women, so important in matters of health and supporting life,[17] but which, until now, has not been adequately analysed in precise researches. In this domain equally, the health professions find themselves directly concerned, notably nurses reflecting on the notion of care and on the difficult identity of their profession.[18] In traditional societies, a certain category of women seems to have a preferential relationship with care: the elderly. Not only are they more available, but also they have acquired with age the necessary knowledge and experience. There are, without doubt, some reasons of a symbolic order to this that have not been adequately considered: illness is often a privileged moment of relation with the past and therefore with age.

FOLK MEDICINE AND RELATIONS WITH THE PAST

One of the ambiguities of the notion of folk medicine is that it is situated both in the past and in the present. To some extent, the folk medicine of today – studied by the anthropologists – is the domestic medicine of yesterday – studied by the historians. To abolish this specification of folk medicine would be to suppress this ambiguity. It would not be necessary to suppress from the analysis all relation to tradition, to the past. For that, it is necessary, indeed, to study ancient domestic-medicine systems with the help of materials left by the folklorists, but it is equally necessary to analyse the recourse to the past, the relation to a past which necessarily is both that of history and of mythology, which renders lively and operative the recourse to tradition.[19]

For several carers, a reflection of this type appears indispensable, in particular in the multi-ethnic context in which most of the eastern countries are found. According to certain of them, before understanding the traditions of others, it is necessary to rediscover our own traditions. In this connection, we may cite the work of continuous education in anthropology effected at Le Havre by Jean Pierre Castelain and Marie Claude Niel.[20] At the end of several years, the nurses reversed the relations with the anthropologists and summoned them to a colloquium in which one of the questions considered was the transformation of their professional practice through anthropological reflection on their own traditions.[21] In fact, whether it is called 'folk medicine' or not, the analysis of popular domestic medicine should belong just as well to anthropology as to the history of disease, but this is far from being the case. It is, however, perhaps one of the strong points of anchorage of the relations between anthropology, history, and healing. One of the roles of the anthropologists, similar to that of the historians, is in effect to be witnesses. One of their tasks is perhaps to reinstate the coherence of threatened cultures by restoring their dignity. On this point too, these researches can be of great importance for the health professionals. Almost everywhere, notably in the United States with B. J. Goode and J. D. Goode,[22] or in Italy with R. Lionetti and the *Revue Antropologia Medica* and the group of medical anthropology of Perouse,[23] some efforts are being made to introduce the anthropological dimension into the heart of clinical medicine. In this case, the anthropologist has a role of passage, of interpreter between several cultures. That can be done only by respecting popular knowledge.

NOTES

1   Laurent Joubert, *Erreurs populaires au fait de la médicine et régime de santé*, 1578.

2   Abbé Thiers, *Traité des Superstitions qui regardent les sacraments selon l'écriture sainte, les décrets des conciles et les sentiments des saints pères et des théologiens*, 2nd edn, Paris, Antoine Dezaillier, 1697.

3   R. Mandrou, *De la Culture populaire aux 17ᵉ et 18ᵉ siècles, la bibliothèque bleue de Troyes*, Paris, Stock, 1964 (2nd edn, Paris, Imago, 1975); G. Bollème, *La bibliothèque bleue: la littérature populaire en France du 17ᵉ au 19ᵉ siècle*, Paris, Julliard, Coll Archives, 1971; P. Slack, 'Mirrors of health and treasures of poor men: uses of the vernacular medical literature of Tudor England', in C. Webster (ed.), *Health, Medicine and Mortality in the Sixteenth Century*, Cambridge, Cambridge University Press, 1979, pp. 237–74; F. Lebrun, *Se soigner autrefois. Médecins, saints et sorciers aux 17ᵉ et 18ᵉ siècles*, Paris, Temps Actuels, 1983; G. Smith, 'Prescribing the rules of health: self-help and advice in late eighteenth-century

England', in R. Porter (ed.), *Patients and Practitioners*, Cambridge, Cambridge University Press, 1979, pp. 249–82.

4 L. Boltanski, *Prime éducation et morale de classe*, The Hague, Mouton, 1969; G. Delaisi de Parseval and S. Lallemand, *L'Art d'accomoder les bébés. Cent ans de recettes françaises de puériculture*, Paris, Le Seuil, 1980.

5 M. de Certeau, D. Julia and J. Revel, 'La beauté du mort', in *La Culture au pluriel*, Paris, 1974: 10/18.

6 De Westphalen, *Petit Dictionnaire des traditions messines*, Metz, 1934; P. Nourry-Saintyves, *L'Astrologie populaire étudiée spécialement dans les doctrines et les traditions relatives à l'influence de la lune*, Paris, Nourry, 1937; A. Van Gennep, *Manuel de folklore français contemporain*, Paris, Picard, 1949.

7 Marcel Bouteiller, *Médecine populaire d'hier à aujourd'hui*, Paris, Maisonneuve & Larose, 1966; 2nd edn, 1987.

8 N. Belmont, *Paroles paiennes. Mythe et folklore*, Paris, Imago, 1986.

9 M. Augé, 'L'anthropologie de la maladie', *L'Homme*, 1986, 97–8: 81–9.

10 A. Bruneton-Governatori, 'La mise par écrit d'un savoir local béarnais au 18ᵉ siècle et ses reprises au 19ᵉ siècle: questions et enseignement', *Reclams*, 1989, 12: 'La tradition médicale en Gascogne'.

11 F. Laplantine, *La Médecine populaire des campagnes françaises aujourd'hui*, Paris, Delarge, 1978.

12 F. Saillant, 'Les recettes de médecine populaire. Pertinence anthropologique et clinique', *Anthropologie et soins*, 1990, 1: 93–114; Saillant and F. Loux, 'Le pain dans les recettes françaises et québéquoises de médecine populaire', Rome, *L'Uomo*, 1991, 1.

13 M. Augé and C. Herzlich, *Le Sens du mal. Anthropologie, histoire, sociologie de la maladie*, Paris, Éditions des Archives Contemporaines, 1983.

14 J. Favret, *Les Mots, la mort et le sort*, Paris, Gallimard, 1977.

15 Saillant and Loux, op. cit. (n. 12).

16 A. Kleinman, *Patients and Healers in the Context of Culture: an Exploration of the Borderland between Anthropology, Medicine and Psychiatry*, Berkeley, University of California Press, 1980.

17 F. Saillant, 'Les soins en péril: entre la nécessité et l'exclusion', *Recherches féministes* (special issue on the health of women), 1991; M. F. Collière, *Promouvoir la vie. De la pratique des femmes soignantes aux soins infirmiers*, Paris, InterEditions, 1982.

18 Collière, op. cit. (n. 17).

19 Belmont, op. cit. (n. 8).

20 J. P. Castelain and M. C. I. Niel (eds), *Anthropologie, soins infirmiers, travail social*, Paris, Éditions de la Maison des Sciences de l'Homme, 1991.

21 Onze travailleurs sociaux et hospitaliers du Havre, 'Anthropologie hors les murs: ethnologues, que faisons nous de votre savoir?', *Cahiers de Sociologie économique et culturelle*, 1987, 7: 131–40.

22 B. J. Goode and J. Delvecchio Goode, 'The meaning of symptoms: a cultural hermeneutic model for clinical practice', in J. Eisenberg and A. Kleinman (eds), *The Relevance of Social Science for Medicine*, Boston, MA, Reidel, 1981, pp. 165–96.

23 T. Seppilli (ed.), 'La medicina popolare in Italia', *La Ricerca Folklorica*, no. 8, 1983.

FURTHER READING

Benoit, J., 'Une anthropologie médicale pour les anthropologues et pour les médecins', *Bulletin d'ethnomédecine*, 1985, 33: 85–95.

Camargo, M. Th. L. de Arruda, *Medicina Popular*, Sao Paolo, Almed, 1985.

Fainzang, S., *Pour une anthropologie de la maladie en France. Un regard africaniste*, Paris, École Hautes Études en Sciences Sociales, 1989.

Genest, S., 'Introduction à l'ethno-médecine, essai de synthèse', *Anthropologie et sociétés*, 1978: 5–28.

Guio Cerzo, Y., 'El influjo de la luna: acerca de la salud y la enfermedad en dos pueblos extremenos', *Asclepio*, 1988, 1: 317–41.

Hand, W. D., *Magical Medicine. The Folkloric Component of Medicine in the Folk Belief, Custom and Ritual of the People of Europe and America*, Berkeley, University California Press, 1980.

Joubert, Laurent, *Erreurs populaires au fait de la médecine et régime de santé*, 1578.

Laget, M. and Uu, C., *D'après le livret de Dom Alexandre. Médecine et chirurgie des Pauvres au 18e siècle*, Toulouse, Privat, 1984.

Lieutaghi, P., *L'Herbe qui renouvelle. Un aspect de la médecine traditionnelle en Haute-Provence*, Paris, Éditions de la Maison des Sciences de l'Homme, 1986.

Mandianes Castro, M., 'La medicina popular Gallega', *Anthropologia (Barcelona)*, 1987, 1: 47–61.

Renzetti, E. and Taiani, R., *Sulla Pelle del Villano, Profili de Terapeuti e Metodi di Cura Empirica nella Tradizione Trentina*, Trente, Museu delle Gente Trentina, 1988.

Romanucci-Ross, L., 'Folk medicine and metaphor in the context of medicalization: syncretics in curing practices', in *The Anthropology of Medicine. From Culture to Method*, New York, Praeger, 1983, pp. 5–19.

Saillant, F., *Cancer et culture. Produire le sens de la maladie*, Quebec, Éditions St Martin, 1988.

Smith, G., 'Thomas Tryon's regimen for women: sectarian health in the seventeenth century', in Smith (ed.), *The Sexual Dynamics of History*, London, Pluto Press, 1983, pp. 47–85.

Soriano, M., *Les Contes de Perrault. Culture savante et traditions populaires*, Paris, Gallimard, 1968; 2nd edn, 1977.

Thiers, Abbé, *Traité des superstitions qui regardent les sacrements selon l'écriture sainte, les décrets des conciles et les sentiments des saints pères et des théologiens*, 2nd edn, Paris, Antoine Dezailler, 1697.

Thomas, K., *Religion and the Decline of Magic. Studies in Popular Beliefs in Sixteenth- and Seventeenth-Century England*, London, Weidenfeld & Nicolson, 1971.

Tissot, S. A., *Avis au peuple sur la santé*, Lausanne, 1761.

Whorton, J. C., 'Traditions of folk medicine in America', *Journal of the American Medical Association*, 1987, 12: 1632–5.

Woodward, J. and Richards, D., *Health Care and Popular Medicine in Nineteenth-Century England*, New York, Holmes & Meier, 1977.

Young, A., 'The anthropologies of illness and sickness', *Annual Review of Anthropology*, 1982, 11: 257–87.

31

ARAB-ISLAMIC MEDICINE

Lawrence I. Conrad

It is often proposed that medicine in the Middle East in medieval times cannot properly be viewed as either an Islamic or an Arab topic of inquiry:[1] the professional textual tradition that arose under Muslim auspices was firmly grounded in the Galenic system of pagan antiquity, and many of the key roles in the rise and development of formal medicine under Islam were played by non-Muslims, and indeed, non-Arabs.[2] Yet it is impossible to deny the central role of both the Arabic and Islamic elements in the medical history of the medieval Middle East, as in most other fields of cultural endeavour and social life.

Throughout the medieval period, the term '*arab*' was generally used to mean 'bedouins', and the ancient Arabs did not identify themselves as 'Arabs' *per se*, but rather as members of particular tribes or clans. When a distinct Arab identity began to emerge in the aftermath of the Arab conquests of the seventh century, it quickly passed beyond considerations of ethnic origin to encompass all those who spoke Arabic as their native tongue and identified with the norms and values of the culture expressed in the Arabic language.[3] The language of the Arabs became the common cultural denominator of the medieval Middle East and was spoken as the *lingua franca* by not only Muslims, but Christians and Jews as well. It thus comes as no surprise to find that just as many of the great works of Arabic historical writing, for example, were authored by historians of Persian origin. Some of the most prominent monuments of formal medical learning were written in Arabic by scholars who hailed from such Persian urban centres as Rayy (al-Rāzī), al-Ahwāz (al-Majūsī), and Hamadhān (Ibn Sīnā). The rise and development of medical scholarship was characterized by an ever sharper focus upon Arabic as the medium for translations and the vehicle for new original work, and once Arabic gained this dominant position it never lost it, even with the revival of Persian and the later emergence of Turkish as literary languages. All of the great classics of the formal medical tradition were written in Arabic, and were aimed at the literate audience from Spain and North Africa across the Middle East itself to lands as far east as India. It is therefore pointless to agonize over the extent to which 'genuine Arabs' or 'the Arabian element' contributed to scientific literature;[4] things 'Arab' were always defined in very broad terms, and scholars of the time would not have denied a particular author's contribution to 'Arab' culture simply because of non-Arab ethnic origin.

A factor of even greater importance was the Islamic faith itself, and here both practical and ideological considerations must be taken into account. On the practical side, the conquests of the seventh and eighth centuries were the work not of vast hordes, but of small armies, and the events associated with this era involved no sharp cultural caesurae or large-scale displacements of population. That is, the leaders of the new empire were, and long remained, a small ruling minority. Indeed, it is probable that Muslims did not become a majority of the population until the mid-ninth century in Persia, the late ninth century in Egypt, Syria, and Iraq, and the tenth century in Spain.[5] Consequently, old traditional customs and practices continued undisturbed.

The ideological side of this coin is that Islam was not a proselytizing faith. The Arab conquerors made no effort to convert non-Muslims, and the Qur'ān granted Christians and Jews protected status as 'People of the Book' (*ahl al-kitāb*), adherents of faiths based on scriptures regarded as directly antecedent to Islam and now superseded by it. Other faiths (especially Zoroastrianism in Persia) were also dealt with leniently, and in general, only overt paganism or deliberate open blasphemy provoked harsh retribution. Indeed, Christianity and Islam shared considerable religious ground in common, and in the medieval period, perceptions of religious difference did not normally precipitate the difficult barriers of 'otherness' which typify modern sensitivities on such issues. In the study of medieval Arab-Islamic medicine, several important lines of tension and cleavage must undoubtedly be taken into account, but these will not be found in the domains of language and religion. To use the phrase 'Arab-Islamic' with reference to this history is rather to evoke the factors outlined above: the emergence and continuing dominance of the Arabic language, and a pattern of broad-ranging social, cultural, and intellectual pluralism focused on the concerns of Muslims, but yet fully capable of accommodating participation by and contributions from adherents of other faiths as well.

THE TRADITIONAL SUBSTRATE

Arabs and their customs were already well-known in the Near East long before the conquests of the early seventh century,[6] but the Arab-Islamic expansion encouraged a far higher degree of cultural and social interaction among the various communities, and it was against the backdrop of this symbiosis that the formal Arab-Islamic medical tradition arose a century and a half later. It is thus important to consider what sort of medicine the Arabs brought with them, and how it compared with other medical traditions in the region.

Arab society in pre-Islamic Arabia upheld a complex structure of well-established medical customs and deeply entrenched beliefs that affected how health and medical problems were perceived and managed.[7] In many ways, such questions were approached from a highly practical point of view, and if someone lapsed from good health – regarded as the natural human condition – popular lore had a host of counter-measures to offer. Materia medica included a broad range of plants and herbs believed to have some specific or general therapeutic value, and it is unlikely that the popular pharmacopoeia of the Middle East in the seventh and eighth centuries was significantly different from that familiar to the area in late antiquity.

Among the Arabs a number of remedies seem to have been particularly prominent. Cumin and caraway seeds were used in numerous medical recipes, the juice of truffles was regarded as good for eye disorders,[8] and 'Indian stick wood' was employed to soothe throat infections. Many preparations were used to counteract disease and relieve its symptoms: soups and broths made with water or milk, thickened with flour and sometimes sweetened to make them more palatable ('ghastly, but good for you'), were recommended for various ills and for relieving grief; a mixture of three parts clarified butter to one part milk was administered to reduce fever; liniments and salves made from the leaves or buds of certain trees were used against skin disorders and as aphrodisiacs; snuff-like errhines (a category subsumed under the rubric of sa'ūṭ) were inhaled through the nose for nasal, sinus, and respiratory problems; date porridge ('ajwa) was given to counter food poisoning, and dates were generally believed to be useful for many ills, particularly those of children.[9]

Inorganic medicaments are not commonly encountered, but there was considerable use of animal products. Certain meats were believed to be good for febrile illnesses, the gall of some animals (especially the wolf) had medical applications, and the milk of the camel and donkey was used in therapy. Camel's urine was widely used to keep the hair clean and for other similar purposes, and it also made its way into medical preparations: drinking it was recommended as generally conducive to good health, and the leaves of the aromatic *arāk* bush (*Salvadora persica*) cooked in camel urine produced a medicine to treat scrofula (whether internally or externally is not known).

As medical procedures, cupping, cautery, and venesection were very widespread, as they had been in earlier times, and medical leeches were also used. The means available to respond to serious physical injury were very limited, however, and such mishaps were often fatal. Broken limbs were massaged, rubbed with salves, and kept immobile to heal; wounds were cleaned with saltwort (high in alkali content), and ashes were used to stop bleeding. Although the Arabs had a detailed vocabulary where externally visible anatomical features of the body were concerned, there was only vague knowledge of the internal organs, and recourse to surgery seems to have occurred only in straightforward cases in which it was an obvious alternative, or when the situation was truly desperate. Haemorrhoids were removed surgically, boils and tumours were often cut out, and intense pain was relieved by making an incision at the point where the allegedly affected organ was believed to be located. Amputation was a last resort in cases of gangrene or other serious infections, and the procedure of Caesarean section was employed, if reluctantly, in cases of difficult labour and doubts as to the safety of the mother and child. (➤ Ch. 41 Surgery (traditional))

Intertwined among these measures was a broad range of beliefs and practices inspired by a deep-seated animism.[10] Deviations from good health were approached as ordinary physical problems to be treated on an empirical basis; but at the same time, they were also attributed to forces regarded as animate entities one had to out-manœuvre, or subject to the power of some greater force, in order to restore or protect one's well-being. Animism of this kind was prominent in many aspects of life, and in medicine the two main entities held responsible for ill health were the *jinn* and the evil eye (*al-ʿayn*). The *jinn* (sing. *jinnī*, from whence the English word 'genie') were minor spirits of the physical world which interacted with human beings in many ways; one could see, negotiate with, outwit, defeat, and even kill a *jinnī*, and they could bring good as well as misfortune and calamity. In popular medicine, however, their activity was seen as uniformly negative, and they were held particularly responsible for epidemic disease, madness, and diseases of children. The evil eye was an entirely malevolent force, which could be summoned by certain gifted persons or called forth with spells, and was suspected in cases of accidental injury or when an individual (as opposed to many persons in an area) suffered from some medical complaint. Even where the *jinn* and the evil eye were not brought into play, medical problems were still regarded in animistic terms. Contagion (*ʿadwā*), for example, was viewed in the same magical context as augury and the roaming spirits of the unavenged dead, and seems to have been viewed as an animate force attached to each specific disease and responsible for spreading it.[11] (➤ Ch. 60 Medicine and anthropology)

Avoidance of illness thus involved not only practical therapeutic measures, but also magical precautions and remedies intended to defeat or ward off malevolent unseen forces. There were incantations and charms for complaints ranging from ulcerated veins to insomnia and night-blindness, and for guaranteeing the growth of good teeth and the survival of the children of women who tended to miscarry. An amulet in the form of a necklace, collar, armband, or bracelet could contain defensive devices ranging from rabbit's feet or fox or cat teeth to the sap of the acacia tree, from ornaments and bells to menstrual rags or bones of the dead. A wide variety of special stones (usually colourful or radiant) were believed to ward off the *jinn* and the evil eye, and phrases used in oral charms could also be written down and worn as talismans. Such devices were sometimes believed to repel weapons, the bite of snakes, and the sting of scorpions, or prevent grief, drunkenness, and physical enfeeblement, in much the same way that they warded off spirits and such ills as fever, migraine, and nosebleed. (➤ Ch. 30 Folk medicine)

The character of the animism inspiring these measures can be seen in several particularly illustrative examples. Epidemic disease in general (*wabā'*) was regarded as the work of the *jinn*, and it was noticed that such human illnesses did not also affect livestock, thereby demonstrating that the *jinn* were lying in wait especially for human victims. The custom that thus arose to deal with this problem was the *tanhīq* or *ta'shīr*, in which a person approaching a town or village suspected to be pestiferous would place the hands behind the ears and bray ten times like a donkey. As donkeys that brayed for no apparent reason were believed to do so because they had seen a *jinnī*, it was felt that the spirits in this case would be tricked into thinking that the person performing the rite was also a beast and therefore not worth infecting.[12] We are also told of a case in which someone drank from the water container used by a leper, for fear that were he to decline the offered container, his obvious effort to avoid infection would draw him to the attention of the 'contagion' of leprosy, which, having noticed him, would rush forth and 'infect' him anyway.[13] Even more telling is a custom according to which a boy suffering from a fever blister on his lip should carry a sieve around on his head, announcing his condition and requesting donations of scraps of food. He would then throw the contents of the sieve out in front of the dogs; as the pustule had originally been attracted to him by the food passing his lip, it would by now have been attracted to the scraps and would be thus transferred to the dogs.[14]

A view of medicine so heavily coloured by such notions was, of course, bound to be dominated by practitioners of the same sort, and here some revealing lines of specialization seem to have prevailed. Cuppers and phlebotomists seem to have been regarded as possessed of particular skills and were paid for their services, but otherwise the more practical medicine seems to have been the common stock and trade of society. Procedures and remedies were generally known and their ingredients were widely available, and in cases where the treatment of an actual case of injury or illness is described, family members (especially women) and friends administered care.

On the other hand, the esoteric dimension of traditional Arab medicine was viewed as a field restricted to certain specialists – a conspicuous category of diviners, seers, befoulers,[15] and charm-purveyors who dealt with medical problems related to the unseen on what was probably a professional basis. Indeed, in pre-Islamic times the Arabic root *ṭ-b-b*, which later came to refer to the administration of formal medical care, has almost always to do with incantation, charms, and amulets – that is, with esoteric matters rather than with the more empirical and practical alternatives. Someone who is *maṭbūb* has not received medical care, but rather has been afflicted by a spell; *ṭibb* is not medicine, but the manipulation of incantations and charms; and a *ṭabīb* is not a doctor, but a purveyor of such religous services.[16] One such practitioner, al-Ḥārith ibn Kalada (*fl.* AD 530–70), became so famous for his activities that he was known as the *ṭabīb* par excellence – '*ṭabīb* of the tribal Arabs'.[17]

For all its prominence, however, the occult medicine was not universally accepted. 'Urwa ibn al-Ward (*fl.* late sixth century), for example, mocks the braying custom of the *ta'shīr* as demeaning and the mark of a coward:

> By my life, were doom's dread to bring it to pass
> That I too should cry out, not one time but ten,
> With the honking sound of the braying ass,
> Then demeaned I would rank with the timid of men.
> May the fear-stricken souls of those who deign
> To perform this ritual no inner peace find;
> Toward Rawḍat al-Ajdād may they journey in vain,
> And on to the grave may the path they tread wind![18]

Another anonymous poet vilified the *ta'shīr*, the use of amulets, and incantations in general as useless.[19] Al-Nābigha al-Dhubyānī (d. *c.*604) poured scorn on the custom of branding healthy camels so that the 'contagion' of mangy camels will not pass to them, comparing this to vilifying the innocent person while the guilty party goes scot-free.[20] That such customs prevailed, then, was not due to universal credulity. More likely, it had to do with the inclination, in the face of long-prevailing custom, to regard the failure of such measures in a specific rather than general sense. That is, if an amulet against the *jinn* failed to protect a villager in an epidemic of smallpox, it was very likely that the individual's death would be explained in specific terms – a poorly made amulet or an extremely powerful *jinnī*; far less common was the overarching conclusion that amulets and talismans in general were useless.[21]

In the early years after the conquests this medical lore continued unchanged; or at least, the rise of Islam at first did nothing to undermine it. Indeed, exponents of the new faith at first had little basis from which to do so. The Qur'ān has almost nothing to say about medicine, aside from a few brief comments assuring that there is no fault in the lame, the blind, or the sick,[22] advising the faithful of how to wash for prayer when they are sick,[23] and asserting that there is curative power in honey.[24] On the other hand, Islamic scripture concedes the existence of the *jinn* and repeatedly refers to their activities in the world.[25] (➤ Ch. 29 Non-Western concepts of disease)

There was likewise no impediment raised against this dual system as it came into contact with medicine as practised by the indigenous communities of the newly conquered provinces. The decline of secular culture in the Near East prior to Islam is a topic to which we will return, but here it is worth noting that even in the heyday of classical Greek medicine there coexisted with it a deeply entrenched tradition of popular medicine.[26] In the Middle East of the seventh century, a similar situation prevailed. Formal scientific learning, including medicine, continued in the eastern church, and especially in the Jacobite and Nestorian monasteries of Syria and Mesopotamia; however, Christians and Jews, no less than their new Muslim overlords, also had a venerable tradition of deep-seated beliefs in the supernatural and its role in medicine and health. Amulets and incantation bowls in Syriac and Jewish Aramaic demonstrate beyond all doubt that, in the fourth to seventh centuries, people commonly resorted to such devices to seek healing and protection from disease.[27] Even more revealing is the composite Syriac *Book of Medicine*, which highlights a society in which some practitioners had a detailed knowledge of the materia medica of Dioscorides (AD *c.*40–*c.*90) and the works of Galen (AD 129–*c.*200/210) and other formal medical writers, but in which people were also wary of the evil eye, convinced of the powers of charms and amulets, and prepared to predict whether or not a seriously ill patient would live based on the 'day of the moon' or whether his or her nail parings would float.[28] On the eve of the Arab invasions, Alexander of Tralles (*fl.* late sixth century) presented medicine in much the same way: an impressive array of Galenic teachings mixed with incantations, charms, and even Jewish and Christian prayers.[29] Though differences on points of detail can often be identified among the various offerings, there are also extraordinary correspondences with what we find in the Arabic sources (for example, animal teeth as amulets, wolf gall and camel urine in recipes, etc.), and most importantly, the basic framework of juxtaposed and intertwined customs of practical and religious medicine is identical.

EARLY ISLAMIC MEDICAL DISCUSSIONS

The seventh and eighth centuries witnessed the gradual development of Islam from its origins as a simple monotheistic creed to a highly articulated religion confronting and resolving a vast array of questions in dogma and theology.[30] As Muslim society moved in this direction, traditional popular medicine became embroiled in controversy over its animistic tenor and a host of customs and practices increasingly regarded as unacceptable.

The imbroglio owed no small degree of its intensity to the fact that in the first centuries after the Prophet's death in AD 632, discussions of all sorts of questions tended to be dominated by claims that Muḥammad (d. 11/632), one of his Companions, or some other eminent early Muslim had authoritatively pronounced on the matter under consideration, either by explicit statement or implicitly through his deeds. Accounts of such pronouncements rapidly multiplied and came to comprise a distinct genre called *ḥadīth*. It comes as no surprise, then, that Muslim proponents of the traditional medicine began to use statements attributed to Muḥammad and other early Muslim figures in efforts to 'update' it in Islamic terms. Traditions alleged to have come from the Prophet related, for example, that 'the evil eye is real', that there was healing power in Muḥammad's breath and saliva, and that the water of the well of Zamzam in Mecca had curative properties. The situation was further complicated by the fact that people were quick to conclude that, as God's word, the Qur'ān too must have magical powers which could be used in charms and incantations. It was claimed, for example, that for a woman having difficulty in labour, certain verses of the Qur'ān should be written on a slate, washed off, and the water given to her to drink. Water prepared using other verses could be sprinkled on a sick person; the *Fātiḥa*, the opening chapter of the Qur'ān, was recommended as a remedy for snakebite (and indeed, for every malady); and verses in general were used against epilepsy and scabies.[31] It would be anachronistic to dismiss all this as crude superstition, for the early Muslims responsible for this material – like the Christian and Jewish exponents of traditional magical practices before them – would have denied that they were dabbling in sorcery, but rather engaged in legitimate medicine entirely within the proper bounds of their religion.

But the difference between medicine and magic, the pious and the blasphemous, depends very much on how such terms are defined and where the boundaries between them are set, and to many other Muslims, all this posed serious problems. At a general level, the use of the Qur'ān for charms and incantations and the presentation of the Prophet as a purveyor of such remedies smacked of sorcery, a grave difficulty in any case. The early opposition to Muḥammad in Mecca had, in fact, dismissed him as deluded and bewitched, and one of the main early priorities of Islam was to eliminate pagan animism, not to tidy it up in a new monotheistic garb (though in some cases this was the result).

More specifically, numerous aspects of the traditional medicine posed significant dilemmas as the tenets of Islam were gradually worked out and elaborated. Here a major problem was the great plague pandemic of 541–749.[32] Early views had attributed the repeated epidemics of this scourge to the *jinn*, set upon the faithful by their enemies. Through the eighth and early ninth centuries, however, this explanation was gradually displaced by arguments intended to refute this old belief, and indeed, to orient the entire problem of epidemic disease within the monotheistic framework of a God who is the ordainer of all things (including disease), and yet just and merciful as well.[33] In other cases, arguments arose over the extent to which traditional medical beliefs contradicted specific points of emerging Islamic law. Wolf's gall and intoxicating beverages, for example, figured in both the formal and popular traditions, but both were anathema in Islamic terms, the first as ritually unclean, the second as specifically disapproved in the Qur'ān. Incantations posed the vexed problem of maintaining a clear distinction between magic and pious pleas for divine succour, and a concerted effort was made to limit these, especially where use of the Qur'ān was concerned, to prayers calling upon God for strength and relief.[34]

As Islamic awareness and influence in society broadened and deepened and became more articulate, the fact that many practices and beliefs were questionable in Islamic terms weakened their authority as part of venerable old custom. This, in turn, made it easier to bring other non-religious arguments to bear against them; and indeed, interesting rhetorical techniques attacking from both perspectives at once seem to have found favour. We are told, for example, that one of Muḥammad's Companions cured a snake-bitten bedouin by reciting the *Fātiḥa*, gathering his saliva, and spitting it on to the bite; when the man and his comrades returned to Medina and related the story to the Prophet, he laughed and said: 'And what gave you the idea that the *Fātiḥa* would serve as a cure?'[35] Here Muḥammad speaks as both the Prophet of Islam and the voice of practical reason. As the Arabic literary tradition developed, the old medical customs were also repeatedly collected and commented upon as bedouin superstition and deluded whimsy, and they were often the basis for proverbs on the theme of futility and ignorance. The great Baṣran littérateur al-Jāḥiẓ (d. 255/868), for example, whose *Kitāb al-ḥayawān* is a mine of valuable information on this process, misses no opportunity to contrast the folkloric and superstitious views of the past to his own more rationalist approach: 'In such fashion', he sardonically comments, 'do they sicken the healthy without curing the sick.'[36]

Several important aspects of these debates merit comment. First, they did not represent any official agenda or the interpretation of an educated élite, though by the ninth century an educated élite was certainly involved in them. The accounts in which these arguments were embedded were in early Islamic times transmitted orally and would have been discussed, as other topics, in mosques, markets, and homes – any place where Muslims tended to congregate. And though the various contributions were at first limited in circulation to the particular region in which they had originated, by the ninth century, Muslims were travelling widely on the 'journey in quest of learning' (the *rihla fī ṭalab al-'ilm*), which ensured that the various shades of opinion would eventually reach most parts of the Islamic world. In sum, these debates were not the preserve of the urban literati, but rather expressed the genuine concerns of society at large.

Second, it is significant that while many practices of the traditional medical folklore were attacked, and medicine *qua* magic was especially condemned, medicine in its practical therapeutic form was distinguished from all this and encouraged. 'Should one go to the doctor (*ṭabīb*)?', one tradition has a man ask the Prophet; and the response is that he should, for 'God sends down no malady without also sending down with it a cure.' In this account, transmitted in many variant forms and one of the most widespread of medical traditions, a sharp distinction is drawn between the old-style *ṭabīb*, the master of spells and charms, and a different kind of *ṭabīb*, one who searches out the cures provided by God, the giver of all things.[37] The critique is aimed not at 'medicine' *per se*, but at specific aspects of it which are repugnant to religious sensibilities. 'Contagion', for example, was denied not because it was regarded as a false medical principle, but because the traditional lore viewed it in animistic terms and so exposed it to attack on religious grounds.[38]

In other cases, considerations of practical expediency prevailed regarding materia medica which were formally excluded as ritually unclean or forbidden by religious law. In one illustrative case, the reader is advised to proceed anyway with such a treatment: 'If one is compelled to use something which has been declared illicit to him, then in his particular case it is not illicit, but allowed.'[39] When it comes to the essential welfare of the believer, matters of formal observance are overruled.

A word must also be said concerning the outcome of these discussions. In some cases, the targeted practices seem to have disappeared, at times almost immediately; there is no trace, for example, of the braying custom of the *ta'shīr* after the rise of Islam, except for comments upon it as a curiosity found in ancient poetry,[40] and a proverb of the type indicated above.[41] In other cases, however, it is clear that the issue remained unresolved, with many customs and beliefs formally disapproved but in practice still widely espoused. Amulets, magic squares, and talismans of all kinds were recommended for protection against the plague, especially in the Black Death of

747–9/1347–9, and the role of the *jinn* in causing epidemics continued as common belief into the twentieth century.[42] Some medical practices used in pre-Islamic times were still to be seen in use in Arabia in the nineteenth and early twentieth centuries,[43] and Syriac collections of Christian charms and amulets against illness and many other kinds of misfortune were still being actively copied out and used a hundred years ago.[44] The debates served to define some new boundaries for the proper domain of medicine, but they did not – and indeed, could not – enforce them.

THE RISE OF THE FORMAL MEDICAL TRADITION

The eastern Mediterranean world into which Islam expanded was a region undergoing profound changes in its passage from late antiquity. The reasons behind these patterns of transformation are complex and controversial, but a few salient features seem beyond doubt. Prolonged warfare between the Byzantine and Sasanian empires had drained the resources of both sides and caused enormous destruction and social disruption; in the case of Byzantium, the strains on fiscal and human resources were made particularly severe by the efforts of Justinian I (r. 524–65) to recover the western domains of the old Roman Empire and his commitment to enormously expensive building programmes. The advent of the bubonic plague in AD 541 marked the beginning of a 200-year cycle of repeated outbreaks that devastated cities, wiped out villages, and in general made for broad-ranging and continuing disruption of everyday life throughout the Mediterranean world and beyond.[45] (➤ Ch. 52 Epidemiology) In the spiritual sphere, christological controversies and related disputes in the lands of Christendom made religion a focus of division and estrangement rather than unity, and in terms of political economy the centuries prior to the rise of Islam were characterized by the displacement of patterns of civic autonomy by increasing interference in and manipulation of municipal affairs in the interest of ever-expanding imperial demands for income.

The effects of these developments were profound. The vitality of cities was seriously sapped, and the disruption of agriculture and village life by plague and prolonged warfare posed grave consequences for all urban centres, which were dependent upon their agrarian hinterlands for both foodstuffs and investment opportunities. Similarly, expanding imperial interference in municipal affairs had the effect of attracting investment away from regional centres to the seat of imperial power in Constantinople. Although it is true that much wealth remained concentrated in local hands, a trend of urban recession is clear from the archaeological record, and seems to have been widespread.[46]

These patterns, in turn, had an important impact on culture and learning. Local languages – Syriac in Syria, Coptic in Egypt – had long been playing more-important roles in Near Eastern society in any case, and their advance was paralleled by a decline in the use of Greek. The provincial immigrants with whom the 'high' culture had flourished ceased to make their way to the great regional centres, and traditional élites and the civil culture they represented were gradually replaced by the church, which, of course, had a very different cultural agenda. The traditional forms of Greek secular culture had disappeared almost entirely by the end of the seventh century.[47]

The fate of classical medicine in the era preceding and immediately following the rise of Islam must be viewed against this background, one in which the classical Greek heritage was being reinterpreted within the framework of shifting interests and priorities. This reassessment had two consequences of particular importance to present concerns, the first having to do with physicians themselves. The literature of the period makes it clear that formal Greek medicine continued to be practised and had representatives in several large towns and cities (especially Alexandria), but these figures seem to have been acting as isolated individuals rather than as part of a living tradition. In the latter sense, medicine was moving into the domain of religion, where disease tested faith and punished sin and the Christian saint or holy man healed and cured all manner of ills by the power of the Lord. An apt commentary on the times may be seen in the image of the physician, weak in faith and unable to cure himself, healed by the ministrations of a saint. (➤ Ch. 61 Religion and medicine)

The second consequence concerned the educational and literary tradition. Teachers such as Asclepius and Palladius were active in the mid- and late sixth century, original scholarship was in the early seventh century still represented by Paul of Aegina (AD c.625–c.690), and formal teaching in Alexandria may have continued after the Arab conquest of Egypt in the 640s.[48] But overall, as interests shifted, the teaching of formal Greek medicine seems to have declined sharply. Certainly, fewer and fewer books of the enormous classical Greek medical Corpus were available for study: such works were not to be found even in the patriarchal library of Constantinople itself,[49] access to copies elsewhere often required extensive inquiry and searching, and only a small sampling of Galen was pursued in depth. (➤ Ch. 14 Humoralism)

It may, of course, be doubted whether the formal classical tradition of medicine had ever displaced popular medicine, folklore, and superstition at any level below that of the educated élite in the first place. But the increasingly dominant role of more spiritually oriented perspectives, coupled with the recession of traditional classical culture, tended to undermine the standing of formal Greek medicine generally. The interesting mix of formal and popular elements evident in the work of Alexander of Tralles (see p. 682), was probably typical of the prevailing trend.

In the centuries following the expansion of Islam, then, forms of cultural expression on all fronts – and in all the monotheistic communities – were characterized by a sharpening focus on religion. In the light of this trend, the rise of a formal medical tradition in Arabic should be expected to reveal definite and fundamental links with spiritual concerns; conversely, it would be unrealistic to expect that it represented some attempt to revive the scientific and philosophical heritage of antiquity for purely utilitarian purposes or for general edification.[50] Though the exponent of secular culture was not, by any criterion, an extinct species in the early medieval period,[51] even the Byzantine Greeks of the seventh and eighth centuries looked back at classical times uneasily and used such terms as 'Hellenes' and 'Hellenism' to refer to the bad old pagan ways and those who adhered to them.[52]

It has often been claimed that Arab-Islamic medicine as a formal tradition harks back to the time of the Prophet Muḥammad himself, and has connections with a Sasanian hospital and academy at Jundīshāpūr in southern Persia. The Prophet's physician al-Ḥārith ibn Kalada travelled twice to Persia, we are told, was trained at Jundīshāpūr, and engaged in a 'dialogue on medicine' with the Sasanian ruler Chosroes Anūshirvān (r. 531–78).[53] In reality, however, there is no evidence that any academy ever existed at Jundīshāpūr. The hospital there was a foundation of early Islamic times, and all of the medieval material on the ancient glories of the town is late in origin and may best be interpreted as baseless literary invention inspired by the eminence of the Bakhtīshū' family of Nestorian physicians, on which more is said on p. 710. Al-Ḥārith figures in the legend because of his reputation as 'ṭabīb of the tribal Arabs'. But, as has been seen above, in al-Ḥārith's own day, ṭabīb meant a worker of charms and spells, and even a cursory examination of the relevant evidence will reveal that in early Islamic times he was an obscure figure about whom little was known – it was not until the late tenth century that material about al-Ḥārith as a physician began to appear in earnest, and over the following 300 years successive accretions of speculation and storytelling promoted him to the formally trained counterpart of the Byzantine and Sasanian court physician.[54]

Aside from the folklore about Jundīshāpūr we have only scanty and dubious information about a limited number of Arab, Greek, Syriac, and Jewish physicians, and seldom with any clear indication as to whether or not they were practitioners of a formal medicine. Viewing the situation from a far clearer vantage point than we now enjoy, Ṣā'id al-Andalusī (d. 462/1070) concluded that formal medicine 'was practised by isolated individuals from among the Arabs',[55] and the state of affairs among Christians and Jews is not likely to have been significantly different.

Already in pre-Islamic times, however, there was some movement toward broadening the foundations of formal medicine. Sergius of Resh-'Aynā (d. 536), for example, translated more than twenty works of Galen into Syriac and also wrote an original monograph on dropsy. In early Islamic times, a prince of the ruling Umayyad family, Khālid ibn Yazīd (d. 85/704), is said by al-Jāḥiẓ to have been active in pursuing the ancient sciences:

> Khālid ibn Yazīd ibn Muʿāwiya was an orator and poet, well-versed in matters of culture and full of learning in the sciences. He was the first to patronize translators and philosophers, kept company with sages and the leading authorities in all the fields of applied learning, and had translations made of books on astrology, medicine, alchemy, military sciences, the various branches of literature, mechanical devices, and the arts.[56]

Perhaps related to this effort was the work of the obscure Māsarjawayh of al-Baṣra, whose translation of the *Pandects* of Ahrun of Alexandria (*fl.* late sixth/early seventh centuries) was made in the mid-Umayyad period and marked the first known Arabic translation of a text from the classical medical tradition. In the related field of philosophy, we hear of Syriac translations of Aristotelian texts by Anastasius of Balad (d. 79/698), Jacob of Edessa (d. 89/708), George, Bishop of the Arabs (d. 106/724), and Theophilus of Edessa (d. 169/785). But all these and similar enterprises were efforts of individuals and limited in their impact. It was not until the early ninth century that the revival of formal medicine began in earnest.

This revival arose from the confluence of three crucial factors which explain both why it emerged when and where it did, and why it involved such prominent roles by non-Muslims. The first of these factors was social and economic, in that the rise of a formal scientific tradition where a firmly grounded popular one already existed may in part be assigned to the growth of an educated élite with broad interests and the financial resources required to fund scholarship, teaching, and the physical production and maintenance of collections of books. This development was especially pronounced in Iraq, where towns such as al-Baṣra and al-Kūfa expanded from primitive garrison camps established by Arab armies in the 630s to become, by the mid- to late eighth century, vast thriving cities where cultural influences from places as remote as India and China were felt, and where the resources made available by officials and wealthy merchants and landowners promoted lively and sophisticated scholarship in a broad range of subjects.[57] The ʿAbbāsid foundation of Baghdad in 145/762 sparked an even greater surge of urban growth: by the mid-ninth century the new imperial capital was a focus of incredible wealth and cultural vitality and, with a population far in excess of one million, perhaps the largest city in the world.[58]

Another key precondition was a specific need which a formal medical tradition could fill, for enterprises of this level of ambition are not the product of some yearning for a revival of ancient glories, especially not those of other peoples, and into the bargain, pagans. And as the early caliphate did not see its role as including guardianship of public health, it is likewise unlikely that the work was underpinned by a concern for the well-being of the general population. In fact, the developments of this period cannot be understood without bearing in mind that this was an era of ubiquitous religious disputation: among Christians, for example, over church law, icons, and Christology; and among Muslims, over issues of dogma and theology and the nature of legitimate political authority. Perhaps most significantly, there was a lively production of polemical and apologetical literature, with both Christians and Muslims seeking to justify their faith against the claims of the other.[59] At the beginning, Muslims were at a particular disadvantage in these exchanges, for while Christians had for centuries been using the tools of classical Greek logic and philosophical argumentation to elevate confessional quarrelling to the level of an art, the defenders of Islam had no prior experience in disputation at this level. It should not be surprising, then, that they began to turn to the same sources of inspiration which their Christian opponents had long been accustomed to use.

At the same time, the atmosphere of confessional disputation left a great deal of common ground between Christians and Muslims. In part, this had to do with the presence of a common enemy, for equal to the threat each presented to the other was the challenge posed to both by the ancient dualist doctrines of Manichaeism. Though the gnostic ideas of Mani did not appeal so much to the common person, they did attract considerable attention from intellectuals, and in the late eighth century the world-view they embodied was espoused by many sophisticated Muslims. Their arguments were cogent ones and, as emerges quite clearly in the formulations of Ibn al-Muqaffaʿ (d. c.140/757), they struck to the very heart of monotheistic religion: a god cannot be omnipotent who stands idly by while his creatures murder his prophets, disobey his will, and throng to the ranks of Satan; a god cannot be just who allows pestilence and famine to ravage the faithful and ruin to spread through his creation; the *creatio ex nihilo* is an absurd doctrine, and hardly less so are the notions of revelation and prophecy; monotheistic scriptures are full of anthropomorphic follies, such as the image of an all-powerful god confined within the limits of his throne. Such propositions brought bitter persecution down on the sect and its members, for not only was Manichaean dualism utterly irreconcilable with the tenets of Islam (and of monotheism in general), its sympathizers were often intellectuals and courtiers who stood (as Ibn al-Muqaffaʿ did) at the heart of the circles then striving to give direction and form to nascent Islamic culture.[60]

Even without the factor of shared enemies, however, there was much commonality between Muslims and Christians in this period. For example, the Qur'ān accepts numerous Old Testament prophets, manifests many biblical parallels, and acknowledges the virgin birth of Jesus and regards him as a prophet. Apart from matters of common religious belief, there were also numerous concerns over identical medical questions being raised at the time: the Muslims' arguments over whether one should flee from the plague (which has, after all, been sent by God) is paralleled by similar concerns discussed by Anastasius of Sinai (d. c.81/700),[61] for example, and just as Muslims disputed predestination and whether one should resort to a physician, the Nestorian Christian Ḥunayn ibn Isḥāq did likewise.[62]

The extent to which medical works could contribute to the religious concerns of the day was considerable. Paradigms for rational inference from empirical data (that is, for formulating proofs for tenets of faith) were to hand on every side, religiously offensive passages were few and easily deleted or revised with minimal damage to the surrounding context, and Galen, in particular, offered powerful evidence for the argument from design: if the parts of the body work together for the benefit of the whole, for example, and accord to some principle of harmony and order, then this necessarily implies a giver of harmony and order – that is, God. It did not pass unnoticed that such formulations provided powerful arguments against Manichaean dualism.

Of equal importance was the fact that, after the Arab conquests, the Arabic language began to spread at the expense of the local and confessional languages. A key indicator, the advent of an Arabic translation of the Gospels, can be dated to the early 'Abbāsid period,[63] and in general, by the ninth century, a working knowledge of Arabic had become essential for anyone engaging in serious scholarly work addressed to audiences beyond the confines of the monasteries. Eventually, even Syriac dictionaries and some histories of the eastern church had to be available in Arabic (that is, bilingually, or in Arabic, sometimes written in Syriac characters) in order for eastern Christians to use them.

In sum, in the ninth century both Christians and Muslims stood to benefit from works that could be used in disputations to defend tenets of their faiths. For the Muslims, this automatically meant works in Arabic, and for Christians, Arabic was rapidly becoming an important medium as well.

The third factor was, of course, a source of intellectual inspiration, a corpus of intellectually systematic material which could serve as a foundation that could be elaborated and expanded. Here, the contribution of the Christian community was crucial, for though books seem to have been scarce in Byzantine lands, they were more plentiful in Egypt, Syria, and Iraq. The main ecclesiastical libraries were large and varied, monasteries kept extensive collections of manuscripts (as they do to this day), and many texts were also in private hands. Such books were regarded as a precious resource not to be denied to others, and a whole battery of scribes could be mobilized to produce copies of works in particular demand.[64] We are often told of how books were borrowed and sent long distances to be read and copied elsewhere – for those inclined to forget to return them, manuscripts often contained anathemas calling down God's wrath upon any negligent borrower. It also seems that Muslim forces raiding Byzantine territory sometimes brought books back with them, probably by specific order of the regime.[65]

The first phase of the Arab-Islamic tradition of formal medicine was thus a major translation movement brought about by a combination of these three factors: an increasingly favourable social and economic climate for the pursuit of advanced scholarship in general; a perceived need among both Christians and Muslims for broader access – that is, in Arabic – to the medical heritage of antiquity, and a pre-existing means of relatively easy access to the required texts. This is not to say, of course, that no scientific considerations – for practical applications or purposes of general edification – had any role to play, but the overwhelmingly religious concerns of the day, undoubtedly the key influence on the articulation of Islamic philosophy at this time,[66] were no less crucial in the development of medicine. This can be seen in the fact that the translation movement, if already underway in the reign of Hārūn al-Rashīd (r. 170–93/786–809), gained decisive impetus during the caliphate of his son al-Ma'mūn (r. 198–218/813–33).

On the personal level, al-Ma'mūn was a sophisticated and learned man; as caliph, he was a ruler confronted with the task of uniting and consolidating his authority over a vast empire suffering from the effects of several seriously divisive difficulties: four years of civil war with his brother al-Amīn (defeated and killed in 198/813), autonomist tendencies in various provinces of a far-flung empire, controversies over influences on nascent Islamic culture and theology, and socio-political problems focusing on fiscal policy and the legitimate sphere of imperial authority. It should come as no surprise, then, that in such a situation the caliph should find common cause with the Mu'tazila, an expanding circle of speculative theologians seeking to articulate Islamic doctrine in a systematic fashion on rationalist foundations, and to mount a defence of Islam capable of meeting on equal terms the intellectual challenges posed by other religious systems. The agenda of the Mu'tazila was in no small part aimed to confront Christianity and Manichaeism, but their activities had other attractions as well. Their insistence on laying a rigorous rational foundation for religious discussions undercut the position of more traditional views asserting the literal authority of religious texts (that is, over the caliph's desire to interpret them according to his own priorities); their receptivity to non-Arab and non-Islamic cultural and intellectual influences opened the way for the foundation of a new culture, Islamic in orientation and articulated in Arabic, but capable of integrating contributions from all the peoples of the empire and from other cultures (especially Byzantium and India) with which they were familiar; and several of their key doctrines, in particular the createdness of the Qur'ān, favoured the aspirations of an absolutist caliph who, advised by an inner circle of select confidants, would himself decide what the nature and content of reform should be.[67]

Such moves immediately provoked a vigorous counter-reaction, and the next fifty years of Islamic history are, in fact, dominated by a storm of controversy over the issues raised by the Mu'tazila. Beginning in the time of al-Ma'mūn, then, those favourable to the Mu'tazila committed extremely high levels of political, social, and financial support to the task of encouraging its exponents and providing them with the materials necessary to support their doctrinal positions and justify them to society at large.

A landmark in these efforts was the establishment in Baghdad in 217/832 of the Bayt al-Ḥikma, where scholars supervised by a series of directors from the renowned al-Munajjim family worked to collect important texts and to translate into Arabic a broad range of non-Arabic and non-Islamic works that could contribute to the tasks set by the regime. The name Bayt al-Ḥikma is usually translated 'House of Wisdom', and the institution itself is often regarded as an indubitable imitation of the 'academy' at Jundīshāpūr.[68] But in consideration of the spirit of the times, the title should rather be taken in its more juridical and dogmatic sense, as suggesting not a pursuit of truth wherever it may lie, but a choice among competing, exclusive, and unequivocal formulations on a given issue, one of which is to be upheld as absolutely true while the others are repudiated as absolutely false. In this sense, the foundation of the Bayt al-Ḥikma, though based on an ongoing library tradition (having nothing whatever to do with Jundīshāpūr), must be seen as marking a major new turn in programme and agenda.

The translation work associated with the Bayt al-Ḥikma was dominated by Christians, by virtue of their knowledge of Greek and Syriac and their prior experience in translation and intellectual debates. Of the various eminent figures involved,[69] the most important was Ḥunayn ibn Isḥāq (d. 260/873), a Nestorian Christian from the southern Iraqi town of al-Ḥīra, long a Christian centre and a focus for Manichaean sympathies in the region. Ḥunayn was himself a Christian theologian, author of works on such subjects as predestination and divine will, the nature of divine unity, the creation of human beings, and how the truths of religion may be known, and translator of the Old Testament into Arabic.[70] His lost treatise on why sea water is salty was almost certainly an anti-Manichaean tract.[71] His interests and abilities exactly reflect the spirit of the times, and the fact that it was possible for him and his circle to play such a major role in the programme pursued by the 'Abbāsids indicates, once again, the common ground between Christians and Muslims and the extent to which Christians could participate in Islamic culture.

Much of what we know about Ḥunayn's activities comes from Ḥunayn himself, in particular his *Letter to 'Alī ibn Yaḥyā*, one of the al-Munajjims, in which he describes his translation technique, comments on past translation work, and enumerates 129 Galenic texts which have now been made available in Arabic by himself and his circle.[72] From this crucial work and comments by him elsewhere, we learn much of importance: accounts of difficult and long-ranging searches for desired books, specifics on the extreme care taken to render texts accurately, and details about the enormous materials – impressive in their range as much as in their bulk – which the translators typified by Ḥunayn were able to produce.

At the same time, however, there is a great deal of fancy and embroidery to be taken into account, both in Ḥunayn's own descriptions of his work and in later accounts of it. He often speaks, for example, of previous translations in extremely disparaging terms, and portrays the authors of these past works as culpably incompetent. The truth of the matter rather seems to lie in the fact that while earlier translators had worked on the paradigm of the Bible, and so were anxious to produce a literal word-for-word rendering, Ḥunayn and his circle recognized that this method often produced a translation intelligible only if one knew the original text (as, in the case of the Bible, people often did), and that, in their case, what was needed was translation which conveyed the sense of the original, if not in the same words or phrasing. Ḥunayn also stresses the intermediary role of Syriac in the translation programme. The part played by Syriac was indeed important in many instances, but in numerous others it is not mentioned at all, and it is worth recalling that the notion that Arabs knew no Greek and Greeks no Arabic is a fantasy of modern Western scholarship – that the opposite was true is manifest from the large number of Greek words which had already made their way into Arabic by the ninth century. Here we may note that the famous Muslim littérateur, al-Mas'ūdī (d. 345/956), refers to Ḥunayn's Arabic translation of the Old Testament as a rendering made directly from the Greek Septuagint and a work 'regarded by many people as the best translation' of it.[73] Finally, it cannot be true that Ḥunayn (as he reports to 'Alī ibn Yaḥyā) made a habit of carefully collating numerous Greek exemplars to produce a correct text before translating, while at the same time (as he repeatedly states in the *Letter*) manuscripts of Greek medical works were extremely rare and attainable only after much searching and enquiry.[74] Such a critical method may have been feasible in the case of the sixteen books of the *Summaria alexandrinorum*, but in many other cases (and perhaps *most* other cases) it would have been out of the question because of the scarcity of Greek manuscripts of the text. The surviving examples of Ḥunayn's translation work clearly establish him as a master, but it is perhaps extreme to credit him as the precursor of modern *Quellenkritik*. In all these cases, and perhaps others, Ḥunayn had an obvious vested interest in ensuring that others should appreciate the difficulty of his work and the level of his achievements.

Finally, later accounts of al-Ma'mūn, Ḥunayn, and the translation movement in general sometimes tended to indulge in glorification which can easily be exposed as the stuff of folklore and legend. The oft-repeated story that al-Ma'mūn obtained texts in the ancient sciences by asking the Byzantine emperor's permission to remove representative copies from libraries in Byzantine lands is at once falsified by the fact that (as we have seen on p. 691) the emperor in those days had very few such books to offer, and it at least needs to be asked whether any Byzantine ruler would have condoned, much less formally authorized, what amounted to the looting of monasteries. Closer examination will reveal that the topos of 'letters/requests to the Byzantine emperor' is a common one in Arabic literature, and that the example of it here is embedded in an anecdote in which Aristotle appears to al-Ma'mūn in a dream – as a result of their conversation al-Ma'mūn suddenly appreciates the importance of the Greek heritage and writes to the Byzantine emperor, etc.[75] We are likewise told that Ḥunayn journeyed in person to Byzantine lands in search of manuscripts, travels about which Ḥunayn himself, we should note, says nothing.[76] It is far more likely that books were obtained by travels to private collections in Syria, Mesopotamia, Persia, and Egypt (repeatedly mentioned by Ḥunayn), through the venerable custom of loans from monasteries (as discussed on p. 691), and occasionally by seizure as booty during Arab campaigns in Asia Minor.

The output of the translation movement was vast in both range and content. Hundreds of Greek texts were rendered into Arabic, these being primarily works by Galen, followed by such authors as Rufus of Ephesus (*fl.* late first century AD), from whom nearly sixty titles appeared in Arabic. Though Greek was by far the tradition preferred for attention, it must be borne in mind that one work may be known under different names in different (or even the same) accounts or lists, and that some titles undoubtedly represent only chapters from what had originally been a single book. Further, works in Syriac, Pahlavi, and Sanskrit were also translated, reflecting, once again, the rich cultural tradition thriving in Iraq in the ninth century AD.[77]

The era of the translators continued into the early eleventh century, but a major change seems to have occurred by about 900. Through the time of Ḥunayn, and so long as the controversy over the issues raised by the Mu'tazila endured, the quest for and translation of ancient texts proceeded at a frenetic pace, encouraged by official sanction, generous patronage, and the immediacy of the debate at hand. But it is again an indication of the close ties between the translation movement and the controversies of its day that with the definitive repudiation of Mu'tazilism by the caliph al-Mutawakkil (r. 232–47/ 847–61), and the resulting sharp drop in theological temperature, the demise of the Bayt al-Ḥikma, and the gradual drying-up of patronage and financial support, the movement could not be sustained at its earlier pace. Although individuals continued to pursue this sort of work on their own, they were just that – individuals. It is revealing that al-Rāzī, for example, writing in the early tenth century and from a position (as director of a hospital in Baghdad) in which access to medical texts would have been easier than for most others, seems to regard the Arabic translations of Greek works as a closed corpus; he knows of those who can read Greek and Syriac, but they are useful to him not for any translation activity, but rather as informants who can answer specific queries when these are put to them.[78]

The impact of the translation movement was enormous, most obviously for the hundreds of ancient texts which it saved for posterity in Arabic. But beyond the factor of quantity was that of selection: the favoured author was always Galen, to no small extent for the reasons suggested above, and as a result it was Galen who set the standard for Arabic medicine in centuries to come. It was his system that prevailed throughout the Islamic lands, and even the works of the Hippocratic Corpus were known primarily through the prism of Galen's commentaries. Further, the translation movement rose to prominence at precisely the time in which Arabic-Islamic literary culture was generating masses of texts in many other subjects. Although we are told nothing about any connection, it is difficult to imagine how the high standards set by the translation movement for assessing, copying, and using manuscript texts could have failed to influence the ways in which Islamic culture in general came to set equally high standards for handling codices in all fields of learning.[79]

The movement also provided the decisive impetus for the revival of formal scientific medicine, in several ways. First, it made Arabic a language in which original scientific scholarship could henceforth proceed. The Arabic of Umayyad times had no formal vocabulary for expressing philosophical or scientific concepts, and no exact terminology for, for example, names of diseases or their symptoms. Such problems are the object of specific comment by Ḥunayn himself.[80] The efforts of the translators, culminating in Ḥunayn and his circle, bequeathed to future generations a mode of scientific discourse in which even the most obscure and complex formulations – not just in medicine but in philosophy and science in general – could be articulated with precision and clarity.[81] This endeavour, which Ullman rightly characterizes as the 'creation of a language', was one in which the translators received little support from professional philologists, who were more concerned to collect and study ancient poetry and elucidate philological difficulties in the Qur'ān.[82] Second, the movement thrust into the arena of emergent Islamic culture a vast array of scholarship of manifest practical utility, and it is to this era that the re-emergence of formal medicine can be traced. The first Islamic hospital, for example, seems to have been founded by Hārūn al-Rashīd, and for formal physicians we need look no further than the ranks of the translators themselves. Ḥunayn is perhaps the most illustrative example, The chronology of his works is largely unknown, but it seems that it was his theological interests which, in the first instance, led him to an interest in medicine as a specialization; he was the son of a pharmacist, but says nothing about any formal medical training, and appears to have learned what he knew from his work as a translator. Eventually, he took to composing his own works, which were often based on classical and late antique models, and to practising medicine himself, eventually becoming court physician to the caliph al-Mutawakkil. Both of his sons followed the same path to medical practice, and the transition from medical translator to medical author and physician appears to have been common. Whatever else remains unclear, however, there can be no doubt that the era of the translators produced a corpus of texts, a revived intellectual tradition, and a core of practitioners upon the foundations of which all subsequent achievements were to be based.

Finally, it must be noted that the translation movement was closely related to the discussions of popular medicine described above (pp. 682–686), in that both were part of the broader debate in early Islamic times over what the content and direction of Islamic culture – in the broadest sense of the term – was to be. Just as discussions of the former decided, through arguments largely pursued in the domain of *hadīth*, how and to what extent the old medical folklore would be accommodated within Islam, the translation movement determined, through its selection of specific works and by its adjustments to offensive or troublesome passages (for example, references to the pagan gods in the Hippocratic Oath) the ways in which ancient literary culture was to play a role in shaping that of Islam. Here it must be noted that while the Bayt al-Ḥikma clearly played a central role in the movement, patronage of translators extended to circles beyond the 'Abbāsid regime to include many private individuals interested in the issues under discussion.[83] The movement thus injected into emergent Islamic thought a profoundly rationalist current which was to dominate formal Islamic medicine (and science more generally) throughout the medieval period, and even to set the standard for what formal medicine was. Physicians knowledgeable in the Greek tradition regarded those who were not as unqualified dilettanti, and this perception was one that came to be widely shared in high society at large. At the same time, the translation movement, in so far as it made concessions to new religious sensibilities, laid the foundations for a medical tradition which was more generally monotheist than specifically Islamic in tone, indicative, again, of the broad concerns motivating the movement in the first place. The tradition thus, on the one hand, always allowed for large-scale participation by non-Muslim practitioners and thinkers, and on the other, manifested a certain ambivalence which often rendered its Islamic credentials suspect. These considerations were all to prove important in the era of efflorescence that followed.

THE FORMAL MEDICAL TRADITION

Although it would be wrong to conceive of a distinct break between the era of the translators and that of the later masters of formal medicine, it is certainly true that the field of medicine *c.*900 was very different from what it had been in the heyday of Ḥunayn fifty years earlier. While the earlier period was dominated by efforts to render what was already known into Arabic, the later period was increasingly devoted to the formulation of new scholarship.

As observed above (pp. 696–697), the early translators were themselves also involved in the creation of original medical literature, and at this early stage they produced mainly specialized treatises on specific topics. Ḥunayn, for example, authored a series of essays on ophthalmology, now known as his *Kitāb al-'ashr maqālāt fī l-'ayn* (*Book of the Ten Treatises on the Eye*). These essays, although sometimes problematic and lacking in their sense of balance between the theoretical and the practical, were pioneering studies into the nature of vision and the workings of the eye, and laid the foundations for future studies which established Arab-Islamic science as the leader in this field in medieval times.[84] A further shift in emphasis away from translation and more toward original scholarly work can be seen in the career of Qusṭā ibn Lūqā (d. 300/912), a Christian from Baalbek and a younger contemporary of Ḥunayn in Baghdad. Qusṭā collected Greek scientific and medical texts and did work as a translator (some seventeen such works are attributed to him by the medieval sources), but most of his career was devoted to his own research in physics, mathematics, astronomy, and especially medicine. Many of the more than sixty titles attributed to him are now lost, but those that survive reflect the thought of a broadly learned scholar able to work on many specialized topics with equal facility, and writing under the patronage of various high officials at the 'Abbāsid court. Lately, some of these works have become available in editions and translations of high quality, including his *Fī ṭūl al-'umr wa-qaṣrihi* ('On Length and Shortness of Life'), *Fī l-bāh* ('On Sexuality'), *Fī i'dā'* ('On Contagion'), and *Fī tadbīr safar al-ḥajj* ('On the Regimen of the Pilgrimage to Mecca').[85]

Many other scholars composed similarly specialized works, and by the late ninth century researchers in medicine had available not only a vast array of ancient texts in Arabic translations of high standard, but also a rapidly expanding corpus of original scholarship pursuing the work of the ancients in new directions. This trend continued for several hundred years and produced many monographs of fundamental importance. One of the most outstanding was the *Fī l-ḥaṣba wa-l-judarī* ('On Smallpox and Measles') by al-Rāzī, to whom we shall return on pp. 699–700. Here, questions of pathology, diagnosis, therapeutics, and materia medica are all brought together into a brilliant analysis, which provided the world's first serious treatment of smallpox (measles is only a secondary concern).[86]

As the sheer quantity of this material increased, the need arose for more synthetic writing that would provide researchers, practitioners, and other interested parties with ready and reliable access to the essential information across the whole range of medical science. The efforts to fill this need gave rise to the most spectacular achievement of medieval Arab-Islamic medicine, the medical compendium.

The appearance of the medical compendia must be viewed within the context of research in other fields in the ninth and tenth centuries, when similar works were being produced in such disciplines as history, lexicography, *belles-lettres*, and Qur'ānic exegesis. In all these disciplines, authors wrote ambitious compendia not just with the aim of collecting what was already known, but also with the intention of pursuing the implications of current knowledge to their appropriate conclusions, filling in gaps, and, in sum, creating a work that would remain authoritative indefinitely.

In medicine, the first great compendium was the *Firdaws al-ḥikma* ('Paradise of Wisdom') by 'Alī ibn Sahl Rabban al-Ṭabarī (wr. *c.*236/850), in which the author (a convert to Islam) sought to collect a *summa*, in more than 350 chapters, of the medical knowledge of his day sufficiently worthy for presentation to the caliph al-Mutawakkil. His sources were Arabic and Persian translations of ancient classics, and his citations include not only such leading Greek personalities as Hippocrates, Galen, and Dioscorides, but also Indian and Persian medical writers.[87]

The early date of al-Ṭabarī's work is indicated by his innocent interweaving of rational and magical lore, and even more by his interest in non-Greek medical traditions. The presence of a considerable body of Indian medical lore in his compendium suggests that, in his view, it was still possible to undertake a unified study of the various medical traditions within an Islamic framework, and hence also that in his day the Greek tradition had not yet gained the authority it was to achieve in the next generation, that of Ḥunayn.[88] And as al-Ṭabarī lived and worked in northern Persia, where the eastern influences would have been quite strong, the possibility of such a synthesis might have seemed very real indeed. As the Greek tradition became ever more influential, however, this receded, and later compendia were entirely dominated by classical and late antique influences.

In the following generation, northern Persia produced another scholar who was one of the greatest Muslim physicians and philosophers of medieval times, Muḥammad ibn Zakarīyā' al-Rāzī (known in the Latin West as Rhazes; d. 313/925). A student of the natural sciences, alchemy, and music in his youth, al-Rāzī travelled from his native Rayy to Baghdad at about the age of 30, and studied medicine. His career saw him rise to the directorships of hospitals in both Rayy and Baghdad, and compose (among 200 other books on medicine, alchemy, philosophy, and other subjects) two works of particular importance. His *Al-Kitāb al-manṣūrī fī l-ṭibb* ('The Manṣūrian Book of Medicine') was composed for and dedicated to the Sāmānid governor of Rayy Manṣūr ibn Isḥāq (d. 302/914–15), and covered the various fields of medicine in ten books. Books I-VI treat such theoretical concerns as diet, anatomy, physiology, general pathology, and materia medica, while the last four books deal with practical matters: diagnosis, therapy, surgery, and special pathology, the chapter on pathology being a famous account which discusses diseases and maladies from head to foot. The work soon came to be regarded as a classic and was extensively used by later authors.[89]

Like many scholars of medieval times, al-Rāzī kept detailed notes and copied bits of texts for which he anticipated some future use. These notes on pathology and therapy seem to represent his 'files', each of these consisting of a quire of pages devoted to a particular subject, and gradually filled as al-Rāzī added quotations and his own observations and notes. When one quire was filled, another would be added, and the result was thus a kind of *aide-mémoire*, well organized at the level of primary subjects, but problematic at any more detailed level. Such a corpus would, of course, not have been compiled with broader circulation in mind, but as was also the case with other Muslim scholars, al-Rāzī's jottings and reflections were gathered together after his death and published. The resulting compendium, called *Al-Ḥāwī fī l-ṭibb* ('The All-Inclusive Work on Medicine'), was a vast book, of which complete copies soon became very difficult to find, but despite its size, problematic organization, and scarcity, it proved to be very influential.[90]

The achievement of the Arabic medical compendium culminates in two works of the tenth and eleventh centuries. 'Ali ibn al-'Abbās al-Majūsī (Haly Abbas, d. late fourth/tenth century) was a native of al-Ahwāz in southern Persia, but apart from this little is known about his personal life. He was attached to the Būyid ruler 'Aḍud al-Dawla (r. 338–72/949–83), and it was to this prince that he dedicated his *Kāmil al-ṣinā'a al-ṭibbīya* ('The Complete Medical Art').[91] Following the example of al-Rāzī, he divided this work into two sections on theoretical and practical medicine, each of which included ten different treatises on specialized topics, and his introduction gives an especially valuable assessment of the development of medicine up to his own day. This was his only medical work, but the *Kāmil* paid greater attention to certain subjects than al-Rāzī had (especially anatomy and surgery), and was both more compact than the vast *Al-Ḥāwī* (and hence easier for the scribe to copy and the scholar to afford) and more comprehensive than the *Manṣūrī*. An eminently practical work, it was so well organized and accessible that it secured al-Majūsī's medical reputation and eventually occupied a place second only to that of the *Qānūn* of Ibn Sīnā.

The talents of Abū 'Alī Ibn Sīnā (Avicenna, d. 428/1037) were already quite evident when he was still a youth, although it may be unwise to trust his own claim that he was practising medicine by the age of 16. It is certain, however, that he was a brilliant student in numerous branches of learning, and that he handed down legal opinions as a jurist and held several govern-ment positions in Persia. His primary interests were philosophy and medicine, and these concerns dominate his bibliography of over 250 titles. In medicine, his great work was his *Al-Qānūn fī l-ṭibb* ('Canon of Medicine'), a vast compendium in five books, written over several stages of his career, which abandoned the theoretical/practical division of al-Rāzī and al-Majūsī.[92] Book I covers what Ibn Sīnā calls 'universals' (*kullīyāt*): medical theory, aetiology, hygiene, therapy, and surgery; Book II is his materia medica, with detailed descriptions of each item and its medical character and applications; Book III discusses diseases from head to foot; Book IV considers general pathology (that is, medical problems which did not belong to Book III), fevers, pro-gnoses, pustules and abscesses, wounds, poisons, surgery, fractures, and obesity and emaciation; and Book V describes compound drugs and thera-peutics. The *Qānūn* covered the various fields of medicine with a precision and thoroughness that gave it authoritative sway over the discipline for hundreds of years, and it ranks as one of the most impressive and enduring achievements of medieval Islamic science. If al-Rāzī would have to be con-ceded as the superior writer in terms of practical utility, Ibn Sīnā would, in the same way, have to be acknowledged as the better theorist, for it was in his *Qānūn* that the ideas and thought scattered through the many works of Galen and his later proponents were drawn together into a definitive system of medicine.

All of the great compendia mentioned above originated in Persia, but important works of this kind were being produced elsewhere as well. One from Islamic Spain merits special attention. Little is known about the Spanish physician Abū l-Qāsim al-Zahrāwī (Albucasis, *fl. c.*330/940), aside from his authorship of a medical compendium organized in thirty treatises and entitled *Al-Taṣrīf li-man 'ajaza 'an al-ta'līf* ('The Recourse of Him Who Cannot Compose [a Medical Work of His Own]'). Its content is similar in some ways to what other compendia offered, but in others it is important specifically because it offers information on topics not always well covered in other works, including surgery, midwifery, the raising and education of children, cooking, weights and measures, psychology, and the flora and fauna of Spain. Its section on surgery is particularly important for its detailed treatment of the subject and its many illustrations of surgical instruments, including what may be the first true scissors.[93]

As the Persian language came to be more extensively used in later medieval times, it was inevitable that medical writers from this part of the Islamic world, who had long played a leading role in Arabic literature, would begin to write important medical works in Persian as well. Of these, two were of particular importance. The *Zakhīra-i Khwārizmshāhī* ('Treasury of the Shāh of Khwārizm') was written by Ismā'īl ibn Muḥammad al-Jurjānī (d. 531/ 1136), the first physician to do all of his scientific writing in Persian. The work was a comprehensive medical encyclopedia in ten books, with many clinical observations from the author's own practice, and covered not only the main topics of medieval Islamic medicine, but also such matters as ancient Greek weights and measures and why physicians die of diseases for which they offer treatments and cures to their patients. Its success was immediate, and as it quickly rose to the status of a classic, it had the further – and ultimately most important – effect of setting an authoritative standard for medical writing in Persian.[94] The second work of particular note for present purposes is the *Tashrīḥ-i Manṣūrī* ('Manṣūrian Anatomy') by Manṣūr ibn Muḥammad ibn Ilyās (wr. 798/1396). This work of descriptive anatomy devoted separate chapters to the skeletal, nervous, muscular, veinous, and arterial systems, and was built around a set of five full-body illustrations showing the layout of each of the five systems under discussion, with some manuscripts bearing additional illustrations of a pregnant woman carrying a foetus in a transverse or breech position, and a second female figure marked to show cautery points. Inaccuracies and abiguities abound in these diagrams, which represent a tradition long predating the time of Ibn Ilyās; however, these representations none the less became very popular, and were often tipped into appropriate places in copies of older texts (for example, the *Qānūn* of Ibn Sīnā), and the emergence of anatomical illustration on such a scale is in itself a development of great importance.[95]

Several important questions may be asked concerning this medical literature, including that of its originality – to what extent did Arab-Islamic medicine make original contributions to medical knowledge, as opposed to simply transmitting what was already known to the ancients? In this regard, we must first observe that originality is not the only factor in judging the importance of a tradition, and to view originality as a criterion of first significance is to impose on medieval times a perspective that is distinctly modern.

This said, numerous aspects of Arab-Islamic medicine were unquestionably original. In ophthalmology, for example, Ḥunayn and his successors added much to medical knowledge of the eye, vision, ailments and diseases involving the eye, and, more generally, to the science of optics. Also important was the contribution to pharmacology. The lands overrun by Arab armies were, of course, full of plants, animals, and minerals not found elsewhere, and the various cultures in these lands had their own systems through which the medical uses and perils of all these were formally set forth. The rise of Arabic pharmacology thus involved the tasks of collating names and descriptions coming into Arabic from Greek, Latin, Syriac, Persian, Sanskrit, and other languages, harmonizing diverse descriptions of their nature and use into one system, generating standards for expressing and comparing weights and measures, and unifying the results of research simultaneously proceeding in botany, zoology, chemistry, toxicology, and materia medica.[96] That this was achieved at all is already a formidable accomplishment, and the result may be judged from the fact that while the materia medica of Dioscorides included only about 850 plants, animals, and minerals, that of Ibn al-Bayṭār (d. 646/1248) listed over 3,000 items, the result of consulting over 250 sources ranging from Dioscorides and Galen to al-Rāzī, Ibn Sīnā, and other Muslim researchers.[97]

It would be possible to continue this list with specific procedures and observations unknown to the ancients, but to pursue this not only falls into the trap indicated on p. 702, but also obscures the fact that perhaps the greatest contribution of Arab-Islamic medicine was that it systematized and unified the field of medicine as never before. The greatness of the contribution of such authors as al-Majūsī and Ibn Sīnā lies not in their originality, but rather in the devastating thoroughness with which they drew together what was known in many discrete fields and harmonized it in such a way that it both made sense intellectually and gave the physician ready access to information needed for practical work, all this within the confines of a single (albeit very large) book.

Another question worth considering is that of the extent to which the formal medical tradition actually shaped and directed medical practice. In this connection, it must be borne in mind that in medieval times most persons were illiterate, that books were always expensive (large ones prohibitively so) and often hard to find, and that medical texts in particular – with their complex argumentation, many non-Arabic terms simply transliterated into Arabic characters, and presumptions of formal background – could make for extremely difficult reading.

We can never know exactly how influential the great classics of formal medicine were at the individual level, but these works clearly not only expressed the medical learning of their day, but also served to shape it. The most obvious indication of this is the enormous effort devoted to disseminating formal medical learning in written form. Many classics of Arab-Islamic literature (for example, numerous historical and literary texts) survive today in only a single manuscript, or have had to be pieced together from multiple incomplete copies. Medical texts, on the other hand, were copied and recopied at a pace which, considering the time, effort, skill, and expense required, can only be described as vast. The case of Turkey is illustrative. Over 5,000 medical manuscripts in Arabic, Turkish, and Persian survive in both public and private libraries in modern Turkey, and cover about 1,000 works by 449 authors.[98] There are more than fifty complete or partial copies of Ibn Sīnā's *Qānūn* (most of them in Istanbul), and copies of the many later commentaries on it are even more numerous.[99] Information of this kind, of course, does not prove that the manuscripts were actually in use, but for the era before the printed book, it is worth knowing that copies of medical works of all kinds were far more numerous than exemplars of texts relevant to other fields.

There are also more specific examples of the formative influence of the medical literary tradition. The existence of a generally accessible and rapidly expanding body of materia medica – the results of work in pharmacology – is evident from the recipes and prescriptions in many medical works, for example, and in the case of ophthalmology it is possible to trace the origins of the Arab-Islamic discipline to the essays of a single author, Ḥunayn ibn Isḥāq. Another example may be seen in the field of surgery, which until the time of al-Zahrāwī was a secondary concern of medicine, if not despised, as in medieval Europe, as the task of cuppers and barbers. The last treatise of the *Taṣrīf*, however, dealt with surgery in detail, with full accounts of surgical procedures and illustrations of surgical instruments, and this discussion, coupled with that of al-Majūsī, played no small role in the ultimate acceptance of surgery as a respectable aspect of the medical profession and laid the groundwork for the pursuit of further study, which culminated in the surgical work in Syria by Abū l-Faraj ibn Yaʿqūb Ibn al-Quff (d. 685/1286), *Al-ʿUmda fī ṣināʿat al-jirāḥa* ('The Pillar Sustaining the Art of Surgery').[100]

The issue of the practical impact of formal medical scholarship is closely related to that of how accessible formal medical learning was in medieval Islamic society. One of the foremost features of the work of the exponents of the formal tradition was their effort to make the results of their research as widely available as possible. Ḥunayn, for example, wrote a book entitled *Al-Masāʾil fī l-ṭibb* ('Questions on Medicine') in which, following a typically classical model, he posed and answered a broad range of questions of the sort for which aspiring physicians or already established practitioners would need cogent advice and information. This work is also known as his *Al-Madkhal ilā l-ṭibb* ('Introduction to Medicine'), and, in fact, many authors wrote introductory manuals (often with exactly this title) aimed at the aspiring novice.

Formal medical writers also sought to make the results of their work accessible to the literate lay person. The Iraqi physician Ibn Buṭlān (d. 455/ 1063), for example, devotes his *Taqwīm al-ṣiḥḥa* ('The Maintenance of Health') to the presentation in terse tabular form of everything he could collect pertaining to the six Galenic non-naturals, and leaves the reader in no doubt as to why he proceeded in this fashion:

> People are dissatisfied at the length to which the learned pursue their dis-
> cussions and the prolixity encountered when these are set down in writing in
> books; what [lay people] need from the sciences is that which will benefit them,
> not the proofs for these things or their definitions.[101]

The example set by this book was followed by others, in particular by the *Taqwīm al-abdān fī tadbīr al-insān* ('The Proper Assessment of Bodies for the Pursuit of Man's Well Being') by Yaḥyā ibn 'Īsā Ibn Jazla (d. *c.*494/ 1100),[102] and the *Zād al-musāfir wa-qūt al-ḥāḍir* ('Provisions for the Traveller and Sustenance for the Sedentary') by the Tunisian Aḥmad ibn Ibrāhīm Ibn al-Jazzār (d. 369/979).[103] Even a Christian physician like Qusṭā ibn Lūqā found no impediment to writing a book of advice on how the Muslim pilgrim could stay healthy and avoid mishaps on his way to Mecca.[104]

The era of the great Arabic medical compendia may be said to have ended with the *Qānūn* of Ibn Sīnā, but these works long continued to be the focus of creative scholarly attention. No fewer than thirteen later authors wrote commentaries on the *Qānūn* of Ibn Sīnā, and these commentaries, in turn, were the bases for super-commentaries and glosses. It has long been custom-ary to devalue these commentaries as works of no independent importance, but apart from the fact that such criticisms seldom show any sign of real familiarity with the commentary literature, there is much evidence that this view is false. 'Alā' al-Dīn Ibn al-Nafīs (d. 687/1288) is an illustrative example of the genre. In his extensive comments on Ibn Sīnā's *Qānūn*, one will find, to be sure, much which belabours rather basic points and adds nothing to medical knowledge; however, this is balanced by a broad range of his own independent comments and observations, including his famous pronounce-ment on the pulmonary circulation of the blood in his commentary on the anatomy of Ibn Sīnā.[105] Such works are undervalued today because the commentary mode of discourse not only makes them appear to be unoriginal to modern scholars, but also has the deleterious effect of fragmenting the main trends of thought into disconnected comments on discrete points of detail. Ibn al-Nafīs's comments on the pulmonary circulation, for example, were a priori unlikely to provoke further discussion, and in fact did not do so. The main utility of works such as his was twofold: to the physician unable to find or afford copies of such massive classics as the *Qānūn*, they offered access to the main arguments and most important points advanced by the masters; while to the student and lay person, they served to convey something of the gist of the tradition in a distilled and more accessible form.

The period was also characterized by the composition of summary handbooks. Many of the manuscripts of these works are obviously well-used copies, and here too the aim and result was to make the main points of the formal tradition accessible to a larger audience. Some of these manuals were written for use by a physician, as in the case of the *Mā lā yasa'u l-ṭabīb jahluhu* ('Those Things of Which Physicians Dare Not be Ignorant') by Yūsuf ibn Ismā'īl al-Kutubī (wr. 711/1311),[106] but others, pursuing a common theme in ancient Greek medicine, were clearly composed for use by the lay person, such as the early *Man lā yaḥḍuruhu l-ṭabīb* ('He Who Has No Physician to Attend Him') by al-Rāzī.[107]

These efforts on the part of the formal medical authorities were paralleled by a trend to appropriate medical learning and to incorporate it into Islamic literary and popular culture as a whole. In the *Al-Kiyāsa fī aḥkām al-siyāsa* ('Principles for Sagacious Conduct of State') by Ibn al-Ṣaydāwī (wr. 884/1479), for example, fully half of the text is taken up by medical advice to the prince: the main epidemic diseases which may devastate his lands, a wide range of endemic afflictions and personal health problems, and the preparation and use of simple and compound drugs.[108] In his cultural encyclopedia *Al-Nuqāya fī l-'ulūm* ('The Select Work on the Sciences'), Jalāl al-Dīn al-Suyūṭī (d. 911/1505) includes medicine and anatomy among the fourteen topics – including Qur'ānic exegesis, theoretical and applied jurisprudence, grammar, calligraphy, and rhetorical skills – of which the educated Muslim should have a thorough knowledge.[109] Especially prominent was the tendency to represent ancient medical personalities as wise and Islamicly unobjectionable sages in a vast range of popular tales and literary narratives, and in one branch of Arabic literature, the category of 'physician' became the focus of a series of literary compendia, culminating in the *'Uyūn al-anbā' fī ṭabaqāt al-aṭibbā'* ('Pristine Sources of Information on the Classes of Physicians'), a collection of notices on almost 400 medical personalities compiled by the Syrian Aḥmad ibn al-Qāsim Ibn Abī Uṣaybi'a.[110] These works appear to be biographical dictionaries of physicians, and they certainly contain a wealth of valuable historical information. But their literary focus is manifest in the entertaining tales and poetry that figure so prominently in them, as also in the fact that, in many cases, genuinely biographical material (for example, birth and death rates, mention of education or professional interests, etc.) is incidental, highly speculative, or absent altogether. The prominence of the anecdotal element has wrought much mischief among researchers who take these works for straightforward biographical compendia, but at the same time indicates one of the major ways in which aspects of medical learning were assimilated into Arab-Islamic culture.

Of even greater importance in this regard is the so-called *Ṭibb al-nabī*, or 'Medicine of the Prophet'. As we have seen on p. 683, traditions ascribed to the Prophet Muḥammad were often used in the formative period to argue over important issues, including questions involving medicine. It was noticed, for example, that formal medicine sometimes prescribed a medicament which would violate Islamic law (for example, the drinking of alcohol or the ingestion of potions made with ritually unclean or forbidden substances), so the question thus arose: does the prohibition apply in the case of the person for whom the substance might provide a cure? In cases when an illness or injury called for amputation, the question arose of what, on the Judgement Day, God would think of a believer who had tried to escape His will by submitting to the procedure. Such issues were addressed not by posing a direct question and then answering it, but rather by recalling a situation in which the Prophet or one of his respected companions had allegedly dealt with that problem or one analogous to it.

By the mid-ninth century, collections of these sayings and stories, the *ḥadīth*, were including chapters devoted to traditions on medicine. Ibn Abī Shayba has the largest collection of this early material, and his student al-Bukhārī includes in his *Ṣaḥīḥ* a more conservative (in both scope and numbers) selection. If Qusṭā is at all representative, it seems that in early Islamic times formal physicians were very chary of this lore,[111] but the *ḥadīth* collections were extremely influential among Muslims in general, and new traditions, addressing new medical questions, continued to be set in circulation. These materials were repeatedly gathered into separate monographs with titles like 'The Medicine of the Prophet', the most comprehensive being the collection by Ibn Qayyim al-Jawzīya (d. 751/1350).[112]

It is often claimed that these works were written to combat Greek-inspired medicine by providing a more Islamicly acceptable alternative, but in fact the 'Medicine of the Prophet' is but the logical outcome of a continuing interest in medical questions among a religiously educated public which already knew the medical chapters and medical traditions in the *ḥadīth* collections. Far from being the targets of special criticism in this literature, Hippocrates, Dioscorides, Galen, Aristotle, and Plato are all quoted as eminent authorities, and the Greek humoral system permeates the 'Medicine of the Prophet' as thoroughly as it does the formal medicine. It is also sometimes claimed that the 'Medicine of the Prophet' is but bedouin superstition in pious Islamic dress, but this too is wrong. As argued above, these traditions reflect, on the one hand, beliefs and customs common at the popular level among all peoples of the early medieval Near East, not just bedouins, or even Arabs; on the other hand, they represent a process of argument in which the old pagan ideas were often specifically repudiated. The 'Medicine of the Prophet' collections combine formal medical axioms, aphorisms, and basic precepts with popular folklore, common-sense traditions, and religious dictums, and they offer a wide range of medical advice and views on the use and efficacy of many items of materia medica. As in the literary compendia on physicians, the process at work is that of Islamic society assimilating formal medicine on its own terms.

MEDICINE IN ARAB-ISLAMIC SOCIETY

Medical and public-health conditions in the pre-modern Middle East were, in general, as bad as they were in other parts of the world before the advent of modern medicine and the implementation of public-health schemes broad enough to affect the lives of the common person. The vast majority of people were peasants in the agrarian hinterlands, and most of the rest of the population in any given area consisted of labourers in urban centres. Such individuals were rendered especially and constantly susceptible to illness and physical mishap by poverty, hunger, and malnutrition. Fractures and other injuries which today threaten little more than prolonged inconvenience and discomfort, in medieval times were often fatal. Endemic diseases such as dysentery, leprosy, malaria, scurvy, tuberculosis, and typhus were widespread, and parasitic infections and eye diseases like trachoma and conjunctivitis were common.

It is often claimed that Middle Eastern towns were cleaner than their European counterparts, but the evidence against this is overwhelming. There were elaborate sewage disposal systems in some towns (al-Fusṭāṭ in Egypt is the most famous example[113]), but the effective disposal of refuse and waste always depends on the availability of huge amounts of water and the existence and efficient functioning of elaborate (and therefore expensive) networks dedicated to the moving of the enormous masses of refuse which are constantly generated by the various activities of human life. In no medieval town were either water supplies or disposal systems ever up to the formidable task confronting them, and we constantly read of how filthy towns were. Garbage was cast into the streets or nearby bodies of water, dead animals were abandoned without proper disposal, and water supplies were often polluted. Domestic animals in both cities and rural villages were often kept in the home with the family, and vermin infestation of homes, clothing, and hair was almost impossible to prevent or combat.[114]

These problems were, of course, most difficult in urban centres, and it was in such places that epidemic diseases wrought great havoc. Medieval sources usually refer to outbreaks of 'pestilence', and without detailed descriptions of symptoms it is impossible to identify the disease in question. Smallpox is sometimes specifically named, but the greatest scourge was undoubtedly the plague, which devastated the Middle East in a series of outbreaks between

541 and 131/749, largely faded away, and then returned with the Black Death in 747–9/1347–9 and recurred on numerous occasions until the advent of modern medicine in the region in the nineteenth century.[115] Plague mortality in the medieval Middle East is as uncertain as for anywhere else, but it is clear that epidemics often wiped out entire families and even villages. In large cities a single outbreak of the disease could certainly kill tens of thousands of people, and in some cases, as in the Black Death, the mortality was even higher. (➤ Ch. 37 Diseases of civilization; Ch. 51 Public health)

To confront the dangers posed by these medical problems, a wide range of medical practitioners and services emerged in medieval Middle East society. It is worth noting that even if one excludes the purveyors of popular folklore, the formal physicians who remain were themselves a very disparate lot. In religious terms, the formative period is marked by the predominance of Christians, with a smaller number of Jews and pagans. The Christians were particularly prominent, not because of their central position in the translation movement, but rather because of the long tradition of medical learning within the ecclesiastical hierarchy. Many leading clergy in the towns were physicians, and in both urban and rural monasteries, many monks also had some medical expertise. Later trends toward conversion largely eliminated the pagan element and significantly diminished the ranks of the Christian practitioners, while increasing numbers of Muslims entered medical practice, and the Jewish element remained (in so far as we can judge such matters) about the same. But as has been stressed above, the rise of Arab-Islamic medicine created a central discipline within Islamic science and culture which, at the same time, allowed for the participation of many non-Muslims. Christians still dominated the medical profession in Palestine in the tenth century, for example,[116] and in Egypt and North Africa Jewish doctors were very prominent throughout the medieval period.[117]

In intellectual terms, physicians again display a great deal of variation. Formal Islamic medicine was largely Galenic in inspiration, but our sources occasionally refer to what appear to be circles of medical thinking that focused on other sources of influence (for example, the *baqāriṭa*, 'Hippocratics', or the *rawāfisa*, 'followers of Rufus [of Ephesus]') or were sufficiently distinctive to gain separate recognition (for example, the *jundīshābūrīyūn*, the '[doctors] of Jundīshāpūr').[118] Physicians also engaged in vigorous debates over what rendered them qualified practitioners. Some felt that formal study with a teacher was essential, while others considered that knowledge of the classics of the medical literary tradition was what mattered; certain authorities stressed the importance of experience and empirical observation, while others saw the key to medical truth in logical skills and formal reasoning. (➤ Ch. 48 Medical education)

The same diversity is evident in professional terms. Many physicians had other occupations which they practised alongside their medical career, and interests in trade and property appear to have been common. The most eminent doctors had often benefited from a very broad education, and in some cases are better known today for their literary careers, though in their own time their prominence had been in the field of medicine. The most extraordinary example of this is perhaps the Andalusian Ibn Ṭufayl (d. *c*.581/ 1185), the influential court physician of the Muwaḥḥids, but known today almost exclusively for his remarkable tale *Ḥayy ibn Yaqẓān*.[119] Such noted scholars as Ibn Durayd (d. 321/933) and Miskawayh (d. 421/1030) were both trained as physicians, but this aspect of their careers has, in modern times, been entirely obscured by their achievements in other fields: poetry and philology in the former case, history and philosophy in the latter. The links between philosophy and medicine were particularly strong, and such figures as al-Rāzī and Ibn Sīnā excelled in both.

These trends highlight the fact that in medieval Islamic times the medical profession was very fluid: there were no specific requirements to fulfil before practice, no fixed curriculum of study or fixed places where one could learn medicine, and no delineated boundaries defining the profession *per se*. One could practise medicine provided that, and so long as, sufficient means of support – patronage or clientele – existed to make it feasible.

There were various ways to prepare for a medical career.[120] In some instances a great doctor seems to have been self-taught. Ibn Sīnā and Ibn Riḍwān, for example, both claimed to have been self-taught and asserted that it was entirely on their own that they absorbed what the formal tradition had to offer. The special pleading in such claims requires that we take them with some reserve, but they do serve to highlight the broad and fluid bounds of the profession and the often unstructured way in which access to it could be gained.

In many cases a physician would be followed into the profession by his son; this practice assured the latter's education without charge, and also guaranteed him immediate access to books, instruments, and clientele. Family lines of medical men were common in all religious communities, but were especially prominent among the Christians. The families of Ḥunayn ibn Isḥāq and Thābit ibn Qurra (d. 288/901) were prominent examples of this pattern, and the most dramatic case is that of Jibrā'īl ibn Bakhtīshū' (d. 152/769) and his descendants. For three centuries, this famous family from Jundīshāpūr produced successive generations of eminent physicians, pharmacists, and translators, and members of the line served as the personal physicians to numerous caliphs and other rulers of Iraq and Persia. Their renown was such that they became the subject of entertaining and didactic anecdotes, many of which were duly collected and recorded in the literary compendia on physicians, and this lore seems to have figured considerably in the growth of the legend attributing an academy and hospital to their native city as early as Sasanian times.

Other physicians gained their education through study with a formal teacher. At first, teachers instructed students in their homes, and Muslims sometimes taught in the mosques, which were centres for education in any case. Once hospitals were widespread, these were the logical places for medical education to be pursued, since patients for examination were immediately to hand and many hospitals had libraries of medical books attached to them. In the thirteenth century AD, great medical schools began to be founded, complete with hospital facilities, libraries, and student living quarters. Even this, however, did not displace the older custom of study in the master's home. Students embarking on formal medical education were very often quite young, reflecting the widespread social norm that viewed a youth's passage to adulthood as the age of 15 or sexual maturity, whichever occurred first. Ḥunayn ibn Isḥāq made his way to Baghdad at the age of 17, Ibn Sīnā began his studies at 16, and Moses Maimonides (d. 601/1204) was only 13 when he embarked on his medical studies.

Teaching methods also seem to have varied. The reading and mastery of medical and other related texts were very important, but while instruction often focused on the sixteen Galenic works in the *Summaria alexandrinorum*, matters of curriculum were entirely at the discretion of the teacher. Mathematics and logic were also studied the novice had available a vast array of general and specialized manuals, *aides-mémoire*, and other introductory materials, supplemented in the later medieval period by the burgeoning commentary literature focused on the *Qānūn* of Ibn Sīnā. These texts were usually memorized and/or read aloud, and class work consisted of sitting for extended periods of time with a master, who would correct misreadings, clarify obscure passages, and pose and answer relevant questions. When a teacher was satisfied with a student's mastery of a text, the student would be granted permission to teach it with the master's formal approval, thus incorporating the new scholar into an exactly known chain of transmitters and scholars (the *silsila* or *isnād*) extending back to the author of the text in question (or even, if the work was a religious text, to God).

Classes were not always the staid dignified sessions portrayed, for example, by nineteenth-century orientalist painters. Then, as now, teachers were sometimes confronted by a challenging and even defiant attitude on the part of their students. During a session held in the presence of the 'Abbāsid vizier Abū l-Qāsim 'Abd Allāh, al-Rāzī proposed that in certain diseases a physician could eliminate within an hour symptoms which had been building up for days or months. This met with amazement and disbelief among the assembled company, which included some practising physicians, so to settle the issue (and at the request of the vizier) he had to write his *Bur' al-sā'a* ('Healing within an Hour').[121] Resolution of such situations was essential, for the eminence of a physician was, in part, dependent on the extent to which students esteemed him and vied to study with him, and dissatisfied students could – and did – easily leave one teacher for another.[122]

Clinical experience was available in hospitals, but exactly how such opportunities were pursued in pedagogical terms is unclear. It seems that physicians used patients to illustrate various maladies and problems to students accompanying them on their rounds, and it is sometimes implied that students would assume certain basic duties. At a practitioner's office in Fāṭimid Cairo, however, a bit more is known: advanced students would undertake preliminary examinations of patients waiting outside and could perform procedures such as simple venesection. (➤ Ch. 40 Physical methods)

It is clear, however, that medical education concentrated on written texts, and many students must have entered medical practice without ever having treated a patient. We must also conclude that practical knowledge of human anatomy was gradually acquired as a doctor's career proceeded, for knowledge of the internal workings and arrangement of the body could only be gained in *ad hoc* ways, as treatment of individual medical complaints required access to internal tissues and organs. Dissection of cadavers was almost always out of the question, as it was abhorrent to both Muslim and Christian sensibilities for two reasons: first, the belief was widespread that the dead can continue to feel pain, and second, it was considered that dissection was tantamount to mutilation and desecration of the dead. Related to both of these views was the eschatological doctrine in both faiths that at the Last Judgment the dead would be summoned before God in their physical bodies, at which time the full horrors of what had been done would be clear to all and accountable before God. In the early medieval period we are told that Yōḥannān ibn Māsawayh (d. 243/857), the teacher of Ḥunayn ibn Isḥāq, dissected monkeys in order to gain information for an anatomical work, one which eventually won great praise.[123] But this was exceptional in the extreme, and even a cursory glance at the illustrations in the *Tashrīḥ-i manṣūrī* of Ibn Ilyās will demonstrate that such knowledge of anatomy as a practitioner might have, would have been gained piecemeal through the course of a career. (➤ Ch. 5 The anatomical tradition)

While it was widely felt that the competence of physicians should be verified, there was, in fact, no regular system of examinations or other qualifying procedures which one had to complete successfully before beginning to work. There are numerous instances in which an authority enumerates all that a physician should know, but such material is prescriptive rather than descriptive, and closer to the mark is an incident recorded by Thābit ibn Sinān concerning his father, the famous physician Sinān ibn Thābit ibn Qurra (d. 330/942). In 319/931, word reached the caliph in Baghdad that one of the common folk had died at the hands of an incompetent doctor, so the ruler ordered that only physicians who had been examined by Sinān should practise medicine in the capital. This entailed a comprehensive examination of physicians in Baghdad, excluding only those who were too eminent to require review of their cases and physicians in the imperial service. About 860 physicians applied during the first year, and among them was an elderly, well-appointed gentleman who, when pressed, confessed that he had had no formal training and indeed, could hardly read and write, but pleaded that Sinān should not deprive his family of the means for their subsistence by denying him permission to practise medicine. Sinān agreed, provided that the man confine himself strictly to simple maladies and ordinary medications. The next day, the man's son also appeared before Sinān, and was also authorized to practise so long as he too confined himself to medical pursuits in which he was unlikely to do any harm.[124] As this episode clearly illustrates, the examination process was aimed not at establishing a uniform standard for admission to medical practice, but rather to ensure that through a very wide range of acceptable practitioners, individuals should not make pretensions to levels of learning and expertise that they did not actually possess.

In a social and professional system with no precise boundaries defining where one passed from unorthodox medicine to fraud and incompetence, the notion of quackery differed from what the term would connote today. Reputable and competent physicians were always concerned about it, as it tended to discredit formal medicine in general and them in particular, or at least to lower formal medicine to the same level as the popular folklore. And as detailed medical knowledge was restricted to very few persons, others, even the highly educated, could be taken in by tricks and fraud.

Overall, Islamic society was prepared to tolerate a very broad range of practitioners and remedies, in the first instance because the more popular lore, if not legitimated in formal intellectual terms, was nevertheless upheld by equally (or even more) compelling structures of authority – the approval of the Prophet, for example, or the compelling sanction of long-established custom. Further, formal remedies were often unavailable in the countryside, where most people lived; in the cities, formal medicine was often beyond the financial means of the common person. And it could not have passed unobserved that if many folk remedies seemed to be ineffective or even dangerous, the same could be said of many of the formal procedures and drugs. (➤ Ch. 47 History of the medical profession)

What society sought to root out was deliberate fraud: the chemist who adulterated drugs with inert ingredients to make a higher profit, the surgeon who pretended to extract a stone, olive pit, or lizard from a boil he had just excised, the doctor who pretended to cure epilepsy by making a cross-shaped incision in the forehead, and so forth.[125] Such practices were completely unacceptable, but these excepted, both society and the governing authorities were willing to tolerate doctors of many sorts so long as they did not practise beyond their knowledge and expertise.

Access to a physician could be had in a number of ways. Doctors received patients in their homes or in a 'surgery', an open shop like most other business establishments in the medieval Islamic city. Wealthy or favoured patients would receive special attention, but most people with medical complaints could expect to wait at the door until the master was available, and in the meantime, be seen by an attendant or student, who might perform a preliminary examination or simple procedure, such as venesection. On many occasions, a messenger would be sent to the doctor with a description of the patient's problem, and on the basis of this (often ambiguous and minimally helpful) account a written prescription would be issued. At other times, a physician could be summoned to a patient's home, even in the middle of the night, although it was expected that transportation and a fee in advance would be provided. If a patient required constant attention or was in a critical condition, the doctor might take the sufferer into his own home until the crisis had passed or the situation was truly hopeless. The documents from the Cairo Geniza (a cache of discarded medieval Jewish documents on a vast range of topics) suggest that doctors must have been very busy and in high demand, for people sought their advice and assistance even for such minor complaints as headaches or constipation.[126]

Medical examinations involved careful questioning of the patient (and sometimes also of family members and servants), examination and palpation of affected body parts, and uroscopy. Doctors were routinely advised to exercise prudent judgement in discussing the case with others, who might thereafter reveal confusing or frightening details to the sufferer, and visitors were also a source of concern as potential busybodies who might contradict the physician's diagnosis and treatment. Second and third opinions were sometimes sought, however, and it was the patient's right to be fully satisfied with the correctness of the doctor's decisions and conclusions. (➤ Ch. 35 The art of diagnosis: medicine and the five senses; Ch. 34 History of the doctor–patient relationship)

Arab-Islamic medicine always gave highest priority to the preservation of good health, but once this had been lost, many means were used to restore it. The vast materia medica of the medieval period included thousands of herbs and drugs, but of these a much smaller number were, of course, the staple of the trade. Medications were often prepared by the actual physician, and some prescriptions provided that if the medication were supplied from elsewhere, it should be taken only in the doctor's presence. If surgery was required, the doctor would have access to a wide range of specialized surgical instruments, the scope and complexity of which are immediately evident from the drawings in the *Taṣrīf* of al-Zahrāwī. For the relief of pain, both numbing drugs and actual anaesthetic agents were available. (➤ Ch. 39 Drug therapies)

Payment of the physician seems to have been due upon conclusion of the case treatment, and fees varied widely according to the means of the patient and the renown of the physician. If the patient died, the family could institute proceedings against the doctor if they felt that the diagnosis had been wrong or the treatment inappropriate. Witnesses and the written prescriptions could be produced in evidence, and if found guilty of malpractice, the unfortunate doctor could be heavily fined and/or barred from further practice. For Christian and Jewish doctors, this system of redress must have posed a serious dilemma, since in Islamic court proceedings the testimony of non-Muslims against Muslims was not accepted.[127] (➤ Ch. 37 History of medical ethics; Ch. 69 Medicine and the law)

It is seldom appreciated how far the influence of Arab-Islamic medicine extended into medieval society. Accounts of private nurses and exotic and expensive treatments give the impression that formal medicine was available only to the wealthy, but there is much evidence of efforts to extend care to less fortunate divisions of society as well. In the cities, doctors were sometimes appointed to visit prisons to tend to persons suffering the effects of the appalling health conditions there, and similar visits were arranged for lunatic asylums as well.[128] Efforts were also made to extend medical care to rural areas, where, in almost all regions and periods in medieval Islamic history, most people lived. In Egypt and Syria in the eleventh and twelfth centuries AD, for example, small towns and large villages all seem to have had at least one, and sometimes more than one, formal physician; and in Iraq a century earlier, specific arrangements were made for medical teams to tour the agrarian hinterland to tend to the needs of the peasantry. References to impassable roads, the need for guides, and raging outbreaks of epidemic disease suggest that these journeys were of considerable danger and difficulty.[129]

Physicians also had other duties to fulfil, some of them quite bureaucratic. Prescriptions were formal legal documents, and recording and filing them seems to have been a major organizational exercise. Doctors were also frequently called upon to make official statements of their findings, as for example, in the case of a leper seeking confirmation of the condition so as to gain access to communal support funds.[130] Jewish physicians were often leaders of their local communities, and Muslims often found themselves in bureaucracy-bound positions such as medical inspector, chief physician of the army, medical superintendent at this or that hospital, and so forth.[131]

The hospital was perhaps the crowning achievement of medieval Arab-Islamic medical practice.[132] These institutions appear to have been generally inspired by the precedent of poor- and sick-relief services offered at Christian monasteries and other ecclesiastical establishments (but not an alleged academy-cum-hospital at Jundīshāpūr), although the Islamic hospital was a far more elaborate medical institution. The first hospital foundation by Muslims is often attributed to the Umayyad caliph al-Walīd (r. 86–96/705–15) and placed in Damascus, but the oldest accounts of the episode in question clearly refer simply to the restriction and feeding of lepers, not to a hospital, and this in the Arabian town of Medina, not Damascus. So far as the extant information allows us to judge, the first Islamic hospital seems to be that founded by Jibrā'īl ibn Bakhtīshū' on the orders of Hārūn al-Rashīd *c*.190/ 805. This was followed by similar constructions elsewhere, and by the twelfth century AD a hospital was an essential feature of any large Islamic town. (➤ Ch. 49 The hospital)

Hospitals were in all known cases established and funded as acts of personal charity and not as matters of state policy, although the founders were most often rulers or highly placed administrators. The founding of a hospital involved formally setting aside the revenues from specified properties as a religious trust (*waqf*) which would defray the costs of providing the services stipulated by the endower. Such endowments were to survive in perpetuity, and as every aspect of the arrangement was spelled out in the endowment deed in minute detail, a great deal is known about several hospitals for which these deeds survive. (➤ Ch. 62 Charity before *c*.1850)

Hospitals were almost always complex institutions, with separate facilities for men and women, in-patient and out-patient departments, and wards for different kinds of diseases and afflictions and different medical procedures (for example, ophthalmological complaints as opposed to the setting of broken bones). Some seem to have specialized to a certain extent, or at least had more than usually prominent facilities for the insane, the poor, or army officers. The hospital precinct usually included kitchen and pharmacy facilities, a mosque or some other place for prayer, and audience or lecture rooms, and very often there was a bath and a library stocked with medical books. The better-endowed hospitals were spectacular places built to the highest architectural standard, with pools, streams of running water, and small groves of trees where patients (and, presumably, staff as well) could relax.

The self-contained medical community so created attracted both students and practising physicians, and association with a leading hospital seems to have been regarded by the public as a sign of particular eminence. Doctors regularly made rounds at the hospitals and seem to have used both patients and library facilities to teach their students. As the hospital was established as a pious act of charity, admission to it was free; in some cases provisions were made not only for poor inmates to receive their treatment, lodging, and board without charge, but also for them to be given a stipend upon discharge, to support them for a time until they could resume their former positions in society.

Impressive as they were as individual institutions, Islamic hospitals should not be regarded as having played the leading role in health care in medieval Islam. They were, in all cases, extremely limited compared to the vast size of the populations they were called upon to serve (in much the same way that a shelter in a modern Western city does not meet the problem of homelessness), and their effective function must always have been rather to demonstrate and promote ideals of compassion and charity and to serve as focuses for the activities and expansion of the medical profession. In so far as it was possible to offer meaningful medical care at all, given the scientific, technological, and logistical limitations of the times, this remained the effective domain of the individual practitioner.

POSTSCRIPT

The medical system described in the foregoing pages survived in the Middle East until the nineteenth century, when it gradually receded before the advance of modern Western medicine. In some cases, this was introduced and promoted by indigenous regimes (as in Egypt), and in others, came with Western economic interests and missionary groups (as in Lebanon, Syria, and Iran). Ironically enough, it is the popular medicine ensconced in the 'Medicine of the Prophet' which has best resisted the challenge of the West. When the great medical classics of al-Majūsī and Ibn Sīnā were first printed in Cairo in the 1870s, this was undertaken as a contribution to medical science, not to the history of Arab-Islamic culture.[133] Even then, however, formal medical practice had already shifted to European practitioners and Egyptians who had studied Western medicine with them, especially at the Qaṣr al-'Aynī Medical School.[134] As Unani medicine, the system created by Ibn Sīnā survives in the Indian subcontinent and other areas where Indian influence is strong, but elsewhere it has been almost entirely overthrown. (➤ Ch. 33 Indian medicine) In Arab lands, what survives of the old Islamic medical heritage is the 'Medicine of the Prophet'; books on it sell in huge numbers (the work of Ibn Qayyim al-Jawzīya is especially popular), and its practical advice is, in many circles, known and followed in detail. Its influence can even be detected outside the region. Surveys among Muslims in Britain, for example, show that the contents of the 'Medicine of the Prophet' are well known, and that many regard it as medically effective. Efforts to show that common ground can be found between it and modern medicine have resulted in numerous monographs and discussions in medical journals in Islamic countries.[135]

The reasons for this survival can be viewed from both a negative and a positive perspective. The negative would have to do with the problems involved in promoting a culturally intrusive, complex, urban-based, and extremely expensive medical system from without, and would take us far from the concerns of this discussion. From a positive perspective, however, it perhaps offers a useful concluding point by drawing our attention to the continuing dynamic interplay between medical systems that compete without gaining absolute mastery, one over the other, and the continuing importance of traditional and religious considerations in a changing world – both of these have been formative factors in the medical history of the Middle East for the past 1,500 years.

NOTES

1 The best introduction to the history of medicine in the medieval Middle East is Manfred Ullmann, *Islamic Medicine*, Edinburgh, Edinburgh University Press, 1978. For other accounts, see Further Reading at the end of this chapter.

2 On medical literature in the medieval Middle East, see Carl Brockelmann, *Geschichte des arabischen Literatur*, 2nd edn, Leiden, E. J. Brill, 1943–9, Vol. I, pp. 231–40; Vol. II, pp. 136–8, 169–70, 189, 213–14, 233, 257, 364–5, 414, 447, 465; see also the further material in the corresponding parts of the *Supplementbände*, Leiden, E. J. Brill, 1937–42; Manfred Ullmann, *Die Medizin im Islam*, Leiden, E. J. Brill, 1970; Fuat Sezgin, *Geschichte des arabischen Schrifttums*, Vol. III: *Medizin – Pharmacie – Zoologie – Tierheilkunde bis ca. 430 H.*, Leiden, E. J. Brill, 1970, pp. 3–340.

3 On these developments, see A. A. Duri, *The Historical Formation of the Arab Nation: a Study in Identity and Consciousness*, trans. by Lawrence I. Conrad, London, Croom Helm, 1987, pp. 4–133.

4 For example, see Edward G. Browne, *Arabian Medicine*, Cambridge, Cambridge University Press, 1921, p. 7.

5 See Richard W. Bulliet, *Conversion to Islam in the Medieval Period: an Essay in Quantitative History*, Cambridge, MA, Harvard University Press, 1979; Michael G. Morony, 'The age of conversions: a reassessment', in Michael Gervers and Ramzi Jibran Bikhazi (eds), *Conversion and Continuity: Indigenous Christian Communities in Islamic Lands, Eighth to Eighteenth Centuries*, Toronto, Pontifical Institute of Mediaeval Studies, 1990, pp. 135–50.

6 See, for example, René Dussaud, *La Pénétration des Arabes en Syrie avant l'Islam*, Paris, Paul Geuthner, 1955.

7 The relevant sources on this subject have not yet been exploited to full advantage. Useful studies are Georg Jacob, *Altarabisches Beduinenleben*, Berlin, Mayer & Müller, 1897, pp. 154–8; Ullmann, op. cit. (n. 1), pp. 1–6. The discussion here is largely based on the materials collected in Ibn Abī Shayba (d. 235/849), al-*Muṣannaf*, 'Abd al-Khāliq al-Afghānī, Bombay, Al-Dār al-salafīya, 1399–1403/1979–83, 7: 359–457; Ibn Abī Sarḥ (wr. 274/887–8), *Kitāb al-rumūz*, ed. S. M. Ḥusayn, in *Révue de l'Académie Arabe de Damas*, 1931, 11:

641–55; Ibn Abī l-Ḥadīd (d. 656/1258), *Sharḥ nahj al-balāgha*, ed. Muḥammad Abū l'Faḍl Ibrāhīm, Cairo, 'Īsā al-Bābī al-Ḥalabī, 1959–64, 19: 372–429.

8   Truffles were not a delicacy; they grew wild in the desert and could be detected and dug up in the late winter months, usually February.

9   Cf. Avner Giladi, 'Some notes on *Taḥnīk* in medieval Islam', *Journal of Near Eastern Studies*, 1988, 47: 175–9.

10 See Julius Wellhausen, *Reste arabischen Heidentums*, 2nd edn, Berlin, Georg Reimer, 1897; Toufic Fahd, *La Divination Arabe: Études religieuses, sociologiques et folkloriques sur le Milieu natif de l'Islam*, Leiden, E. J. Brill, 1966; and more generally, Hamilton A. R. Gibb, *Studies on the Civilization of Islam*, Boston, MA, Beacon Press, 1962, pp. 176–87.

11 See Ernst Seidel, 'Die Lehre von der Kontagion bei den Arabern', *Archiv für Geschichte der Medizin*, 1913, 6: 81–93; Lawrence I. Conrad, *Epidemic Disease in Formal and Popular Thought in Early Islamic Society*, Berlin, Walter de Gruyter, 1992.

12 For a detailed discussion of this custom, see Conrad, ibid.

13 Ibn Sa'd (d. 230/844), *Kitāb al-ṭabaqāt al-kabīr*, ed. by Eduard Sachau *et al.*, Leiden, E. J. Brill, 1904–40, Vol. IV.1: 86–7.

14 Ibn Abī Sarḥ, op. cit. (n. 7), p. 647.

15 Here referring to the *munajjis*, one who knew which unclean things could be used to ward off which spirits, spells, and illnesses.

16 Ancient Arabic poetry frequently speaks of the practitioner of *ṭibb* as identical to the purveyor of charms and incantations, or *ruqā*, and the medieval commentaries regard this correspondence as a matter of common knowledge. See, for example, *Dīwān al-hudhalīyīn*, edited in the recension of al-Sukkarī (d. 275/888) by 'Abd al-Sattār Aḥmad Farrāj and Maḥmūd Muḥammad Shākir, Cairo, Maṭba'at al-Madanī, 1385/1965, 1: 236, 3rd verse and the commentary; Abū l-Faraj al-Iṣfahānī (d. 356/967), *Kitāb al-aghānī*, ed. by Naṣr al-Hūrīnī, Cairo, Dār al-ṭibā'a, A. H. 1285, 10: 136, 8th verse. Cf. also the revealing and early accounts in Ibn Hishām (d. 218/833), *Sīrat Rasū Allāh*, ed. by Ferdinand Wüstenfeld, Göttingen, Dieterische Universitäts-Buchhandlung, 1858–60, I.1, 188; Ibn Abī Shayba, *Muṣannaf*, 7: 387–9 nos. 3569–70. Cf. also Felix Klein-Franke, *Vorlesungen über die Medizin im Islam*, Wiesbaden, Franz Steiner Verlag, 1982, pp. 8–13.

17 See, for example, Ibn Sa'd, *Ṭabaqāt*, 5: 371–2; Ibn Abī Shayba, *Muṣannaf*, 7: 452 no. 3769.

18 'Urwa ibn al-Ward, *Dīwān*, ed. by Karam al-Bustānī, Beirut, Dār Ṣādir, [n.d.], p. 46.

19 Ibn Abī Sarḥ, op. cit. (n. 7), p. 646.

20 Al-Nābigha al-Dhubyānī, *Dīwān*, ed. by Fawzī Khalīl 'Aṭawī, Beirut, Al-Sharika al-lubnānīya li-l-kitāb, 1969, p. 83, 3rd verse.

21 See Lawrence I. Conrad, 'The social structure of medicine in medieval Islam', *Bulletin of the Society for the Social History of Medicine*, 1985, 37: 14.

22 Sūrat al-Tawba (9), v. 91; Sūrat al-Nūr (24), v. 61; Sūrat al-Fatḥ (48), v. 17. See Arthur J. Arberry, *The Koran Interpreted*, Oxford, Oxford University Press, 1964, pp. 190, 360, 533.

23 Sūrat al-Nisā' (4), v. 43; Sūrat al-Mā'ida (5), v. 6; = Arberry *The Koran Interpreted*, Oxford, Oxford University Press, 1964, pp. 79, 100.

24 Sūrat al-Naḥl (16), v. 69; = Arberry, op. cit. (n. 23), pp. 265–6.

25 See the materials collected in Paul Arno Eichler, *Dschinn, Teufel und Engel im Koran*, Leipzig, Verlag der Buchhandlung Klein, 1928.

26 This phenomenon has recently been highlighted in the excellent study by Vivian Nutton, 'Healers in the medical market place: towards a social history of Graeco-Roman medicine', in Andrew Wear (ed.), *Medicine in Society: Historical Essays*, Cambridge, Cambridge University Press, 1992, pp. 15–58.

27 There is a vast literature on this material. See, for example, Victor Paul Hamilton, 'Syriac incantation bowls', unpublished Ph.D. thesis, Brandeis University, 1971; Joseph Naveh and Shaul Shaked, *Amulets and Magic Bowls: Aramaic Incantations of Late Antiquity*, 2nd edn, Jerusalem, Magnes Press, 1987. Stimulating new approaches in interpretation are suggested in various studies by Erica Hunter, such as her 'Saints in Syriac anathemas: a form-critical analysis of role', *Journal of Semitic Studies*, 1987, 32: 83–104.

28 E. A. Wallis Budge (ed.), *Syrian Anatomy, Pathology and Therapeutics, or 'the Book of Medicines'*, London, Oxford University Press, 1913.

29 Alexander of Tralles, *Oeuvres médicales d'Alexandre de Tralles*, ed. by F. Brunet, Paris, Paul Geuthner, 1933–7.

30 For an excellent account of this process, see Andrew Rippin, *Muslims: their Beliefs and Practices*, Vol. I: *The Formative Period*, London, Routledge, 1990.

31 Aspects of this are discussed in Ibn Abī Shayba, *Muṣannaf*, 7: 373, 374, 385–6, nos. 3515, 3518–20, 3559–61, 3564.

32 See Michael W. Dols, 'Plague in early Islamic history', *Journal of the American Oriental Society*, 1974, 94: 371–83; Lawrence I. Conrad, 'The plague in the early medieval Near East', unpublished Ph.D. thesis, Princeton University, 1981.

33 On the course of these discussions, see Conrad, op. cit. (n. 11).

34 These were Sūrat al-Fātiḥa (1), and the *mu'awwadhatān*, the last two chapters, Sūrat al-Falaq (113) and Sūrat al-Nās (114); = Arberry, pp. 1, 668–9.

35 Al-Bukhārī (d. 256/870), *Al-Jāmi' al-ṣaḥīḥ*, ed. by Ludolf Krehl and T. W. Juynboll, Leiden, E. J. Brill, 1864–1908, 4: 61, *Ṭibb* no. 33.

36 Al-Jāḥiẓ, *Kitāb al-ḥayawān*, ed. by 'Abd al-Salām Muḥammad Harun, Cairo, Muṣṭafā al-Bābī al-Ḥalabī, 1384–9/1965–9, 1: 17.

37 Ibn Abī Shayba, *Muṣannaf*, 7: 359 no. 3465. For other variants in the later authoritative collections, see A. J. Wensinck, *Concordance et indices de la tradition musulman*, Leiden, E. J. Brill, 1936–88, 2: 156b–157a.

38 Conrad, op. cit. (n. 11).

39 Ibn Abī Shayba, *Muṣannaf*, 7: 451 nos. 3764–5.

40 For example, al-Jāḥiẓ, *Ḥayawān*, 6: 358–9.

41 Al-Maydānī (d. 518/1124), *Majma' al-amthāl*, ed. by Muḥammad Muḥyī l'Dīn 'Abd al-Ḥamīd, Cairo, Maṭba'at al-sunna al-muḥammadīya, 1374/1955, 2: 42a no. 2591.

42 These beliefs are discussed in detail in Michael W. Dols, *The Black Death in the Middle East*, Priceton, Princeton University Press, 1977, pp. 117–42.

43 These were often commented upon by travellers and explorers. Particularly

interesting accounts are John Lewis Burckhardt, *Notes on the Bedouins and Wahábys*, London, Colburn & Bentley, 1831, Vol. I, pp. 90–6; Vol. II, pp. 61–2; William Gifford Palgrave, *Narrative of a Year's Journey through Central and Eastern Arabia (1862–63)*, London and Cambridge, Macmillan, 1866, Vol. II, pp. 1–37; H. R. P. Dickson, *The Arab of the Desert*, 2nd edn, London, George Allen & Unwin, 1951, pp. 505–15.

44   Hermann Gollancz (ed.), *The Book of Protection*, London, Oxford University Press, 1912.

45   See Lawrence I. Conrad, 'The plague in Bilād al-Shām in pre-Islamic times', in Muḥammad 'Adnān al-Bakhīt and Muḥammad 'Aṣfūr (eds), *Proceedings of the Symposium on Bilād al-Shām during the Byzantine Period*, Amman, University of Jordan, 1986, Vol. II, pp. 143–63; Conrad, op. cit. (n. 32).

46   See, for example, the case of Syria, as elaborated in two important studies by Hugh Kennedy, 'From polis to *Madina*: urban change in late antique and early Islamic Syria', *Past and Present*, 1985, 106: 3–27; 'The last century of Byzantine Syria: a reinterpretation', *Byzantinische Forschungen*, 1985, 10: 141–83.

47   These patterns of change are well described in John F. Haldon, *Byzantium in the Seventh Century: the Transformation of a Culture*, Cambridge, Cambridge University Press, 1990, pp. 348–75, 425–35.

48   'Alī ibn Riḍwān (d. c.460/1067) states that before the accession of the Umayyad caliph 'Umar ibn 'Abd al-'Azīz (r. 99–101/717–20), the prince encouraged certain Alexandrian physicians to convert to Islam; when he became caliph, education passed to Antioch and Ḥarrān. See the extended passage cited in A. Z. Iskandar, 'An attempted reconstruction of the late Alexandrian medical curriculum', *Medical History*, 1976, 20: 249. This statement is often taken as meaning that the Alexandrian 'medical school' continued in existence until the reign of this caliph. However, apart from the fact that the passage in question says nothing of the sort, it must be borne in mind that no earlier authority knows anything about this, and that by the time of 'Alī ibn Riḍwān it had become absolutely typical for 'Umar ibn 'Abd al-'Azīz to be exalted as the only true Muslim ruler of the fallen Umayyad house, and thus to be credited with all kinds of virtues, initiatives, and achievements of which earlier sources, despite their own detailed treatment of him, know absolutely nothing.

49   See Paul van den Ven, 'La patristique et l'hagiographie au concile de Nicée de 787', *Byzantion*, 1955–7, 25–7: 325–62; and the seminal study of Cyril Mango, 'The availability of books in the Byzantine Empire, AD 750–850', in *Byzantine Books and Bookmen*, Washington, DC, Dumbarton Oaks, 1975, pp. 29–45.

50   Cf. the parallel observation by Richard Walzer, concerning Islamic philosophy, in his *Greek into Arabic: Essays on Islamic Philosophy*, Oxford, Bruno Cassirer, 1962, p. 35.

51   Witness, for example, the great bulk of thoroughly 'worldly' poetry written in Arabic, and the translation of Homer into Syriac by Theophilus of Edessa in the early or mid-eighth century.

52   See Averil Cameron, 'New themes and styles in Greek literature: seventh–eighth centuries', in Cameron and Lawrence I. Conrad (eds), *The Byzantine and Early*

Islamic Near East, Vol. I: *Problems in the Literary Sources*, Princeton, NJ, Darwin Press, 1992, p. 88.

53   See, for example, Cyril Elgood, *A Medical History of Persia and the Eastern Caliphate*, Cambridge, Cambridge University Press, 1951, pp. 46–50, 66; Heinz H. Schöffler, *Die Akademie von Gondischapur. Aristoteles auf dem Wege in den Orient*, Stuttgart, Artemis, 1979.

54   On Jundīshāpūr, see Lawrence I. Conrad and Vivian Nutton, *Jundīshāpūr: from Myth to History*, where the material on al-Ḥārith is also discussed; see also G. R. Hawting, 'The development of the biography of al-Ḥārith ibn Kalada and the relationship between medicine and Islam', in C. E. Bosworth *et al.* (eds), *Essays in Honor of Bernard Lewis: the Islamic World from Classical to Modern Times*, Princeton, NJ, Darwin Press, 1989, pp. 127–40.

55   Ṣāʿid al-Andalusī, *Ṭabaqāt al-umam*, ed. by Ḥayāt Bū-ʿAlwān, Beirut, Dār al-ṭalīʿa, 1985, pp. 126–7.

56   Al-Jāḥiẓ, *Faḍl Hāshim ʿalā ʿAbd Shams*, preserved in Ibn Abī l-Ḥadīd, *Sharḥ nahj al-balāgha*, 15: 258. Cf. also al-Nadīm (wr. *c.*377/987), *Kitāb al-fihrist*, ed. by Riḍā-Tajaddud, Tehran, Maṭbaʿat Dānishgāh, 1391/1971, pp. 303, 304, 419.

57   See, for example, Charles Pellat, *Le Milieu baṣrien et la formation de Ǧāḥiz*, Paris, Adrien-Maisonneuve, 1953; Hichem Djaït, *Al-Kūfa: Naissance de la ville islamique*, Paris, G.-P. Maisonneuve et Larose, 1986.

58   On Baghdad, see Robert McC. Adams, *Land Behind Baghdad*, Chicago, IL, University of Chicago Press, 1965, pp. 84–102; Jacob Lassner, *The Topography of Baghdad in the Early Middle Ages*, Detroit, MI, Wayne State University Press, 1970, esp. p. 160 (population).

59   See G. J. Reinink and H. L. J. Vanstiphout (eds), *Dispute Poems and Dialogues in the Ancient and Medieval Near East*, Leuven, Peeters, 1991.

60   On the Manichaeans in general, see Samuel N. C. Lieu, *Manichaeism in the Later Roman Empire and Medieval China*, 2nd edn, Tübingen, J. C. B. Möhr, 1992. Their impact in Islamic society is discussed in Michelangelo Guidi, *La lotta tra l'Islam e il Manicheismo*, Rome, Fondazione Caetani per gli studi Musulmani, 1927; Johann Fück, *Arabische Kultur und Islam im Mittelalter*, Weimar, Hermann Böhlaus Nachfolger, 1981, pp. 258–71.

61   Anastasius of Sinai, *Quaestiones et Responsiones*, PG 89, cols. 765A-B.

62   See Samīr Khalīl, 'Maqālat "Fī l'ājāl" li-Ḥunayn ibn Isḥāq', *Al-Mashriq*, 1991, 65: 403–25.

63   See Lawrence I. Conrad, 'Theophanes and the Arabic literary tradition: some indications of intercultural transmission', *Byzantinische Forschungen*, 1990, 15: 31–3.

64   See Anastasius of Sinai, *Hodegos*, PG 89, cols. 184–5. It is to be noticed that the context here is that of confessional polemics.

65   Ṣāʿid al-Andalusī, for example, speaks of 'ancient books' being brought back by Muslim troops 'from Ankara and other places in Roman territory'; see his *Ṭabaqāt al-umam*, p. 101.

66   See Walzer, op. cit. (n. 50), pp. 175–200, on the philosopher al-Kindī (d. 256/870), a contemporary of the translation movement.

67   On the reign of al-Maʾmūn, with the various cultural matters discussed above,

see the important study by M. Rekaya in his article 'al-Ma'mūn', in *EI²*, Leiden, E. J. Brill, 1991, 6: 331–9.

68 See, for example, Dominique Sourdel, 'Bayt al-Ḥikma', in *EI²*, Leiden, E. J. Brill, 1960, 1: 1141a.

69 Lucien Leclerc refers to more than a hundred translators known to have been active during the reign of al-Ma'mūn; see his *Histoire de la médecine arabe*, Paris, Ernest Leroux, 1876, Vol. I, p. 154.

70 See the list and discussion in Samīr, op. cit. (n. 62), pp. 413–14; also Paul Nwyia, 'Actualité du concept de religion chez Ḥunayn ibn Isḥāq', in Gérard Troupeau (ed.), *Ḥunayn ibn Isḥāq*, Leiden, E. J. Brill, 1975, pp. 313–17.

71 See Ibn Abī Uṣaybi'a, '*Uyūn al-anbā*', 1: 200. The Manichaean argument under attack would have been that the existence of vast oceans full of salt water shows that the physical world does not reflect an all-encompassing divine plan (because God creates useless things), or that the monotheists' God is an unjust trifler, creating useless salt water in unlimited supply, while along the very shores of these seas His worshippers suffer from drought and thirst. Arguments over such issues were, in fact, very common.

72 See Gotthelf Bergsträsser, *Ḥunain ibn Isḥāq über die syrischen und arabischen Galen-Übersetzungen*, Leipzig, F. A. Brockhaus, 1925; also his edition and translation of a different recension of the work in his *Neue Materialien zu Ḥunain ibn Isḥāq's Galen-Bibliographie*, Leipzig, F. A. Brockhaus, 1932.

73 Al-Mas'ūdī, *Al-Tanbīh wa-l-ishrāf*, ed. by M. J. de Goeje, Leiden, E. J. Brill, 1894, p. 112.

74 Cf., for example, Bergsträsser, op. cit. (n. 72), p. 47, no. 115, a case in which searching all through Mesopotamia and across Syria and Palestine as far as Alexandria in Egypt failed to locate even *one* complete Greek manuscript of the text in question.

75 Ibn Al-Nadīm, *Fihrist*, pp. 303–4.

76 Cf. Walzer, op. cit. (n. 50), p. 118, for a similar reservation: Ḥunayn would not have needed to go to Byzantium to learn Greek.

77 See Ullmann, op. cit. (n. 1), pp. 15–20; Sezgin, op. cit. (n. 2), Vol. III, pp. 172–202.

78 Such, at least, is my reading of his *Treatise on the Smallpox and Measles*, trans. by William Alexander Greenhill, London, Sydenham Society, 1848, p. 28.

79 See, for example, Franz Rosenthal, *The Approach and Technique of Muslim Scholarship*, Rome, Pontificum Institutum Biblicum, 1947; Johannes Pedersen, *The Arabic Book*, trans. by Geoffrey French, Princeton, NJ, Princeton University Press, 1984, pp. 20–88; and especially Walzer, op. cit. (n. 50), pp. 70–3.

80 For example, in his *Kitāb al-nuqaṭ*, ed. by Louis Cheikho in *Al-Mashriq*, 1922, 20: 373. Cf. also his marginalia to his translation of Galen's *On Medical Experience*, ed. and trans. by Richard Walzer, London, Oxford University Press, 1944, pp. 37 (text), 114 (trans.).

81 The dramatic difference between the way Ḥunayn's contemporary al-Kindī expressed sophisticated philosophical ideas, and the way these same concepts were articulated by thinkers of the following century, is a vivid illustration of this. An essay on the eye by one of Ḥunayn's teacher's, the *Daghal al-'ayn* of Yōḥannān ibn Māsawayh (d. 243/857), is an obvious reflection of the problems

(awkward sentence structures, excessive and obscure use of loan words from Greek, Syriac, and Pahlavi) involved in scientific expression in a language which yet lacks the means to articulate such ideas clearly. See P. Prüfer and M. Meyerhof, 'Die Augenheilkunde des Jûḥannâ ibn Mâsawaih', *Der Islam*, 1916, 6: 217–56.

82 Ullmann, op. cit. (n. 1), p. 9.

83 See Ibn Abī Uṣaybiʿa (d. 668/1270), '*Uyūn al-anbāʾ fī ṭabaqāt al-aṭibbāʾ*, ed. by August Müller, Königsberg, A. Müller, and Cairo, Al-Maṭbaʿa al-wahbīya, 1882–4, Vol. I, pp. 203–6.

84 *The Book of the Ten Treatises on the Eye ascribed to Ḥunain ibn Isḥāq*, ed. and trans. by Max Meyerhof, Cairo, Government Press, 1928.

85 See G. Haydar (ed. and trans.), 'Das Buch über die Kohabitation und die für ihre Ausübung notwendigen körperlichen Voraussetzungen', unpublished Ph.D. thesis, Erlangen-Nürnberg, 1973; Martin Pelster (ed. and trans.), '*Die Abhandlung des Qusṭā Ibn Lūqā über die Länge und Kürze des Lebens und die Physiognomie der Langlebigen*', unpublished Ph.D. thesis, Universität Mainz, 1985; Hartmut Fähndrich (ed. and trans.), *Abhandlung über die Ansteckung von Qusṭā Ibn Lūqā*, Stuttgart, Deutsche Morgenländische Gesellschaft, 1987; *Qusṭā Ibn Lūqāʾs Medical Regime for the Pilgrims to Mecca*, ed. and trans. by Gerrit Bos Leiden, E. J. Brill, 1992.

86 See n. 78.

87 *Firdaws al-ḥikma*, ed. by M. Z. Siddiqi, Berlin, Charlottenburg, 1928.

88 On this Indian material see Alfred Siggel, *Die indischen Bücher aus dem Paradies der Weisheit über die Medizin des ʿAlī ibn Sahl Rabban aṭ-Ṭabarī*, Wiesbaden, Franz Steiner Verlag, 1951. In the period just prior to the reign of al-Maʾmūn there were several prominent Indian physicians at the ʿAbbāsid court. See Ibn Abī Uṣaybiʾa, '*Uyūn al-anbāʾ*, 2: 33–5.

89 The Arabic edition and Latin translation of the *Manṣūrī* prepared by Johann Jacob Reiske and published posthumously in Halle in 1776 is practically impossible to access. On the Arabic manuscripts. and Latin translation and commentaries, see Sezgin, op. cit. (n. 2), pp. 281–3.

90 Al-Rāzī, *Al-Ḥāwī fī l-ṭibb*, Hyderabad, Dāʾirat al-maʿārif al-ʿuthmānīya, 1374–90/1955–70. A valuable collection of clinical extracts from the text has been published by Max Meyerhof, 'Thirty-three clinical observations by Rhazes (circa 900 AD)', *Isis*, 1935, 23: 321–56.

91 Al-Majūsī, *Kāmil al-ṣināʿa al-ṭibbīya*, Cairo, Al-Maṭbaʿa al-amīrīya, A. H. 1294.

92 Ibn Sīnā, *Al-Qānūn fī l-ṭibb*, Cairo, Al-Maṭbaʿa al-amīrīya, A. H. 1294.

93 This section has been edited and translated by M. S. Spink and G. L. Lewis, *Albucasis on Surgery and Instruments*, London, Wellcome Institute for the History of Medicine, 1973.

94 See Cyril Elgood, *A Medical History of Persia* and the Eastern Caliphate, Cambridge, Cambridge University Press, 1951, pp. 214–8; Ullmann, op. cit. (n. 2), p. 161.

95 A critical edition and translation of the *Tashrīḥ-i Manṣūrī* is presently in preparation by Andrew Newman, and Emilie Savage-Smith is engaged in a detailed study of the tradition of anatomical illustration which the diagrams in this text represent.

96 Apparently this was a particular concern of al-Rāzī himself, who devoted a special work to such problems. See Ibn Abī Uṣaybiʻa, '*Uyūn al-anbāʾ*', 1: 318.

97 Ibn al-Bayṭār, *Al-Jāmiʻ li-mufradāt al-adwiya wa-l-aghdiya*, Cairo, Al-Maṭbaʻa al-amīrīya, A. H. 1291.

98 See Ekmeleddin Ihsanoglu, *Fihris makhṭūṭāt al-ṭibb al-islāmī bi-l-lughāt al-ʻarabīya wa-l-turkīya wa-l-fārisīya fī maktabāt Turkīyā*, Istanbul, Research Centre for Islamic History, Art and Culture, 1984.

99 Ibid., pp. 54–76, no. 43.

100 Ibn al-Quff, *Al-ʻUmda fī ṣināʻat al-jirāḥa*, Hyderabad, Dāʾirat al-maʻarif al-ʻuthmānīya, 1356/1937.

101 Ibn Buṭlān, *Taqwīm al-ṣiḥḥa bi-l-asbāb al-sitta*, ed. and trans. by Hosam Elkhadem, Leuven, Peeters, 1990, pp. 71 (Arabic), 146 (trans.).

102 *Arabic Medicine in the Eleventh Century as Represented in the Works of Ibn Jazlah*, ed. and trans. by Joseph Salvatore Graziani Karachi, Hamdard Academy, 1980.

103 An edition of the first three of the seven books of the text has recently been published by Muḥammad Suwaysī and al-Rāḍī al-Jāzī, Tunis, Al-Dār al-ʻarabīya li-l-kitāb, 1986, but on the basis of defective manuscript materials. A complete edition and English translation of this important work is currently in preparation by Gerrit Bos. The title of the book may seem to imply that it was written for travellers, but what is meant is that whether one is constantly travelling or never ventures from home, this is the book to have on hand.

104 Cf. n. 42.

105 Max Meyerhof, 'Ibn an-Nafis (XIIIth cent.) and his theory of the lesser circulation', *Isis*, 1935, 23: 100–20; Abdul-Karim Chéhadé, *Ibn an-Nafis et la découverte de la Circulation pulmonaire*, Damascus, Institut Français de Damas, 1955.

106 See Ullmann, op. cit. (n. 2), p. 285. The essay remains unpublished.

107 Al-Rāzī, *Man lā yaḥḍuruhu l-ṭabīb*, Delhi, Maṭbaʻ Jaʻfarī, [n.d.]. Rufus of Ephesus and Oribasius had both written similar works, and in early Islamic times ʻĪsā ibn Māssa (d. c. 275/888) also wrote on this subject. See Sezgin, op. cit. (n. 2), Vol. III, pp. 65, 154, 258.

108 Ibn al-Ṣaydāwī, *Al-Kiyāsa fī aḥkām al-siyāsa*, Khalidi Library (Jerusalem), Ms. Ar. 1184, fols. 49r–68r.

109 Al-Suyūṭī, *Al-Nuqāya fī l-ʻulūm*, lithographed in Bombay, A. H. 1309, with the author's own commentary, *Itmām al-dirāya fī tafsīr al-Nuqāya*, on the margin.

110 See n. 83.

111 See Qusṭā ibn Lūqā, *Kitāb fī l-iʻdāʾ* (Abhandlung über die Ansteckung), p. 12, nos. 4–5.

112 Ibn Qayyim al-Jawzīya, *Al-Ṭibb al-nabawī*, ed. by Shuʻayb al-Arnaʾūṭ and ʻAbd al-Qādir al-Arnaʾūṭ, Beirut, Muʾassāsat al-risāla, 1402/1982. An English translation of this work is in preparation by Penelope Johnstone. For a representative example of the genre in translation, see Cyril Elgood, 'Tibb ul-Nabbi or Medicine of the Prophet, being a translation of two works of the same name', *Osiris*, 1962, 14: 33–192.

113 See George T. Scanlon, 'Housing and sanitation: some aspects of medieval public service', in A. H. Hourani and S. M. Stern (eds), *The Islamic City: a Colloquium*, Oxford, Bruno Cassirer, 1970, pp. 179–94.

114 On these problems, see Conrad, op. cit. (n. 32), pp. 388–412.

115 On the plague, see Conrad, op. cit. (n. 32); Dols, *The Black Death in the Middle East*, op. cit. (n. 42).

116 See al-Muqaddasī (wr. *c.*375/985), *Aḥsan al-taqāsīm fī ma'rifat al-aqālīm*, ed. by M. J. de Goeje, Leiden, E. J. Brill, 1906, p. 183.

117 S. D. Goitein, *A Mediterranean Society: the Jewish Communities of the Arab World as Portrayed in the Documents of the Cairo Geniza*, Los Angeles and Berkeley, University of California Press, 1967–88, Vol. II, pp. 240–72.

118 See, for example, Ibn al-Nadīm, op. cit. (n. 75), p. 350; Ibn Buṭlān, *Taqwīm al-ṣiḥḥa*, p. 74.

119 See Lawrence I. Conrad (ed.), *The World of Ibn Ṭufayl: Interdisciplinary Perspectives on Ḥayy ibn Yaqẓān*.

120 Of the numerous studies on medical education in medieval Islam, the best is Gary Leiser, 'Medical education in Islamic lands from the seventh to the fourteenth century', *Journal of the History of Medicine*, 1983, 38: 48–75.

121 See al-Rāzī, *Bur' al-sā'a*, ed. by Paul Guigues, in *Al-Mashriq*, 1903, 6: 396.

122 See Goitein, op. cit. (n. 117), p. 248.

123 Ibn Abī Uṣaybi'a, *'Uyūn al-anbā'*, 1: 178.

124 Ibid., *'Uyūn al-anbā'*, 1: 222; Ibn al-Qifṭī (d. 646/1248), *Ta'rīkh al-ḥukamā'*, ed. by Julius Lippert, Leipzig, Dieterich'sche Verlagsbuchhandlung, 1903, pp. 191–2.

125 See al-Rāzī, *Miḥnat al-ṭabīb*, ed. by A. Z. Iskandar, in *Al-Mashriq*, 1960, 54: 487–92.

126 Goitein, op. cit. (n. 117), p. 241.

127 These matters are discussed in detail in Ibn al-Ukhūwa (d. 729/1329), *Ma'ālim al-qurba fī aḥkām al-ḥisba*, ed. with English abstract of contents by Reuben Levy, London, Luzac, 1938, pp. 56–9 (abstract), 203–9 (text).

128 See, for example, Ibn Abī Uṣaybi'a, *'Uyūn al-anbā'*, 1: 221–2.

129 See Goitein, op. cit. (n. 117), p. 241; Ibn Abī Uṣaybi'a, *'Uyūn al-anbā'*, 1: 221.

130 See H. D. Isaacs, 'A medieval Arab medical certificate', *Medical History*, 1991, 35: 250–7.

131 A number of interesting diplomas investing such officials in office have survived in various literary texts. See, for example, Horst-Adolf Hein, *Beiträge zur ayyubidischen Diplomatik*, Freiburg, Klaus Schwarz Verlag, 1971, pp. 154–8; Ibn Ḥijja al-Ḥamawī (d. 837/1434), *Qahwat al-inshā'*, Khalidi Library (Jerusalem), MS Ar. 968, fols. 8r–12v, 12v–13r, 71v, 96r–97r, 169v–170r.

132 There is as yet no satisfactory history of the Islamic hospital. See Aḥmad 'Īsā, *Ta'rīkh al-bīmāristānāt fī l-islām*, Beirut, Dār al-ra'id al-'arabī 1401/1981; also his earlier and less detailed account in his *Histoire des Bimaristans (hôpitaux) à l'époque islamique*, Cairo, Imprimerie Paul Barbey, 1928.

133 Ullmann, op. cit. (n. 1), p. 52.

134 For indications of the patterns for such changes, see LaVerne Kuhnke, *Lives at Risk: Public Health in Nineteenth-Century Egypt*, Berkeley and Los Angeles, University of California Press, 1990; Amira el-Azhary Sonbol, *The Creation of a Medical Profession in Egypt, 1800–1922*, Syracuse, Syracuse University Press, 1991.

135 A most interesting example is Muḥammad 'Alī al-Bār, *Al-'Adwā: bayna l-ṭibb wa-ḥadīth al-Muṣṭafā*, Riyadh, Al-Dār al-sa'ūdīya li-l-nashr wa-l-tawzī', 1401/

1981. The book deals with the sensitive topic of contagion, denied in Prophetic tradition but, of course, a central truth of modern Western medicine.

FURTHER READING

Browne, Edward G., *Arabian Medicine*, Cambridge, Cambridge University Press, 1921.

Conrad, Lawrence I., *Epidemic Disease in Formal and Popular Thought in Early Islamic Society*, Berlin, Walter de Gruyter, 1992.

Dols, Michael W., *The Black Death in the Middle East*, Princeton, NJ, Princeton University Press, 1977.

——, *Medieval Islamic Medicine: Ibn Riḍwān's Essay 'On the Prevention of Bodily Ills in Egypt'*, Los Angeles and Berkeley, University of California Press, 1984.

Dunlop, D. M., *Arab Civilization to AD 1500*, London, Longman, 1971.

Elgood, Cyril, *A Medical History of Persia and the Eastern Caliphate*, Cambridge, Cambridge University Press, 1951.

Jacquart, Danielle and Micheau, Françoise, *La Médecine arabe et l'occident médiéval*, Paris, Maisonneuve et Larose, 1990.

Klein-Franke, Felix, *Vorlesungen über die Medizin im Islam*, Wiesbaden, Franz Steiner Verlag, 1982.

Leclerc, Lucien, *Histoire de la médecine arabe*, Paris, Ernest Leroux, 1876.

Meyerhof, Max, *Studies in Medieval Arabic Medicine*, ed. by Penelope Johnstone, London, Variorum, 1984.

Rahman, Fazlur, *Health and Medicine in the Islamic Tradition: Change and Identity*, New York, Crossroads, 1989.

Rosenthal, Franz, *The Classical Heritage in Islam*, trans. by Emile and Jenny Marmorstein, London, Routledge & Kegan Paul, 1975.

——, *Science and Medicine in Islam*, Aldershot, Variorum, 1990.

Sezgin, Fuat, *Geschichte des arabischen Schrifttums*, Vol. III: *Medizin – Zoologie – Tierheilkunde bis ca. 430 H.*, Leiden, E. J. Brill, 1970.

—— (ed.), *Beiträge Geschichte der arabisch-islamischen Medizin*, Frankfurt, Institut für Geschichte der arabisch-islamischen Wissenschaften, 4 vols, 1980-.

Ullmann, Manfred, *Islamic Medicine*, Edinburgh, Edinburgh University Press, 1978.

——, *Die Medizin im Islam*, Leiden, E. J. Brill, 1970.

Young, M. J. L., Latham, J. D. and Sergeant, R. B. (eds), *Religion, Learning and Science in the 'Abbasid Period* (Cambridge History of Arabic Literature, Vol. III), Cambridge, Cambridge University Press, 1990.

32

CHINESE MEDICINE

Francesca Bray

Traditional Chinese medicine is often described as ancient and unchanging, holistic and natural.[1] A trained doctor practising in a Shanghai hospital is as likely as a mystical California health enthusiast to insist that Chinese medicine has remained essentially unchanged since the writing of the *Yellow Emperor's Inner Canon of Medicine* over two thousand years ago,[2] and that in stark contrast to Western biomedicine, Chinese medicine is gentle, uses only 'natural' substances, and treats body, mind, and soul as one. This conceptualization is to some extent a conscious or unconscious exercise in marketing, the dramatic differentiation of a product which today has to survive the competition with Western, professionalized, scientific biomedicine. At the same time, the long history of Chinese medicine provides some grounds for the terms of the contrast, in the form of enduring attitudes towards time and knowledge, and towards the human body and its metaphysical, political, social, and environmental place. (➤ Ch. 2 What is specific to Western medicine?)

Over the centuries, the system of medical beliefs and practices that originated in China and continued to develop there absorbed many outside influences, from India, Tibet, Central and South-East Asia, and – since the later nineteenth century – from the West. And as the Chinese language, Chinese Buddhism, and Confucian ideology were adopted by other East Asian élites, so too was Chinese medicine, absorbing, superseding, or co-existing with local systems of healing.

Tracing the external influences on Chinese medicine precisely is not easy, for the evidence is mostly circumstantial at best. It has been suggested that the bloodletting and needling techniques from which acupuncture therapy developed had their origins in Central Asian shamanic curing.[3] Buddhism, which came to China in the first century AD from India via Central Asia, brought with it beliefs concerning the soul and salvation which encouraged adherents to provide charitable care for the sick; during the medieval period, the poor might find relief in monastic hospitals or receive free prescriptions at charitable dispensaries. Indian medical theories of physiology and the nature and origins of disease were not easily reconciled with Chinese ideas; however, some see the influence of Ayurvedic or even Galenic classifications in the use of such categories as 'hot' and 'cold' in Chinese materia medica.[4] (➤ Ch. 33 Indian medicine) The use of Buddhist charms and recitations was incorporated into classical therapy. Buddhist concepts of aetiology allowed for treatment by surgery, and during the medieval period surgical operations for cataract were performed, though probably not on a large scale.[5] Many of the most important drugs in the Chinese materia medica were introduced or imported from abroad: for instance, ginseng from Korea; cassia from Tonkin; musk from Tibet; liquidambar, camphor, cardamom, and cloves from South-East Asia; costus, catechu, and zedoary from the Indian subcontinent; aniseed, saffron, storax, frankincense, and myrrh from the Persian and Arab world, Africa, and the Mediterranean. The relations between Chinese medicine and modern Western medicine will be dealt with in the final section (see pp. 745–9).

Chinese medicine was probably introduced to Korea with Buddhism some time prior to the sixth century AD, and it seems that Buddhist priests from the Korean kingdom of Paekche introduced it to Japan soon afterwards. It is known as *hanui* in Korea today, and as *kanpo* in Japan.[6] The medical beliefs and practices of China and the states that now constitute Vietnam have been closely intertwined for over two millennia. The flow of migrants from south-east China which began in the sixteenth century brought Chinese medicine to Taiwan, the Philippines, and much of South-East Asia, and then in the nineteenth and twentieth centuries, to the Americas. In all these areas, Chinese medicine still flourishes today alongside Western medicine, as it does in the People's Republic of China.

The influence of Chinese medicine on the West was small, at least until very recently. Missionaries and travellers to the Far East acquainted Europeans with some of the ideas and techniques of Chinese medicine, including acupuncture, in the seventeenth and eighteenth centuries. But they were not received with great enthusiasm, for by then European thinkers were absorbed in 'the mechanick Principles invented, or revived, by our Modern Virtuosi'.[7] However, by the early nineteenth century, acupuncture began to enjoy quite a vogue, especially in France; it continued to be regularly practised by a number of specialists even before the recent boom.[8] Variolation against small-pox was well established in China by the seventeenth century, and was also practised in Korea, Japan, and southern Asia. Despite claims for Chinese influence, it has been cogently argued that Jennerian vaccination was developed quite independently of the Chinese practice of variolation.[9]

Of course, over time and across the world, Chinese medicine has undergone significant changes: changes in ideas, in scope, in technique, and in efficacy; changes in institutions, and in social and political context. But it is important to bear in mind that Chinese medical thinkers and practitioners did not share modern Western notions of the historical 'progress' of knowledge; furthermore, even today, Chinese medical thought has not undergone the transition to a positivist science as biomedicine has done. Perhaps that is one of its chief sources of strength in the face of the competition.

THE MEDICAL CORPUS AND THE CONSTITUTION OF KNOWLEDGE

Classical medicine was studied, developed, and practised largely by educated males, treating clients who came mostly from the upper and middle strata of urban society. Most ordinary people had recourse to folk or religious healers of whose knowledge and practices we know very little.

Almost all our knowledge of the internalist history of classical Chinese medicine comes from medical or closely related specialist texts: texts on medical theory; the classification, diagnosis, and treatment of diseases (including collections of individual physicians' cases); drug use and collections of medical prescriptions; and compendia of plant and non-plant drugs with their medical, dietary, and other uses. Some ten thousand specialized medical works are estimated to survive now, at the end of the twentieth century.[10]

Archaeology has contributed significantly to our fragmentary knowledge of medicine in early China. While scattered references to healing practices in the divination inscriptions of the Shang dynasty of about 1300 BC constitute our only source of knowledge for that period, references to medical topics abound in the written works of the Zhou period (c.900 to 221 BC). Recent discoveries of medical and cosmological texts in Han tombs dating from just before the present era have thrown light not only on the range of medical practice of the time, but also on the process of constitution of the medical canon.[11] As well as these crucial discoveries, some instruments and containers of drugs have been found in tombs from the Han dynasty and later, and there are also some famous bas-reliefs and paintings depicting medical themes.[12]

Biographies of famous physicians are to be found in dynastic and local histories as well as in separate collections. Dynastic histories, lineage or monastic records, and legal codes provide information on medical institutions and charities,[13] formalized training and examinations,[14] and forensic medicine;[15] while diaries, collections of anecdotes and stories, medical case histories, and novels,[16] provide incidental information about the social context and ideological role of medicine. From the mid-nineteenth century, accounts by Westerners, particularly by missionaries (who were often doctors too), provide rich information, especially on popular medical ideas and health practices, supplemented in more recent years by ethnographic studies.[17]

The earliest Chinese medical texts extant today are about twenty-two centuries old, and are presumed to include even older materials. It seems that several very different types of medical belief and treatment existed then, perhaps characteristic of different regions. For instance, there is an ancient tradition that treatment with acupuncture was typical in eastern China, while exercising was typical in the central region. The medical works discovered in 1973 in a tomb dated 168 BC at Mawangdui in Hunan (which in Han times was considered the far south of China) include several texts on moxibustion, gymnastics, and dietetics, as well as works on demonological medicine, drug prescriptions, and childbirth, but nothing at all on acupuncture. On the other hand, the formularies of roughly the same period discovered at Wuwei, Gansu (north-west China) in 1972, contain drug prescriptions and mention acupuncture techniques as well as moxibustion.[18]

China was politically unified in 221 BC. The early emperors of the Han dynasty (206 BC–AD 220) were actively concerned with establishing a political, philosophical, and cosmological orthodoxy, and during this period we see the emergence of a medical canon that constitutes the theoretical basis for the 'high classical tradition' of medicine,[19] and the frame of reference for all subsequent medical debate.

The central works in the classical medical tradition are the *Inner Canon*, the *Divine Husbandman's Materia Medica*,[20] the *Canon of Problems*,[21] and the *Treatise on Cold-Damage Disorders*.[22] The first two works are canonical in status, that is to say they are considered to contain a revelation of the wisdom of legendary sages. Later and lesser mortals could only hope to attain partial understanding of this fundamental knowledge: any educated person interested in medicine would know these works by heart, and while hundreds of commentaries have been written on the canons, they are works of explication, not of criticism. The last two works were indispensable classics, which again any physician would be expected to know almost by heart, but they contain human knowledge acquired through experience, not divine revelation, and such knowledge could be called into question, revised, or even superseded.

The books of the *Inner Canon* are principally concerned with the physiological constitution of the body, including the circulation of *qi* (see pp. 737–8), with health and the onset and progression of disease, and with therapy through needling (whether bloodletting or acupuncture).

The *Canon of Problems* takes up eighty-one 'difficult issues' in the *Inner Canon*, relating mostly to diagnosis and needling therapy, and offering, according to Unschuld, 'a virtually complete system of medical care that also includes a detailed discussion of physiology, aetiology, and pathology'. He characterizes the work as '*the* classic of the medicine of systematic correspondence'.[23] Its importance as an adjunct to the *Inner Canon* was unquestioned up until the Song dynasty (960–1279), but thereafter, where divergences occurred between the two works, medical authors assumed that the writer of the *Canon of Problems* had simply failed to understand the *Inner Canon*.[24]

The *Treatise on Cold Damage Disorders* deals with the diagnosis and treatment of a broad category of diseases caused by external cold factors, *shanghan bing*, 'roughly equivalent to the acute infectious febrile disorders of modern medicine'.[25] Diagnosis is guided by Six Warps theory (see p. 739), and treatment is not by needling, but by drugs. Details are given for the preparation of 113 prescriptions, many of which are still in use in the twentieth century.[26] In the late seventeenth century, Japanese medical theorists extended the methods of diagnosis and treatment of the *Treatise* to include all types of diseases, not only those generated by external factors, and the work remains central to the practice of *kanpo* in Japan today.[27] But the *Treatise* is concerned more with diagnosis and therapy than with the aetiology of disease. Chinese physicians began in the twelfth century to refine *shanghan* theory into a theory of heat-factor disorders, *wenre bing*, in an attempt to distinguish more clearly between disorders of different aetiology. The move gathered strength and coherence during the seventeenth century, a period of wars, rebellions, and economic disruption resulting in a change of dynasty. There was a wave of serious epidemics, and dissatisfaction with the limitations of cold-damage theory in coping with these outbreaks led to the publication of a series of works on heat-factor disorders, chief of which was the *Wenre lun* of Ye Tianshi (*c*.1740), which uses the 'triple burners' *san jiao* system (see p. 739) to classify such disorders.[28]

The *Divine Husbandman's Materia Medica* contains a description of the characteristics and properties of 347 vegetable, animal, and mineral drugs, classified into three classes: upper, middle, and lower. The upper class of drugs was mild and cumulative in action, promoting health and longevity; the use of the stronger lower class of drugs was a response to the onset of disease. This longevity-oriented classification was abandoned in later materia medica for systems more directly based on the curative qualities of drugs, categorized according to a system of correspondences between *yin yang* and *wu xing* (see p. 736). Thousands of materia medica, some universal, some local in scope, have been produced over the centuries. The greatest of these works is universally acknowledged to be the late sixteenth-century *Bencao gangmu*, modern editions of which will be found on every East Asian physician's desk. Though not the largest of these works, the *Bencao gangmu* contains information on 1,892 drugs.[29] (➤ Ch. 39 Drug therapies)

Why has Chinese medicine retained these ancient texts as the core of its creed, rather than rejecting and replacing them with a constantly evolving new body of knowledge, as has happened in European medicine since the

Renaissance? Is it because the variants of Chinese medical theory are fundamentally coherent, or because the Chinese mind is not troubled by inconsistency? Were Chinese physicians concerned mainly with abstract theory and
thus indifferent to empirical evidence that might have encouraged the disman-
tling of the ancient system, or were theory and praxis interdependent? Can
we speak of Chinese medicine as a science, in the sense that it is concerned
with discovering the fundamental principles that govern the natural world, or
is it more aptly described as a philosophy of the cosmos, whose undoubted
therapeutic effects must be seen more often than not as psychosomatic? How
was Chinese medical knowledge constituted, and what did it represent?

In the work of some very distinguished scholars, including Needham and
many of the historians of medicine working in the People's Republic or
Taiwan, we see a sustained attempt to produce a Whiggish history of Chinese
medicine, which demonstrates a progressive winnowing of the grains of
science from the chaff of superstition. It is assumed that Chinese physicians
evolved theories (such as the heart as a pump) that fit into the evolutionary
and universal history of medicine which has culminated in modern biomedicine.[30] Others – and this is a point of view that seems to be most popular
among Western medical scientists and practitioners with a superficial familiarity only with a few techniques of Chinese medicine – dismiss it as an
inchoate muddle of poetic but unscientific claptrap which could not possibly
work except on the indoctrinated. (Remember the heated controversies about
acupuncture anaesthesia.) This view is taken still further by people (usually
Westerners) who portray Chinese medicine as mystical, eternal, and thereby
closer to the deep truths of Nature than any mere empirical science. The
most insight into the history of Chinese medicine comes from scholars who
are able to avoid the tendency towards orientalism inculcated by a training
either in modern Western science or in strict Marxism–Leninism.

To understand the history of Chinese medical thought, at least until the
present century, it helps to remember that it is a *classical* system of knowledge.
That is to say, the central role of such basic concepts as *yin yang* and *wu
xing* (see p. 736) remained unchanged, even if their meanings and their
precise relations to natural phenomena could be redefined. The canonical
works and classics were considered the fundamental guides to understanding
the human body and its relations to the cosmos.

> [A]n author's [or physician's] historical predecessors were his colleagues in
> recapturing what the sagely revelators of the archaic golden age had already
> understood.... Some authors were quite aware of the growth in knowledge
> and in sophistication of method over the centuries; but the current apex of that
> slow upward curve did not in their minds approach the mastery attained by
> the sages and lost when the golden age ended. All of a physician's great
> predecessors coexisted in his mind.[31]

Chinese thinkers were not, as is sometimes alleged, indifferent to inconsistency or contradiction. The inconsistencies of both theory and practice within and between the canonical works were addressed as early as the third century AD by the *A-B Canon*,[32] and by the *Canon of the Pulse*,[33] the first in a long series of works that justified or rationalized divergences. Underlying this predisposition towards reconciling differences was the belief that they would disappear or be revealed as irrelevant given a sufficiently deep comprehension of the philosophy expressed in the classics. Focusing on different aspects of the fundamental workings of the cosmos could produce different theories, and the visible effects of these workings could be interpreted in various ways according to the theory chosen and the level at which it was applied – in Unschuld's phrase, according to the pattern of knowledge selected.[34] The utility of one pattern did not invalidate the existence of other patterns, nor did its failure to explicate a particular phenomenon invalidate it. As Sivin points out, 'Chinese [medical] theories were large and well-articulated structures that related clinical experience to the underlying reality revealed by what we would call philosophical reasoning', but the nature of the concepts fundamental to this philosophical reasoning (*yin yang* and *wu xing*) was such that, like the four elements of Western medicine, 'no failure to accord with experience could have proven them invalid'.[35]

Recent attempts to accommodate traditional Chinese medical thought, practice, and education to the challenge of contemporary science and biomedicine will be mentioned in the final section on 'Coexistence with Western medicine' (pp. 745–9).

MACROCOSM AND MICROCOSM

Chinese medical theories have been founded on the belief that the human body represents a microcosm of the natural and social world. Bodily processes follow patterns which are the same as those governing the workings of nature. The human body cannot be reduced to an isolated system, whether a machine or a test-tube full of chemicals – it is inseparable from the cosmos. To explain health and disorder the *Inner Canon* repeatedly invokes the triad of Heaven, Man, and Earth; its reasoning is paralleled in most works of political and natural philosophy:

> A human body is the counterpart of a state. . . . The spirit [the body's governing vitalities, *shen*] is like the monarch; the Blood *xue* is like the ministers; the *qi* is like the people. Thus we know that one who keeps his own body in order can keep a state in order. Loving care for one's people is what makes it possible for a state to be secure; nurturing one's *qi* is what makes it possible to keep the body intact. . . . [T]he perfected man allays catastrophe before it happens, and cures illness before it has developed.[36]

734

Health depends on harmony within the body, with the environment, and with the moral order; successful curing depends on understanding how this harmony can be restored, and 'the challenge to the physician is as much philosophical as technical'.[37]

The core of *classical* Chinese medical theory concentrates on the body as a natural phenomenon influenced by a natural environment. Ill health can be brought on either by some internal disruption or by external pathogens such as cold, damp, or contagion. In most ordinary people's minds, however, social or supernatural factors were just as likely responsible. During the Shang period (*c.*1300 BC), it seems that most illness was believed to be triggered by ancestral displeasure,[38] and even today, one avoids causing offence to one's ancestors for fear of being punished by sickness or bad luck. Pestilence and plague might also result from human sin or from the ruler's evil behaviour disrupting the cosmic order. Such signs of having forfeited the Mandate of Heaven entitled righteous men and women to overthrow the dynasty; rebellions were often led by religious sects obsessed with attaining not only moral but also bodily health and purity, through diet, meditation techniques or exercises, or mass-healing ceremonies conducted by a charismatic leader.[39] (➤ Ch. 60 Medicine and anthropology)

In the three or four hundred years before the founding of the Han (*c.*600–200 BC), much individual sickness was attributed to evil spirits or evil 'wind', which disturbed, possessed, or drove out the soul;[40] cures could be effected by exorcism or by drugs, and charms or talismans helped ward off such attacks. Children have an especially fragile attachment to their souls and are very vulnerable. To this day, a major medical category of children's disorders is called 'fright'. Although the emphasis on supernaturally caused disorders declined through the centuries, most medical works still recognized their existence. In the twentieth century, physicians no longer practise exorcisms, but diviners and priests do so routinely.[41] Until extremely recently, 'ritual remained the therapy of first resort for the majority of Chinese'.[42] (➤ Ch. 29 Non-Western concepts of disease)

From the first systematic formulations of cosmological principles and patterns around 200 BC, the processes and effects of an illness – if not always its ultimate causes – were seen by physicians as determined by those principles and following those patterns. Chinese natural philosophy does not deal in essences, absolutes, or geometrical regularities, but rather in relations, processes, and complex cycles or patterns of transformation.

The stuff of which the natural world consists is *qi* (or *ch'i*), which has been variously translated as 'air', 'vapours', 'finest matter influences', 'pneuma', 'energy', and so on, but since it does not correspond to any single Western concept, it is best left untranslated.[43] In natural philosophy, *qi* can be understood as something that stimulates a process of transformation, or as a vector or medium for such a process. *Qi* fills the cosmos; life comes from an accumulation of *qi*, and death from its dissipation; in certain contexts *qi* can be understood as 'vital energies'. A person must nurture the 'orthopathic' *qi* which regulates bodily functions, preserving good health. But *qi* can also disrupt: 'pathogenic' *qi* triggers illness, and the nature of the pathogenic *qi* determines its course.

One fundamental concept for analysing the patterning and distribution of *qi* is *yin yang*. To *yin* are attached a complex series of attributes that Westerners sometimes think of as polar opposites of the attributes of *yang*: female–male, dark–light, cold–hot, and so on. But these concepts are always relative. In any one phenomenon *yin* and *yang* are interrelated and changing cyclically: a baby's *qi* is more *yin* than an adult's, an old person's than a young person's, and a woman's than the *qi* of a man of the same age. *Yin yang* structures patterns in space and time. *Yang* is more exterior, *yin* more interior. As pathogenic *qi* penetrates the outer *yang qi*, which constitutes the defences of the body, it reaches the inner regions of *yin qi* on which the body depends for nourishment and growth, thus becoming more dangerous. A disorder, like any natural process, will go through active *yang* phases and latent *yin* phases: after a *yang* illness peaks, it will enter a *yin* phase for which a different kind of treatment is required. *Yin yang* relations are fundamental, extremely complex, and can be understood at very different levels. As the famous physician Zhang Jiebin wrote in 1624: 'In diagnosis and therapy it is essential to consider *yin yang* first; it is the organizing principle of the medical art. If there is no error with regard to *yin* and *yang*, how can therapy be deficient?'[44]

The term *wu xing*, Five Phases, regularly used to be translated as 'five elements', but it does not correspond to the Greek notion of elements at all: rather, the action of *qi* can be divided into distinct but interrelated categories.[45] The Five Phases are wood, fire, earth, metal, and water. Each phase is characterized by a type of action or interaction; in a physiological context, wood denotes a phase of growth and of branching development, fire a phase of rapid upward dispersal. Each phase is manifested in a characteristic colour, flavour, emotion, physiological system, bodily secretion, etc. The theory of how these phases and their manifestations interrelate is generally known in English as the theory of systematic correspondence: the Five Phases naturally give rise to each other in the order mentioned above (the order of 'mutual production'), and a sequence of 'mutual restraint' also occurs: wood, earth, water, fire, metal. The normal physiological phases proceed according to the order of mutual production, while pathological processes are transmitted through the sequence of mutual restraint.

PHYSIOLOGY

The human body is a microcosm whose processes, normal and abnormal, are patterned by the universal characteristics of *qi, yin yang*, and the Five Phases. It is contained and separated from the outer environment by a skin which is not impermeable, but is patterned with interstices through which pathogens can penetrate.

The *qi* within the body has two components, which in English are often referred to as *vital substances*, but which are processual as much as material. The *yang* component, likewise called *gi*, represents the capacity for or vectors of action and transformation; the *yin* component, called *xue* (literally 'blood', though in classical medicine its meaning is much broader), represents the capacity for or vectors of circulation, nourishment, and growth. Another vital substance is often translated as 'essence', *jing*, which encompasses both the nourishing forces and substances derived from food, and the reproductive forces and substances (including semen) necessary for procreation.

The vital substances circulate through the body in regular cycles along the circulation tracts, *jing luo* or *jing mai*. These tracts include the anatomically identifiable blood vessels and the invisible tracts along which *qi* in its various manifestations circulates (in many cases corresponding to nerve pathways).[46] The circulation tracts connect the visceral systems of function.

Before the full elaboration of the theory of systematic correspondence, the conception of tracts and viscera was much closer to that of Western anatomy. (➤ Ch. 5 The anatomical tradition) Early texts identify certain tracts with blood vessels; others chart the precise location and dimensions of the viscera.[47] But Chinese physicians were not interested in the notion of the body as a machine, nor was exact anatomical knowledge of the organs necessary as medical theory shifted from a material to a processual perspective. On the other hand, efforts were repeatedly made to extend knowledge of the circulation tracts.[48]

According to classical medical theory, there are five *yin* visceral systems (cardiac, hepatic, splenetic, pulmonary and renal), and six *yang* systems (gall-bladder, stomach, large intestine, small intestine, urinary bladder, and *san jiao*/'triple burner'). The *yin* systems produce, transform, regulate, and store *qi, xue*, and *jing*; the *yang* systems receive and process food to produce them, and transport and excrete the detritus.[49] Despite the superficial correspondence between most of these systems and Western anatomical organs like the heart, lungs, and liver, the primary conceptual focus is on the nature of and interrelations between their functions; the 'triple burner', which only came to analytical prominence rather late in the history of Chinese medicine, does not correspond even superficially to any anatomical entity, yet has a very clearly defined range of functions.[50] The relations between the visceral systems, the ways in which the functioning or malfunctioning of one affects the others, have to be understood in terms of the theory of systematic correspondence. Because of the systemic relationship between the viscera and the associated senses, organs, emotions, secretions, etc., no Cartesian separation between mind and body is possible in Chinese medical thought. (➤ Ch. 7 The physiological tradition)

HEALTH AND DISORDER

When *qi* is circulating normally through the body, harmony and balance prevail, external pathogens are warded off, and the person enjoys good health. This harmony is maintained through moderate and appropriate behaviour. There are many ways for an individual to activate, nourish, and develop *qi*: through diet, exercise, preventative acupuncture or moxibustion, meditation, or even sexual techniques. Such methods not only improve the health but extend the life-span, and some even aim at immortality.[51]

Disorder, *bing* results from an imbalance of *yin* and *yang*, causing disruption of the circulation and functioning of *qi*, which then impairs or distorts the normal transformative functions of the vital fluids and the visceral systems. Stagnation, blockage, accumulation, or depletion of *qi* or *xue* in one of the visceral systems will affect its function and spread through the organism in a pattern dictated by phase dynamics and modified by the constitution of the sufferer. In the early, *yang* phases of a disorder, it is possible to treat the imbalance and disruption and restore the patient to health. Once it reaches the life-threatening *yin* phases, the damage to the system may be irreversible, and a physician may refuse to take on the case.

A disorder can be caused either by the incursion of an external pathogen, or by an internally generated imbalance generally occasioned by a departure from moderation. While 'excesses' are the more frequent problem, moderation precludes both excess and abstinence – gynaecological disorders are as characteristic of nuns and widows as they are of married women prey to their husbands' unbridled lust; a lack of appropriate emotion can be as harmful as its excess. Pent-up anger, melancholy, or resentment are often at the root of female disorders.[52] External pathogens, conceptualized as noxious *qi*, include heat, cold, damp, the ingestion of poisonous substances, fright (for children), or even intercourse with ghosts. The individual manifestation and course of a disorder is shaped not only by the nature of the pathogen, but also by the constitution and behaviour of the individual sufferer, which influences the phase dynamics of the disorder. The range of disorders caused by one particular type of pathogen – cold-damage disorders, for example – thus followed a general pattern but had a wide range of possible variations at each stage in its development. Handbooks of diagnosis and treatment often classified disorders for purposes of convenience by symptoms rather than by causes, but no disorder could be cured unless its fundamental cause was thoroughly understood.

The biomedical concept of disease, a universal bodily response to a specific pathogen, which can be cured by eliminating the pathogen, is largely absent from Chinese medicine. However, in the seventeenth century, a wave of epidemics, where a single disorder followed exactly the same course in hundreds of invididuals, led physicians to postulate the existence of certain specific types of pathogenic *qi*, which entered the body through the nose and mouth, and which in the case of some disorders such as tuberculosis or smallpox could be passed on by contact with patients or their kin – a radically new concept close to the Western one of infectious or contagious diseases,[53] but one that remained of explanatory value for only a limited category of disorders. (➤ Ch. 16 Contagion/germ theory/specificity)

DISORDER MANIFESTATIONS AND DIAGNOSIS

When a patient consulted a physician, the physician had to identify the nature of the disorder and the stage of development it had reached before beginning to consider the best form of treatment. Very often, the root cause of the problem would be obscured in a plethora of complex and even contradictory symptoms. It was also crucial to understand the constitution and background of the patient, since this would influence both the natural course of the disorder and the response to treatment.

In determining the manifestation type of a patient's disorder, the physician reduced the complexity of symptoms past and present to a manageable set of dynamic characteristics – the fundamental cause, the level of penetration of the pathogen, how the *qi* was affected, which visceral systems were impaired or threatened. Perhaps the most popular system for determining the manifestation type was and remains the 'Eight Rubrics', first outlined in the *Inner Canon*, which pairs four sets of contradictory terms, inner–outer, cold–hot, depletion–repletion, and *yin–yang*.[54] Another important system is the 'Six Warps', first developed in the *Treatise on Cold Damage*, which classifies manifestations according to the degree of penetration of the pathogenic *qi*.[55] This approach was developed in the seventeenth and eighteenth centuries by heat-factor disorder theorists into a four-level classification based on the location of symptoms among the 'triple burners', *san jiao*.[56]

As diagnostic techniques, the earliest medical texts emphasize pulse-taking as well as the observation of other physical and emotional signs. Pulse-reading is fundamental because it provides information about the circulation of *qi* and thus indicates the basic imbalances in the body and how the visceral systems are affected. Pulse-taking techniques were steadily elaborated into a complex art, the radial pulse of the wrist being palpated at three different depths at each of three locations, and classified according to strength, length, fullness, texture, rhythm, etc. Pulses in other parts of the body might also be taken.[57]

Observation of the patient's complexion, breathing, emotional state, temperature, pain or discomfort, sensory or motor problems, eating and excreting patterns, and so on is also crucial. Deep-lying visceral effects are discernible at many other levels. Disorders of the hepatic system, for instance, are manifested in the condition of the eyes and sinews, and are associated with outbursts of anger; renal disorders affect the ears and bones as well as the sexual and procreative capacities, and elicit feelings of apprehension. Thus mental or emotional disorders are construed as symptoms rather than as diseases in themselves.[58]

The physician elicits a case history from the patient and the family, and is interested not only in incidents or behaviour patterns that might be considered immediate causes of the disorder (exhaustion, exposure to cold, melancholy, over-eating, etc.), but also in establishing any short- or long-term cyclical patterns in the symptoms (regular onset of insomnia, cycles of fever or of pain, patterns of loss of appetite, long-term difficulties in conception or childbearing, etc.). The elements of diagnosis have been continually elaborated from earliest times to the present. A systemization of diagnosis based on tongue examination, for example, appeared in the late nineteenth century.[59] The last few decades have seen the incorporation of temperature measurement, blood count, blood-sugar levels, and so on into case histories. Nevertheless, the fundamentals of the 'Four Methods of Examination' remain interrogation, visual inspection, auditory and olfactory examination, and palpation (centred on pulse-taking).[60] Even though a contemporary physician may include biomedical elements like blood pressure as symptoms in his case history, the diagnosis will still be conceived and expressed in the strict classical terms: repletion or depletion of *yin* or *yang*, affecting the circulation and function of *qi*, and centred in one of the visceral systems. (➤ Ch. 34 History of the doctor–patient relationship; Ch. 35 The art of diagnosis: medicine and the five senses)

THERAPY

Effective therapy combines two aspects: it eliminates the pathogenic *qi* and counters its effects, while at the same time building up the orthogenic *qi* that constitutes the body's own defences.

For almost any disorder manifestation there will be several recommended therapies for the physician to choose from. The dangerous symptoms of an acute disorder (such as coma, breathing problems, inability to absorb nourishment) must be treated at once before underlying problems of imbalance can be systematically tackled, but the choice of treatment at any stage must always take these fundamental problems into account. For instance, although certain *yin* drugs are highly efficacious in reducing acute fever, if the fever is a manifestation of a *yang* depletion, the use of *yin* drugs would simply worsen the disorder. The choice of therapy must take into account not only the nature of the disorder, but also the constitution of the patient and other factors, such as the season and the weather. The physician will adjust the therapy step by step as the disorder is gradually brought under control. At the first stages, this may require several changes of treatment within a few hours; later phases may continue unchanged for days, weeks, or even months.

Given the way in which Chinese medicine conceptualizes disorders, almost all disorders must be treated as 'internal', *neike*: even skin disorders or wounds can be understood and treated in terms of systematic correspondence. Problems of the eyes must be cured through treatment of the hepatic system, problems of the bones through treatment of the renal system. A disorder of a visceral system can only be cured by restoring the balance of *yin* and *yang*, not by removing the diseased organ. 'External medicine', *waike*, which uses external remedies, is of secondary importance since it involves only the (literally) superficial treatment of symptoms. Apart from a short period predating the theory of systematic correspondence, surgery was not included in mainstream Chinese medicine.[61]

Chinese medicine today is often characterized in contrast to Western medicine as 'gentle', slow in its effects, and more suitable to the treatment of chronic than acute disease. Until very recently, however, no such choice between medical systems existed. Chinese physicians routinely dealt with acute disease in the past, and not infrequently do so today.[62] And far from always being gentle and free from side-effects, the therapies may well be as drastic and immediate in their effects as the bleeding and purges that constituted the principal forms of treatment in the pre-modern West.

A physician may prescribe one or a combination of therapies. By far the most important in classical Chinese medicine is the prescription of drugs. Drug action has been classified in numerous ways; some of the principal categories are drugs that replenish depleted *qi* or blood, those that disperse pathogenic *qi*, unblock obstructed orthopathic *qi*, act as sudorifics or as purgatives, expel cold, or clear heat.[63] In very rare cases, a single drug may be prescribed: for instance, an infusion of pure ginseng to counter the shock of a severe haemorrhage. Most prescriptions, *fang*, include a combination of drugs in carefully specified proportions: perhaps a strong dose of a powerful 'principal' drug to break up congealed blood, smaller quantities of a 'leading' drug to help direct the principal drug to the affected visceral system, one 'auxiliary' drug with a dispersing action which complements that of the principal drug, and another auxiliary that tempers the principal drug's potency, preventing undesirable side-effects.

There are thousands of well-known *fang*, some of which have been in use for centuries or even millennia. Some could be purchased ready-made, as patent medicines. Some were kept strictly secret, handed down within a family through generations. (An eleventh-century emperor graciously made public a secret family cure after he had cured his prime minister of debilitating headaches: the grateful patient asked if he might include the prescription in a collection he was compiling for the use of the common people.) A physician would usually modify a prescription, changing or adding ingredients to fit the conditions of the case. Some medicines were taken as pills or powders made up by the physician or the pharmacist; others were taken as syrups, decoctions, or infusions prepared at home, the dried ingredients being made up and sold in packets, each containing enough for the patient's family to prepare a day's supply.

Second in importance to drug therapy were acupuncture and moxibustion, a technique involving the burning of small pellets of dried wormwood on points on the skin. (The smoke of wormwood and other aromatics was popularly known to drive away all kinds of noxious influences, including insects and ghosts as well as pathogenic *qi*.) Both acupuncture and moxibustion involve the stimulation of key nodal points along the *qi* circulation tracts; they unblock obstructions of *qi*, redirect it to depleted viscera, and eventually restore the regular circulation necessary to good health. Nowadays, the scars left by direct moxibustion are considered unsightly and potential sources of infection, and heat is more usually applied indirectly to the skin. Meanwhile, acupuncture techniques have been developed to include the electrical stimulation of the needles and its use for local anaesthesia.[64]

Social convention required that the physical contact between physicians and their genteel patients be kept to a minimum, especially in the case of females (who remained concealed behind a screen during the consultation, and sometimes only communicated with the physician through their husbands or maidservants). It is not surprising, then, that drug therapy was the most common treatment prescribed by physicians, though many also performed acupuncture. There were also acupuncture specialists who did not prescribe drugs. And many lay people were familiar enough with the main circulation tracts to perform some acupuncture or moxibustion within the family; popular almanacs usually devote several chapters to such techniques. Massage, though it could be prescribed by physicians, would not be performed by them; there were lower-class specialists, including bone-setters and female masseurs, who also acted as midwives. During childbirth, the male physician might be in a separate room, preparing medicines and giving instructions for massage or acupuncture through an intermediary to the midwife. A good midwife could even turn a child in the womb to avoid a breech delivery, as well as help the mother with her contractions. But we also hear of cases where an impatient midwife knelt on the pregnant woman's belly to hasten delivery, causing a stillbirth.[65]

THE SOCIAL RELATIONS OF HEALING

Classical Chinese medical thought was secular if cosmological, but most Chinese people believed that illness was caused not only by natural imbalances but also by malevolent ghosts, disgruntled ancestors, offended gods, karma, and sin. The previous account of Chinese medical thought and practice is derived from the written tradition, which obviously privileges an erudite and philosophical approach both to sickness and cure.

The hagiography of the medical corpus depicted two kinds of successful healer. One is the so-called 'Confucian physician', *ruyi*, a scholar of good family who studied the medical arts as an extension of philosophy, in a spirit of benevolence, perhaps because he wanted to help a sick parent. He might also apply his talents to healing other sick people, but his main role in life was that of a civil servant and gentleman, so (ideally at least) he did not earn money by this practice.[66] This kind of healer acquired knowledge mainly through studying texts by himself, and then through personal experience. One wonders how many of his early patients were cured – case histories and biographies do not record failures.

The second hero of the medical corpus was the so-called 'hereditary physician', *shiyi*. He came from a line of doctors, so his training would include apprenticeship as well as book-learning. Such families often came to fame by specializing in certain types of disorder, or having some 'secret prescription' handed down from father to son. Ethics required that these physicians refrain from overcharging their patients, or from abandoning them if they took a turn for the worse. (It was crucial to be able to diagnose a hopeless case at once, in which event it was legitimate to refuse to take it on.) Some seem to have had the status of regular family doctors receiving an annual salary from well-to-do clients. Ideally, they were expected to treat poor patients free.[67]

These two categories of healer clearly did not constitute a profession. Perhaps the nearest to professional physicians were those who took the medical examinations instituted by the state at various periods from the ninth century, and who then served as state medical officers.[68] But they did not constitute a self-regulating body, and although they included a hierarchy of court physicians, as well as provincial yamen and army physicians, their social and intellectual status was not usually high, and they seldom figure prominently in the medical hagiography.

The medical corpus also refers to a whole range of would-be healers who are generally dismissed as incompetents or quacks, 'vulgar doctors', *yongyi*, or 'itinerant doctors', *lingyi*, as well as priests, shamans, acupuncturists, masseurs, and the dreaded 'six kinds of old women', *liu po*. When these people appear in the medical corpus, it is generally because a patient has consulted them unsuccessfully and has eventually decided to see a proper physician, who then effects a cure. The low status of these healers in the medical corpus derives from a number of factors. They were neither scholars nor philosophers nor gentlemen – their knowledge of cosmology was probably limited, many of them were low class, and some were even female. More importantly, they did not have the kinds of disciples or clients who were able to publish their collected case studies or inscribe stelae in their memory. I would also suggest that the more physical or social contact there was between healer and patient, the more likely the healer's skills were to be dismissed.

The case of women healers is interesting since it indicates that the status of healers is not necessarily related to the social importance of their role. Women healers are generally depicted both in medical texts and in other writings (including novels[69]) as illiterate, ignorant, and unscrupulous, though in texts on childbirth their importance is often acknowledged. Physicians themselves recognized the difficulty of communicating effectively with female patients. Despite official male reservations about their integrity, large numbers of women (midwives, wet-nurses, etc.) served the health-care needs of the women of the imperial palace.[70] The Korean state even introduced formal medical training for women in the fourteenth century, when it was strenuously promoting the neo-Confucian ethos by which unrelated men and women were to be completely segregated. These women were of very low social status, many of them slaves.[71] Though it was unusual for women healers to have formal medical training, they were relied upon by women of all classes for their own illnesses and those of their children, and possibly by lower-class men too.[72] (➤ Ch. 38 Women and medicine)

Case histories show that sick people were likely to seek help serially or simultaneously from a whole range of healers, and that if dissatisfied, they would dismiss even a high-status physician. Women and the uneducated were more likely to turn to religious healers than were male scholars. There may be parallels with the contemporary Korean situation, where women often take their family or male relatives' problems to the diviner or shaman.[73] Religious healing retains its importance throughout East Asia today, and has even shown a resurgence in the People's Republic of China. Kleinman, in a study of Taiwan carried out in the 1970s, indicated that patient satisfaction with treatment by religious healers was significantly higher than satisfaction with either Chinese- or Western-style doctors, the last being lowest on the scale, perhaps because their clients' expectations were unrealistically high.[74]

ORGANIZED MEDICINE

The earliest hospices and charitable medical services in China were probably those established by Buddhist monasteries in the early centuries of our era. But Confucians also took the provision of health services seriously: there was a cosmological link between the health of the body politic and the health of the common people, and assuring the health of one's inferiors was a demonstration of one's fitness for power.

Buddhist monasteries were nationalized in the ninth century, during the Tang dynasty, and the imperial authorities assumed responsibility for their infirmaries for the indigent. They also promoted the publication and free distribution of prescriptions, and set official prices for medicines. Such state initiatives continued throughout the Song and Yuan, when the government also sponsored the compilation of materia medica and established charity pharmacies and clinics in numerous magistratures throughout China.[75] The Ming imperial authorities lost interest in such claims to political legitimacy, although they did attempt to distribute money and medicine to the sick during epidemics, often on a huge scale. During an epidemic in the capital in 1587, it was reported that 109,590 sick people received free medicine.[76]

The decline of government medical services during the late Ming (c.1500–1644) coincided with a steady rise in private medical charities. The wealthy and educated élite of such rich areas as the Lower Yangzi were the first to establish charitable dispensaries and clinics. During the late Ming and Qing (1644–1911), similar institutions came into being throughout the empire, often founded not by the gentry but by prosperous commoners, for whom such activities constituted a legitimating claim to prestige.[77]

COEXISTENCE WITH WESTERN MEDICINE

Until the nineteenth century, Chinese medicine more or less matched its European counterpart in efficacy and authority. The Chinese emperors allowed very restricted access to Westerners, and few Chinese physicians had any knowledge of European medicine. Japanese scholars did have access to Western sciences through the Westerners who were allowed to live in the port of Nagasaki, and from the eighteenth century 'Dutch scholarship' (*rangaku*) flourished. Japanese *rangaku* physicians became interested in anatomy and surgery, and introduced Jennerian vaccination in 1824. Its astonishing success helped undermine the authority of *kanpo*, and schools of Western medicine began to appear.[78] But international politics were still more important than scientific merit in effecting this change. By 1850, both Japan and China were forcibly confronted with the terrifying strength of the Western powers. Humiliating defeat or its threat convinced many people of the total bankruptcy of their traditional culture, and Western medicine became symbolic of modernity.

The Meiji government decided officially to adopt the German system of medical training in 1869, and while it did not ban *kanpo* altogether, over the next fifteen years it introduced increasingly rigorous restrictions on its practice, while establishing an effective state system of Western medical education and services. Western-style doctors in Japan were badly trained and few in number during the early Meiji period, but the success of inoculation in controlling the rampant epidemics helped establish the credentials of Western medicine rapidly.[79] (➤ Ch. 52 Epidemiology) By the beginning of the twentieth century, there were three imperial and eleven other state colleges of Western medicine in Japan, which by 1912 had trained 63 per cent (14,552) of the physicians currently in practice.[80] When the Japanese government annexed Taiwan and Korea, in 1895 and 1910, respectively, it established similar policies there; the ban on speaking any language other than Japanese was a further blow to those trained in Chinese medicine. (➤ Ch. 48 Medical education)

In all three nations, Chinese medicine has made a come-back in the post-war period, together with other kinds of cultural revivalism: a luxury they could presumably afford once they had shown their capacity to modernize economically. Chinese medicine remains separate and largely private, although it has now become professionalized. Standardized training (including basic training in anatomy and physiology) is offered in private medical colleges and hospitals, many of which contain equipment and research laboratories designed to establish the scientific bases of Chinese medicine (see pp. 748–9). Perhaps the clearest proof that Chinese medicine is now acceptable even to the state is the fact that both Japan and Korea recently included a range of Chinese medical prescriptions and treatments in their list of valid claims on medical insurance.[81]

The Chinese became familiar with Western medicine through the missionaries, who were able to set up all over China after the treaties of 1860. Many reformers held Chinese medicine partly responsible for China's defeats:

> The hollow-breasted and hump-backed, the pale-faced and slender-limbed, consequently the devastating epidemic, the high death rate, the lack of strong character and national morale, the pessimistic belief in destiny... the award of the very title of "The Far Eastern Sick Person" – these are the direct gifts of the old-style medicine to China.[82]

But others felt it would be better to reform and modernize Chinese medicine rather than to ban it. In any case, the weak government of the late Qing was in no position to effect Mieji-style reforms. The chief impulse for change came not from the state but from the hated foreigners, in particular the Chinese Medical Missionary Association (founded in 1886), which, together with the Rockefeller-funded Chinese Medical Commission, attempted to standardize the medical education and services offered by some sixty different

Protestant societies. (➤ Ch. 61 Religion and medicine) These services included the 'union medical colleges', established in Peking (Beijing) and other major cities between 1903 and 1912. But by 1913, there were still only 500 Chinese medical students receiving training in all the mission services throughout China.[83] A number of Chinese received medical training in Japan at that period, among them the famous writer Lu Xun.

The government of Republican China (1911–49), despite its often precarious hold on the reins of power, had ambitious plans to establish a modern state medical system. In 1926, about 100 cities had Western-style medical practitioners or hospitals, and in 1928, after the worst of the war-lord struggles, the relatively stable Nationalist government centred at Nanjing used them as a nucleus for a complex hierarchical structure of health institutions, which administered medical education, epidemic prevention, health centres, and hospitals from the capital and provincial level right down to county clinics and village paramedics. Providing rural health care was a high priority, and the Central Field Health Service of Nanjing was much influenced by Yugoslav rural health reforms in developing its programmes. Village health workers were given a few weeks' intensive training, including basic hygiene, the diagnosis and treatment of standard minor illnesses, immunization against smallpox, typhoid, and diphtheria, and referral of serious illnesses to higher authorities.[84] The whole system was premissed on the pre-eminence of Western medicine. There was an attempt to eliminate Chinese medicine, against which both practitioners and cultural conservatives protested vigorously, after which an Institute for National Medicine was founded.[85] But although Chinese medicine was not banned, it certainly suffered from the competition.

The unremitting turmoil of the Republican period, including the devastation caused by the Japanese invasion, meant that this elaborate centralized health system seldom functioned effectively except in very restricted areas. But interestingly, despite the claims of the new Communist state that it had totally rejected the corrupt past, the Nationalist health-care structure was adopted almost unchanged by the new regime. The main difference was that under the People's Republic, Chinese medicine was integrated into this system. Science was the key to the future, yet nationalistic sentiment combined with anti-bourgeois principles gave Chinese medicine a new symbolic authority, leading to professional parity with Western medicine. At the top of the scale of practitioners, since the mid-1950s, not only are Chinese-style physicians required to have a basic training in Western-style medicine, but the converse is also true. Indeed, in the late 1950s, when China was desperately short of skilled medical practitioners, 'up to 2,000 doctors at a time were withdrawn from regular medical practice for three years of full-time study of traditional medicine'. Moreover, the government devoted a large portion of its health budget to providing hospitals, clinics, and medical schools for Chinese medicine.[86] The famous 'barefoot doctors' of the 1960s and 1970s were, who as an institution are largely modelled on the rural health workers of the 1930s, differed most obviously in that their skills included basic acupuncture and a knowledge of Chinese materia medica.[87]

The balance between Western and Chinese medicine has fluctuated in the People's Republic over the years, often in tune with ideological shifts. The notion of a 'syncretic medicine', which would combine the best features of Western and Chinese medicine, was first advanced in the 1920s and has become popular again in Chinese medical and philosophical circles.[88] Given the complete lack of theoretical and empirical overlap between the two systems, this project seems doomed to failure. But great efforts are being made not just in the People's Republic, but throughout East Asia to establish an experimental, scientific basis for Chinese medicine, thus establishing it as a valid competitor to biomedicine.

At one level, there has been a marked historic shift from functionalism to materialism in the understanding of Chinese medical concepts, accompanied by a tendency to reduce Chinese technical terms to the biomedical equivalents. Thus the term *xue* in classical medicine includes a whole range of meanings, only one of which more or less corresponds to the biomedical concept of 'blood'. While most contemporary practitioners still recognize this distinction, there is an increasing tendency to use the two interpretations interchangeably.

Materialism provides a basis for explaining Chinese medical theory and therapeutics in Western scientific terms, applying the methods of the experimental laboratory: first, the location and nature of the acupuncture tracts have been investigated, and an explanation of the effects of acupuncture anaesthesia given in terms of the synthesis of endorphins;[89] second, numerous investigations of the pharmacological effects of Chinese drugs, alone and in combination, have been carried out (though nobody has yet scientifically proven the value of ginseng). This yearning towards science tends to produce a selective and partial approach to traditional theory and praxis, whereby elements that can be 'scientifically' proven are given central prominence, while those that cannot are marginalized or even dismissed as 'superstitious' or 'feudal remnants'. This attitude has produced, as mentioned earlier, a fair amount of positivist history of Chinese medicine, and it is also affecting current education and praxis.

The classical conception of knowledge continues to shape the thinking of contemporary Asian practitioners of Chinese medicine at one level: neither in Beijing nor Tokyo nor Seoul can a physician be trained without becoming acquainted with the works of the canon. One important change, however, relates to language education. Classical Chinese is no longer an essential element of education in East Asia. Many physicians can read the classical works only in modern translation, if available. Those who can still read the originals may be tempted to project contemporary meanings (often heavily influenced by biomedicine) on to classical terms. Physicians may only become acquainted with the classical works and the traditions of exegesis through excerpts or quotations in modern textbooks.[90] In the People's Republic and Taiwan, the emphasis on practice and empiricism means that many practitioners receive at best a very superficial training in the theoretical rationales underlying therapy.[91]

Finally, Chinese medical practitioners used to reinforce their prestige by their skills with the book and the writing-brush; now they are turning to the technical trappings of Western medicine. Traditional physicians wear white coats and carry stethoscopes. Acupuncturists prominently display electric sterilizing machines. A Korean *hanui* hospital uses CAT-scans to supplement traditional diagnostic methods; a doctor explains that it resssures the patients. Meanwhile, in a small traditional drugstore nearby, the young resident doctor has just installed a leather stretcher with straps and flashing dials, which vibrates patients with back trouble until the sweat runs and their skin turns grey. Then he prescribes traditional drugs for them. His patients tell me that they prefer Chinese medicine because it is gentle and has no side-effects; he tells me he has bought the machine because the more he hurts them, the more good they believe he has done.

NOTES

1   For purposes of simplicity I use here a single system of romanization, *pinyin* (the official system used in the People's Republic of China), except where other systems such as Wade-Giles are used by the authors of works cited.

There are no standard translations for the titles of Chinese medical works, let alone for medical terminology. Here I have mostly adopted the translations suggested by Nathan Sivin in two works: *Traditional Medicine in Contemporary China*, Ann Arbor, Center for Chinese Studies, University of Michigan, 1988; and 'A cornucopia of works for the history of Chinese medicine', *Chinese Science*, 1989, 9: 29–52. However, I must alert the reader to the fact that they often differ from those used by other writers, including such authorities as Needham and Lu, Unschuld, or Porkert.

Many of the most fundamental studies of Chinese medicine are, of course, written in Chinese, Japanese, or Korean, but here I refer to secondary sources in Asian languages only where no satisfactory work on that topic exists in a Western language. Frustrated Asian scholars should consult the works cited in the main bibliography, which provide ample polyglot references.

Where dates given for the composition of a work seem to cover unreasonably long periods, this is usually because the date is recorded simply as a certain reign-period, some of which were several decades in length.

2   *Huangdi neijing*, the most authoritative source of traditional medical doctrine. Traditionally ascribed to the legendary Yellow Emperor, recent scholarship suggests that it is the work of several authors compiled in the first century BC or early

first century AD. However, the two books which form the core of the canon, the 'Basic questions' (*Suwen*) and the 'Divine pivot' (*Lingshu*), did not exist in their present form before the eighth century (Sivin, op. cit, (n. 1) 1988, pp. 5–6, 88–9).

3   Paul D. Buell, 'The *Yin-shan cheng-yao*, a Sino-Uighur dietary: synopsis, problems, prospects', in Paul U. Unschuld (ed.), *Approaches to Traditional Chinese Medical Literature*, Dordrecht, Kluwer, 1989, p. 109. D. C. Epler, citing Miyashita, sees it as part of a Chinese shamanic tradition: 'Bloodletting in early Chinese medicine and its relation to the origin of acupuncture', *Bulletin of the History of Medicine*, 1980, 54: 337–67.

4   Buell, op. cit. (n. 3).

5   Paul U. Unschuld, *Medicine in China: a History of Ideas*, Berkeley, University of California Press, 1985, ch. 6.

6   Kim Tu-chong, *Hankuk uihak si* [*History of Korean medicine*], Seoul, T'anku Press, 1981; Margaret Lock, *East Asian Medicine in Urban Japan: Varieties of Medical Experience*, Berkeley, University of California Press, 1980; Yasuo Otsuka, 'Chinese traditional medicine in Japan', in Charles Leslie (ed.), *Asian Medical Systems: a Comparative Study*, Berkeley, University of California Press, 1976, pp. 322–41.

7   Pierre Bayle, *Nouvelles de la république des lettres*, quoted in Lu Gwei-Djen and Joseph Needham, *Celestial Lancets: a History and Rationale of Acupuncture and Moxibustion*, Cambridge, Cambridge University Press, 1980, p. 286.

8   Ibid., pp. 269–302.

9   Angela K. C. Leung, 'Organized medicine in Ming-Qing China: state and private medical institutions in the Lower Yangzi region', *Late Imperial China*, 1987, 8, 1: 143 no. 41.

10 Sivin, op. cit. (n. 1), 1988, p. 16.

11 For example, Donald J. Harper, 'The *Wu shih erh ping fang*: translation and prolegomenon', unpublished Ph.D. thesis, University of California, Berkeley; A. Akahori, 'The interpretation of classical Chinese medical texts in contemporary Japan', in Unschuld, op. cit. (n. 3), pp. 19–28.

12 For example, C. Y. Chen, *History of Chinese Medical Science*, Hong Kong, Chinese Medical College, 1968, pp. 36, 47.

13 For example, Leung, op. cit. (n. 9).

14 Joseph Needham, 'China and the origin of qualifying medical examinations', in Needham, *Clerks and Craftsmen in China and the West*, Cambridge, Cambridge University Press, 1970, pp. 379–95; Robert P. Hymes, 'Not quite gentlemen? Physicians in the Sung and Yuan', *Chinese Science*, 1987, 8: 9–76.

15 Sung Tz'u, *The Washing Away of Wrongs: Forensic Medicine in Thirteenth-Century China*, trans. by Brian E. McKnight, Ann Arbor, University of Michigan Press, 1981.

16 Wilt Idema, 'Diseases and doctors, drugs and cures: a very preliminary list of passages of medical interest in a number of traditional Chinese novels and related plays', *Chinese Science*, 1977, 2: 37–63.

17 For example, Mechtild Leutner, *Geburt, Heirat und Tod in Peking: Volskultur und Elitekultur vom 19. Jahrhundert bis zum Gegenwart*, Berlin, Dietrich Riemer Verlag, 1989; also see various articles in Arthur Kleinman, Peter Kleinstadter *et. al.* (eds), *Medicine in Chinese Cultures: Comparative Studies of Health Care in Chinese and Other Societies*, Washington, DC, John E. Fogarty Center for Advanced Study in the Health Sciences, 1975; Kleinman, *Patients and Healers in the Context of*

Culture: an Exploration of the Borderland between Anthropology, Medicine and Psychiatry, Berkeley, University of California Press, 1980; Kristofer Schipper, 'Seigneurs royaux, dieux des epidémies', *Archives de sciences sociales des religions* 1985, 59 (1): 31–40; Paul Katz, 'Demons or deities? – the *Wangye* of Taiwan', *Asian Folklore Studies*, 1987, 46: 197–215.

18   Akahori, op. cit. (n. 11), pp. 19, 20; U. Engelhardt, 'Translating and interpreting the *Fu-ch'i ching-i lun*', in Unschuld, op. cit. (n. 3), p. 131; Donald J. Harper, 'A Chinese demonography of the third century BC', *Harvard Journal of Asiatic Studies*, 1985, 45 (2): 459–98.

19   Sivin, op. cit. (n. 1), 1988, p. 44.

20   *Shennong bencao jing*, an anonymous work, late first or early second century AD. The word *jing* was added by an editor at a later date to indicate the canonical status of the work. The original work has not survived, but the famous physician and alchemist Tao Hongjing wrote an annotated commentary on the work, the *Bencao jing jizhu* (*c.*500), and the text is reconstructed in the *Xinxiu bencao* (Rev. Materia Medica) of Su Jing, completed 650/659.

21   *Huangdi bashiyi nan jing*, 'Canon of problems in the [Inner Canon of the] Yellow Emperor', an anonymous work probably compiled in the first century AD. Translated and annotated by Paul U. Unschuld, as *Medicine in China: Nan-ching, the Classic of Difficult Issues*, Berkeley, University of California Press, 1986.

22   *Shang han za bing lun*, 'Treatise on cold damage and miscellaneous disorders', attributed to Zhang Zhongjing (and supposedly composed *c.*196–220), though this attribution has often been questioned. Translated with annotations by Catherine Despeux as *Shanghanlun. Traité des 'coups de froid'*, Paris, Éditions de la Tisserande, 1985. See also Dean C. Epler, 'The concept of disease in an ancient Chinese medical text, the *Discourse on Cold-Damage Disorders (Shang-han Lun)*', *Journal of the History of Medicine and Allied Sciences*, 1988, 43: 8–35.

23   Op. cit. (n. 21), 17, 3.

24   P. U. Unschuld, 'Terminological problems encountered and experiences gained in the process of editing a commentated *Nan-ching* edition', in Unschuld, op. cit. (n. 3), p. 100.

25   Sivin, op. cit. (n. 1), 1988, p. 84.

26   Despeux, op. cit. (n. 22), p. 9.

27   Otsuka, op. cit. (n. 6), p. 328; Lock, op. cit. (n. 6) pp. 54, 129.

28   Sivin, op. cit. (n. 1), 1988, pp. 87, 402 ff.

29   Li Shizhen, *Systematic Materia Medica*, compiled 1552–1593 and first printed in 1596; see Paul U. Unschuld, *Medicine in China: a History of Pharmaceutics*, Berkeley, University of California Press, 1986, pp. 145–69. This work deals admirably with the complex history of Chinese materia medica.

30   Lu and Needham, op. cit. (n. 7), pp. 30 ff., argue that in the *Inner Canon* and the *Canon of Problems* the heart and lungs were considered to pump blood and *qi* through the body; Sivin, op. cit. (n. 1), 1988, pp. 438 ff., demonstrates that this is a misunderstanding.

31   Sivin, ibid., p. 25.

32   Huangfu Mi, *Huangdi jiayi jing*, completed 256/282. It drew on three extant works of the Yellow Emperor tradition to provide a consistent anthology of the theory underlying acupuncture therapy.

33 Wang Shuhe, *Mai jing*, *c.*280. It drew on the *Inner Canon*, the *Canon of Problems*, the *Treatise of Cold Damage Disorders*, and other early works to provide a comprehensive treatment of diagnosis and therapeutics.

34 Op. cit. (n. 21), p. 7.

35 Sivin, op. cit. (n. 1), 1988, p. 20.

36 Ge Hong, *Baopuzi neipian* [Inner chapters of the Master who Holds to Simplicity], written AD *c.*320, quoted in Sivin, op. cit. (n. 1), 1988, pp. 58–9.

37 Ibid., p. 57.

38 Unschuld, op. cit. (n. 5), ch. 1.

39 For example, K. Schipper, 'Millenarismes et messianismes dans la Chine ancienne', *Actes du 26ᵉ Congres d'études chinoises*, Rome, ISMEO, 1978; Schipper, op. cit. (n. 17); Katz, op. cit. (n. 17).

40 Unschuld, op. cit. (n. 5), ch. 2.

41 Kleinman, op. cit. (n. 17). On an earlier period where the professional distinction was not yet clear, see Kenneth J. DeWoskin (trans.), *Doctors, Diviners, and Magicians of Ancient China*, New York, Columbia University Press, 1983.

42 Sivin, op. cit. (n. 1), 1988, p. 21.

43 Joseph Needham *et al.*, *Science and Civilisation in China*, Cambridge, Cambridge University Press; Vol. II on philosophical concepts, and Vol. IV, chs 2–5 on alchemy. Manfred Porkert, *The Theoretical Foundations of Chinese Medicine: Systems of Correspondence*, Cambridge, MA, MIT Press, 1974, pp. 168 ff; Sivin, op. cit. (n. 1), 1988, pp. 45–59.

44 Ibid., p. 62.

45 Ibid., p. 75.

46 Ibid., pp. 133 ff, 249–72.

47 Ibid., p. 136; Unschuld, op. cit. (n. 5), pp. 78–9.

48 Lu and Needham, op. cit. (n. 7), pp. 13–169.

49 Porkert, op. cit. (n. 43), pp. 112–12; Sivin, op. cit. (n. 1), 1988, pp. 213–36; Ted J. Kaptchuk, *The Web that has No Weaver: Understanding Chinese Medicine*, New York, Congdon & Weed, 1983, pp. 50–77.

50 Sivin, op. cit. (n. 1), 1988, pp. 125 ff.

51 Needham *et al.*, op. cit., (n. 43), Vol. V chs 2–5 on alchemy and the search for longevity and immortality; see also, *inter alia.*, Livia Kohn in co-operation with Yoshinobu Sakade (eds), *Taoist Meditation and Longevity Techniques*, Ann Arbor, Michigan University Press, 1989.

52 Charlotte Furth, 'Blood, body and gender: medical images of the female condition in China, 1600–1850', *Chinese Science*, 1986, 7: 43–66.

53 Sivin, op. cit. (n. 1), 1988, p. 151; Leung, op. cit. (n. 9).

54 Sivin, op. cit. (n. 1), 1988, p. 331.

55 Sivin, op. cit. (n. 1), 1988, pp. 398 ff.

56 Sivin, op. cit. (n. 1), 1988, p. 402.

57 Sivin, op. cit. (n. 1), 1988, pp. 314–26; Kaptchuk, op. cit. (n. 49), pp. 158–74.

58 Hans Agren, 'The conceptual history of psychiatric terms in traditional Chinese medicine', in Li Guohao *et al.* (eds), *Explorations in the History of Science and Technology in China*, Shanghai, Chinese Classics, 1982, pp. 573–82; Arthur Kleinman and Joan Kleinman, 'Somatization: the interconnection in Chinese society among culture, depressive experiences, and the meanings of pain', in Arthur

Kleinman and Byron Good (eds), *Culture and Depression*, Berkeley, University of California Press, 1985, pp. 429–90; Martha Li Chiu, 'Insanity in imperial China: a case study', in Arthur Kleinman and Tsung-yi Lin (eds), *Normal and Abnormal Behaviour in Chinese Culture*, Dordrecht, Reidel, 1981, pp. 75–94.

59 Sivin, op. cit. (n. 1), 1988, p. 175; Kaptchuk, op. cit. (n. 49), pp. 147–9.

60 Sivin (1988), op. cit. (n. 1), pp. 291–328; Kaptchuk, op. cit. (n. 49), pp. 138–77.

61 See Unschuld, op. cit. (n. 5), p. 151, on the lack of successors to the famous third-century AD physician, Hua Tuo, who is said to have removed a diseased gall-bladder as well as performing other surgical operations (DeWoskin, op. cit. (n. 41), pp. 140 ff.).

62 For an example of contemporary treatment of acute fever in a child, see the case described in Sivin, op. cit. (n. 1), 1988, pp. 421–5. For the alleged success of Chinese physicians in curing large numbers during epidemics, see Leung, op. cit. (n. 9), pp. 137, 146.

63 Sivin, op. cit. (n. 1), 1988, pp. 177–96; Beijing Medical College, 'Chinese materia medica', *Dictionary of Traditional Chinese Medicine*, Hong Kong, Commercial Press, 1984, pp. 138–227; Judith Farquhar, *Knowledge and Practice in Chinese Medicine*, Chicago, IL, Chicago University Press.

64 The most complete account of acupuncture and moxibustion past and present is Lu and Needham, op. cit. (n. 7), but it has been criticized for reading biomedical concepts too freely into Chinese medical thought: see, for example, Sivin, op. cit. (n. 1), 1988, pp. 437–40.

65 Leutner, op. cit. (n. 17).

66 Hymes, op. cit. (n. 14).

67 Paul U. Unschuld, *Medical Ethics in Imperial China: a Study in Historical Anthropology*, Berkeley, University of California Press, 1979.

68 Needham, op. cit., and Hymes, op. cit. (n. 14).

69 Idema, op. cit. (n. 16).

70 Victoria B. Cass, 'Female healers in the Ming and the lodge of ritual and ceremony', *Journal of the American Oriental Society*, 1986, 106 (1): 233–40.

71 Kim, op. cit. (n. 6).

72 Leung, op. cit. (n. 9), p. 153, citing the sixteenth-century scholar Lü Kun.

73 Laurel Kendall, *Shamans, Housewives, and Other Restless Spirits: Women in Korean Ritual Life*, Honolulu, University of Hawaii Press, 1985.

74 Kleinman, op. cit. (n. 17), p. 331.

75 Leung, op. cit. (n. 9), pp. 135–6.

76 Leung, op. cit. (n. 9), p. 141.

77 Leung, op. cit. (n. 9), p. 156.

78 Lock, op. cit. (n. 6), p. 61; Otsuka, op. cit. (n. 6), p. 334.

79 Lock, op. cit. (n. 6), p. 62.

80 AnElissa Lucas, *Chinese Medical Modernization: Comparative Policy Continuities, 1930–1980s*, New York, Praeger, 1982, p. 39.

81 For example, Lock, op. cit. (n. 6), p. 169.

82 Chang Tsung-Liang, *'Old Style' Versus 'Modern' Medicine in China*, Shanghai, 1926, p. 9; quoted in Ralph C. Croizier, 'The ideology of medical revivalism in modern China', in Leslie, op. cit. (n. 6), p. 343.

83 Lucas, op. cit. (n. 80), pp. 42 ff.

84 Lucas, op. cit. (n. 80), ch. 4.
85 Croizier, op. cit. (n. 82), p. 345.
86 Croizier, op. cit. (n. 82), p. 349.
87 *A Barefoot Doctor's Manual: the American Translation of the Official Chinese Paramedical Manual*, Philadelphia, PA, Running Press, 1974.
88 Croizier, op. cit. (n. 82), p. 344.
89 Lu and Needham, op. cit. (n. 7), pp. 260 ff.
90 Sivin, op. cit. (n. 1), 1988, p. 27; Farquhar, op. cit. (n. 63).
91 Paul U. Unschuld, 'The social organization and ecology of medical practice in Taiwan', in Leslie, op. cit. (n. 6), pp. 300–21; Croizier, op. cit. (n. 82), p. 353.

FURTHER READING

A Barefoot Doctor's Manual: the American Translation of the Official Chinese Paramedical Manual, Philadelphia, PA, Running Press, 1977.

Kleinman, Arthur, Kleinstadter, Peter *et al.* (eds), *Medicine in Chinese Cultures: Comparative Studies of Health Care in Chinese and Other Societies*, Washington, DC, John E. Fogarty Center for Advanced Study in the Health Sciences, 1975.

Kleinman, Arthur, *Patients and Healers in the Context of Culture: an Exploration of the Borderland between Anthropology, Medicine and Psychiatry*, Berkeley, University of California Press, 1980.

——, *Social Origins of Distress and Disease: Depression, Neurasthenia and Pain in Modern China*, New Haven, CT, Yale University Press, 1986.

Leslie, Charles (ed.), *Asian Medical Systems: a Comparative Study*, Berkeley, University of California Press, 1976.

Lock, Margaret, *East Asian Medicine in Urban Japan: Varieties of Medical Experience*, Berkeley, University of California Press, 1980.

Lu Gwei-Djen and Needham, Joseph, *Celestial Lancets: a History and Rationale of Acupuncture and Moxa*, Cambridge, Cambridge University Press, 1980.

Lucas, AnElissa, *Chinese Medical Modernization: Comparative Policy Continuities, 1930s–1980s*, New York, Praeger, 1982.

Ohnuki-Tierney, Emiko, *Illness and Culture in Contemporary Japan: an Anthropological View*, Cambridge, Cambridge University Press, 1984.

Porkert, Manfred, *The Theoretical Foundations of Chinese Medicine: Systems of Correspondence*, Cambridge, MA, MIT Press, 1974.

Sivin, Nathan, *Traditional Medicine in Contemporary China, a Partial Translation of Revised Outline of Chinese Medicine (1972) with an Introductory Study on Change in Present-Day and Early Medicine*, Ann Arbor, Center for Chinese Studies, University of Michigan, 1987.

Unschuld, Paul U., *Medicine in China: a History of Ideas*, Berkeley, University of California Press, 1985.

——, *Medicine in China: a History of Pharmaceutics*, Berkeley, University of California Press, 1986.

——, *Medicine in China: Nan-ching, the Classic of Difficult Issues*, Berkeley, University of California Press, 1986.

33

INDIAN MEDICINE

Dominik Wujastyk

PREHISTORY AND THE INDUS VALLEY

There is extensive archaeological evidence from all parts of the South Asian peninsula for the presence of humans from the Lower Palaeolithic Stone Age onwards. The first settled agricultural communities seem to have appeared at the end of the Pleistocene, about ten thousand years ago. A marked increase in the use of grains of cereal type is indicated in eastern Rajasthan from about 7000 BC, accompanied by the development of mud-brick architecture, and the domestication of cattle, sheep, and goats.

During the second half of the fourth and the early part of the third millennium BC, developments took place around the course of the Indus river that were to lead to the Mature Indus civilization, which flourished during the middle and late third millennium. Archaeologists have pointed to the concurrence of three factors which brought the Indus civilization to its maturity: the pre-existence in the region of many incipient urban trading communities; the rich natural environment offered by the Indus river system, a great river flowing through a desert, which inevitably reminds us of Egypt and Mesopotamia; and finally, the stimulus of contacts with other societies outside the Indus system, including those of Central Asia and Mesopotamia.[1]

Excavations of the impressive Indus cities of Harappa, Mohenjo-daro, and Lothal have revealed an elaborate and refined civilization, and continuing archaeological work shows that the Indus culture stretched across a far greater area of northern India than was once realized, through a system of smaller villages and settlements that were linked to the cities by trade and shared artefacts. The period of the Mature Indus civilization shows us an evolved urban society with clearly drawn class divisions and roles. No doubt healers of some type existed, perhaps coinciding with the religious functionaries.

However, the script of this civilization remains undecipherable at present, in spite of many promising attempts using modern techniques of decipherment, and the lack of access to the surviving written records impedes interpretation of the archaeological artefacts.

One may point to the large, central water tanks or communal baths that exist in the main cities and postulate religious or secular rites of cleansing. It certainly seems that hygiene was highly regarded, since the houses in Harappa, Mohenjo-daro, and Lothal often have separate bathrooms with drainage to covered culverts that run beneath the city streets. Several statues, toy models, and images survive, representing plants, animals, and presumed deities, and in many cases it is tempting to draw parallels with later Vedic developments in the historical period. For example, there are images of what looks like a Pipal (Skt. *pippala, aśvattha*) leaf, which was of importance in the materia medica of later Indian medicine.[2] But while the Indus script remains unread, such conjectures concerning cultural continuity must remain tentative in the extreme.

During the middle of the second millennium BC, the Indus civilization declined. The cities seem to have fallen into disuse, and the populations to have migrated to outlying villages. The causes for this decline are subject to strenuous debate today by archaeologists, geologists, linguists, and historians, but they probably include environmental changes affecting the river courses and the climate,[3] and perhaps the collapse of an over-rigid hieratic system of centralized government in the face of declining economic prosperity.

MEDICINE IN THE VEDIC TEXTS

During the latter part of the second millennium BC, the eastward migrations of the Indo-European peoples reached South Asia.[4] The sacrificial liturgy of these peoples was memorized wholesale by families of hereditary priests (Skt. *brāhmaṇa*). By extraordinary feats of memory and tradition, these hymns have reached us today in much the same form as they existed *c.*1200 BC. This body of Sanskrit liturgical literature is called *veda*, 'the knowledge'. The subject matter of these hymns is religious and includes the praise and worship of the gods, and prayers for health, long life, and many sons. From them, we are able to deduce obliquely some information about health and healing in these early times. It must be stressed that there is no such thing as 'Vedic medicine' in any unified sense. All we can do is scour the surviving liturgical texts for insights into the healing practices of the time.[5]

The picture that emerges is – perhaps unsurprisingly, given the nature of our sources – one of a magical and religious approach to the causes of disease and to remedies. Several deities were ascribed particular healing powers, including the Aśvins, twin horsemen and divine physicians, cognate with the Roman Dioscuri. Diseases could be caused by evil spirits or by external accident, and rituals involving incantations (Skt. *mantra*), penances, and prayers were used to placate the suprahuman beings who brought disease upon people. Plants too were recognized for their healing powers. In general, internal diseases like *yákṣma* (consumption) and *takmán* (fever, particularly associated with the onset of the monsoon) were believed to have magical and demonic causes, while broken bones, wounds, and other external afflictions were ascribed to their more obvious mundane causes. Poisons were evidently known and used.

A superficial knowledge of anatomy is revealed. The Vedic rites included animal and human sacrifice, and in this connection the ritual texts include some lists of anatomical parts.

A simple form of surgery is described, in which a reed was used as a catheter to cure urine retention.[6] Cauterization with caustic substances and resins was used to prevent wounds from bleeding. In many places, the texts refer to water as a potent healing substance, but it is unclear whether it was to be drunk, sprinkled on the patient, or used for bathing.

MEDICINE AMONGST THE EARLY HETERODOX ASCETICS

The religion of Vedic ritual continued to embody the orthodox religion of north India in the latter half of the first millennium BC, and it has continued to do so to some extent even today. However, a number of other religious groups sprang up in opposition to what was seen as a sterile, mechanistic religion. Generally speaking, these heterodox groups sought to internalize religious values to a greater extent than was demanded by Vedic ritual, and to live a life of ethical, rather than solely sacramental, integrity. The best known such groups was the Buddhist *saṅgha* (community), founded by Gautama Śākyamuni, but there were others such as the followers of Mahāvīra (later called the Jains), and of Makkhali Gosāla (the Ājīvikas, now extinct), as well as many independent ascetics (Skt. *śramaṇa*). Amongst these groups a new kind of medical practice evolved. The evidence we have comes mainly from the Buddhist canonical texts, which contain important medical information.[7]

The monastic rule governing Buddhist monks (Pāli *vinaya*) laid down that their few possessions should include five basic medicines: clarified butter, fresh butter, oil, honey, and molasses.[8] As the Buddhist *saṅgha* evolved, the list of medical prerequisites grew to include numerous foods and a large pharmacopoeia. There is archaeological evidence from about the fourth century AD that some Buddhist monasteries included a sick-room, which may have evolved into a more formal hospital.[9] Initially, the monks' healing activities were aimed at the care of their fellow monks, but by the middle of the third century BC, the monasteries were beginning to serve the lay community.

Of particular interest for the history of Indian medicine are the close similarities that exist between the Buddhist texts and the later āyurvedic texts in some lists of herbs, salts, and other medicines, as well as in specific treatments. This is in contrast to the medicine of the Vedic texts, which is not generally similar to āyurveda. The evidence points to the āyurvedic texts having grown, at least partly, from the ascetic milieu.[10] This seemingly simple fact has long been obscured because scholars have taken at face value the āyurvedic texts' own strenuous assertions that they are derived from the Vedic tradition. But something quite complicated seems to have happened to this tradition, and research has not cleared up all the issues yet. Recent work has discerned in the classical compendia of Caraka and Suśruta a core of world-affirming, pragmatic realism amounting to an early scientific attitude, which has been subjected to a secondary process of religious over-coding.[11] Texts which were originally dedicated wholly to the accurate observation and description of disease, and to healing by whatever means were effective, have been recast in the framework of a dialogue between primeval Hindu sages and gods, and a pedigree has been clumsily prefixed to the works that traces the descent of the science of medicine back to the gods themselves.

Some of these ideas are still, perhaps, somewhat speculative. But the role of the ascetic communities of the fourth century BC onwards, and in particular that of the Buddhist *saṅgha*, must now be recognized as a vital part of the early evolution of āyurveda.

ĀYURVEDIC MEDICINE

The classical system of Indian medicine is called, in Sanskrit, *āyurveda*: 'The knowledge (Skt. *veda*) for longevity (Skt. *āyus*)'. One ancient etymological definition of the science runs as follows: 'It is called '*āyurveda*' because it tells us (*vedayati*) which substances, qualities, and actions are life-enhancing (*āyuṣya*), and which are not.'[12]

Āyurveda is a broad system of medical doctrines and practices, with both preventive and prescriptive aspects. It consists of a great deal of excellent practical advice concerning almost every imaginable aspect of life, from cleaning the teeth, to diet, exercise, regimen, and so on. Āyurveda's theoretical foundation is a doctrine of three bodily humours (wind, bile, and phlegm), somewhat analogous to the ancient Greek teachings of Hippocrates and Galen (AD 129–*c*.200/210), and seven bodily constituents (chyle, blood, flesh, fat, bone, marrow, and semen). (➤ Ch. 14 Humoralism) Its medicines are mainly herbal and it teaches a broad range of therapies including enemas, massage, ointments, douches, sudation, and surgery. From the end of the first millennium AD, metallic compounds began to come into medical use, but these remained on the periphery of the āyurvedic pharmacopoeia; opium, too, was introduced, probably from Islamic sources, as an effective cure for diarrhoea. Throughout the classical texts the emphasis is on moderation: whether it be in food, sleep, exercise, sex, or the dosage of medicines, it is vital to stay within the limits of reasonable measure and balance.

SOURCE TEXTS

The textbooks of āyurveda are written in the classical Sanskrit language, although many are today available with translations into modern Indian languages (especially Hindī), and some have been translated into European languages. The earliest surviving texts date from the first centuries of the Christian era, although, as we have seen, there is evidence that a system which could be called āyurveda was developing from perhaps as early as the fourth century BC. However, extravagant claims that āyurveda dates from thousands of years BC can be firmly discounted. Such claims are frequent, and arise from nationalism, religious fundamentalism, a partisan attachment to romantic ideas of India's spiritual heritage, and other such causes. They are not supported by scholarly historical research. Likewise, several English translations, intending to glorify India's past achievements, only make it seem ridiculous by falling into the trap of presenting ancient and medieval Indian medicine as though it foreshadowed all modern discoveries. Āyurveda's real history is impressive enough and does not benefit from proleptic scientism.

There are numerous Sanskrit texts devoted to expounding the traditional system of Indian medicine, āyurveda. The earliest of these texts, by many centuries, are the *Caraka Saṃhitā* and the *Suśruta Saṃhitā*. The Sanskrit word *'saṃhitā'* means 'compendium', and 'Caraka' and 'Suśruta' are proper names. So these titles translate as 'Caraka's Compendium' and 'Suśruta's Compendium'. A third ancient text, the *Bheḷa Saṃhitā* has survived to modern times in only a single damaged manuscript,[13] and it has yet to be critically edited and translated.

The tradition of the *Caraka Saṃhitā* is associated with north-western India, and in particular the ancient university of Takṣaśilā: Chinese sources place Caraka at the court of the famed first-century Scythian king Kaniṣka; the *Suśruta Saṃhitā* is said to have been composed in Benares. We do not know the exact date of composition of these two works. Prior versions of them may date as far back as the time of the Buddha, that is, the early fourth century BC.[14] At the end of several chapters, the texts themselves explicitly declare that they have been supplemented, edited, and partially rewritten by later authors, whose dates run up to about the eighth century AD. The published Sanskrit texts available today represent the works in the form which they had reached during the latter half of the first millennium AD. The *Caraka Saṃhitā* and the *Suśruta Saṃhitā* are both long texts: one continuous English translation of the former is over 1,000 pages long,[15] and a translation of the latter is over 1,700 pages long.[16] These two texts form the cornerstone of āyurveda. Although there are many other texts on āyurveda, these two provide the foundation of the system, and are constantly referred to and paraphrased in other texts.

Later texts of great importance include the *Aṣṭāṅgahṛdaya Saṃhitā* of Vāgbhaṭa (AD c.600), the *Rugviniścaya* of Mādhavakara (AD c.700), the *Śārṅgadhara Saṃhitā* of Śārṅgadhara (c. early fourteenth century), and the *Bhāvaprakāśa* of Bhāvamiśra (sixteenth century) Mādhava's work broke new ground in its rearrangement of medical topics according to pathological categories, and set the pattern of subject arrangement that was followed by almost all later works on general medicine. Śārṅgadhara is important as the first author to discuss in Sanskrit several new foreign elements, including the extensive use of metallic compounds, an idea of respiration, diagnosis and prognosis by pulse, and opium.

There is some variation between north and south India regarding the popularity of āyurvedic texts. Broadly, the *Caraka Saṃhitā* is more popular in the north, while the *Aṣṭāṅgahṛdaya Saṃhitā* is more popular in the south. This regional variation is revealed both by the geographical distribution of surviving manuscripts, and by the location of surviving living traditions of oral medical literature, such as the tradition of the *aṣṭavaidya* brahmins in Kerala.[17] A small medical digest called the *Vaidyajīvana*, written by Lolimbarāja in the late sixteenth century, became extraordinarily popular all over India, perhaps because of the beauty of the ornate classical metres in which its verses were cast: it has a dozen Sanskrit commentaries, and has been translated into many modern Indian languages. A well-known aphorism, 'a doctor by a hundred stanzas' refers jocularly to the fact that anyone can become a doctor by learning the *Vaidyajīvana*.[18]

BASIC TENETS

Both the *Caraka Saṃhitā* and the *Suśruta Saṃhitā* emanate from a single tradition of medicine: that is, their general views and doctrines are in consonance, and the theoretical basis of medicine presented in the texts is identical. The *Caraka Saṃhitā* is distinguished by its long reflective and philosophical passages: why twins are not necessarily identical (4.2),[19] what evidence there is for the doctrine of reincarnation (1.10), definitions of causality (3.8), etc. The *Caraka Saṃhitā* has proved to be of great interest to historians of India's philosophical traditions, since it contains doctrines associated with the philosophical schools of *sāṃkhya* and *vaiśeṣika*, yet predates their standard texts.[20] The *Suśruta Saṃhitā* contains extensive descriptions of sophisticated surgical techniques: eye operations (6.1–17), removal of foreign bodies (1.26), plastic surgery on the face (1.16), etc., which either do not appear in the *Caraka Saṃhitā* at all, or not in such detail.

The *Caraka Saṃhitā* (and similarly the *Suśruta Saṃhitā*) contains a vast accumulation of medical and indeed general information, including: the merits of a measured diet and of smoking herbal mixtures (1.5, 3.2); the pharmacological characteristics of a huge range of plants and vegetables (1.27, 3.1); aetiology and characteristics of various diseases (2.1–8, 3.6–7); epidemics (3.3); methods of examination of the patient (3.4, 3.8); anatomy (3.5, 4.7); nosology (3.6–7); philosophical topics about human life and spirit (4.1, 4.5); conception, embryology, the care of the newborn, and growth (4.2–4, 4.6, 4.8); prognosis (5.1–12); stimulants and aphrodisiacs (6.1–2); description and treatment of fever, heated blood, swellings, urinary disorders, skin disorders, consumption, insanity, epilepsy, dropsy, piles, asthma, cough and hiccup, etc. (6.3–18); cupping, bloodletting and the use of leeches (6.14, 29); proper use of alcohol (6.24); disorders of paralysis, lockjaw, and rheumatism (6.27–29); properties of nuts, vegetables, and other material medica (7.1–12); and the use of enemas (8.1–7, 8.10–12). This heavily abbreviated list is intended just to give a feel for some of the topics covered.

The medicines described in the *Caraka Saṃhitā* and the *Suśruta Saṃhitā* contain a broad array of animal, vegetable, and mineral substances. An estimate of prescribed items in the *Caraka Saṃhitā* shows 177 substances of animal origin (including snake dung, fumes of burnt snake, the milk, flesh, fat, blood, dung, or urine of several animals such as horse, goat, elephant, camel, cow and sheep, the eggs of sparrow, pea-hen and crocodile, beeswax and honey, soup of various meats, etc.), 341 substances of plant origin (including seeds, flowers, fruit, tree-bark, leaves, etc.), and 64 items of mineral origin (including ash, various gems, silver, copper, salt, clay, tin, lead, gold, glass, orpiment, sulphur, etc.).[21]

It is worth noting in this context that several substances in these lists, such as dung and urine, are not necessarily considered shocking in the Indian rural context. To orthodox Hindus, the consumption of meat or wine (both also recommended in the texts) would be a far more horrifying prospect than the admixture of animal dung in a medical recipe. The cow, in particular, is a holy animal for Hindus, and all its products, including milk, urine, and dung, are considered auspicious and purifying. It is normal practice in Indian villages for a housewife to begin the day by smearing the floor of her home with cow dung, which is seen as having disinfectant properties.[22] Cow dung is also commonly used as fuel for cooking-fires. Furthermore, in three cases out of four, animal dung is prescribed for external use (including fumigation); urine is prescribed externally about twice in every three recipes.

The *Caraka Saṃhitā* contains several passages extolling the virtues of the good doctor:

> Everyone admires a twice-born [brahmin] physician who is courteous, wise, self-disciplined, and a master of his subject. He is like a guru, a master of life itself. On completing his studentship a physician is said to be born again: the title 'doctor' [Skt. *vaidya*] is earned, not inherited. On completing his studentship a spirit, be it divine or heroic, enters firmly into him because of his knowledge: that is why the physician is called 'twice-born.' ... For someone being dragged into death's realm by savage diseases, no benefactor, either religious or worldly, can match the person who holds out life. There is no gift to compare with the gift of life. The practitioner of medicine who believes that his highest calling is the care of others achieves the highest happiness. He fufils himself.[23]

Quacks are condemned:

> Attired in doctors' outfits, they wander the streets looking for work. As soon as they hear someone is ill, they descend on him and in his hearing speak loudly of their medical expertise. If a doctor is already in attendance on him, they constantly harp on that doctor's failings. They try to ingratiate themselves with the patient's friends with jokes, confidences, and flattery. They put it about that they won't want much money ... but when they fail to avert the illness they point out that it was the patient himself who lacked equipment, helpers, and the right attitude.[24]

Caraka also presents an 'Oath of Initiation', which has often been compared with the Hippocratic Oath. During a rite of initiation at the beginning of a pupil's tutelage in āyurveda he had to swear to live a celibate life, to speak the truth, to eat a vegetarian diet, to be free of envy, and never to carry arms; he was to subject himself to his teacher completely, except where this would bring him into conflict with higher ethical values; he was to work day and night for the relief of his patients, and was never to desert them, nor take advantage of them sexually; he was to withhold treatment from enemies of the king, wicked people generally, and from women who were unattended by their husbands or guardians; he was to visit the patient's home only in the company of a mutual acquaintance, and was to treat as totally confidential any privileged information acquired concerning the patient's household.[25]
(➤ Ch. 37 History of medical ethics)

IN PRACTICE

The diagnostic and practical aspects of āyurveda depended on a thorough knowledge of the Sanskrit texts. The good physician (Skt. *vaidya*) memorized a vast amount of material, which consisted largely of medical verses giving correspondences between the three humours, wind, bile, and phlegm (Skt.

vāyu, pitta, śleṣman), and the different symptoms, diseases, herbs, and treatments. When confronted with a patient, the *vaidya* performed an examination and took into account the symptoms, and verses would spring to his mind which encapsulated the patient's condition. These verses would trigger the memory of further verses that contained the same key combinations of humoral references, and presented a prognosis and treatment.[26] The *vaidya* was operating in a rich semantic field of correspondences, offering innumerable possibilities for diagnosis and treatment. The āyurvedic schemes of substances, qualities, and actions offered the physician an excellent combination of the freedom to act and a structure within which to exercise choice. It is important to see the practice of āyurveda in the context of oral traditions, in which vast amounts of memorized textual material is 'recreated' orally in order to suit particular circumstances, while nevertheless remaining true to the fundamental meaning of the text.[27]

Of course, āyurveda had (and has) its poor practitioners, and the texts face up to the problem of bad doctors. To be good at āyurveda required not only years of training as a youngster, but also native intelligence and sensitivity.[28] But in the absence of a centralized system of qualification and testing, *vaidyas* were judged by reputation alone, and Sanskrit literature contains sharply satirical passages about dangerously ill-qualified physicians.[29]

SURGERY

The *Suśruta Saṃhitā* tends to be known for its extensive chapter on surgery, which retains its power to impress us even today. Caraka, too, has brief descriptions of surgical techniques, but the *Suśruta Saṃhitā* goes into much greater detail, describing how a surgeon should be trained, and exactly how various operations should be done. There are descriptions of ophthalmic couching, cutting for stone, removal of arrows and splinters, suturing, the examination of dead human bodies for the study of anatomy, and much besides. Suśruta claims that surgery is the most ancient and most efficacious of the eight branches of medical knowledge.[30] It is certain that elaborate surgical techniques were practiced in Suśruta's circle, but there is little evidence to show that these practices persisted beyond the time of the composition of the text. Some of them may have survived as caste skills, isolated from the mainstream of āyurvedic practice. For example, a description of the couching operation for cataract survives in the ninth-century *Kalyāṇakāraka* by Ugrāditya,[31] and texts based on the *Suśruta Saṃhitā* copy out the sections on surgery along with other material. But there is no evidence from other historical sources that the sophisticated surgery described by Suśruta was actually pracised by *vaidyas*. Medical texts do not contain any development of surgical ideas, nor do any genuinely ancient or medieval surgical instruments survive. Surgery is not described in literary or other sources, except as science fiction. It may be that as the caste system grew in rigidity through the first millennium AD, taboos concerning physical contact became almost insurmountable and *vaidyas* may have resisted therapies that involved cutting into the body. Against this it may be argued that examination of the pulse and urine gained in popularity, as did massage therapies. But whatever the reasons, the early efflorescence of sophisticated surgical knowledge seems to have been an isolated phenomenon.

There is, however, one famous historical event which is often cited as evidence that Suśruta's surgery was widely known even up to modern times. In March 1793, an operation took place in Poona which was to change the course of plastic surgery in Europe. A Maratha named Cowasjee,[32] who had been a bullock-driver with the English Army in the war of 1792, was captured by the forces of Tipu Sultan, and had his nose and one hand cut off. After a year without a nose, he turned to a man of the brickmakers' caste, near Poona, to have his face repaired. Thomas Cruso and James Trindlay, British surgeons in the Bombay Presidency, witnessed this operation (or one just like it), and appear to have prepared a description of what they saw, together with a painting of the patient and diagrams of the skin-graft procedure. These details, with diagrams and an engraving from the painting, were published at third hand in London in 1794.[33] The description showed that the anonymous brickmaker had performed a magnificent skin graft and nose reconstruction, using a technique that was superior to anything the English surgeons had ever seen. The technique was taken up in Europe and is still known as the 'Hindu method' today.

This would at first sight seem to be a triumphant vindication of the historical persistence of Suśruta's surgery. But there are several puzzling elements to the story that belie this initial impression. One of the most important is that the rhinoplasty operation is not described in any detail in the *Suśruta Saṃhitā*. The Sanskrit text says:

> Now I shall carefully describe how to repair a severed nose. Take the leaf of a tree, of the same measure as his nose, and append it. The same size should be cut from the side of the cheek. Now it is attached to the end of the nose. With care the physician should scratch it and then swiftly tie it up with a clean bandage. After checking that it is properly joined, he should raise it and attach two reeds. Then he should powder it with sandal wood, liquorice and collyrium. Covering it completely with white cotton he should sprinkle it several times with the oil of sesame seeds. Once his digestion is over, the man should be make to drink ghee, anointed and purged, according to the rules. That repair should become healed; if there is half of it left, it should be cut again. If, however, it is small, one should try to stretch it, and one should even out any excess flesh.[34]

The Sanskrit text of this passage is brief and laconic, and certainly not detailed enough to be followed without an oral commentary and practical demonstration. Also, no surviving manuscript of the text contains any illustration. In fact, there is no tradition of anatomical manuscript illustration in India at all. In other words, it would not be possible for the tradition to have persisted purely textually.

Furthermore, as a member of the brickmakers' caste, the surgeon who performed the Poona operation was not a traditional physician or *vaidya*, and probably knew no Sanskrit at all. He had the skill in his hands, not in his head. And the skill that he had would probably have been specific to his caste, or even family. Maybe it was indeed an extraordinary survival of a technique from Suśruta's time, but in that case it was transmitted by means wholly outside the learned practice of traditional Indian physicians.

There is also no clear evidence from any other historical sources that such operations were ever performed in medieval times. Indeed, the contrary is true (see p. 772). Whatever the not-inconsiderable complications that surround this case, it demonstrates the presence of a major medical practice in the late eighteenth century appearing apparently from nowhere, millennia after being invented and laconically sketched out in the ancient texts. (➤ Ch. 41 Surgery (traditional))

INOCULATION

Before the nineteenth century, inoculation – the deliberate infection of a healthy patient with a dose of smallpox – was the only means of protection from smallpox. The patient was prepared beforehand to be in the best possible health, and was kept quarantined and in a controlled environment, in the hope that the smallpox episode would be mild. If the patient survived, and many did, he or she would thereafter be immune to smallpox. The practice of inoculation first became known to European science after Lady Mary Wortley Montague (1689–1762) observed market women practising it in Constantinople. She had the courage to have her own children inoculated, and returned to England in 1717 to preach the new technique. It was to provoke a terrific controversy, which took on political and theological overtones, and grew stronger until the discovery by Edward Jenner (1749–1823) of vaccination in 1796 rendered inoculation obsolete. Nevertheless, for a considerable time, inoculation, with all its inherent dangers, was the only known defence against smallpox.

Inoculation was current in Turkey in the early eighteenth century; there is evidence that it may have been brought there from China. (➤ Ch. 32 Chinese medicine) It is interesting, then, to find a detailed account by a renowned English surgeon in 1767, describing the widespread practice of inoculation in Bengal.[35] There is also some evidence to push the Indian practice of inoculation back further, to 1731.[36] Once again, there is a historical paradox here: there is not the slightest trace of this important and effective treatment in any of the Sanskrit medical treatises. Smallpox was certainly recognized in āyurvedic texts, where it is called *masūrikā* ('lentil' disease) and was treated after a fashion. But of inoculation there is absolutely no mention. The link between theory and practice is broken once again.

After smallpox vaccine was introduced to India in 1802, a rumour was started in 1819 by an article in the *Madras Courier*, a popular daily newspaper, to the effect that there existed an ancient Sanskrit text describing in detail the process of vaccination. This proved, it was argued, the superiority of ancient Indian science, and that 'there is nothing new under the sun'. Unfortunately, this rumour gained currency and was republished in books and encyclopedias across Europe all through the nineteenth century, and it even surfaces today. Carefuly literary research has shown, however, that no such Sanskrit text exists, and that the whole affair was almost certainly triggered by the excessive zeal of British vaccination propagandists, who composed tracts on vaccination in local languages and probably in Sanskrit too. One of these tracts appears to have been so convincing that the belief was born of an ancient Indian knowledge of the technique.[37]

These cases, rhinoplasty and inoculation, demonstrate that in the history of Indian medicine, all is not what it seems. Techniques in the texts fell into disuse, while new discoveries were widely practised apparently without impinging on the traditional medical establishment. Perhaps this situation is not entirely unlike that of today, with the growing popular acceptance of alternative medicine which is often ignored by the medical establishment.

This is not to deny that there was a strong core of continuity throughout the tradition. A great deal of what is practised by āyurvedic physicians in Indian villages today is derived directly from the classical schools of medicine which were so creative nearly two thousand years ago, and this practice has been the basis of health care in India in all that time. Yet time affected the tradition of Indian medicine just as it affects all things.

CHANGE AND CONTINUITY

It has long been presupposed by historians of Indian medicine that the āyurvedic tradition was static, that later texts merely elaborated a unified theory already present in the earliest texts, the *Caraka Saṃhitā* and the *Suśruta Saṃhitā*. This view of āyurveda was partly due to the fact that these two texts present themselves as timeless bodies of celestial knowledge, containing no programme for development or change, and partly because it conformed to uncritical ideas of India as the home of timeless truths. The idea that āyurveda never evolved also flourished for the simple reason that the research needed to discover evidence of change in the tradition is very difficult, and very detailed. It requires that a vast body of medieval Sanskrit medical literature be read, and that detailed indexes of diseases, therapies, diagnostic techniques, etc., be compiled.

While the most famous texts of the system, mentioned above (pp. 759–60), are indeed homogeneous to a great extent, Meulenbeld's recent pioneering researches into the history of Sanskrit āyurvedic literature have revealed that many authors refused to submit to the orthodox point of view, and stuck to their own ideas.[38] Many new diseases were identified and described in the course of time. For example, from the sixteenth century we find syphilis (Skt. *phiraṅgaroga*, 'foreigners' disease') described in texts like Bhāvamiśra's *Bhāvaprakāśa*; it was treated with mercury. From the eighteenth century onwards, we find texts including descriptions of diseases clearly borrowed from Western medicine. Other diseases that were described in early texts disappear from the literature.

Developments also took place in the field of diagnostics. The detailed and systematic examination of urine (Skt. *mūtraparīkṣā*) is a relatively late development, dating from about the eleventh century. The examination of the pulse (Skt. *nāḍīparīkṣā*) is never found in Sanskrit texts before about the thirteenth century, but it subsequently became a diagnostic method of first resort. A diagnostic technique called 'examination of the eight bases' (Skt. *aṣṭasthānaparīkṣā*), which meant a routine for examining the pulse, urine, faeces, tongue, eyes, general appearance, voice, and skin of the patient, began to appear in texts from the beginning of the sixteenth century. (➤ Ch. 35 The art of diagnosis: medicine and the five senses)

New prognostic methods also came into use. For example, from about the sixteenth century, a technique was developed whereby a drop of oil would be placed in the surface of a patient's urine. The remaining span of the patient's life would be read from the way the oil spread out.[39]

In therapy, one of the most noticeable changes over the centuries was the explosive growth of standardized compound medicines (Skt. *yoga*). A *yoga* normally consists of a large number of ingredients, and is described in terms of its effect against a particular disease or ailment. Its therapeutic use speaks against the view that each patient was treated holistically, as a person in relation to his or her environment, with certain habits, disposition, etc. Although such ideas are certainly present in the early texts, the growth of the use of *yogas* speaks for much more standardized therapeutic methods, with generalized medicines targeted at diseases, over the heads of the patients, so to speak. This development has continued today with the growth of a large pharmaceutical industry devoted to the manufacture of standardized āyurvedic medicines. Most āyurvedic medicines in the twentieth century are of this type, and it is rare to find a practitioner who will prescribe and prepare a medicine specific to a particular patient, as the old texts recommend. Also noticeable is the increasing use in the tradition of astrological, alchemical, and frankly magical methods of healing.

Finally, the enormous Indian pharmacopoeia was subject to far-reaching changes. Meulenbeld has categorized these as follows:[40] the decline of knowledge with respect to the identity of medicinal substances; the change of identity of plants designated by means of a particular name; the appearance of new names and synonyms; the use of substitutes for drugs which had become rare; the introduction of new drugs. The study of this subject is beset by difficulties, but many examples of all these cases can be cited.

Indian āyurvedic medicine certainly changed over the centuries, and in non-trivial ways. The study of these changes is still nascent, but promises to be full of interest. Āyurveda is the 'great tradition' of indigenous Indian medicine, the Sanskritic, literate system that received royal patronage. There are other 'great' traditions in this sense: the Siddha system of the Tamils, and the Yūnānī system of Islam. There is also a whole range of therapies traceable in the subcontinent, from folk medicine and shamanism through astrology to faith healing. We can do no more than mention some of these.

SIDDHA MEDICINE

In south India, a system of medicine evolved in the Tamil-speaking areas that was different in certain conceptions from āyurveda. Known as Siddha medicine (Tamil *cittar*), this was – and is – primarily an esoteric alchemical and magical system, apparently strongly influenced by tantric thought and āyurveda, about which very little has been written.[41] It is marked by a greater use of metals, in particular mercury, than is the case in āyurveda, and holds particular reverence for a substance called *muppū*, which is believed to hold potent powers for both physical and spiritual transformation.[42] Taking the pulse is more prominent as a diagnostic procedure in Siddha medicine than in āyurveda, and it has been suggested that āyurvedic pulse diagnosis – which was not common before the late thirteenth century – was borrowed from Siddha medicine.[43] The semi-legendary founders of Siddha medicine include Bogar, who is believed to have travelled to China, teaching and learning alchemical lore. Other legends include stories of a Siddha called Rāmadevar 'who travelled to Mecca, assumed the name Yakub, and taught the Arabians the alchemical art'.[44]

ASTROLOGICAL MEDICINE

From the earliest times, āyurveda treated a range of children's diseases as being due to the malign influence of celestial demons (Skt. *graha*, 'seizer'), who were believed to attack children and to afflict them with a range of symptoms.[45] The Sanskrit word *graha* was later used to mean 'planet', and although *grahas* are clearly described as celestial beings in the *Suśruta Saṃhitā*, the later evolution of rites for planetary propitiation are clearly aimed at the same types of influence.

The literatures of Indian astrology (Skt. *jyotiḥśāstra*) and religious law (Skt. *dharmaśāstra*) include texts for pacifying the planets, as well as prognostications regarding such matters as pregnancy, the sex of unborn children, the interpretation of dreams, sickness, and death.[46] Private booklets containing invocations for pacifying the planets, as well as prayers and rituals for safeguarding children were not uncommon.[47] As an ancient and influential treatise on law and conducts says, 'One desirous of prosperity, of removing evil or calamities, of rainfall (for crops), long life, bodily health and one desirous of performing magic rites against enemies and others should perform a sacrifice to planets.'[48]

A work exemplifying the close relationship between medicine and astrology as therapeutic systems is the *Vīrasiṃhāvaloka* by Vīrasiṃha, composed in AD 1383, probably in Gwalior. It treats the aetiology and therapy of groups of diseases from three distinct points of view: that of astrology, that of religion,[49] and that of medicine.

Even today, Indian astrologers and physicians are expected to provide charms and prayers to ward off evil influences from the planets and elsewhere. The parts of the body are conceptually equated with the constellations and planets in a complex scheme of relationships and influences, and the astrologer 'reads' this structure of symbols in order to understand the patient's problem and to suggest such remedies as amulets, penances, and prayers, as well as herbal decoctions.[50] A breathtaking variety of omens has formed a compelling element in the daily life of Indians for millennia, and many of these have to do with health and sickness.[51] General bookshops in India frequently stock numerous texts on astrology and healing for popular consumption.[52]

It is worth noting that the Bower manuscript, one of the oldest surviving Indian codices, contains not only important examples of fifth-century medical literature, but also a text on divination by dice.[53] Considered as a cluster of related texts, the Bower manuscript shows us a cross-section of the concerns of a fifth-century healer, who was specially interested in medicinal uses of garlic, elixirs for eternal life, the treatment of eye diseases, herbal medicines, butter decoctions, oils, aphrodisiacs, the care of children, and spells against the bite of the cobra, as well as the aforementioned divinations.

SHAMANISTIC HEALING

Sudhir Kakar has written engagingly of a number of shamanistic and folk healers in modern India, and it is certain that such practices have been common there since earliest times.[54] In fact, there are clearly elements within āyurveda itself that stem from such folk traditions. Patients with a range of beliefs about devils and spirit possessions visit such practitioners. It is interesting to note that shamans are not opposed to recommending patients to cosmopolitan clinics if they recognise an ailment such as an ulcer or high blood pressure.[55] (➤ Ch. 30 Folk medicine)

FOREIGN INFLUENCES

THE COMING OF ISLAMIC MEDICINE

Yūnānī Ṭibb is the name given to the medical practice brought to India with Islam, which began to have a major impact on India starting with the Afghan invasions of Gujarat in the early eleventh century. The word *yūnānī* (sometimes spelt *ūnānī*) is an Indian representation of the name 'Ionian'. Yūnānī medicine is the system founded on that of Galen and in particular as interpreted in the work of Avicenna (AD 980–1037), *Al-Qānūn fī l-ṭibb*. Yūnānī medicine is still very much alive in India today, and it is fascinating to consider that a fundamentally Galenic medicine is still in contemporary practice. (➤ Ch. 31 Arab-Islamic medicine).

As might be expected, Yūnānī medicine and āyurveda have influenced each other, especially in the realm of materia medica. Although the primary languages of Yūnānī medicine are, of course, Persian and Arabic, there are even Sanskrit texts on Yūnānī. For example, the eighteenth-century work *Hikmatprakāśa* was written in Sanskrit by the pious Hindu Mahādevadeva.[56] Yūnānī medicine postulates four basic humours, as opposed to āyurveda's three, and Yūnānī medicine is more oriented towards the treatment of patients in hospitals. The major difference between these systems, however, is in their clientele. Broadly, Yūnānī physicians treat Muslim patients, and āyurvedic physicians treat Hindus.

THE PORTUGUESE AND DUTCH

In the first half of the sixteenth century, the Portuguese arrived in Goa. The first medical book printed in India – and only the third book printed there

– was the *Coloquios dos Simples, e Drogas he Cousas Mediçinais da India* ... or *Colloquies on the Medical Simples and Drugs of India* by Garcia d'Orta (1490–1570), printed in Goa in 1563. D'Orta gathered a mass of material from the local physicans, and learned as much as he could of their methods, even competing with them for rich clients.[57] There was a free and fertile exchange of medical ideas between the Portuguese and the Indians for much of the rest of the sixteenth century; however, despite this promising beginning, the relationship declined, and during the early decades of the seventeenth century the Portuguese introduced restrictions that effectively outlawed Hindu physicians.

The Dutch East India Company officials showed great interest in the local flora and fauna of the Malabar coast from the end of the seventeenth century onwards. Heinrich van Rheede (1637–91), who was appointed Governor of the Dutch possessions in 1667, prepared a magnificent series of twelve folio volumes, published between 1686 and 1703 in Amsterdam, which contained nearly 800 plates of Indian plants, a work much admired by Sir William Jones (1746–94). Other works of a similar scale were produced, including that of van Rheed's appointee to Ceylon, Paul Herman (1646–95), whose herbarium and *Museum Zeylanicum* were major sources of the 1747 publication of Linnaeus (1707–78), *Flora Zeylanica*.[58]

THE BRITISH

The British arrived in India at the beginning of the seventeenth century, in the form of the East India Company. The influence of 'John Company' grew steadily over the succeeding years until a flurry of battles and political acquisitions at the start of the nineteenth century projected the company into the position of *de facto* government in large parts of India. In 1858, the company was dissolved, and India was placed directly under the British Crown. The history of British medicine during this period belongs to the larger context of colonial and imperial medicine and the birth of tropical medicine, but some remarks should be made here about the interaction between British and indigenous physicians. (➤ Ch. 58 Medicine and colonialism; Ch. 24 Tropical medicine)

During the seventeenth century, there were relatively few English traders in India, and like the Portuguese and the Dutch before them, they faced a completely new set of health problems there. They were keen to learn from the local *vaidyas* and *hakīms*, and local remedies and regimens were often adopted. Missionaries were particularly active in both teaching and learning from indigenous practitioners, a task made easier by their mastery of local languages. (➤ Ch. 61 Religion and medicine) For their part, the Indians were particularly interested in British surgeons since, in spite of the early evidence of the *Suśruta Saṃhitā*, surgery had passed almost completely out of practice amongst *vaidyas*. The French traveller J. B. Tavernier (1605–89) reported in 1684 that once when the King of Golconda had a headache and his native physicians prescribed that blood should be let in four places under his tongue, nobody could be found to do it, 'for the Natives of the Country understand nothing of Chirurgery'.[59] Two hundred years later, Sir William Sleeman (1788–1856) observed:

> The educated class, as indeed all classes, say that they do not want our physicians, but stand much in need of our surgeons. Here they feel that they are helpless, and we are strong; and they seek our aid whenever they see any change of obtaining it.[60]

A persistent factor encouraging the British physicians to adopt Indian methods was the sheer difficulty and expense of shipping medical supplies from Europe. When the *British Pharmacopoeia* was formalized in 1858, the idea of a formal and legally enforceable standard for drugs took hold, and caused many British physicians in India to grow increasingly critical of the crudeness of indigenous drugs. Yet in the 1860s, economic pressures forced the Medical Department of the Bengal Presidency to declare that indigenous drugs should be used wherever possible.[61] In the longer term, feelings against Indian medicine hardened, in common with attitudes to all indigenous skills and sciences, and after official Government support for Indian medicine ceased in 1835, āyurvedic and Yūnānī physicians were thrown back on their own private resources for training and practice.[62]

THE CONTEMPORARY PICTURE

In India, āyurveda had been the main system of professional health care for the bulk of the population for at least two millennia. This even continued under the British Raj, which initially encouraged the study of āyurveda alongside British medicine when medical colleges were founded in Bengal and elsewhere. But with the change of British educational policy, after Lord Bentinck's educational reforms of 1835, and the suppression of āyurvedic teaching in state-funded medical colleges, Government support for āyurvedic training ceased. However, āyurvedic physicians continued to practise, although their training was reduced to the traditional family-apprenticeship system and privately sponsored colleges. With the rise of the Indian independence movement, all indigenous traditions received strong support from nationalists. Since independence in 1947, the Indian Government has oscillated between a commitment to modern cosmopolitan medicine and the necessity of grappling with the unavoidable fact that āyurvedic medicine is widely accepted, especially in rural areas, and remains strongly identified with

India nationalistic sentiments.[63] The Indian Government has sponsored a number of commissions and studies regarding national health-care provision, with widely varying outcomes.

The current situation is complicated, but the basic fact is that after much debate over several decades the Indian Government recognizes a place for āyurvedic medicine in its overall health policy. It has become clear, for example, that modern cosmopolitan medicine has not been very successful in penetrating the countryside, and that, by contrast, āyurvedic practitioners are more likely to work in villages. This view was encouraged by the Ramalingaswami report of 1980, which promoted several ideas along the lines of the Chinese 'barefoot doctor' schemes, and was accepted as Government policy.

In 1970, the Indian Parliament passed the Indian Medicine Central Council Act, setting up a Central Council for Āyurveda, thus recognizing and controlling āyurveda, and providing for accredited colleges and standardized qualifications. In the 1990s government-accredited colleges and universities provide professional training and qualifications in āyurveda. This training includes some basic education in Western cosmopolitan methods, family planning, and public health. Graduates of such institutions are recognized by the Government in so far as they may be employed as the third medical officer at Primary Health Centers, and as community health volunteers. Many run successful clinics in urban as well as rural settings. In 1983, there were approximately 100 officially accredited āyurvedic training colleges in India, many attached to universities.

The standard recognized āyurvedic qualifications, and the time taken to acquire them, are:

BAMS: Bachelor of Āyurvedic Medicine and Surgery. A 5½-year degree course including six month's internship. Also known as Āyurvedācārya.
MD Āyu.: Doctor of Medicine in Āyurveda. A three-year postgraduate degree course open to BAMS or equivalent degree-holders only.
Ph.D.: Doctor of Philosophy. A research degree course of two further years.

These qualifications normally involve some clinical experience. Several āyurvedic colleges are attached to hospitals and clinics, where students serve internships. Some colleges, for example the respected Gujarat Āyurveda University, offer an introductory familiarization course in āyurveda, which is typically a three-month certificate course for graduates of modern medicine and postgraduates of allied sciences.

However, private āyurvedic practitioners also prescribe modern cosmopolitan medicines and treatments, often at the insistence of their patients, and this tends to happen with varying degrees of impunity. For example, many people regard the injection to be a powerful, almost magical cure for most ailments, regardless of the substance injected. Separate vernacular tracts exist which extol the virtues of 'injection therapy',[64] and the physician is often under pressure to provide injections, even if only of water. In the course of a 1970s study of fifty-nine indigenous practitioners in Panjab and Mysore, researchers were surprised to find that 75 per cent of the drugs being used were modern cosmopolitan medicines such as antibiotics. The same study uncovered an underground system of health care providing the bulk of local medical treatment and a pervasive but previously unrecognized system of medical education.

> The professors are the drug detail men from the pharmaceutical companies.... The junior faculty are the pharmacists in the cities. Each pharmacist has a continuing class of practitioners scattered throughout the neighbouring villages. The practitioner will drop into the pharmacist's shop and say, 'I am seeing a lot of conjunctivitis these days. What do you have that's good?'
>
> The indigenous practitioners of Ludhiana District had organized an association and had monthly meetings to discuss clinical cases and new treatments.[65]

Government control of indigenous medicine – where it exists at all – continues to be highly pragmatic and based on local political decisions. The idea that āyurvedic physicians deal purely in innocuous herbs, roots, and therapeutic massage is a grossly simplified representation of what really happens in indigenous medical circles today.

CONTEMPORARY PLURALISTIC MEDICINE

Today in India, the patient, or indeed the healthy person, may take any of many available paths towards greater health. There exist physicians of cosmopolitan medicine, āyurveda, and Yūnānī, as well as others we have not mentioned such as homoeopaths, naturopaths, traditional bone-setters, yoga teachers, massage and enema therapists, faith-healers, famous gurus, traditional midwives, and the wandering specialists who remove the wax from ears. The variety is overwhelming, both as a subject of study, and as a subjective experience. (➤ Ch. 28 Unorthodox medical theories; Ch. 29 Non-Western concepts of disease; Ch. 60 Medicine and anthropology)

NOTES

1 Bridget and Raymond Allchin, *The Rise of Civilization in India and Pakistan*, Cambridge, Cambridge University Press, 1982, pp. 221 ff.

2 Ibid., p. 215.

3 Hermann Kulke and Dietmar Rothermund, *A History of India*, rev. edn, London, Routledge, 1990, pp. 30–3.

4 For an excellent discussion of these migrations see Colin Renfrew, *Archaeology*

and Language: the Puzzle of Indo-European Origins, 2nd edn, London, Penguin, 1989.

5 See K. G. Zysk, *Religious Healing in the Veda*, Philadelphia, American Philosophical Society, 1985.

6 Ibid., pp. 70–1.

7 Jyotir Mitra, *A Critical Appraisal of Āyurvedic Material in Buddhist Literature*, Varanasi, Jyotirlok Prakashan, 1985; K. G. Zysk, *Asceticism and Healing in Ancient India: Medicine in the Buddhist Monastery*, New York, Oxford University Press, 1991, chs 2 and 3.

8 Ibid., p. 40.

9 Mitra, op. cit. (n. 7), pp. 44 ff.

10 Mitra, op. cit. (n. 7), pp. 117–19, *passim*.

11 Debiprasad Chattopadhyaya, *Science and Society in Ancient India*, Calcutta, Research India Publications, 1977.

12 *Caraka Saṃhitā* 1.30.23.

13 A. C. Burnell, *A Classified Index to the Sanskrit MSS in the Palace at Tanjore*, London, Trübner, 1880, p. 63b.

14 For recently revised judgements concerning the date of the Buddha see Heinz Bechert, 'The date of the Buddha reconsidered', *Indologica Taurinensia*, 1982, 10: 29 ff.

15 Shree Gulabkunverba Ayurvedic Society, *The Caraka Saṃhitā... with Translations in Hindi, Gujarati and English*, Vol. V: *English Translation*, Jamnagar, Gulabkunverba Ayurvedic Society, 1949.

16 Kaviraj Junja Lal, Bhishagratna, *An English Translation of the Sushruta Samhita, Based on an Original Sanskrit Text*, 3 vols, Calcutta, Bhaduri, 1907–16.

17 Francis Zimmermann, *Le Discours des remèdes au Pays des Épices*: enquête sur la médicine hindone, Paris, Payot, 1989, pp. 40–8, *passim*.

18 The aphorism (Skt. *śataślokena paṇḍitaḥ*) is reported by M. Seshagiri Sastri in his *Report on a Search for Sanskrit and Tamil Manuscripts for the Year 1896–97*, no. 1, Madras, Government Press, 1898, p. 26.

19 References are to the chapters (Skt. *sthāna*) and sections (Skt. *adhyāya*) of the texts.

20 See, for example, Antonella Comba, 'Medicine e Filosofia', *La Medicina Indiana (Āyurveda)*, Turin, Promolibri, 1991, pp. 35–77.

21 See Priyadaranjan Rây and Hirendra Nath Gupta, *Caraka Saṃhitā (a Scientific Synopsis)*, New Delhi, National Institute of Sciences of India, 1965, Tables 1–3.

22 See I. Julia Leslie, *The Perfect Wife*, Delhi, Oxford University Press, 1989, pp. 59–61.

23 *Caraka Saṃhitā* 6.1, pāda 4, verses 51–3, 60–2.

24 *Caraka Saṃhitā* 1.29, verse 9.

25 *Caraka Saṃhitā* 3.8.13–14.

26 Francis Zimmermann, 'Logic and cuisine', *The Jungle and the Aroma of Meats: an Ecological Theme in Hindu Medicine*, Berkeley, University of California Press, 1987, ch. 5; Zimmermann, 'Ethnoscience et rhétorique', op. cit. (n. 17), ch. 4.

27 A.B. Lord, *The Singer of Tales*, Cambridge, MA, Harvard University Press, 1960.

28 Guido Majno presents several interesting vignettes reconstructing the *vaidya* at

work in *The Healing Hand: Man and Wound in the Ancient World*, Cambridge, MA, Harvard University Press, 1975, pp. 271–304.

29 For example, the *Narmamālā* of Kṣemendra (2.68–81), cited by A. L. Basham, 'The practice of medicine in ancient and medieval India', in Charlie Leslie (ed.), *Asian Medical Systems: a Comparative Study*, Berkeley, University of California Press, 1976, pp. 30–1.

30 *Suśruta Saṃhitā* 1.1.15–19.

31 Cited in G. J. Meulenbeld, 'The surveying of Sanskrit medical literature', in Meulenbeld (ed.), *Proceedings of the International Workshop on Priorities in the Study of Indian Medicine*, Groningen, University of Groningen, 1984, p. 67 n. 76. R. H. Elliot describes the activities of contemporary couchers in *The Indian Operation of Couching for Cataract*, London, Lewis, 1917, although he never witnessed the operation personally, and all his descriptions are at second hand.

32 Puzzlingly, this is a Parsee name.

33 *Gentleman's Magazine and Historical Chronicle*, 1794, 64 (2): 883, 891, 892.

34 *Suśruta Saṃhitā* 1.16.28–33.

35 J. Z. Holwell, *An Account of the Manner of Inoculating for the Smallpox in the East Indies*, London, 1767.

36 Ro. Coult in Calcutta, letter to Dr Oliver Coult, 10 February 1731, giving 'An account of the diseases of Bengall'. Ff. 271v–272r of Add. MS 4432 of the Royal Society Papers in the British Library, published in Dharampal, *Indian Science and Technology in the Eighteenth Century*, Delhi, 1971, pp. 141 ff., 276.

37 D. Wujastyk, 'A pious fraud: the Indian claims for pre-Jennerian smallpox vaccination', in Wujastyk and G. J. Meulenbeld (eds), *Studies on Indian Medical History*, Groningen, Forsten, 1987, pp. 139–67.

38 See G. J. Meulenbeld, 'The surveying of Sanskrit medical literature', in Meulenbeld, op. cit. (n. 31), pp. 37 ff; and his forthcoming opus, *A History of Sanskrit Medical Literature*, London, Royal Asiatic Society.

39 This practice was reported at the end of the seventeenth century by John Ovington, *A Voyage to Suratt in the Year 1689*, London, Jacob Tonson, 1696, pp. 351 ff.

40 Meulenbeld, op. cit. (n. 31), pp. 48–56.

41 S. V. Subramanian and V. R. Madhavan, *Heritage of the Tamils Siddha Medicine*, Madras, International Institute of Tamil Studies, 1983; Guy Mazars, 'Les textes médicaux tamouls', in Meulenbeld, op. cit. (n. 31), pp. 123–9; Kamil V. Zvelebil, *The Poets of the Powers*, London, 1973.

42 Kamil V. Zvelebil, 'The ideological basis of the Siddha search for immortality', in *South Asian Digest of Regional Writing*, Vol. VIII, *Sources of Illness and Healing in South Asian Regional Literatures*, Heidelberg, University of Heidelberg, 1979, pp. 1–9; D. M. Bose, S. N. Sen and B. V. Subbarayappa (eds), *A Concise History of Science in India*, New Delhi, Indian National Science Academy, 1971, pp. 335–8.

43 E. Valentine Daniel, 'The pulse as an icon in Siddha medicine', in Daniel and Judy F. Pugh (eds), *Contributions to Asian Studies*, Vol. XVIII: *South Asian Systems of Healing*, Leiden, Brill, 1984, pp. 115–26.

44 Bose, Sen and Subbarayappa, op. cit. (n. 42), p. 318.

45 *Suśruta Saṃhitā* 6.27–37, 60–62.

46 David Pingree, *Jyotiḥśāstra: Astral and Mathematical Literature*, Wiesbaden, Harrassowitz, 1974, pp. 110 ff.

47 For example, Wellcome MS Sanskrit α 456.

48 Nārāyaṇa Rāma Ācārya (ed.), *Yājñavalkyasmṛtiḥ*, 5th edn, Nirṇayasāgaramudraṇālaya, Bombay, 1949, 1.295, p. 103; cited in P. V. Kane, 'Individual Śāntis', *History of Dharmaśāstra (Ancient and Mediaeval Religious and Civil Law)*, 2nd edn, BORI, Pune, 1977, Vol. V, part II, ch. 21, pp. 748–814.

49 Actually, *karmavipāka*, the ripening of deeds performed in former lives.

50 Judy Pugh, 'Concepts of person and situation in North Indian counseling: the case of astrology', in Daniel and Pugh, op. cit. (n. 43), pp. 85–105.

51 Pingree, op. cit. (n. 46), ch. 4.

52 Such texts as J. N. Bhasin, *Medical Astrology: a Rational Approach*, New Delhi, Sagar, 1986; and Jagannath Rao, *Principles and Practice of Medical Astrology*, New Delhi, Sagar, 1972.

53 A. F. R. Hoernle (ed. and trans.), *The Bower Manuscripts*, Calcutta, Archaeological Survey of India, 1893–1912. The dicing text appears to be in a different handwriting from the medical tracts, but this does not necessarily mean that it was not part of a single handbook.

54 Sudhir Kakar, *Shamans, Mystics and Doctors: a Psychological Inquiry into India and its Healing Traditions*, London, Unwin, 1984; see also O. P. Jaggi, *Folk Medicine*, Delhi, Atma Ram, 1973.

55 The first case is described in Kakar, op. cit. (n. 54), p. 97; the second is a personal observation.

56 Described in Meulenbeld, *History*.

57 T. J. S. Patterson, 'The relationship of Indian and European practioners of medicine from the sixteenth century', in Meulenbeld and Wujastyk, op. cit. (n. 37), p. 120.

58 Bose, Sen and Subbarayappa, op. cit. (n. 42), p. 401.

59 Jean-Baptiste Tavernier, *Travels in India*, London, 1684, book 1, part 2, p. 103.

60 W. H. Sleeman, *Rambles and Recollections of an Indian Official*, London, Constable, 1893, Vol. I, p. 130.

61 P. Bala, 'State policy towards indigenous drugs in British Bengal', *Journal of the European Āyurvedic Society*, 1990, 1: 171.

62 See Brahmananda Gupta, 'Indigenous medicine in nineteenth- and twentieth-century Bengal', in Leslie, op. cit. (n. 29), pp. 369 ff.

63 See, for example, the strongly supportive remarks on āyurveda published by the Government of India in its *Report of the Sanskrit Commission, 1956–1957*, Delhi, Government of India Press, 1958, pp. 214–16.

64 For example, Śivadyālu Gupta, *Sacitra- Ādhunika Injekśan Cikitsā* [Illustrated Modern Injection Therapy], Vārāṇasī, Kṛṣṇadāsa Akādamī, 1983.

65 Carl E. Taylor, 'Primary health care in India: relationships with indigenous systems', in *Science and Technology in South Asia: Proceedings of the South Asia Seminar II, 1981–1982*, Philadelphia, PA, Department of South Asia Regional Studies, 1985, pp. 77–89.

FURTHER READING

Bhishagratna, Kaviraj Junja Lal *An English Translation of the Sushruta Samhita, Based on an Original Sanskrit Text*, 3 vols, Calcutta, Bhaduri, 1907–16.

Chattopadhyaya, Debiprasad, *Science and Society in Ancient India*, Calcutta, Research India Publications, 1977.

Jeffery, Roger, *The Politics of Health in India*, London, University of California Press, 1988.

Jolly, Julius, *Indian Medicine*, 2nd rev. edn, New Delhi, Munshiram, 1977.

Kulke, Hermann and Rothermund, Dietmar, *A History of India*, rev. edn, London, Routledge, 1990.

Ramalingaswami, V., *Health for All: an Alternative Strategy*, Report of the Indian Council of Social Science Research and Indian Council of Medical Research Joint Study, 1980.

Rây, Priyadaranjan and Gupta, Hirendra Nath, *Caraka Saṃhitā (a Scientific Synopsis)*, New Delhi, National Institute of Sciences of India, 1965.

Rây, Priyadaranjan, Gupta, Hirendra Nath and Roy, Mira, *Suśruta Saṃhitā (A Scientific Synopsis)*, New Delhi, Indian National Science Academy, 1980.

Renfrew, Colin, *Archaeology and Language: the Puzzle of Indo-European Origins*, 2nd edn, London, Penguin, 1989.

Sharma, Priya Vrata, *Caraka-Saṃhitā: Agniveśa's Treatise Refined and Annotated by Caraka and Redacted by Dṛḍhabala*, 3 vols, Varanasi, Chaukhambha Orientalia, 1981–5.

Zimmerman, Francis, *The Jungle and the Aroma of Meats: an Ecological Theme in Hindu Medicine*, Berkeley, University of California Press, 1987.

——, *Le Discours des remèdes au Pays des Épices: enquête sur la médecine hindoue*, Paris, Payot, 1989.

Zysk, K.G. *Religious Healing in the Veda*, Philadelphia, PA, American Philosophical Society, 1985.

——, *Asceticism and Healing in Ancient India: Medicine in the Buddhist Monastery*, New York, Oxford University Press, 1991.